NUTRITION IN THE COMMUNITY

The Art and Science of Delivering Services

FOURTH EDITION

Anita L. Owen
Patricia L. Splett
George M. Owen

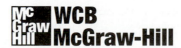

WCB
McGraw-Hill

Boston   Burr Ridge, IL   Dubuque, IA   Madison, WI   New York   San Francisco   St. Louis
Bangkok   Bogotá   Caracas   Lisbon   London   Madrid
Mexico City   Milan   New Delhi   Seoul   Singapore   Sydney   Taipei   Toronto

WCB/McGraw-Hill

A Division of The McGraw·Hill Companies

NUTRITION IN THE COMMUNITY: THE ART AND SCIENCE
OF DELIVERING SERVICES, FOURTH EDITION

This book is printed on acid-free paper.

2 3 4 5 6 7 8 9 0 KGP/KGP 9 3 2 1 0 9

ISBN 0–8151–3311–1

Vice president and editorial director: *Kevin T. Kane*
Publisher: *Colin H. Wheatley*
Senior developmental editor: *Kassi Radomski*
Senior marketing manager: *Pamela S. Cooper*
Project manager: *Terry Routley*
Senior production supervisor: *Mary E. Haas*
Designer: *Kiera M. Cunningham*
Compositor: *Shepherd, Inc.*
Typeface: *10/12 Times Roman*
Printer: *Quebecor Printing Book Group/Kingsport*

Cover image: *Tatjana Krizmanic*

*The cover was inspired by an actual market in New York City located on the far-west side of
Manhattan in Harlem. The artist found herself mesmerized by the market, and the lively
neighborhood around it. The Fairway Market has foods from all over the world, as well
as locally grown produce. As you can see, it also has bulk bins, a deli, and butcher counters.
The Fairway Market does not sell alcohol, but it does roast its own coffee in the store.*

Library of Congress Cataloging-in-Publication Data

Owen, Anita Yanochik, 1937–.
    Nutrition in the community : the art and science of delivering
services / Anita L. Owen, Patricia L. Splett, George M. Owen.—4th ed.
      p.   cm.
    Third ed. / Reva T. Frankle. St. Louis: Mosby, © 1993.
    Includes index.
    ISBN 0–8151–3311–1
    1. Nutrition policy.   2. Community health services.   I. Splett,
Patricia L.   II. Owen, George M.   III. Frankle, Reva T.   Nutrition
in the community.   IV. Title.
TX359.F7   1999
363.8'56—dc21   98–5962
                              CIP

www.mhhe.com

CONTENTS

PREFACE

The fourth edition arrives at a time when we are inundated with change of every kind in demographics, technology, health care, economics, and society. All of these changes are combined with a tidal wave of information. In this edition, we address the central issue in meeting the challenge of the future, while providing the guidelines for successful navigation on the sea of change around us. This text helps give context to the future. It can be an invaluable tool to those seeking to move forward and to embrace change and explore tomorrow. The fourth edition isn't just a formula for survival in a bewildering changing world, it is a blueprint for the community nutrition professional to thrive in it.

For any agent of change to be effective, it is necessary to understand the past and the present. During the 1970s when the first edition was published (1978), the traditional health care concerns of regulation, cost containment, accessibility, quality, and continuity were emphasized. When the second edition was published in 1986, the focus shifted from legislative and technological issues to methods of disease prevention and health promotion. The pursuit of health, as reflected by an individual's personal awareness in nutrition, physical activity, stress management, and overall individual lifestyle were often major items of the public health agenda, as emphasis moved from illness to wellness. In 1993, when the third edition was published, the issues of resource allocation, inequalities and inequities in health care, and the new economics of health care were being discussed. These issues centered around the creation of incentives for keeping people well by emphasizing prevention and health promotion practices. In the twenty-first century the issues that must be addressed to keep people healthy include services that are adequately constituted and financed to meet community needs, access to affordable quality health care, essential health information, and healthy and safe environments.

AUDIENCE

This book is designed for undergraduate and graduate students; practitioners such as dietitians, nutritionists, nurses, physicians, physicians assistants, health educators, social workers, physical therapists, and community workers; and others interested in community nutrition. The fourth edition will assist students to understand the complexities of developing effective programs and services to improve the health and nutrition for all segments of society.

THE CONTEXT OF HEALTH

To prepare community nutrition professionals to shape their future, the authors of this text developed a model describing what constitutes health. The model is called *the Context of Health*. The basic assumption of the model is that health with its many dimensions, has four fundamental attributes. These attributes include human biology such as genetics, growth, and development; behavior and lifestyle include food selection and consumption patterns, physical activity, and coping skills; the environment addresses social and physical attributes such as family income and employment, and the food supply; and the health care system involves issues such as availability, access, and quality. Thus, health results from the interaction of biology, behavior (lifestyle), the environment, and health care. Each of the four factors provides different types of opportunities for interventions to prevent disease and promote health. The model is carried throughout the text, visually demonstrating how each chapter contributes to the context of health.

ORGANIZATION OF THE TEXT

To lay the cornerstone for *Nutrition in the Community, the Art and Science of Delivery Services,* we begin with the driving forces that shape community nutrition practice (Section I). We first address the most important societal and health trends that play a major role in health and nutritional well-being of the community. These trends are similar to the top of a funnel—they address the broad perspectives of issues facing Americans today and act as a gateway to the twenty-first century. The vital role that community nutrition professionals play in protecting the health of the public is described. This section is a primer for the community nutrition professional because it defines the roles and responsibilities required to function effectively in the nutrition arena.

The application of nutrition science to dietary recommendations for people is covered. In addition, dietary guidance, which is the information used by the community nutrition professional to foster healthful food choices, is described as the "blueprint for action" for practitioners.

Section II covers the nutrition interventions required to keep people healthy across the life cycle. Guidelines are presented for each age group to assist the community nutrition professional to deliver quality nutrition services.

Section III demonstrates how managing strategically can make a difference in the quality and quantity of nutrition services and programs provided. In addition to the planning and implementation phases, evaluating nutrition services and managing and obtaining resources are deliberated.

Section IV address the question—What is Needed to achieve effective community nutrition programs? This section provides practitioners with a set of tools to refine their practice. Communicating effectively is a skill required at all levels of practice. Working in cross-cultural and multicultural settings offers sage advice for the practitioner. To practice effectively in the next century, ethics will become a very important issue. No text would be complete without discussing nutrition around the world, because we truly are a global village with instant communication to any part of the world. Thinking in the fu-

ture tense will assist community nutrition professionals to identify how much we need to resolve, how much we need to accomplish, and how we can help form a healthy future for our communities.

NEW TO THIS EDITION

The fourth edition of *Nutrition in the Community, The Art and Science of Delivering Services,* incorporates several new features designed to enhance student learning and understanding.

Context of Health Model

This unique model, presented as the first figure in each chapter, addresses the four attributes of health and nutritional well-being, which include human biology, lifestyles, environment, and health care. Adjacent to the model is a visual depicting how the content of each chapter contributes to the context of health. The context of health provides continuity throughout the text to enhance the community nutrition professionals understanding of the issues.

Case Studies and the Expert Speaks

Each chapter has a case study or an expert speaks commentary that highlights the objectives of individual chapters and offers practical application of the material covered in the chapter.

New Chapters and Expanded Coverage

To meet the needs of the expanding role of the community nutrition professional, four new chapters have been included in the fourth edition: Effective Communications, Ethics in Community Nutrition, The Global Village: Nutrition Around the World, and Entering an Era of Dynamic Change in Health and Nutrition.

Several chapters have expanded coverage of timely topics. These include the following:

- In the community assessment (chapter 3), an epidemiologic approach is used to address nutritional status.
- Product innovation and food safety are included in the chapter on the Changing and Dynamic Food Supply (chapter 6).
- Women's health is covered in chapter 10, Nutrition in Adult Years, and in chapter 20, The Global Village: Nutrition Around the World.
- Grantsmanship is included in the chapter on budgeting (chapter 16).

PEDAGOGY

The following pedagogical features are employed to enhance the usefulness of this text by students and faculty:

Core Concepts: Each chapter begins with an opening paragraph that provides an overview of the chapter.

Objectives: The major learning objectives for each chapter are stated to reinforce their significance for students.

Key Words (new): To learn the terminology of community nutrition professionals, key words are cited with a page number on which they appear or are defined in the chapter.

Context of Health Model (new): Continuity of the learning process for students is facilitated by use of the model as figure 1 in each chapter.

Implications for Community Nutrition Professionals (new): This section acts as a summary of the chapter and also discusses application to community nutrition professionals.

Case Studies and the Expert Speaks (new): Case studies are based on issues, programs, and services. The Expert Speaks sections offer advice and counsel from professionals in their respective fields. Each chapter has either a Case Study or an Expert Speaks section.

Community Nutrition Professionals in Action (new): Study questions and projects are provided in each chapter for undergraduate students.

Going One Step Further (new): This section in each chapter includes advanced projects for graduate students.

Additional Information (new): Professionals societies develop statements, scientific status summaries, and position papers to clarify an issue in which the particular society has expertise. The topics of these papers and references are included in relevant chapters.

Quotes (new): Each chapter opens with a quote that captures the content of the chapter.

References: Each chapter contains up-to-date references, many published in the middle or late 1990s.

ACKNOWLEDGMENTS

Numerous individuals have made significant contributions to this edition. Without their experience, guidance, and advice, this book would not have been completed. Receiving continual feedback from colleagues, practitioners, and students helped us develop a truly teachable textbook.

CONTRIBUTING AUTHORS

A special thanks and public acknowledgment is made to the contributing authors who provided chapters, materials, consultation, and their precious time.

Marci K. Campbell, PhD, RD
Head, Center for Study Development and Learning,
University of North Carolina

Harriet H. Cloud, MS, RD
Professor Emeritus, Sparks Center,
University of Alabama-Birmingham

Jean Hankin, DrPH, RD
Professor of Public Health and Nutrition Researcher,
Cancer Center of Hawaii

Penny Kris-Etherton, PhD, RD
Professor, Department of Nutrition,
Pennsylvania State University

Jeanne P. Goldberg, PhD, RD
Associate Professor of Nutrition and Communications;
Director, Center on Nutrition Communications,
Tufts University

Shiriki Kumanyika, PhD, MPH, RD
Professor and Head,
Department of Human Nutrition & Dietetics,
University of Illinois at Chicago

M. Elizabeth (Beth) Kunkel, PhD, RD
Professor, Department of Food Sciences,
Clemson University

Christiaan B. Morssink, MA, MPH
Sociologist, Health Planner, and PhD Candidate,
University of Illinois at Chicago

Lori Roth-Yousey, RD, MPH, LN
Nutrition Consultant, North Branch, Minnesota

Susan G. Sherman
Center for Study Development and Learning,
University of North Carolina

Madeleine Sigman-Grant, PhD
Professor and MCH Nutrition Specialist, University of Nevada,
Reno at Cooperative Extension in Las Vegas

Laura S. Sims, PhD, MPH, RD
Professor, Department of Nutrition and Food Sciences,
University of Maryland

CASE STUDIES AND THE EXPERT SPEAKS

A unique feature of this book is the collection of insightful Case Studies and expert opinion commentaries entitled the Expert Speaks. We thank the experts whose outstanding and substantive articles highlight this text:

Elsa Ramirez Brisson, MPH, RD
Supervising Public Health Nutritionist,
Monterey County Area Agency on Aging

Kathy Cobb, MS, RD, CD/N
Senior Nutrition Consultant,
State of Connecticut Department of Public Health

Nancy R. Conner, Judge (Retired)
Court of Limited Jurisdiction, Maricopa County, Arizona;
Member, Ethics Training Team

Ruth M. Dow, PhD, RD, LD, FADA
Graduate Coordinator of Nutrition, School of Family &
Consumer Science,
Eastern Illinois University;
Program Director, Alfalit (Spanish for Literacy,
Basic Education, Nutrition, Community Development)
International, Inc., Miami FL

Ted Fairchild, PhD, MPH, RD
President, Fairchild and Associates, Los Angeles, California

Susan Finn, PhD, RD
Director, Nutrition Services, Ross Laboratories

Constance J. Geiger, PhD, RD
President, Geiger & Associates

Jeanne P. Goldberg, PhD, RD
Associate Professor of Nutrition and Communications;
Director, Center on Nutrition Communications,
Tufts University

Dayle M. Hayes, MS, RD, LD
Nutrition Consultant, Billings, Montana

Jennifer P. Hellwig, MS, RD
Tufts University

Sheryl L. Lee, MPH, RD
Chief, Office of Nutrition Services,
Arizona Department of Health Services

Christiaan B. Morssink, MA, MPH
Sociologist, Health Planner, and PhD Candidate,
University of Illinois at Chicago

Mary Naglah, PhD, RD
Pennsylvania State University

Sharon Sass, RD
Community Education Nutrition Consultant,
Office of Nutrition Services,
Arizona Department of Health Services

Jerry Soechting, MS, RD
Public Health Nutrition, St. Paul–Ramsey County Department
of Public Health Community Nutrition Services

McGraw-Hill selected an experienced group of professors to review the third and fourth editions. We appreciated their many excellent suggestions, which had an influence on various aspects of the fourth edition. Our special thanks to the following persons:

Nancy Cotugna, Dr.P.H.
University of Delaware

Mary Darling, PhD, MPH, RD
University of Minnesota

Jeanette Endres, PhD, MPH, RD
Southern Illinois University

Hazel Forsythe, PhD
University of Kentucky

Diana Spillman, PhD, LD, RD
Miami University of Ohio

OTHER CONTRIBUTORS

A work of this kind involves the assistance and expertise of many individuals and organizations who contributed in various ways to its completion. Our heartfelt thanks to the following:

The American Dietetic Association, Chicago, IL
Harold Holler, RD, Governance Team,
Association Management Group

Association of Public Health State & Territorial
   Nutrition Directors, Washington, DC
Executive Director

Institute of Food Technologist, Chicago, IL
Joyce A. Nettleton, DSc, RD, Director, Science Communications;
Ellen S. Sullivan, Science Communications Manager

Brigham and Women's Hospital, Boston, MA
Mary Ellen Collins, MEd, RD,
Director, Department of Nutrition;
Alice McCarley, MS, RD,
Director, Dietetic Internship, Department of Nutrition;
Katherine D. McManus, MS, RD,
Manager, Clinical Nutrition, Department of Nutrition;
Connie R. Roberts, MS, RD,
Manager, Nutrition Consultant Services and Wellness Program

Department of Nutrition, Pennsylvania State University
Assistance with Chapter 10 (Nutrition in the Adult Years) was
provided by Valerie Fishell, MS, research associate;
Julie Haines, MS, RD, research associate;
Kristin Moriarity, MS, research associate;
Mary C. Naglak, PhD, RD, (Case Study);
Brenda Nestor, MS, RD,
graduate student (Nutrition Professional In action)

Carol Boushey, MPH, PhD, RD
Assistant Professor, Department of Animal Sciences, Food
and Nutrition, University of Southern Illinois

Ruth Bowling, MS, RD
Board of Directors, The Colorado Center for Human Nutrition

Johanna Dwyer, DSc, RD
Professor, Department of Medicine and Nutrition,
Tufts University School of Medicine; Senior Scientist, USDA
Human Nutrition Research Center on Aging;
Director, Francis Stern Nutrition Center

Philip J. Garry, PhD
Professor and Director, Clinical Nutrition Program,
University of New Mexico

Karen Glanz, PhD, MPH
Professor, Department of Epidemiology,
Cancer Center of Hawaii, University of Hawaii

Krista Jordheim, MPH, RD
Nutritionist, Children's Health Care, Minneapolis

Morrisa Miller, MPH, RD
Nutrition Director, Yavapai County Health Department

Kristen Tomey
Research Assistant, Department of Human Nutrition & Dietetics,
University of Illinois at Chicago (assistance with Chapter 18)

Jane Grant Tougas
Marketing Communication, J.G.T. Ideas

Faye L. Wong, MPH, RD
Associate Director of Diabetes Education,
Division of Diabetes Translation,
Center for Disease Control and Prevention

Karen Zelenak, MPH, RD
Director, Strategic Planning and Policy Development,
Washington County Department of Health, Environment
and Management

ABOUT THE AUTHORS

The authors of the fourth edition have been practitioners of the art and science of nutrition for a combined total of over a 100 years. They have practiced in public health, hospitals, long-term care, industry, academe, research and development, and government. This experience provides a rich mix of expertise from being on the "firing line" in most areas of nutrition, medicine, and the community.

ANITA L. OWEN, MA, RD, is one of the leading consultants in nutrition and health communications and is recognized both nationally and internationally as a nutrition practitioner and leader in public health, industry, academe, and professional associations. She has gained national recognition in the field of public policy through her work as one of the major architects of the Special Supplemental Nutrition Program for Women, Infants and Children (WIC). Her career in nutrition has spanned nearly thirty-five years. Currently, she is president of Owen & Owen, Ltd., a consulting firm specializing in nutrition and health communications. Full time positions she has held include Senior Vice President, Nutrition Education and Research, National Dairy Council, and Manager, Nutrition, Nabisco Brands, Inc. Her many years of service at the Arizona Department of Health Services included positions as Chief of the Nutrition Bureau, Chief of the Chronic Disease Control Section, and Assistant Director, Community Health Services. Owen's service to professional associations is extensive. She has been president of both the American Dietetic Association (ADA) and the American Dietetic Association Foundation (ADAF) and she was president of the Association of State and Territorial Public Health Nutrition Directors. She is the recipient of numerous awards and honors, including the 1991 Copher Award, the highest honor given by the American Dietetic Association to one of its members, and the 27th Lenna Frances Cooper Memorial Lecturer by the ADA. She also received the first Award of Excellence in Community Nutrition given by the ADAF and the Ross Award for Distinguished Service in Maternal and Child Health Care, Western Branch, American Public Health Association.

PATRICIA L. SPLETT, MPH, PhD, RD, FADA, is a recognized researcher, practitioner, consultant, and teacher. A specialist in cost-effectiveness analysis, she has written more than forty articles on the cost and outcomes of nutrition and health care interventions. Throughout the United States and Canada, she has lectured on the cost, effectiveness, and quality of nutrition care services. Through Splett and Associates, Dr. Splett provides consultation to public health, industry, government, and health care organizations. She authored *The Effectiveness and Cost Effectiveness of Nutrition Care: A Critical Analysis with Recommendations,* which was published as a supplement to the *Journal of the American Dietetic Association.* Dr. Splett was a member of the faculty of the School of Public Health at the University of Minnesota for sixteen years. During six of those years, she served as the Chair of Public Health Nutrition. Under Dr. Splett's direction, nontraditional graduate programs for employed nutritionists and registered dietitians were implemented in the areas of management and health promotion.

GEORGE M. OWEN, MD, is both a pediatric researcher and practitioner and an educator of physicians and dietitians. He is known worldwide for his investigations concerning the growth, body composition, and iron nutrition of infants and children, and for his pioneer research on nutritional status of preschool children. Dr. Owen has held major positions in pediatrics and nutrition throughout his career. At Bristol-Myers Squibb/Mead Johnson, he served as Medical Director for International Nutrition. At the University of Michigan, he was Professor and Director, Human Nutrition Program, School of Public Health; Professor of Pediatrics; and a Fellow of the Center for Human Growth and Development. He was also Professor of Pediatrics and Director, Clinical Nutrition Program, University of New Mexico and Ohio State University. He has published over 100 papers in pediatric and nutrition journals. Dr. Owen served on the Committee on Nutrition, American Academy of Pediatrics and on the Food and Nutrition Board, National Academy of Sciences. He has also served on the editorial boards of the *American Journal of Clinical Nutrition* and the *American Journal of Public Health.* Dr. Owen is a member of the Society for Pediatric Research, the American Pediatric Society, and the European Society for Pediatric Research, and in 1997, he was selected as an Honorary Member of the American Dietetic Association.

LAYING THE CORNERSTONE
ENVIRONMENTAL FORCES INFLUENCING COMMUNITY NUTRITION PRACTICE

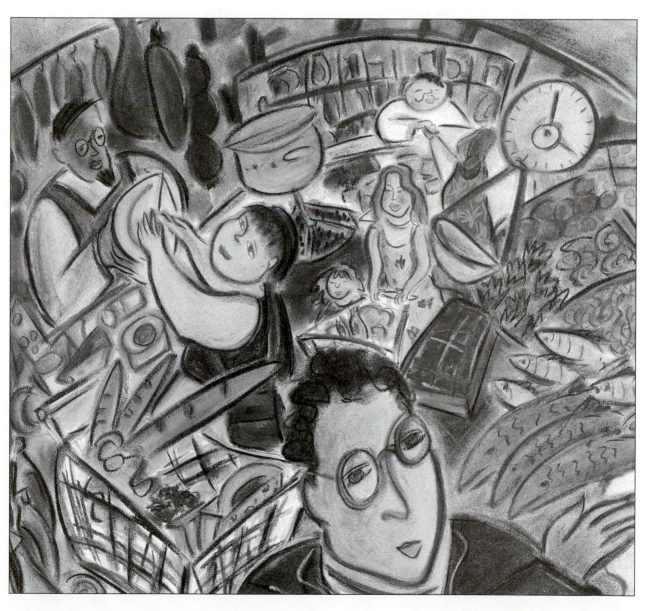

CHAPTER ONE

SOCIETAL AND HEALTH TRENDS
IMPLICATIONS FOR COMMUNITY NUTRITION PROFESSIONALS

*Through scientific discovery and technological innovation,
we enlist the forces of the natural world to solve many
of the uniquely human problems we face—feeding
and providing energy to a growing population, improving human
health, taking responsibility for protecting
the environment and the global ecosystem.*

—President Bill Clinton

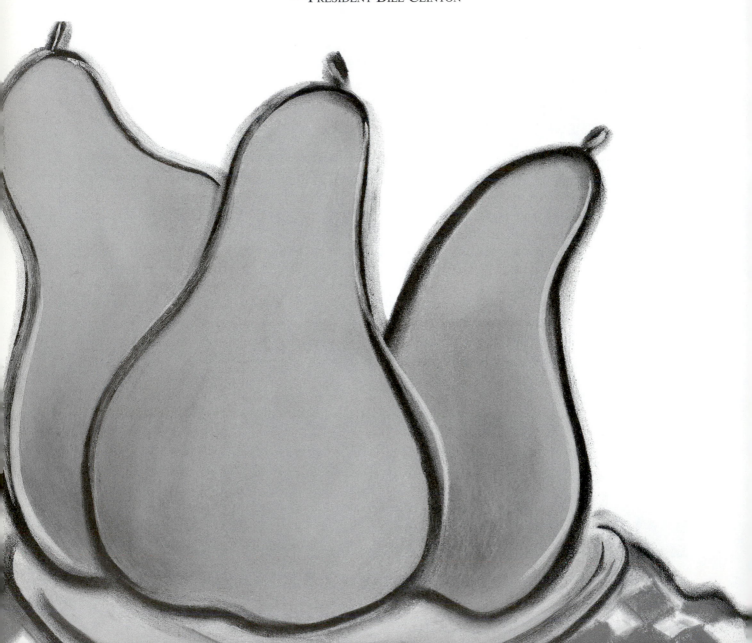

Core Concepts

Environmental forces including societal and health trends have a strong influence on the needs and wants of a community. In this era of rapid change, understanding the factors that contribute to these changes is key to working effectively in the community. The health status of an individual or community is determined by four interacting factors: biological background, self-determined behavior or lifestyle, the environment including social and physical attributes, and the health care system. These factors play a major role in our efforts to deliver health and nutrition interventions that will make a positive change in health status.

Objectives

When you finish chapter one, you should be able to:

~ Identify the major societal trends affecting communities including health and health care, demographics, lifestyle, food, nutrition, and technology.

~ Compare and contrast the societal and health trends described to the trends in the community in which you work or live.

~ Define the "context of health" and determine how it applies to community nutrition.

~ Identify the nutrition-related health status of the U.S. population.

~ Discuss critically the nutritional quality of the U.S. diet.

~ Discuss critically the food and nutrition trends in the United States.

Key Words

Word	Page Mentioned
Community nutrition professional	4
Context of health	4
Income inequities	7
Baby boomers	9
Generation X	9
Health behavior	14
Source of nutrition information	14
Integrated health care	15
Managed health care	15
Information technology	15

In the twenty-first century, we as **community nutrition professionals** will be faced with unlimited opportunities and enormous challenges. No century in human history has experienced so many social transformations as our present century. Just in the last decade, we have seen stunning technological innovations, unprecedented economic opportunity, surprising political reform, a great cultural rebirth, and a health care revolution.

Clearly, the organizational landscape of health care delivery is being rearranged in the United States today. Ultimately, the new system should provide appropriate care in a seamless continuum that uses limited resources most effectively. The way the new health care hybrids grow and develop in the early years has important implications for the health and health care of Americans for years to come. How this arrangement progresses has important implications for community nutrition professionals* as they work to promote optimal nutritional status and maintain health in the populations they serve. Community nutrition professionals will also need to understand that lifestyle, environment, and biological background are as important as the health care delivery system itself.[5] Only by understanding all these factors can the challenges of the twenty-first century be met.

THE CONTEXT OF HEALTH

To help community nutrition professionals meet these challenges, this text is based on a model for health called the **context of health.** This model is composed of a set of factors that interact together to determine the nutritional well-being and health status of individuals and populations. These factors include:

- Biological background
- Lifestyle choices
- The environment
- The health care system

An individual's biological background includes heredity, development, and resistance to disease. This biological background interacts, throughout life, with the individual's environment, which can include pollution, disease, stress, and poverty and the individual's lifestyle choices. The resulting health status and whether

disease develops is affected by the individual's access to the health care system, and by that system's quality.

This interplay of biology, lifestyle, environment, and health care is the **context of health** illustrated in figure 1.1. Each of the four factors of this model provides different opportunities for intervention to prevent disease and promote health. For example:

- Adequate nutrition improves immune function, decreasing susceptibility to infectious agents in the environment.
- Genetic background may reveal a familial risk of heart disease, but individual lifestyle choices in diet and exercise may modify this risk.
- Environmental conditions such as pollution and crowding may increase exposure to disease-causing agents, but improved access to health care services such as immunization can prevent some diseases, while diagnostic and treatment services can prevent advancement to greater disability and early death.

An assessment that takes into account this context of health is the first step toward addressing the nutritional and health problems of a community. To better understand where we are today, we look first at the history of public health.

THE PUBLIC'S HEALTH: A LOOK AT THE NEXT CENTURY

Over the past century, many of the world's major infectious diseases such as pneumonia, diphtheria, and smallpox have been brought under control.[21] In 1900, however, the top three causes of death were all infectious diseases, and they accounted for nearly one third of all deaths (figure 1.2). Presently, the top three causes of death are all chronic diseases, and among them they account for nearly two thirds of all deaths[17] (figure 1.3). Changes in lifestyle, advances in surgical techniques, and new drugs have helped to reduce mortality from heart disease, hypertension, and diabetes, but these disorders remain challenges for the twenty-first century.

Heart Disease

As figure 1.3 shows, in 1994 heart disease was the leading cause of death in the United States. Nonmodifiable risk factors of coronary heart disease are genetics and increasing age. Lifestyle, however, also plays a major role in the development of this disease. Modifiable risk factors include elevated total and low-density lipoprotein

---

*In this text "community nutrition professionals" includes public health nutritionists, community nutritionists, and community dietitians. Other health care professionals are also included in this term when they are involved in promoting the nutritional well-being of communities.

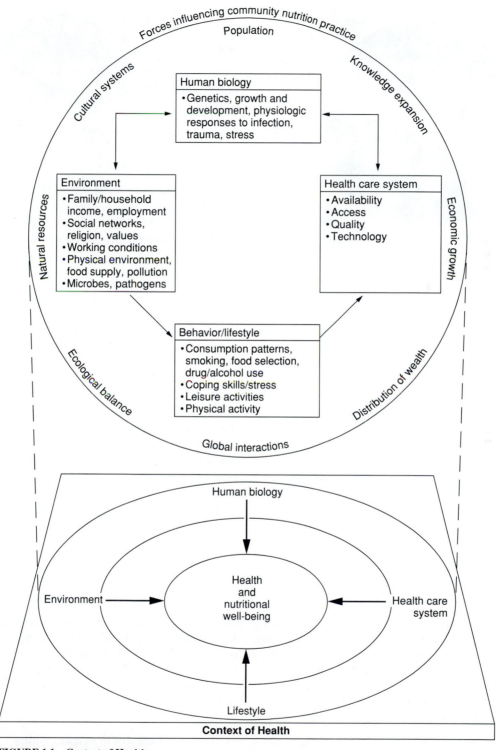

FIGURE 1.1 Context of Health
The forces that influence community nutrition practice.

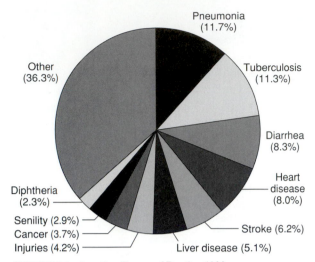

FIGURE 1.2   Leading Causes of Death—1900

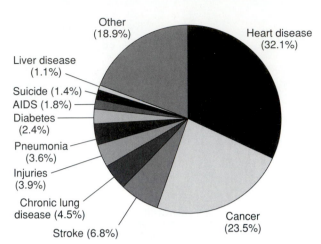

FIGURE 1.3   Leading Causes of Death—1994

cholesterol levels, hypertension, cigarette smoking, excessive weight, and long-term physical inactivity. Americans appear to be making some lifestyle changes: between 1960 and 1991, the proportion of adults age twenty to seventy with high serum total cholesterol levels decreased steadily. However, intakes of total fat and saturated fatty acids remain above recommended levels for a large segment of the population.[16]

Stroke

Each year, 500,000 Americans suffer a stroke and 150,000 of these people die each year. However, the death rate from stroke has fallen by 25 percent over the last decade.[17] Again, lifestyle changes decrease risk: reducing hypertension, maintaining healthy weight, reducing stress, and moderating sodium intake are preventive measures.

Hypertension

Although the prevalence of hypertension has decreased since 1960, hypertension remains a major public health problem. As many as 50 million Americans have elevated blood pressure and take antihypertensive medications.[21] Early detection and treatment is important in controlling hypertension, as is maintaining healthy weight, reducing stress, and sometimes, restricting sodium intake.

Diabetes

Sixteen million Americans have diabetes mellitus, which increases the risk of heart attack, kidney disease,

stroke, blindness, and a variety of other complications. Recent studies have shown that intensive management of diabetes can significantly delay the development of serious complications by as much as fifteen years.[6]

Overweight and Obesity

Significantly more American adults, adolescents, and children were overweight in 1996 than in the period between 1975 and 1980.[18] The association of overweight with many chronic diseases and adverse health outcomes makes this statistic a cause for public health concern. Americans spend more than $33 billion a year on schemes to lose weight, yet their success rate is very low.

Cancer

Along with genetics, lifestyle may play a role in most forms of cancer. It has become increasingly apparent that certain dietary factors either promote or inhibit cancer. Among the carcinogens that can initiate cancer development are radiant energy, chemical agents, and biological agents. Many single nutrients may have cancer-inhibiting properties. These anticarcinogens include antioxidants, certain phytochemicals, and dietary fiber.[31]

Low-Birthweight Infants

More than 250,000 low-birthweight infants are born each year. These infants have an increased risk of death and neurodevelopmental conditions, learning disorders, behavior problems, and lower respiratory tract infections. Factors associated with low birthweight include younger and older mothers, low socioeconomic status, low weight gain during pregnancy, smoking, and substance abuse. Many states have implemented programs for high-risk pregnant women to encourage early and continuous health care, adequate nutrition, and social supports to prevent low birthweight and its complications.

HIV Infection/AIDS

More than 1 million Americans are infected with HIV, the virus that causes AIDS. Some drugs, such as AZT (azidothymidine) have been found to slow the progress of the disease, and combining AZT with other drugs is considerably more effective than single-drug therapy. The HIV/AIDS patient's quality of life can be enhanced by nutritional supplementation. Nutrition intervention is an essential component of the management of individuals with HIV/AIDS. HIV infection and AIDS are discussed in greater detail in chapter 12 "Clients with Special Needs."

FACTORS AFFECTING HEALTH STATUS IN THE NEXT CENTURY

To this point, our discussion has identified some major nutrition-related problems that have challenged community nutrition professionals over the years. As we look to the next century, demographics and food habits will affect the health and nutritional status of the population.[14] Information on the nutritional quality of the U.S. diet can help to identify high-risk areas (box 1.1).

A comparison of dietary trends among racial and socioeconomic groups in the United States revealed that in 1965, dietary quality was very different between racial and socioeconomic groups: Whites of high-socioeconomic status ate the least healthful diets, and Blacks of low-socioeconomic status ate the most healthful diets. When surveyed between 1989 and 1991, the diets of all groups had improved and were relatively similar. Fat consumption decreased over time in all groups. Intake of fruits and vegetables changed little over time, except for an increase among Blacks of medium socioeconomic status. Consumption of grains and legumes increased over time among Whites of medium- and high-socioeconomic status and declined among Blacks of low-socioeconomic status.[23]

Demographic Trends

Examining dietary trends from the perspective of changing demographics can be very enlightening. Household income and composition, culture, as well as health insurance coverage, determine much of the lifestyles of individuals in those households. A Census Bureau report, How We're Changing: Demographic State of the Nation, 1996, provides a glimpse of trends and issues facing Americans today that will also influence the nature and delivery of nutrition services in the next century.[1] Following is an overview of recent and possible future demographic trends.

Americans Living Below the Poverty Level Poverty income guidelines are determined by the Department of Labor and are adjusted yearly. The poverty level for a family of four was $14,800 in 1994. That year, the number of persons below the official poverty level dropped to 38.1 million from the 1993 number of 39.3 million (table 1.1), and the poverty rate also decreased. The number of poor people varied by race and ethnic origin (figure 1.4).

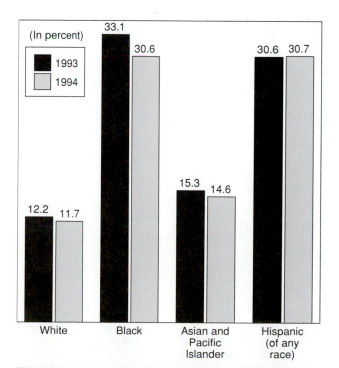

FIGURE 1.4 Poverty Rates by Race and Hispanic Origin
From Bureau of the Census, U.S. Department of Commerce: *How we're changing: demographic status of the nation, 1996,* Special Studies Series P23-91, Washington, DC, 1996, U.S. Government Printing Office.

BOX 1.1

WHAT IS THE NUTRITIONAL QUALITY OF THE U.S. DIET?[16]

- Energy balance remains a problem. About one third of adults and one fifth of children and adolescents are overweight.
- Although intakes of fat, saturated fatty acids, and cholesterol have decreased, they remain above recommended levels for a large proportion of the population.
- Median sodium intakes are higher than recommended values for most Americans six years of age and older.
- Median calcium intakes from food are below recommended values for several segments of the population; many Americans are not getting the calcium they need to maintain optimal bone health.

- Median iron intakes from food are below recommended values for young children and females between twelve and fifty-nine years of age.
- Fewer than one third of American adults consume the recommended five to nine servings of fruits and vegetables per day; average daily intake of fruits and vegetables, when contributions from mixed dishes are included, is about four servings.
- Some Americans do not always get enough to eat. About 9 to 13 percent of low-income people experience some degree of food insufficiency.

TABLE 1.1
Census Highlights
Social and Economic Issues

Median U.S. household income was virtually unchanged from 1993 to 1994	$32,264 32,041	1994 1993
Median household income by region in 1994	$34,926 34,452 32,505 30,021	Northeast West Midwest South
Number of Americans living below poverty level declined in 1994	38.1 million 39.3 million	1994 1993
Number of divorced Americans has more than quadrupled since 1970	17 million 4 million	1994 1970
Divorce rate leveled off and rate of out-of-wedlock births slowed		1990 and 1995
In 1994, there were 23 million immigrants in United States (9% of the total population)	6 million 1 million	Mexican Filipinos
Child care Provided by relatives Nurseries and preschools Family day care	41% 31% 17%	

Cost of child care	Per week	Percentage of income
Two-parent families	$78	7
Single-parent families	61	12
Poor families	50	18

Adapted from Bureau of the Census, U.S. Department of Commerce: *How we're changing: demographic status of the nation, 1996, Special Studies Series P23-191, Washington, D.C. 1996, U.S. Government Printing Office.*

More than 63 percent of related children in single-mother households were poor, compared with about 12 percent of comparable children in two-parent families.

Income Inequities The rich have gained in share of national income, and the poor have lost since World War II.[2] Between 1947 and the 1960s, poor and middle-class families were getting a growing share of the nation's wealth. Then the trend reversed and the gap between rich and poor has steadily widened. In 1994, the richest one fifth of American households got 46.9 percent of national income; the poorest one fifth of families got 4.2 percent.

Lack of Health Insurance Coverage In 1994, 15 percent of the population had no form of health insurance. However, the percentage of poor persons without health insurance was almost double that number (29 percent). In 1994, 20 percent of part-time workers had no health insurance compared with 16 percent of full-time workers and 13 percent of persons who did not work. In each of these groups, the percentage uninsured was much higher among poor persons.

Child Care More than half the mothers of young children are employed outside the home. In 1994, care for preschoolers was provided primarily by relatives (41 percent). Where child care was provided by outside sources, two-parent families spent more on child care than did single-parent families (12 percent of their gross income versus 7 percent). Poor families spent about 18 percent for child care.

Immigrants in the United States In 1994, there were 23 million immigrants in this country, representing 9 percent of the total population. That is the highest level since the beginning of World War II. Nearly half of all immigrants were Hispanic. Mexicans were the largest group, with 6 million, and Filipinos were the second largest, with 1 million.

Lifestyle Influences on Dietary Choices Recognizing changing demographics within a community, and understanding how household dynamics change over the adult years, will determine the direction community nutrition professionals take when designing and implementing nutrition interventions. The changes in family composition reported by the U.S. Census Bureau significantly influence consumer purchasing behavior and attitudes toward health and nutrition. The traditional nuclear family household is no longer the norm (table 1.2). In 1990, nearly one in every four households was a person living alone, ranging from affluent, young, single professionals to elderly people with relatively low, fixed incomes.

Households headed by single mothers more than doubled and, surprisingly, those headed by single fathers more than tripled over the last decade. The number of family households has decreased, while the number of nonfamily members living together as a household has increased. Time for food preparation in these households is limited. As a result, fast foods, take-out, and other forms of convenience foods appeal to this segment of the population.

BABY BOOMERS AND GENERATION X

Two specific population groups that will profoundly influence the lifestyle, health, and nutrition of Americans are the **baby boomers**—more than 77 million Americans born between 1946 and 1964—and their children—the so-called "**Generation X**," now aged eighteen to twenty-nine.

Baby Boomers—A Massive Demographic Shift

In 1996, the first of more than 77 million baby boomers turned fifty. Over the next decade, people aged fifty to sixty will comprise the fastest-growing portion of the U.S. population, although they will not become a majority of those aged fifty to seventy-four until 2005.

Ethnic Profile Change

The ethnic and racial profile of the older population will also change as the boomers age.[4]

- From 1990 to 2050, the older Hispanic population will triple, from 5.1 to 15.6 million.
- In that same time period, the proportion of elderly African-Americans will more than double, from 2.5 to 9.6 million.

TABLE 1.2
Households of the 1990s

Type	1994	1990	1970	Percentage change 1970–1994
Total households	97,107*	93,347	68,401	+53
Families	68,490	66,090	51,456	+33
Married couples	53,171	52,317	44,728	+19
with children < 18	25,085	24,537	25,522	−2
no children < 18	28,117	27,780	19,196	+47
Single mothers				
with children < 18	7,647	6,599	2,858	+168
no children < 18	4,759	4,290	2,642	+80
Single fathers				
with children < 18	1,314	1,153	341	+285
no children < 18	1,599	1,731	887	+80
Nonfamily households				
Female living alone	14,171	13,950	7,319	+94
Males living alone	9,440	9,049	3,532	+167

*In thousands

Adapted from Bureau of the Census, U.S. Department of Commerce: *Household and family characteristics,* Washington, D.C., 1994.

• Older Americans of other racial origins (Asians, Pacific Islanders, Native Americans, Eskimos, Aleuts) will increase from 500,000 to 5 million.[4]

Health Status

Most baby boomers will have better health in their sixties and seventies than did previous generations, because they have had better prenatal care, immunizations, and nutrition. They have also had better health habits as adults, including lower rates of smoking, more time spent exercising, and greater awareness of the benefits of preventive health measures and a healthier diet. They also want more products and services that promote health.[4]

Some Vulnerable Boomers

The 1992 Consumer Expenditure Survey examined per capita income and expenditures for various types of baby-boomer households, and found that single-parent boomers seem to be the most vulnerable economically.[29] Single-parent boomer households (mostly women) were more likely to receive welfare and food stamp income than other forms of public as-

sistance. Because they are less likely to receive earned income, they will be at a disadvantage in later years[8] (see figure 1.5). This fact is significant for community nutrition professionals, who will be working with this generation.

"Generation X"—Baby Boomers' Babies

The segment of consumers now aged eighteen to twenty-nine has been labeled "Generation X." Born between 1966 and 1976, they represent 21 percent of the population. Members of this group have greater expectations than their counterpart baby boomers did.[11] Persons aged eighteen to twenty-four are the most likely to lack health insurance.[20] The economic prospects for this generation differ as well. Although wages do reflect seniority and experience, overall wages have dropped. Median full-time weekly wages ($285) of men aged sixteen to twenty-four fell by $29 per week between 1983 and 1992; income for women of the same group fell from $277 to $267. The types of jobs available also have changed. The shift to a service economy, with generally lower wages and limited benefits, has affected this generation more than any other. Health prospects and em-

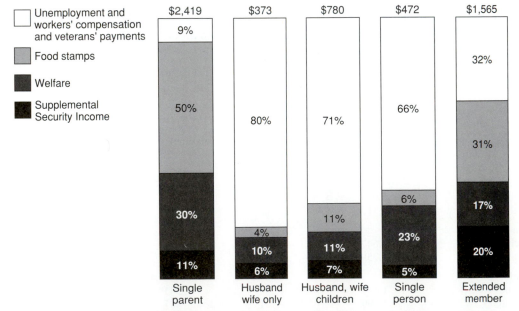

FIGURE 1.5   Dollar Shares of Public Assistance Received by Consumer Units Headed by Baby-Boomer Respondents, 1992
From Dinkins JM: Per capita income and expenditures of baby-boomer households. *Family Economic and Market Review,* 3: 27–39, Washington, DC, 1995.

ployment prospects are also poorer for this generation. A 15 percent decline in physical fitness activities puts this group at risk of becoming overweight; the prevalence of overweight has increased in all racial and ethnic groups. This generation will present a real challenge to community nutrition professionals.

SPENDING PATTERNS IN AMERICAN FAMILIES

The community nutrition professional who works with families to help them purchase nutritious foods needs to know how much money is available. Figure 1.6 shows the breakdown of U.S. household expenses; the average U.S. metropolitan household spends half its income on shelter, utilities, transportation, and food.[19]

MEDIA INFLUENCES ON CHILDREN'S EATING PATTERNS

Community nutrition professionals need to be aware of how the media influences children, who in turn influence family decisions on food choices. In 1995, 38.2 million children watched about twenty-one hours of TV per week.[13] Although the number of hours of TV

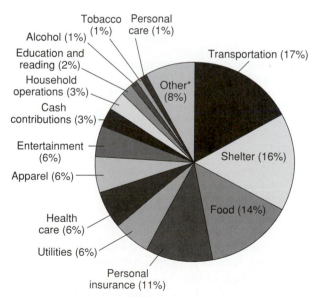

FIGURE 1.6   The Spending Pie
Percentage distribution of estimated average spending by category for households in metropolitan areas, 1993. America's hottest markets. Reprinted with permission. © 1996 American Demographics, Ithaca, New York.

watching has decreased from twenty-four hours in 1990, the number of watchers—the children's market—has increased by almost 3 million. Nearly half of all commercials advertise food, with a high percentage of food commercials aired during children's programs. The foods most frequently advertised are those high in fat, sugar, and salt. The message from these food commercials has a primary emotional and psychological appeal, with little basis in sound nutrition.[30] It has been demonstrated that television influences the eating habits and thus the nutritional status of children in three significant ways:

- Television advertising influences family food purchases and the snacking pattern of young children.
- The use of food as depicted by television programs show food being used for many activities other than satisfaction of hunger.
- The few overweight children used in television programs suggests that inappropriate use of foods has no impact on health or nutritional status.
- The relation between increased television viewing and increased snacks.[7,30]

NUTRITION AND FOOD TRENDS

In past generations, a person could expect to eat about the same foods, cooked the same way, as their parents and grandparents had. That is no longer the case. Today, as with the rest of our lives, the world of food and nutrition is constantly changing. New techniques enhance food. New methods of distribution bring more kinds of foods to more people. People from differing cultures bring their own unique tastes into the marketplace. From "eating healthy" to combining different cuisines, many changes are happening and will continue to happen in the world of food. Take a look at table 1.3 to see the changes that have occurred just in the last half century.[27]

The Food-Health Connection

One of the most exciting developments for the future of food is an increased awareness about the connection between food and health. Increasingly, people are changing (or talking about changing) their diets to maintain or improve their health. According to the thirteenth annual *Prevention Index Survey,* the number of Americans who try to eat a healthful diet and who regularly participate in strenuous exercise has not changed over the past

TABLE 1.3
"Healthy Eating" Approaches from the 1940s to the 1990s

1940s

- Americans are on a meat-eating binge after World War II, consuming 155 pounds per person per year by 1947.
- Milk, cheese, and eggs are in; bread, cereal, potatoes, and beans are out.
- Animal fat is considered a good source of energy.
- The government issues recommended daily allowances outlining minimum nutrients, then later releases a pie chart featuring the Seven Basic Food Groups.
- The government mandates that all commercial yeast-raised baked goods be vitamin-fortified.
- J. I. Rodale's *The Organic Food Front* makes a case for chemical and pesticide-free farming.

1950s

- Protein is king.
- Government issues the Basic Four Food Groups—dairy, vegetables and fruits, meats, breads and cereals—along with recommended daily dietary allowances.
- People consume large amounts of dairy products and highly marbled meats.
- Salt restriction is considered unnecessary by health experts.
- Food faddist, Adele Davis, author of *Lets Eat Right and Keep Fit,* prescribes eating fertile eggs, unpasteurized milk, and toxic doses of vitamins. Her error-ridden book sells in the millions, spawning the growth of self-help health food and vitamin supplement markets.

1960s

- We enter "the high point" of instant food, quick food, and space-age food.
- Julia Child's first cookbook, *Mastering the Art of French Cooking,* leads to her PBS cooking show, which launches the home-gourmet market.
- Researchers link salt to high blood pressure.
- Sugar gets the blame for hyperactivity in children (since disproved).
- Weight Watchers is founded.
- In 1964, Dr. Herman Taller's *Calories Don't Count* espouses eating tons of fat to stay thin (since disproved).
- Food faddist Adele Davis is called the nation's most notorious purveyor of nutrition misinformation by Harvard nutritionist Jean Mayer.

1970s

- Dishes swim in sour cream, whipped cream, cream cheese, margarine, hollandaise, and moray sauces.
- Baby boomers just coming of age love sweets and lack sophistication.
- Ralph Nader associate Michael Jacobson forms the Center for Science in the Public Interest, a Washington, D.C.-based food safety and nutrition watchdog organization.
- Two more fad diets: *Dr. Atkin's Diet Revolution,* a high-fat, high-protein, low-carbohydrate diet and Herman Tarnower's *The Complete Scarsdale Medical Diet* promote meals with no sugar, no potato or flour-based starches, and no dairy fats.

1980s

- Consumers eat nouvelle cuisine—long, pretty bites of strange food on big plates prepared by big name chefs.
- California cuisine is big.
- Government issues its first "Dietary Guidelines for Americans."
- Salt is considered a health hazard despite widely recognized inconsistencies in research.
- A study shows that sugar calms children's hyperactivity by causing release of serotonin in the brain. Sugar-induced illnesses are called fad diagnoses.
- Marketing of cholesterol-free food still high in saturated fat contributes to consumer confusion.

1990s

- Bean cuisine, rustic breads, and more healthful foods are in.
- Red meat consumption is down.
- Fat-free is the battle cry.
- The USDA food pyramid still depends on meat and dairy for much of its protein but recommends no more than 30 percent of calories from fat.
- Trans-fatty acids (TFAs) controversy rages. TFAs are found in margarine and processed foods.
- Oat bran miracle is questioned in the *New England Journal of Medicine*—sales plummet.
- Sugar is back in good graces, approved for use in diabetic diets. Tooth decay is the only sugar-related health problem.
- Moderate use of salt and alcohol are recommended in the 1995 reissue of HHS/USDA "Dietary Guidelines for Americans."
- Exercise is discussed in "Dietary Guidelines for Americans."
- New government thinking: Food is not just food, it is one of life's greatest pleasures.

several years[24] (table 1.4). However, the 1996 Food Marketing Institute trends report[28] shows that consumers continue to be less than satisfied with the healthfulness of their diet. Seventy-four percent believe their diet could be somewhat healthier; 7 percent say their diet is as healthy as it could possibly be. Almost all (97 percent) are changing their eating habits to ensure a healthy diet—an increase from 1995. Because

food preferences are closely tied to individual cultures and tastes, however, people will always eat certain foods regardless of their lack of nutritional value. Community nutrition professionals and other communicators need to teach their clients that it is necessary to strike a balance between the two extremes.

The most important attribute for selecting food continues to be taste, followed by nutrition, price, and

TABLE 1.4
Trends in Some Key Aspects of Diet and Nutrition

	Percent who say they "try a lot" to follow each guideline		
	1995	1994	1983
Get enough vitamins and minerals in foods or in supplements	58	59	63
Eat enough fiber from grains, cereals, fruits, and vegetables	57	54	59
Avoid eating too much fat	52	53	55
Get enough calcium in foods and supplements	50	52	50
Avoid eating too much salt or sodium	48	47	53
Avoid eating too many high-cholesterol foods such as eggs, dairy products, and fatty meats	45	45	42
Avoid too much sugar and sweet food	37	40	51
Avoid foods that contain additives, such as colorings and artificial flavorings	27	30	NA
Avoid caffeine in beverages such as coffee, tea, and certain soft drinks	25	26	NA

Note: NA means not applicable.
From The prevention index: a report card on the nation's health. *Prevention,* Emmaus, PA, 1996 Rodale Press, p.14. Used with permission.

product safety. Nutrition and product safety increased in importance for shoppers questioned in the 1996 survey.[28] Some 58 percent of consumers are very concerned about nutrition, primarily fat content. Salt and cholesterol are lesser concerns, and concern about sugar remains unchanged. Concern for calories, vitamins, and minerals is significantly increased over the previous year (figure 1.7). Four out of ten consumers assume responsibility for buying nutritious foods. Shoppers say that product labeling and nutrition education are important factors in food selection.[28]

Food, Health, and Reality

The National Livestock and Meat Board compared what Americans think they eat to what they actually consume.[10] This study found that perception is not reality when it comes to eating. Although most Americans report that their diets closely reflect the recommendations of the Food Guide Pyramid, in actuality all segments of the population underconsume foods in the vegetable, fruit, breads, and milk groups and overconsume fats, oils, and sweets. On average, the meat group is the only food group consumed in appropriate amounts. The imbalance of other foods shows that dietary recommendations are

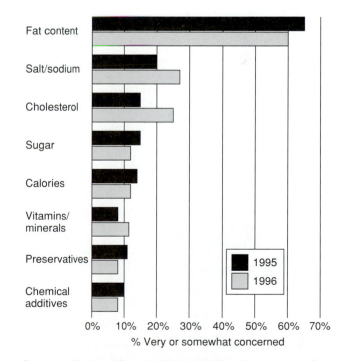

Concern with fat, sodium, and cholesterol heads consumers' lists.

FIGURE 1.7   Consumers Top Nutrition Concerns
Adapted from *Trends in the U.S.: consumer attitudes and the supermarket,* Washington, DC, 1996, Food Marketing Institute. Used with permission.

not being met (see figure 1.8). This survey shows that Americans may lack accurate knowledge of serving sizes, in addition to not recognizing sources of hidden fat in their diet.[10]

Why Is There a Nutrition Gap? What We Know and What We Do

A national survey conducted in 1997 by The American Dietetic Association (ADA) found that most Americans (79 percent) believe nutrition is important to health, yet only 39 percent say they are doing all they can to eat healthfully. Americans say food labels impact purchasing decisions, although they are not reading labels as often.[22]

Americans' behavior, attitudes, and knowledge of nutrition and health issues, their **health behavior,** continue to be affected by perceived and real obstacles. Fear of giving up favorite foods (40 percent), confusion and frustration over nutrition studies and reports (23 percent), and the belief that a balanced diet takes too much time (21 percent) rank as top inhibitors to healthful eating.

Age and gender are related to people's efforts to enjoy a balanced diet and physical activity. Women (42 percent) are more likely than men (36 percent) to say they are doing all they can to achieve a healthful diet, while older Americans (55 percent of those fifty-five years and older) are more likely to strive to eat well than those who are younger (28 percent of twenty-five to thirty-four year olds). Also, women (51 percent) more than the men (32 percent) perceive the Food Guide Pyramid as an important nutrition education tool to be useful in helping make food choices. Men (47 percent), on the other hand, are more likely than women (40 percent) to make an effort to get regular activity.

Knowledge and Source of Information

The ADA's survey shows that the media plays a vital role in educating Americans about food, nutrition, and health. Fifty-seven percent count television news programs as their largest **source of nutrition information**—up from

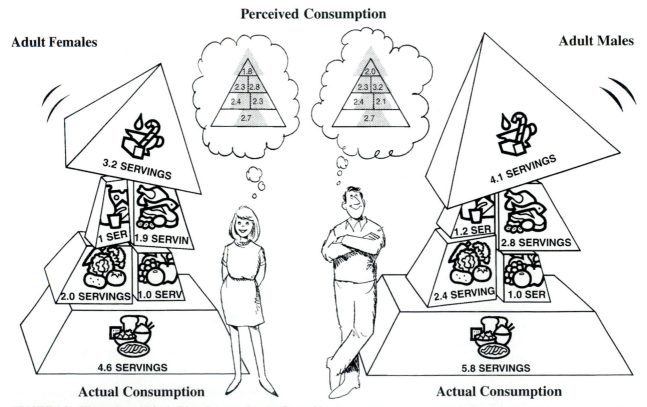

FIGURE 1.8   Women's and Men's Diets Compared to the Pyramid
From *Eating in America: a dietary pattern and intake report,* Chicago, 1994, National Cattlemen's Beef Association. Used with permission from the National Cattlemen's Beef Association.

forty-two percent two years ago. Although television now is the largest source of information, it is judged as "very valuable" by only 24 percent of people. Dietitians and physicians are viewed as the most valuable sources (both at 52 percent) followed by specialty health and nutrition magazines (39 percent), nurses (38 percent), and women's magazines (26 percent). Newspaper sources of nutrition information were rated "very valuable" by 21 percent of the respondents.[22]

Restaurants and Food Service: Impact on Food Consumption

Today's consumers know about a wide variety of foods and cuisines, but fewer people prepare meals from scratch than in the past. This fact is fueling the trade in restaurants and take-out food service. By the year 2000, over three quarters of a million locations will be offering food service in the United States. Sales will reach over $350 billion, or 4.5 percent of U.S. gross domestic product.[25] This is a very important statistic for community nutrition professionals who work with consumers.

Restaurants, supermarkets, and other take-out outlets have become an extension of the kitchen. Consumers are spending more of their money (an estimated $80 to $100 billion) on foods that are either fully prepared or easily assembled meal components ("home meal replacements").[26] By the year 2000, the spending power of minority groups will increase by approximately $300 billion, giving them increased economic power to influence new choices of foods and services.[3]

HEALTH CARE REFORM: THE NEW WORLD OF MANAGED CARE

Another major trend that will directly affect community nutrition professionals and the people they serve is health care reform. The future of the health care industry can be summarized in one word: integration. For years health care in the United States has been fragmented, and focused primarily on treating illness. But today's providers are attempting to prevent illness by organizing **integrated health care** delivery systems that include prevention, and provide a continuum of care.

Under an integrated delivery system, an individual would have one organization to deliver all health care needs. That organization would include major components, such as a primary care center or physician group,

hospital, outpatient specialty services, and home health agency. These entities could combine the organization, financing, and delivery of health care in ways that respond to the demographics identified above as well as the economic conditions present in differing regions of the country. See chapter 4 for a complete discussion of this topic.

As **managed health care** develops, community nutrition professionals will have to be vigilant about the direction they take, because it will certainly affect health and nutrition in the next decade and the way nutrition services are designed and delivered.

TECHNOLOGY TRANSFORMATION

To keep abreast of the societal and health trends described in this chapter, the community nutrition professional must be fully cognizant and knowledgeable about **information technology.**[12,15] As we move more rapidly into a service and knowledge economy, changes will affect all of us. One primary change will be rise of information technology (infotech), or the combination of computer networking and telecommunications. These interconnected technologies are moving out across the nation to reshape how jobs are done, from farm to factory, from office to hospital. By the year 2010, this spread of technology will bring about many changes. Peter Drucker, a business writer, has coined the phrase "knowledge worker" to describe the newly emerging dominant work group in our society.[9] This worker will require a good deal of formal education, and the ability to acquire and to apply theoretical and analytical knowledge. The Case Study by Dayle Hayes (page 18 in this chapter) "Using Information Technology to Enhance Community Nutrition Practice" is an excellent example of the use of technology to meet the community's nutrition needs.

Community nutrition professionals will need to be cognizant of these consumer trends to identify priority needs and to develop interventions that enable consumers to make appropriate food choices and achieve health and nutritional well-being.

IMPLICATIONS FOR COMMUNITY NUTRITION PROFESSIONALS

Evolving societal and health trends provide the context for community nutrition activity. Community nutrition professionals must be aware of general trends affecting the nation as a whole, as well as of specific trends that occur in the professional's community. Understanding issues affecting our society and the community's nutrition and health trends is a vital first step. Diet-related conditions increase the risk of some acute and chronic diseases and affect overall health status. It is important to know the nutrition-related health status of the populations as well as the nutritional quality of the diet. This information will help target populations in need of nutrition interventions.

Examining dietary practices from the perspective of demographic trends can provide a snapshot of people's lifestyles. Lack of health insurance, poverty, income inequities, and divorce rates are some of the information that is necessary in assessing a community.

Consumers have gotten the message that food and nutrition have an influence on their health. As a result, Americans are eating less fat and more grain products. Consumers' lists of attributes for selecting food continue to be taste first, then nutrition, followed by price and product safety. The changes in the health care system supposedly will provide a "seamless health care system." How this will affect community nutrition professionals in the twenty-first century is a question for debate.

Now that we have layed one part of the cornerstone, including environmental and health trends, it is time to build more.

COMMUNITY NUTRITION PROFESSIONALS IN ACTION

- Review the local paper for a period of two weeks to determine the health and nutrition issues covered. According to the reports, what groups or agencies are involved in the issues? Do the local, state, or federal public health agencies have a visible role?
- Compare and contrast the nutrition-related health status of the U.S. population and the nutritional quality of the U.S. diet. What changes should consumers make in their eating patterns to lower the risk of chronic disease?
- Utilizing the list of topics discussed in the demographic trends section, determine how your community compares to the national statistics. Contact the local economic security department or state planning agency to find this information.
- Complete a survey of your family and friends to determine where they obtain nutrition advice. What sources do they consider most accurate and valuable to improve their diets?

- From the survey data presented in the chapter, summarize the most important findings. How could you find out if these concerns hold true for your community?
- Is the growth in take-out foods evident in your community? How may this affect the nutrient value of consumers' diets?
- Visit a local health food store and make a list of the five most highly advertised products in the store. Look at the ingredients and then the health claims. Determine if these claims are warranted.

GOING ONE STEP FURTHER

- Track five periodicals such as *American Demographics, The Futurist, Food Technology,* a national news magazine, and a popular women's magazine. Determine the major health and nutrition information presented in these periodicals. Consider how reported economic, demographic, or lifestyle trends will affect the health and nutritional status of the population you serve. Use the information to become more aware of the context of health.
- Interview a restaurant manager about customers' interest in the health aspects of food. Determine what percentage of patrons are ordering healthy foods. What type of requests are made? How has the menu changed in recent years or months? How does present customer behavior contrast with that of customers the past five years?

REFERENCES

1. Bureau of the Census, U.S. Department of Commerce: *How we're changing: demographic status of the nation, 1996,* Special Studies Series P23–191, Washington, DC, 1996, U.S. Government Printing Office.
2. Bureau of the Census, U.S. Department of Commerce: *Income inequities,* Washington, DC, 1996, U.S. Government Printing Office.
3. Cetron MJ, DeMicco FJ, Williams JA: Restaurant rennaissance: current and future trends in food service, *The Futurist*:8–12, 1996.
4. Chernoff R: Baby boomers coming of age: nutrition in the 21st century, *J Am Diet Assoc* 95:650–654, 1995.
5. Dever AGE: *Community health analysis: global awareness at the local level,* Gaithersburg, MD, 1991, Aspen Publishers, p. 23.
6. The Diabetes Control and Complication Trial (DCCT) Research Group: The effect of intensive treatment of diabetes on the development and progression of long-term

complications in insulin-dependent diabetes mellitus, *N Engl J Med* 329:977–986, 1993.

7. Dietz WH, Gortmaker SL: Do we fatten our children at the TV set? Obesity and television viewing in children and adolescents, *Pediatrics* 75:807, 1985.

8. Dinkins JM: Per capita income and expenditures of baby boomer households, *Family Economic and Market Review* 8(3):27–39, 1995.

9. Drucker PF: Managing in a time of great change, Dutter, NY, 1995, Truman Talley Books.

10. *Eating in America: a dietary pattern and intake report,* Chicago, 1994, National Cattlemen's Beef Association.

11. Fay WB: Understanding growth & market research, 5:54–55, 1996.

12. Hayes D: Cyberspace 101: Taking a ride on the information highway, DBC Dimension, *Quarterly Newsletter of Dietitians in Business and Communications* (Winter):1–2, 1996.

13. Hazelton JL: Kiddie consumers, *The Arizona Republic* 25 April 1996, p. E 1.

14. Institute of Medicine: *Opportunities in nutrition and food sciences,* Washington, DC, 1994, National Academy Press.

15. Kolasa KM: New developments in nutrition education using computer technology, *J Nutr Educ* 28:7–13, 1996.

16. Life Sciences Research Office, Federation of American Societies for Experimental Biology: *Third report on nutrition monitoring in the US,* Washington, DC, 1995, Superintendent of Documents, U.S. Government Printing Office, 1995.

17. McGinnis MJ, Foege WH: Actual causes of death in the US, *JAMA* 270:2207–2211, 1993.

18. Meisler JG, St. Jeor S, Shapiro A, Wynder EL: American Health Foundation roundtable on healthy weight, *Am J Clin Nutr* 63(Suppl): 409 S–477 S, 1996.

19. Mogelonsky M: America's hottest markets, Ithaca, NY, 1996, American Demographics.

20. National Institute on Drug Abuse: *National household survey on drug abuse: population estimates 1988,* DHHS Publication No. ADM 89-1636, Washington, DC, 1988, Department of Health and Human Services.

21. National Research Council: *Diet and health: implications for reducing chronic disease risk,* Washington, DC, 1989, National Academy Press.

22. *Nutrition trends survey 1997,* Chicago, 1997, The American Dietetic Association.

23. Popkin BM, Siega-Riz AM, Haines PS: A comparison of dietary trends among racial and socioeconomic groups in the US, *New Engl J Med* 335:716–720, 1996.

24. *The Prevention index: a report card on the nation's health.* Emmaus, PA, 1996, Prevention Magazine, Rodale Press Inc.

25. Saporito B: What's for dinner, *Fortune* 1312:50–64, 1995.

26. Sloan AE: Take out takes off, *Food Technology* 49:38, 1995.

27. Trager J: *The food chronology,* New York, 1995, Henry Holt Publishers.

28. Trends in the U.S.: Consumer attitudes and the supermarket 1996, Washington, DC, 1996, Food Marketing Institute.

29. U.S. Department of Labor Bureau of Labor Statistics: Consumer expenditure survey 1992, Washington, DC, 1992, Interim Survey Public Use Tapes and Documentation.

30. Windhauser MM and Windhauser JW: A nutritional evaluation of food and beverage products as advertised to children on Saturday morning television, *J Am Diet Assoc* 91:A-83, 1991.

31. Willett WC: Micronutrients and cancer risk, *Am J Clin Nutr* 59(Suppl): 1162 S–1165 S, 1994.

CASE STUDY

USING INFORMATION TECHNOLOGY TO ENHANCE COMMUNITY NUTRITION PRACTICE

BY DAYLE HAYES, M.S., R.D.

NUTRITION CONSULTANT, BILLINGS, MONTANA

DESCRIPTION

This case study describes the use of information technology in planning, developing, implementing, and evaluating a school-based nutrition project in Montana. It is designed to illustrate the numerous ways that technology can be used by nutrition professionals to enhance community education programming.

The case involves a contract project between the Montana Office of Public Instruction (OPI) School Food Services and a nutrition consultant (the author) to produce a nutrition education kit. The kit, entitled *Team Up for Fun, Food and Fitness,* was designed for school food managers to use in promoting the USDA Food Guide Pyramid during a schoolwide nutrition event. This project occurred, as described, during the fall of 1996 and throughout 1997.

METHODOLOGY/TEACHING OBJECTIVES

The major focus of this case is how technology can enhance community nutrition practice. It explores a variety of issues, including how to:

- Survey existing nutrition resources through professional electronic networks
- Access nutrition information for professionals on the World Wide Web
- Utilize e-mail to expedite communication among reviewers of nutrition material
- Promote the availability of accurate nutrition information on the Internet
- Use videoconferences and interactive video networks for nutrition training
- Collect evaluation data for nutrition programs via electronic means

The material presented here can be used in a variety of ways. As homework, students can be assigned to search for specific nutrition information and resources on the World Wide Web. This same activity can also be conducted in a computer lab as a group activity, where students are assigned to compare the effectiveness of different search engines (e.g., Yahoo) in locating food and nutrition sites. Students could also be required to subscribe to, participate in, and monitor one or more professional nutrition listservs (e.g., Mealtalk). Any of these activities could provide extensive material for class discussions on the appropriate use of technology in community nutrition practice.

THE CASE

In Montana, OPI contracts with Montana State University (MSU), Department of Health and Human Development to coordinate USDA's Nutrition Education and Training (NET) Program and Team Nutrition activities. From offices at MSU in Bozeman, Katie Bark, R.D., provides nutrition education materials and training to food service personnel in schools and communities across the state. She also facilitates Team Nutrition activities and coordinates school-based programs with other local, state, and federal nutrition programs.

In the fall of 1996, with funding from a USDA grant, OPI School Food Services contracted with an independent nutrition consultant (Dayle Hayes, M.S., R.D., in Billings, 140 miles from Bozeman) to develop a ready-to-use packet of materials and information. The kit was specifically designed to assist Team Nutrition Schools with hosting a schoolwide nutrition event and help all schools with their nutrition efforts. Ms. Bark served as supervisor for the project. The primary audience for the kits was school food service managers, who would then "team up" with educators, parents, children, and other community resources to promote the Food Guide Pyramid.

The objectives of the *Team Up for Fun, Food and Fitness* kit were to:

- Support healthy food and fitness choices for families
- Expand the variety of foods that kids enjoy

BOX 1.2

SAMPLE LISTSERVS FOR FOOD AND NUTRITION PROFESSIONALS
- FoodTalk (Cooperative Extension Service, Nebraska): To subscribe, send an e-mail message to: listserv@unlvm.unl.edu. Leave the subject section blank and in the message section, type: subscribe foodtalk. DO NOT include an e-mail signature in the body of the message section.
- Fn_spec (Food and Nutrition Specialists, Purdue): To subscribe, send an e-mail message to: almanac@ecn.purdue.edu. In the message section, type a 1-line lowercase message: subscribe fnspec_mg.
- MEALTALK (Child Nutrition Programs, USDA): To subscribe, send an e-mail message to: majordomo@nal.usda.gov. In the message section, type: subscribe mealtalk yourname <your e-mail>
- NETTALK (Nutrition Education and Training, USDA): To subscribe, send an e-mail message to: majordomo@nal.usda.gov. In the message section, type: subscribe nettalk firstname lastname <your e-mail address>
- Public Health Nutrition (Univ. of Washington): To subscribe, send an e-mail to: listproc@u.washington.edu. In the message section type: subscribe PHNUTR-L your name

SAMPLE WEB SITES FOR FOOD AND NUTRITION PROFESSIONALS
- American Dietetic Association ~ http://www.eatright.org/
- Dietetics Online ~ http://www.dietetics.com/
- Food and Nutrition Information Center ~ http://www.nalusda.gov/fnic/
- Healthy School Meals ~ http://schoolmeals.nalusda.gov:8001/team.html
- Wheat Foods Council ~ http://www.wheatfoods.org/

SAMPLE WEB SITES FOR TEACHERS, KIDS AND FAMILIES
- Dole 5 A Day ~ http://www.dole5aday.com
- Fun Foods for Kids ~ http://www.nppc.org/funfood.html
- Kids Health ~ http://www.kidshealth.org/kid
- Nutrition Expedition ~ http://www.fsci.umn.edu/nutrexp
- PearBear Healthy Kids ~ http://www.usapears.com/pears/pbbear.htm

---

- Encourage kids to eat more fruits, vegetables, and grains
- Promote the enjoyment of lower fat foods
- Motivate schools and communities to work together for kids' health

In developing the kit, Dayle Hayes sought to utilize existing resources rather than "reinvent the wheel." She teamed up with two other nutrition professionals Terry Egan, M.S., extension agent with the Expanded Food and Nutrition Program (EFNEP), and Michele Taylor McMullen, M.S., M.A., R.D., nutrition instructor at Montana State University-Billings (MSU-B) to search for appropriate existing materials. Their search involved actual resource libraries at MSU and EFNEP, as well as *an electronic search* of nutrition web sites and requests for information posted on *Internet listservs* for nutrition and school food service professionals. From a local hospital site, Hayes, Egan, and McMullen also participated in a *downlinked videoconference* in which the USDA showcased the recently released Team Nutrition Community Action Kit.

These resources produced numerous ideas for existing educational activities, menus and materials that were incorporated into the first draft of the kit. The draft text was forwarded, via *electronic mail,* to Katie Bark in Bozeman and the Office of Public Instruction in Helena. Suggestions, additions and corrections to the text were returned to Hayes by *e-mail.* The draft logos from a graphic designer in Bozeman were also transmitted by e-mail to the involved parties around the state.

Hayes and McMullen searched the World Wide Web for consumer-oriented *web sites.* Using several different *search engines,* they were able to locate numerous sites that offered food, fun, and fitness information for teachers, parents and children. A selection of these sites, with *web site locators (URLs)* and brief descriptions, was included in the kit under the heading *Five Fabulous Web Sites.*

Technology was also important in promoting the *Team Up for Fun, Food and Fitness* kit and in training school food service and cooperative extension staff in the use of the kit. Prior to distribution, Katie

Contents of the Kit:

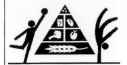

Team Up for Fun, Food and Fitness
How to Celebrate the Food Guide Pyramid
with a "Pyramid Power" Event

- Introduction: Team Up for Fun, Food and Fitness
- Checklist for Fun, Food and Fitness
- Team Players: Looking for Talent in All the Right Places
- Games and More Games
- Sources for Games and Other Nutrition Materials
- Prizes and More Prizes
- Five Fabulous Web Sites
- Menus of Champions
- Getting the Word Out
- Sample Press Release
- Winning Decorations
- Kit Evaluation
- Flyer: Fit Families Have More Fun
- Flyer: Pyramid Power Invitation
- Flyer: Team Thank You

Developed by:
Dayle Hayes, MS, RD, Nutrition Consultant, Billings, Montana
Terry Egan, MS, MSU Extension Service-EFNEP Extension Agent, Yellowstone County
Michele Taylor McMullen, MS, RD, Instructor, MSU-Billings

Project Supervisor:
Katie Bark, RD, Nutrition Education and Training Program, Bozeman

With thanks to:
Montana Beef Council: Charlene Schuster, Helena ~ (406) 442-5111
Montana Pork Producers Council: Sue Huls, Bozeman ~ (406) 994-3595
Montana Wheat & Barley Committee: Cheryl Tuck, Great Falls ~ (406) 761-7732
Western Dairy Council: Judy Barbe, Thornton, Colorado ~ (800) 274-6455

Bark discussed kit availability and use during an interactive videoconference with regional Team Nutrition training leaders through the METNET (Montana Education Telecommunications Network) system. The complete kit was posted in the METNET *bulletin board* so that educators and food service personnel, and other school staff could access all text and graphics electronically. The kit evaluation form was also posted on the METNET bulletin board so that users could fill out the form and send their feedback to the NET office electronically.

SOME QUESTIONS

- How could this community nutrition project have been further enhanced through the use of technology? What technologies have been developed since this project period (1996 to 1997) that could now be utilized in planning, development, implementation, or evaluation of an updated *Team Up for Fun, Food and Fitness* kit?
- What additional World Wide Web nutrition sites are available for professionals and consumers? How can Internet users distinguish between sites that

contain science-based nutrition information and those that promote unproven products or nutrition misinformation?

- What additional listservs, bulletin board systems, and videoconferences can be accessed by food and nutrition professionals? How can professionals quickly and easily learn about the availability of these resources?

- Where can food and nutrition professionals obtain the training and savvy they need to utilize technology on projects like this one?

- What are some of the advantages and disadvantages of current information technologies? How can food and nutrition professionals balance the opportunities and challenges of using these technologies in community nutrition practice?

CHAPTER TWO

THE ART AND SCIENCE OF COMMUNITY NUTRITION

*The history of public health might well be written as a record
of successive redefining of the unacceptable.*
—SIR GODFREY VICKERS

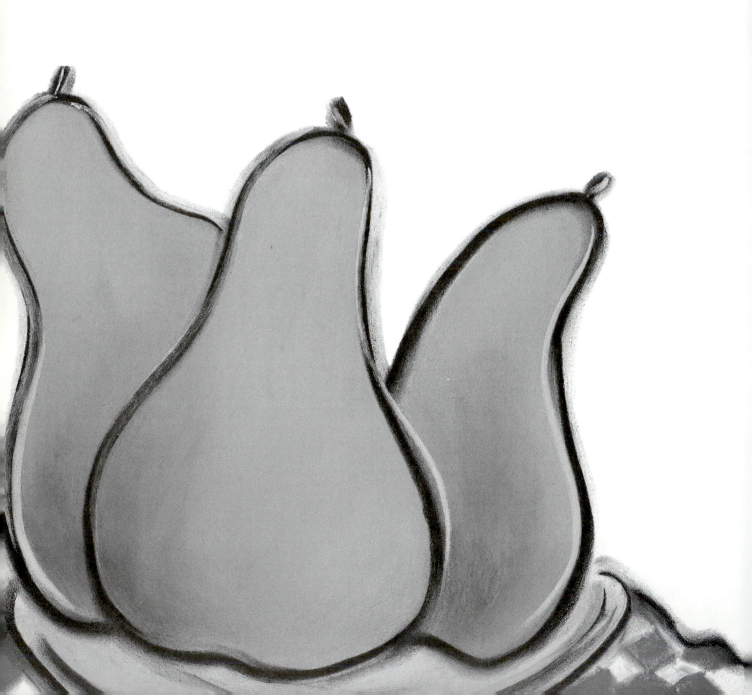

Core Concepts

Public health is the science and art of preventing disease and promoting and protecting the health of the community. This is accomplished through three core functions: assessment, policy development, and assurance. Community nutrition professionals play a vital role in this process. Because of their knowledge of food, nutrition, and health, community nutrition professionals develop systems that address nutrition needs throughout the life cycle. They are advocates for the needs of vulnerable groups. In addition, they provide nutrition intervention at the primary, secondary, and tertiary levels of prevention.

Consensus among scientists has developed about the role of diet in the cause and prevention of chronic disease. Interpreting and applying scientific findings related to diet and disease for people is done through dietary guidance. Dietary guidance tools including the *Guidelines for Americans,* the *Food Guide Pyramid,* and *Nutrition Facts* food labels are based on the most current application of science and help people to make food choices that promote health and prevent disease.

Objectives

When you finish chapter two, you should be able to:

~ Apply the definitions of health promotion, health protection, and disease prevention to the community in which you live.
~ Cite examples of primary, secondary, and tertiary prevention in public health and public health nutrition.
~ Describe the work of public health nutritionists and give examples of nutrition interventions that you have observed in operation in your community.
~ Describe the development of the Health Objectives for the Nation and indicate the priority areas to be achieved by the year 2000.
~ Define the basis for dietary guidance in the United States.
~ Discuss critically the use of RDA and DRI.
~ Differentiate between the Food Guide Pyramid and the Basic Four Food Groups.
~ Identify the key changes in food labeling and indicate how these changes benefit the consumer.
~ Cite the basis for health claims on the food label.

Key Words

THE ROLE OF PUBLIC HEALTH IN AMERICAN COMMUNITIES

To define public health as we know it today, it is first necessary to discuss the concept of health itself. Health has been defined by the World Health Organization (WHO) as a state of complete physical, mental, and social well-being, not the mere absence of disease or infirmity.[2] The WHO concept has been a major impetus in changing beliefs about the context of health.

In chapter 1, health and its context was described as having four fundamental factors: environment, lifestyle, human biology, and health care systems. Figure 2.1 presents a contemporary model for health and its attributes. The model depicts how public health fits into the context of health and it demonstrates how science is applied to dietary guidance to improve the health and nutritional well-being of the community.

Community Defined

A **community** consists of interdependent social units composed of individuals that transact a common life. Within a community, there may be several subgroups with varying norms, but some agreed on commonalities, values, and language. As a complex social group functioning with norms of behavior and organization of resources, the community regulates both the environment and behavior.[4]

A community can be defined by geographical (city, county, or state), political (voting district), or organizational boundaries (employees of Ford Motor Company or students and staff of Metro University), or by heritage or ethnic group or by shared interest or concern (the arts community). All communities have norms, values, and a system of organization.

Official government agencies are assigned the responsibility for overseeing the health of people in communities, usually defined geographically. They include local (public health departments or county hospitals), state (departments of agriculture, education, environment, health, social services and transportation), or federal (the United States Public Health Service [USPHS] is the lead agency for community health efforts).

Other critical participants in the community health system include clinical medicine (public and private clinics and hospitals and managed care organizations, voluntary health agencies (the American Cancer Society and the American Heart Association), schools and universities (education and research), business (chambers of commerce) and industry (Kraft and Nabisco), professional associations (the American Dietetic Association and the American Medical Association), community organizations (churches and Hunger Coalitions), and third-party payers (Medicare and Medicaid and insurance companies).

Defining Public Health

Public health is an organized effort to shape the environment to promote and protect the health of all people in the community. In 1920, Winslow enunciated what became the known and most widely accepted definition of public health[14,40] (see box 2.1). Winslow's definition is still very applicable today.

A more recent definition of public health was developed for the *Future of Public Health* report in 1988.[14] The definition that evolved is "Public health is what a society does collectively to assure the conditions in which people can be healthy." To protect the public's health, government funds are allocated to federal, state, and local public health agencies. The core functions of these agencies are **assessment, policy development, and assurance** .[40]

Assessment　Assessment consists of regularly and systematically collecting, assembling, analyzing, and making available information on the health of the community. This includes statistics on health status, community health needs, and epidemiology and other studies of health problems. Public health agencies have a very important role in this effort because they have the assessment expertise to track the health of populations and the distribution of problems and risk factors.

Policy Development　Public health agencies serve the public interest in the development of comprehensive public health policies by promoting use of a scientific knowledge base in decision making about public health problems and their causes and strategies for intervention, and by leading in developing public health policy. For example, the Dietary Guidelines for Americans were based on scientific knowledge linking nutrition to chronic disease.

Assurance　Public health agencies assure their constituents that services necessary to achieve agreed on goals are provided by encouraging actions by other entities (private, voluntary, or public sector), by requiring

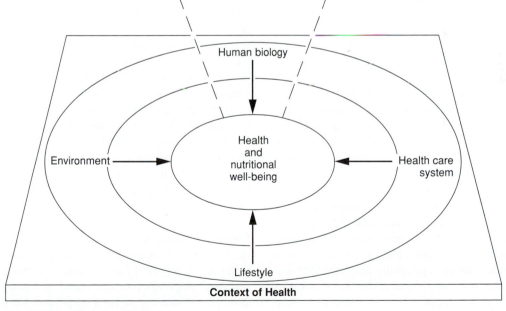

FIGURE 2.1   Context of Health
How public health fits into the context of health.

BOX 2.1

PUBLIC HEALTH IS THE SCIENCE AND ART OF

- Preventing disease
- Prolonging life
- Promoting health and efficiency through organized community effort for:
  - Sanitation of the environment
  - Control of communicable diseases
  - Education of the individual in personal hygiene
  - Organization of medical and nursing services for the early diagnosis and prevention of disease
  - Development of the social machinery to ensure everyone a standard of living adequate for the maintenance of health, organizing these benefits so as to enable all citizens to realize their birthright of health and longevity.

such action through regulation, or by providing services directly. The latter includes provision of essential personal health services to high-risk groups such as prenatal care to low-income women.

Health Objectives for the United States

One of the most significant events in public health was the development of the Health Objectives for the Nation. It provided a blueprint for action on the major health problems that the United States faces. Development of these objectives began in the 1970s with input from major health organizations in the United States. After two years of discussion and deliberation, the document *Promoting Health/Preventing Disease: Objectives for the Nation 1990* was released.[38] A decade later, **Healthy People 2000:** *National Health Promotion and Disease Prevention Objectives* was published.[36] This document includes twenty-two priority areas under the general headings of health promotion, health protection, preventive services, and surveillance. Nutrition is covered under health promotion. The year 2000 priority areas expanded on the 1990 objectives with the addition of topics such as HIV infection and cancer. The emphasis shifted to prevention of disability and morbidity and greater attention to improvement in the health status of definable population groups at highest risk of premature death, disease, and disability.

In the 1995 mid-course review of the health objectives, new objectives were added and new special population targets were included. Modifications to the year 2000 objectives were made because of new baseline data.[37] This process of defining and tracking progress toward national health objectives is on-going. Readers should refer to emerging documents with objectives for 2005 and 2010.

Positive Trends   Figure 2.2 provides an overview of the tremendous strides the United States has made over the past two decades in reducing mortality due to heart disease and strokes. As shown in the figure, between 1972 and 1992, the coronary heart disease (CHD) death rate declined about 49 percent, and the stroke death rate dropped about 58 percent. Preventive lifestyle improvements and better control of the risk factors for cardiovascular disease have been the major factors in the reductions. Key to the success has been the focus on science-based strategies in which research findings are translated and applied to clinical and public health practice. Despite these gains, heart disease continues to be the leading cause of death in the United States, and stroke is the third leading cause. The disease toll among minority populations continues to be a concern, as they have not experienced the same levels of improvement in risk factor control.

Unmet Challenges   Rates of overweight and obesity are increasing in most segments of the population. Objectives for physical activity and fitness address this problem. An objective presented in *Healthy People 2000* is "to increase at least 30 percent the proportion of people age six years and older who exercise regularly, preferably daily, in light to moderate activity for at least 30 minutes per day."[37] To help consumers meet their physical fitness needs, the *Surgeon General's Report on Physical Activity and Health* was released in July 1996.[32] The report is based on extensive review of the current data on exercise and longevity. The report

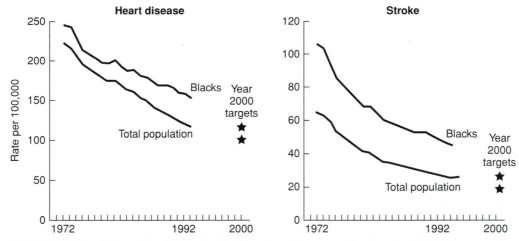

FIGURE 2.2   Age-Adjusted Death Rates for Coronary Heart Disease and Stroke in the United States
From National Heart, Lung, and Blood Institute (NHLBI), National Institutes of Health (NIH), Heart Memo, Washington, DC, Fall, 1995.

clearly states that a sedentary lifestyle is unhealthy, and that exercise will reduce the risk of dying from coronary heart disease. Physical activity also reduces the risk of developing diabetes, hypertension, and colon cancer, fosters healthy muscles, bones, and joints, enhances mental health, and helps maintain function and preserve independence in older adults. There is virtually unanimous agreement that we need to get our country more physically active. Some of the problem areas include:

- Sixty percent of adults in the United States are not active enough.
- Only 22 percent of people meet at least the minimum exercise guidelines of 30 minutes of moderate activity each day most of the week.
- Thirty-four percent are sedentary.
- Fifty-four percent exercise sporadically.
- From the ninth to the twelfth grades, participation in physical education drops from 100 percent to 50 percent.

Canadian Experience with Health Promotion and Disease Prevention   "Optimal health for Canadians can only be achieved when greater efforts are made in health promotion and prevention of illness and when nutrition is an integral part of these." This is the approach taken by Health-Welfare Canada as they developed Canada's Guidelines for Healthy Eating.[9] The Canadian government also has developed Achieving Health for All: A Framework for Health Promotion. Through this effort, they hope to strengthen their community-based

health services. The focus of these national efforts include the following:

- Reduce inequities in access to and use of the health care system.
- Change unhealthy behavior by increasing preventive strategies.
- Enhance individuals' ability to deal with chronic illness and disabilities.

Nielsen has indicated that adopting a health promotion focus based on Achieving Health for All can mean a change in direction for many Canadian community nutrition professionals.[22] It can mean moving away from a traditional caregiver role to one of facilitator, educator, and advocate. It means moving away from past emphasis on individual risk reduction to prevention, and toward the future of a multifactorial, global, community-based approach.

Health Promotion, Health Protection, and Disease Prevention

The major strategies for achieving national, state, and local health objectives are health promotion, health protection, and disease prevention. Health promotion is the science and art of helping people change their lifestyles in the direction of optimal health.[26] The focus of health promotion is lifestyle and behavior. Because personal choices have a powerful influence on health, when behavior changes positively, health improves.

Health-enhancing behaviors include obvious immediate behaviors that affect physical and emotional health, such as exercising regularly; eating nutritious foods; managing stress well; and avoiding tobacco, excess alcohol, and drugs. Health promotion programs will be most successful if they take into account the individual's level of readiness to change. With this definition of health promotion, it is important to consider the dimensions of optimal health. Most definitions and programs focus on the physical dimensions, addressing fitness, nutrition, and risk factors for disease (such as hypertension or elevated serum cholesterol) and to a lesser extent, the emotional dimension, especially stress management. Although these dimensions are crucial to an effective health promotion program, they often neglect the social, spiritual, and intellectual dimensions of health. Ideally, optimal health is a balance of physical, emotional, social, spiritual, and intellectual health.[4]

Health Protection

Health protection includes environmental and regulatory measures to confer protection on large population groups. An example of this is community food codes for institutional feeding.

Disease Prevention

Disease prevention includes screening and clinical preventive services to eliminate unnecessary disease, disability, and premature death caused by acute and chronic diseases and injury associated with environmental home and workplace hazards. Disease prevention strategies include improved access to clinical preventive services such as maternal and child health, cancer screening, and diabetes control. Across the continuum from health to disease, health promotion, health protection, and disease prevention can be directed to three levels of **prevention—primary, secondary, and tertiary.**[15] Figure 2.3 illustrates these levels of prevention.

Primary Prevention   Primary prevention activities promote health and provide specific protection against the onset or incidence of a health problem. They prevent a problem from affecting people in the first place. Primary prevention efforts work to change the environment and the community, as well as family and individ-

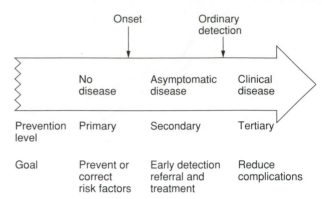

FIGURE 2.3   Three Levels of Prevention

ual lifestyles and behaviors, to enhance and maintain a state of optimal health. Examples include nutrition campaigns such as the "5 a Day for Better Health," the promotion and support of breast-feeding, and food safety training for food service workers.

Secondary Prevention   Secondary prevention refers to activities concerned with the early diagnosis and treatment of health problems. Interventions are designed to reduce risk among those who may be more susceptible to health problems because of their family history, lifestyle, environment, or age. Secondary prevention includes screening detection, early diagnosis, treatment, and follow-up. Examples include cholesterol screening and referral, nutrition screening initiatives, and nutrition therapy. These interventions may be offered by a public health agency or by a community group involved in health care delivery.

Tertiary Prevention   Tertiary prevention refers to minimizing existing disability through treatment and rehabilitation efforts. Tertiary prevention helps to limit further negative effects of existing conditions. These interventions are frequently provided by specialty clinics or rehabilitation centers as part of the medical care system. Examples include nutrition services for children with special health care needs and diabetes management.[4,15]

Types of Intervention

Public health interventions can be categorized into three intervention types: **individual-based interventions, community-based interventions,** and **systems-based interventions** as described below and outlined in table 2.1.

TABLE 2.1
Nutrition Intervention Matrix

	Primary	Secondary	Tertiary
Individual	Breast-feeding support	Nutrition education for high-risk WIC clients	Medical nutrition therapy for clients with special health care conditions
Community	"5 A Day" campaign	Cholesterol screening clinic with referral	Computer bulletin board for chronic disease interest group
	Congregate dining for seniors	"Shape Up America"	
System	School lunch menus required to meet the Dietary Guidelines	Registered dietitian required team member in diabetes management standards of care	Legislation to mandate payment of nutrition service for diabetes, hypercholesterolemia, and obesity
	Folic acid fortification of foods	Fat and calorie labels	New regulations for folate fortification of certain foods

Individual-Based Interventions   Individual-based interventions focus on creating changes in the knowledge, behavior, or health outcomes of individuals, either singly or in small groups. They are typically seen as direct service to clients. Examples include one-to-one counseling, home health visits, prenatal classes, emergency medical response for an injury, pregnancy testing, case management, and respite services.

Community-Based Interventions   Community-based interventions focus on creating changes in populations. They are directed toward groups or subgroups of persons within the community. Examples include immunization clinics, media campaigns to eat more fruits and vegetables, lodging inspections, bike paths, worksite health promotion programs, and health fairs.

Systems-Based Interventions   Community nutrition professionals are also involved in systems-based interventions, which focus on creating change in organizations, policies, laws, or structures. The focus is not directly on individuals or communities but on the system that serves them. Examples include revised school lunch recipes to reduce fat content, food labeling laws, requiring a registered dietitian (RD) on the health care team, improving access to health care, and improving emergency medical services response time.

Nutrition Intervention   Nutrition intervention is defined as a purposefully planned activity, program, policy, or other action that is designed with the intent of changing a behavior, risk factor, environmental condition, or aspect of health status for an individual, target group, community, or the population at large.[17] It includes a range of planned change efforts designed to improve the nutritional status of the population. It requires skills in planning, implementing, and evaluating community nutrition programs and services. Nutrition intervention also includes effective communication, advocacy, and political action to bring about individual, community, and system changes.

PUBLIC HEALTH NUTRITION'S RICH HISTORY

The historical perspective of public health nutrition is rich with events throughout history that have greatly influenced public health practice. The chronology of events from 1900 through 1996 have been described.[6,7] During the twentieth century, demographic changes; advances in nutrition science and technology; and social, political, and economic changes have influenced the growth and development of public health nutrition. Some adverse changes have included the high rates of disease and death among mothers and children, food shortages during the wars, and the continuing presence of poverty and hunger. A positive change has been the greater recognition of the benefits of health promotion and disease prevention.

In contrast to those of the 1920s, the 1950s policy makers boasted about the abundance and quality of the American food supply.[6] In this decade, health problems related to dietary excesses such as obesity, diabetes, heart disease, and hypertension were identified as emerging public health problems. This brought about employment of nutritionists in chronic disease programs.

The 1960s increased nationwide awareness of nutrition issues and refocused attention on the maldistribution of the nation's food supply. In 1968, the publication "Hunger USA" and the CBS documentary "Hunger in America" drew public attention to the problems of malnutrition in the United States.[35] This led to the appointment of the Senate Select Committee on Nutrition and Human Needs in 1968 and the White House Conference of Food, Nutrition and Health in 1969. During the same period, two major surveys funded by the federal government— the Preschool Nutrition Survey and the Ten-State Nutrition Survey—were carried out.[28,33] As a result of the White House Conference and the findings from the surveys, food assistance programs were expanded.[35] One of the most effective programs began in 1972. The Child Nutrition Act provided funding to start the food program now known as the Special Supplemental Nutrition Program for Women, Infants and Children (WIC).

During the 1970s, the USDA also implemented the Expanded Food and Nutrition Education Program (EFNEP). In 1977, the Child Nutrition Act authorized funding for Nutrition Education Training (NET). The 1979 Surgeon General's report "Healthy People," specifically cited nutrition and diet among the significant factors affecting the health of the population.[38]

Public Health Nutrition

It is appropriate to define nutrition before we discuss public health nutrition. Nutrition is the science and art that deals with human health as it is affected by food nutrients and related dietary factors. The scope of this definition is very comprehensive. It includes the processes by which a safe, adequate supply of food and essential nutrients is processed, ingested, digested, absorbed, assimilated, metabolized, and eliminated by the human body so that growth, physical and mental development, reproduction, and productive living may occur.[6] There is compelling evidence for the interrelation of key nutrients and food components to human health, physical and mental development, reproduction, and active productive living. Research increasingly relates dietary excesses and imbalances to today's serious chronic diseases.

Public health nutrition is an integral component of *public health*. It is defined as the application of nutrition through an organized community effort to improve or maintain optimum nutritional health of the population and targeted subgroups. Public health nutrition efforts are primarily focused on health promotion and disease prevention but may address therapeutic and rehabilitation services when these needs are not adequately met by other parts of the health care system.

Public health nutritionists play a major role in delivering services at the primary and secondary levels of prevention. Discussion about the difference between public health and community health is relevant as we begin to define the role of the community nutrition professional. The terms public health nutritionist, community nutritionist, and community dietitian all appear under the community nutrition professional title. The distinction is that the public health nutritionist functions in an official government health agency, whereas the community nutritionist or dietitian functions in a broader context of the public and private sectors, such as public and private school systems, and USDA cooperative extension units.

The term community nutrition professional is used throughout this text to include both public health nutritionists and community nutritionists or dietitians because they use similar information and skills. For the purposes of this section, the discussion centers on the role of the public health nutritionist since it has been a well-defined and recognized specialty since early in the century. Information on public health nutrition is particularly helpful to students since the mission, functions, and responsibilities of public health nutritionists are clearly delineated.

A study of the classification of public health nutrition personnel indicates a continuum of functions.[6] Some public health nutritionists focus primarily on population-based interventions for health promotion and disease prevention and are highly involved in administration and policy setting. Others focus on provision of direct nutrition care of clients and are primarily engaged in nutrition education and counseling. The range of functions also results in a career ladder within the field of community nutrition (see figure 2.4).

Recommended educational, professional, and experience guidelines are available to assure that public health nutrition personnel possess the requisite knowledge, skills, and ability to serve the community. Public health nutritionists employed as supervisors or managers of nutrition programs generally have a master's degree with preparation in biostatistics, epidemiology, and environmental sciences; in health program planning, management, and evaluation; and in advanced

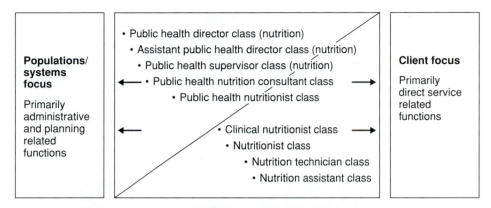

FIGURE 2.4   Major Focus of Public Health Nutrition Teams Positions
From Dodds JM, Kaufman M, editors: *Personnel in public health nutrition for the late 1990s: a comprehensive guide*. Washington, DC, 1991, Public Health Foundation. Used wih permission.

human nutrition.[6] For the managerial and professional series, licensure as a nutritionist (LN) or dietitian (LD) is the recommended professional credential in states that have licensure. In states without licensure laws, dietetic registration (RD) with the Commission on Dietetic Registration (The American Dietetic Association) is recommended.

The work of public health nutritionists is supported by a host of other health and social service professionals, such as physicians, nurses, and social workers. Public health nutrition is integrated into the work of many governmental and nongovernmental agencies and organizations at the local, state, national, and international levels.

The public health nutritionist promotes optimal nutritional status of the population by taking a leadership role in identifying nutrition-related needs of the community, planning and conducting interventions, mobilizing resources to meet needs, and evaluating outcomes as a member of a multidisciplinary team in an "official" public health agency. A comprehensive public health nutrition system should address:

- Nutrition needs across all ages and stages of the life cycle
- Advocacy for the needs of vulnerable groups
- Primary, secondary, and tertiary prevention
- Leadership advocacy and management oversight to assess, set policy, and assure that necessary services are available

Much of the work of the public health nutritionist centers around community assessment, followed by planning, implementation, and evaluation of nutrition interventions.

Knowledge and Skills Required to Function in Public Health

Community nutrition professionals functioning in public health must understand the following elements of nutrition and health:

- Science of food and nutrition and its roots in basic science
- Production and distribution of the food supply
- Safe preparation of food for consumption in the home, day-care center, school, worksite, or commercial eating establishment
- Advertising and marketing of food
- Utilization of food and nutrients by the human body to satisfy its needs in states of health or disease throughout the life cycle
- Interaction of food choice with multiple economic, political, geographic, social, cultural, psychological, and health factors that influence food selection
- Interactions with a broad range of health professionals, policy makers, advocates, and media communicators as well as the general public[6]

Community nutrition professionals working in public health agencies and other community settings must be experts in normal and clinical nutrition and must be competent in bringing about change in eating behavior. In addition to addressing population-based needs, the community nutrition professional must possess the following knowledge and skills in public health.[6]

- Policy, planning, and administration (knowing the community political structure and using skills in planning, organizing, managing, and evaluating community nutrition service systems to change eating behavior through organized community effort)

- Biostatistics (having skills in collecting, analyzing, and reporting demographic, health, and food composition data)
- Epidemiology (understanding health and disease distribution patterns in the population and studying trends over time)
- Environmental science (understanding the biological and chemical factors that influence the quality and safety of the air, water and food supply)

Community nutrition professionals function in a variety of settings and direct interventions to individuals, groups, and systems in the community. Settings include federal, state, city, or county government-operated public health departments. Community nutrition professionals are also employed in neighborhood or comprehensive health centers, hospitals, ambulatory care centers, HMOs, home health agencies, and specialized nutrition projects. They are also employed in a variety of community and human services agencies, as well as cooperative extension and public school systems.

Future Training Needs in Public Health Nutrition

A survey was undertaken to determine the future training needs of public health nutrition professionals in 2005.[27] The participants indicated that in the year 2005, the most important public health issues, and their nutritional implications will be (in descending order of importance):

- An increasingly elderly population, with more emphasis on health care and nutrition needs of this group
- Prevention and control of chronic diseases and increasing focus on nutrition risk factors

- Increasing poverty, with nutrition and health problems resulting from inadequate resources to purchase food and health care
- Health promotion and diseases prevention throughout the life cycle and increasing populations of color and need for cultural competency and sensitivity skills

As public health nutrition prepares for the third millenium, many changes are needed in public health nutrition practice to address the identified issues. The most important knowledge areas and skills projected to be a routine part of public health nutrition in 2005 are shown in table 2.2.

A master's degree in public health nutrition was ranked as the most important credential for work as a public health nutritionist. However, numerous community nutrition professionals with a range of knowledge and skills will be necessary to assist communities in promoting and maintaining the nutritional health of its members. Considering the pace of change, all community nutrition professionals need on-going training to strengthen their skills to meet the coming challenges of both today and tomorrow.[27,13]

DIETARY GUIDANCE FOR AMERICANS
RDAs as the Basis

Government **dietary guidance** activities are designed to help Americans choose diets that promote good health. Dietary recommendations have been in existence since the first recommended dietary allowances (**RDA**s) were published in 1943. The objective of the first edition of the RDAs, published during World War II,

TABLE 2.2
Most Important Knowledge Areas and Skills in Public Health Nutrition in 2005

• Effective communication skills, including public speaking, dealing with mass media, writing for all audiences, counseling, and using new technologies	• Greater cultural sensitivity and skills to develop culturally relevant programs and services; bilingual practitioners
• Knowledge and skill in health care policy and food and nutrition policy	• Knowledge of health promotion and disease prevention, including knowledge of theories and interventions
• Sound nutrition knowledge base, including understanding of the relation of nutrition to health and disease throughout the lifespan	• Coalition-building skills
	• Knowledge about community food systems and food needs of the community, including food products
• Management and public administration skills, including program planning and evaluation skills	• Knowledge of behavioral change strategies
	• Understanding of legislative and political processes

From Olmstead-Schaefer M, Story M & Haughton B.: "Future Training Needs in Public Health Nutrition." Copyright The American Dietetic Association. Reprinted by permission from JOURNAL OF THE AMERICAN DIETETIC ASSOCIATION, Vol 96:282-3.

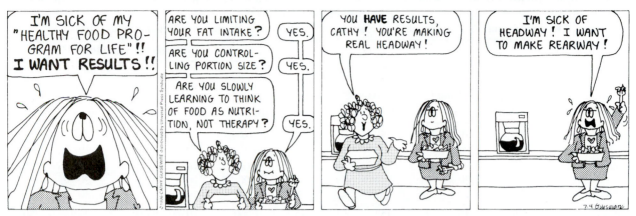

was to "provide standards to serve as a goal for good nutrition."[19] Because the RDAs are intended to reflect the best scientific judgment on nutritional allowances for the maintenance of good health and to serve as the basis for evaluating the adequacy of diets of groups of people, the RDAs have been revised periodically to incorporate new scientific knowledge and interpretation.

RDAs are defined as:

> The levels of intakes of essential nutrients that, on the basis of scientific knowledge, are judged by the Food and Nutrition Board to be adequate to meet the known nutritional needs of practically all healthy persons.[19] The RDA for all nutrients except energy (calories), are set two standard deviations above the estimated mean level required for each particular age and gender group (see table 2.3). If the population nutrient requirement follows a normal distribution pattern, adding two standard deviations (SDs) to the average requirement provides an "allowance" to cover the nutrient needs of most (98 percent) individuals in the population.[3,19] Individuals with special nutritional needs are not covered by the RDAs.

Use and Implications of the RDAs

Since the RDAs have been widely used as a basis for nutrition recommendations and dietary guidance, it is important to understand their appropriate applications and limitations. Three points are of particular importance:

• The recommended allowances for nutrients are amounts intended to be consumed as part of a normal diet. If the RDAs are met through diets composed of a variety of foods derived from diverse food groups rather than by supplementation or fortification, such diets will likely be adequate in all other nutrients for which RDAs cannot currently be established.

• RDAs are neither minimal requirements nor necessarily optimal levels of intake. It is not possible with the available data to establish optimal RDAs at this time. RDAs are safe and adequate levels reflecting the state of knowledge concerning a nutrient, its bioavailability, and the variation among the U.S. population. The safe and adequate levels incorporate margins of safety intended to be sufficiently generous to encompass the presumed variability in requirements among people.

• Although RDAs are most appropriately applied to population groups, a comparison of an individual's nutrient intakes, averaged over a sufficient length of time, to the RDAs allows an estimate to be made about the possible risk of deficiency or excess for that individual.

From the original application of RDAs as a guide for advising on nutrition problems in connection with national defense, the RDAs have come to serve many useful purposes. Table 2.4 describes ten major uses of the RDAs.[31] In the past, the RDAs were the only values available to health professionals for planning and assessing diets of individuals and groups and for making judgments about inadequate or excessive intakes. However, the RDAs were not ideally suited for many of these purposes. The Food and Nutrition Board and the Institute of Medicine of the National Academy of Sciences have established a committee to revise the RDAs. The committee is called the Scientific Evaluation of Dietary Reference Intake (**DRI**).[18] They are establishing new reference values.

TABLE 2.3

Food and Nutrition Board, National Academy of Sciences—National Research Recommended Dietary Allowances,[a] Revised 1989

Designed for the Maintenance of Good Nutrition of Practically All Healthy People in the United States

Category	Age (years) or condition	Weight[b] (kg)	Weight[b] (lb)	Height[b] (cm)	Height[b] (in)	Protein (g)	Fat-soluble vitamins Vitamin A (μg RE)[c]	Vitamin D (μg)[d]	Vitamin E (mg) α-TE)[e]	Vitamin K (μg)	Vitamin C (mg)
Infants	0.0–0.5	6	13	60	24	13	375	7.5	3	5	30
	0.5–1.0	9	20	71	28	14	375	10	4	10	35
Children	1–3	13	29	90	35	16	400	10	6	15	40
	4–6	20	44	112	44	24	500	10	7	20	45
	7–10	28	62	132	52	28	700	10	7	30	45
Males	11–14	45	99	157	62	45	1,000	10	10	45	50
	15–18	66	145	176	69	59	1,000	10	10	65	60
	19–24	72	160	177	70	58	1,000	10	10	70	60
	25–50	79	174	176	70	63	1,000	5	10	80	60
	51+	77	170	173	68	63	1,000	5	10	80	60
Females	11–14	46	101	157	62	46	800	10	8	45	50
	15–18	55	120	163	64	44	800	10	8	55	60
	19–24	58	128	164	65	46	800	10	8	60	60
	25–50	63	138	163	64	50	800	5	8	65	60
	51+	65	143	160	63	50	800	5	8	65	60
Pregnant						60	800	10	10	65	70
Lactating	1st 6 months					65	1,300	10	12	65	95
	2nd 6 months					62	1,200	10	11	65	90

[a]The allowances, expressed as average daily intakes over time, are intended to provide for individual variations among most normal persons as they live in the United States under usual environmental stresses. Diets should be based on a variety of common foods to provide other nutrients for which human requirements have been less well defined.

[b]Weights and heights of reference adults are actual medians for the U.S. population of the designated age, as reported by NHANES II. The use of these figures does not imply that the height-to-weight ratios are ideal.

The term dietary reference intakes (DRIs) is new to the field of nutrition. It refers to a set of at least four nutrient-based reference values that can be used for planning and assessing diets and for many other purposes. The development of DRIs replaces the periodic revision of RDAs—which were last (tenth edition) published in 1989. The dietary reference intakes—estimated average requirements (EARs), adequate intakes (AIs), and tolerable upper intake levels (ULs)—are a complete set of reference values. Each type of DRI has specific uses.[25] (See box 2.2).

A new format has been established for the release of DRIs. The DRI will appear in installments dealing with groups of nutrients. The Institute of Medicine is reviewing RDAs for the full spectrum of nutrients in a seven-stage project to be completed in the year 2000. The August 1997 release was the first of these and deals with calcium, phosphorus, vitamin D, and fluoride. The new calcium guidelines compared to the old RDAs are shown in box 2.3. The new guidelines have different age categories, nutrient measures, and recommended intake levels.[21]

DIETARY GUIDELINES FOR AMERICANS

The 1995 Dietary guidelines provide sound advice to help consumers make food choices for an active and healthful life and are based on overwhelming scientific consensus on the link between nutrition and health.[16]

—EILEEN KENNEDY, MARCH 1996

The Dietary Guidelines for Americans provide the basis for federal nutrition policy and education activities. They translate science into sound advice for healthy Americans age two years and over about mak-

Water-soluble vitamins						Minerals						
Thia-min (mg)	Ribo-flavin (mg)	Niacin (mg NE)[f]	Vita-min B$_6$ (mg)	Folate (µg)	Vita-min B$_{12}$ (µg)	Cal-cium (mg)	Phos-phorus (mg)	Mag-nesium (mg)	Iron (mg)	Zinc (mg)	Iodine (µg)	Sele-nium (µg)
0.3	0.4	5	0.3	25	0.3	400	300	40	6	5	40	10
0.4	0.5	6	0.6	35	0.5	600	500	60	10	5	50	15
0.7	0.8	9	1.0	50	0.7	800	800	80	10	10	70	20
0.9	1.1	12	1.1	75	1.0	800	800	120	10	10	90	20
1.0	1.2	13	1.4	100	1.4	800	800	170	10	10	120	30
1.3	1.5	17	1.7	150	2.0	1,200	1,200	270	12	15	150	40
1.5	1.8	20	2.0	200	2.0	1,200	1,200	400	12	15	150	50
1.5	1.7	19	2.0	200	2.0	1,200	1,200	350	10	15	150	70
1.5	1.7	19	2.0	200	2.0	800	800	350	10	15	150	70
1.2	1.4	15	2.0	200	2.0	800	800	350	10	15	150	70
1.1	1.3	15	1.4	150	2.0	1,200	1,200	280	15	12	150	45
1.1	1.3	15	1.5	180	2.0	1,200	1,200	300	15	12	150	50
1.1	1.3	15	1.6	180	2.0	1,200	1,200	280	15	12	150	55
1.1	1.3	15	1.6	180	2.0	800	800	280	15	12	150	55
1.0	1.2	13	1.6	180	2.0	800	800	280	10	12	150	55
1.5	1.6	17	2.2	400	2.2	1,200	1,200	320	30	15	175	65
1.6	1.8	20	2.1	280	2.6	1,200	1,200	355	15	19	200	75
1.6	1.7	20	2.1	260	2.6	1,200	1,200	340	15	16	200	75

[c]Retinol equivalents. 1 retinol equivalent = 1 µg retinol or 6 µg β-carotene.
[d]As cholecalciferol. 10 µg cholecalciferol = 400 IU of vitamin D.
[e]α-Tocopherol equivalents. 1 mg d-α tocopherol = 1 α-TE.
[f]NE (niacin equivalent) is equal to 1 mg of niacin or 60 mg of dietary tryptophan.

ing food choices that promote health and prevent disease.[5,23] In contrast to RDA and RDI, which are nutrient-based recommendations, the Dietary Guidelines are food-based recommendations. The U.S. Senate Select Committee on Nutrition and Human Need held hearings in 1977 on diet and nutrition. As a result of those hearings, the committee issued Dietary Goals for the United States (the McGovern Report).[39] This was a forerunner of the first Dietary Guidelines for Americans published in 1980 in the form of a consumer bulletin available in English and Spanish. The National Nutrition Monitoring and Related Research Act of 1990 requires that the Secretaries of USDA and HHS jointly publish a report entitled Dietary Guidelines for Americans every five years. The report must contain information and guidelines on diet and nutrition for the general public and must be based on the prepon-

derance of scientific and medical knowledge current at the time of publication.

Changes in 1995 Dietary Guidelines for Americans

The 1995 Dietary Guidelines reinforce the earlier version but there are some important conceptual changes. The 1995 guidelines committee acknowledged that "eating is one of life's greatest pleasures." They indicate that food choices depend on history, culture, and environment as well as on energy and nutrient needs. People also eat foods for enjoyment. Family, friends, and beliefs play a major role in the ways people select foods and plan meals. The guidelines bulletin describes some of the many different and pleasurable ways to combine foods to make healthful diets.[5,23]

TABLE 2.4
Uses of the Recommended Dietary Allowances (RDAs)

Use	Examples	Comments on the use of RDAs
Food planning and procurement	Use to develop plans for feeding groups of healthy people	Use as an appropriate nutrient standard for a period of at least a week, but also use as one of many food planning criteria; should be adjusted as group varies from RDA reference individual
	Use for food purchasing, cost control, and budgeting	Use as an appropriate nutrient standard with knowledge of such factors as food composition, availability, acceptability, and storage changes and losses
Food programs	Serve as a basis for the nutritional goal for feeding programs	Use as a standard for nutritional quality of meals along with other food selection criteria
	Provide the nutritional standard for the Thrifty Food Plan, the basis for allotments in the Food Stamp Program	Use as a guideline along with other food selection criteria
	Provide nutritional guidelines for food distribution programs	Use as a standard for nutritional quality of food packages
Evaluating dietary survey data	Evaluate dietary intake of individuals	Use as a standard for evaluating dietary status, but not for evaluating individual nutritional status
	Evaluate household food use	Use as a benchmark to compare households and to identify nutrient shortfalls
	Evaluate national food supply (food disappearance data)	Use only as a benchmark for comparison over time and to identify nutrient shortfalls
Guides for food selection	Develop and evaluate food guides and family food plans	Use along with other food selection criteria
Food and nutrition information and education	Provide guidelines for obtaining nutritious diets	Use as a point of reference; becomes more useful to consumers when translated into food selection goals
	Use as a basis for educators to discuss individuals' nutrient needs	Use in combination with information in the text accompanying the RDA table and with recognition that the RDAs are for reference individuals
	Evaluate an individual's diet as a basis for recommending specific changes in food patterns and/or dietary supplements	Use to identify nutrient shortfalls and as a tool to assess nutrient contribution of diet; do not use in prescriptive manner
Food labeling	Provide basis for nutritional labeling of foods	Use as a basis for labeling standards (U.S. RDA); such standards should not be used to determine nutritional intake of individuals or groups
Food fortification	Serve as a guide for fortification for general population	Use as a guide, but such other factors as food consumption patterns and contribution to the total diet must also be considered
Developing new or modified food products	Provide guidance in establishing nutritional levels for new food products	Use in combination with information or probable products; use within the context of the total diet
Clinical dietetics	Develop therapeutic diet manuals	Use to assess the nutritional quality of modified diets
	Plan modified diets	Use as a starting point along with information on the patient's nutritional status and individual needs
	Counsel patients requiring modified diets	Use as one basis for advice on food selection
	Plan menus and food served in institutions for the developmentally disabled	Use as a starting point, but modify for individual's developmental status and body size
Nutrient supplements and special dietary foods	Use as a basis to formulate supplements and special dietary foods	Use as a basis in developing infant formulas and other oral supplements or foods, but also consider nutrient bioavailability and nutrient balance; cannot be used as the only guide for parenteral feeding products

BOX 2.2

DIETARY REFERENCE INTAKES*

EAR (estimated average requirement): the intake that meets the estimated nutrient need of 50 percent of the individuals in that group

RDA (recommended dietary allowance): the intake that meets the nutrient need of almost all (97 to 98 percent) of individuals in that group

AI (adequate intake): average observed or experimentally derived intake by a defined population or subgroup that ap-

pears to sustain a defined nutritional state, such as normal circulating nutrient values, growth, or other functional indicators of health

UL (tolerable upper limit): the maximum intake by an individual that is unlikely to pose risks of adverse health effects in almost all (97 to 98 percent) individuals.

---

*Refers to daily intakes, averaged over time.
Source: Nutrition Reviews 1997;55:327–331.

BOX 2.3

NEW CALCIUM GUIDELINES (INSTITUTE OF MEDICINE GUIDELINES)
Milligrams of Calcium per Day

OLD		NEW	
Age	**RDA**	**Age**	**AI**
Up to 6 months	400	Up to 6 months	210
6 months to 1 year	600	6 months to 1 year	270
1 to 3	800	1 to 3	500
4 to 6	800	4 to 8	800
7 to 10	800	9 to 13	1,300
11 to 14	1,200	14 to 18	1,300
15 to 18	1,200	19 to 30	1,000
19 to 24	1,200	31 to 50	1,000
25 to 50	800	51 to 70	1,200
51 and older	800	71 and older	1,200

From *The nation's health,* Washington, DC, 1997, American Public Health Association.

Emphasis on Total Dietary Patterns

The 1995 Dietary Guidelines emphasize more clearly than previous editions the importance of a person's overall dietary pattern. To that end, the wording of the 1995 guidelines bulletin moves away from discussion of individual foods, focusing instead on broader food choices that contribute to variety, proportionality, and moderation in the total diet. In addition to their emphasis on the total diet, the 1995 Dietary Guidelines convey the message that foods are the preferred form of consuming nutrients. The 1995 Dietary Guidelines are presented in figure 2.5, which depicts the cover of the consumer bulletin which is distributed widely to the public. It is available in English and Spanish versions. This idea is reinforced by a discussion of other healthful substances present in foods but not in dietary supplements. Examples of situations (e.g., during pregnancy) in which dietary supplements may be needed are also provided. In consideration of various dietary patterns, vegetarian diets are mentioned.

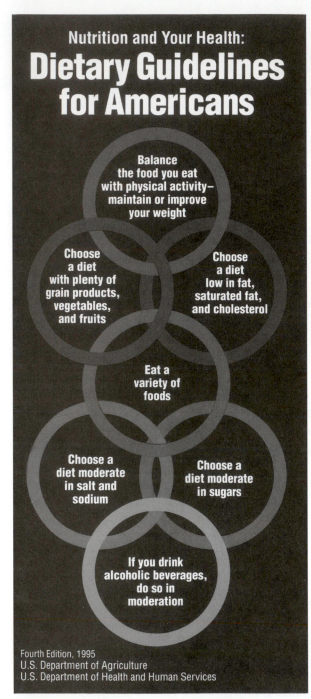

FIGURE 2.5   1995 Dietary Guidelines for Americans

Attention to Physical Activity

The 1995 edition places new attention on physical activity. The guideline in the top position is "Balance the food you eat with physical activity—maintain or improve your weight." For the first time, this guideline emphasizes both diet and physical activity. In addition, the weight guideline now stresses both maintenance and weight loss. The previous weight guideline, "Maintain a Healthy Weight," was based on the presumption that a healthy weight could be achieved and maintained. The committee concluded that although maintenance of a healthy weight is a reasonable goal for persons already within the healthy weight guidelines, the high rate of relapse after weight loss suggest that this goal may be impossible for the large number of overweight people in the United States. The new guideline therefore emphasizes the importance of weight maintenance as a more realistic goal that people are more likely to attempt. The weight guideline eliminates a higher weight standard for older adults used in the previous edition. In the 1995 guidelines text, the same healthy weight range applies to all adults. This range is depicted in the guidelines bulletin as a chart with three categories: healthy weight, moderate overweight, and severe overweight.

Eat a Variety of Foods

The variety guideline is placed at the center, linking all other guidelines, in the new graphic representation (see figure 2.5). To clarify the message of variety and provide educational tools for putting the guidelines into practice, the **Food Guide Pyramid** and **Nutrition Facts label** have been incorporated into the 1995 bulletin.[8,34]

Choose a Diet with Plenty of Grain Products, Vegetables, and Fruits

This guideline was moved up to third place in the bulletin to emphasize its increasing importance. Grains are mentioned first to ensure more consistency with the ordering of food groups in the Food Guide Pyramid. The bulletin's text offers a more detailed discussion of fiber, vitamins, minerals, and other food components that are important for health.

Choose a Diet Low in Fat, Saturated Fat, and Cholesterol

American diets have improved with respect to this guideline, but more improvement is needed. The guideline continues the previously recommended levels for intake of fat and saturated fat: no more than 30 percent of total energy and less than 10 percent of energy, respectively. The Nutrition Facts label is referenced in the text to help illustrate how one can calculate the 30 percent energy from fat limit for a 2,000 kcal diet. The **Daily Value** of 300 mg of cholesterol from the Nutrition Facts label is also cited. This linkage of concepts in the bulletins text with the Nutrition Facts Label illustrates the 1995 edition's focus on providing practical information and tips for consumers.

For the first time, the text of the Dietary Guidelines indicates that children between the ages of two and five years should gradually decrease fat intake so that by school age they are consuming no more than 30 percent of calories from fat. This recommended gradual transition in fat intake is intended to guard against an abrupt and overzealous dietary fat restriction that might compromise energy intake in the preschool-aged child.[1]

Choose a Diet Moderate in Sugars

In addition to the change in wording of the guideline itself, the discussion of this guideline was modified to include mention of sugars and weight maintenance. The text explains that simply avoiding sugars will not correct overweight.

Choose a Diet Moderate in Salt and Sodium

Refinements in the text of this guideline draw on the growing scientific evidence that calcium and potassium intakes, in addition to sodium intake, weight maintenance, and alcohol intake, interact and affect blood pressure. The Nutrition Facts label Daily Value for sodium of 2,400 mg is also referenced as a guide to consumers.

If You Drink Alcoholic Beverages, Do So in Moderation

Although the wording for this guideline is the same as that in the 1990 edition, there are some subtle differences in the text. First, the tone is less negative and the discussion mentions that moderate alcohol intake may enhance enjoyment of meals and offer some protection from coronary disease. Children and adolescents have been moved to the top of the list of persons who should not drink alcohol.[1]

Considerations for Future Dietary Guidelines

The Advisory Committee on Dietary Guidelines for 1995 made several recommendations for future revisions. The

committee recommends that the development and publication of material giving practical advice on both family food management and congregate feeding. Particular attention should be given to the needs of the elderly.[5] They recommended continued support of national nutrition and health surveys including the assessment of food consumption of individuals and families because such information is the basis for sound dietary guidance. Since very young children are excluded from the guidelines, it is recommended that dietary guidelines for children including those less than two years of age be developed.[5]

Dietary Guidance Developed by Health Professional Organizations

Several professional and voluntary health organizations develop dietary recommendations for the public based on their particular concerns, for example, the American Cancer Society's Eat Smart guidelines (1993). The American Academy of Pediatrics has issued statements on cholesterol for children under two years of age (1992) and the use of cow's milk for infants (1992). The American Heart Association issued guidelines for adults in 1988 and the American Dental Association issued nutrition guidelines for children and adults (1983). Nutrition professionals have a major role in assisting consumers to follow the guidelines to promote good health.

Canada's Approach to Guidelines for Healthy Eating

Nutrition has long been recognized in Canada as a key factor in promoting good health and preventing disease. National guidelines have been the cornerstone of nutrition policies for almost fifty years.[32] In 1987, Health-Welfare Canada initiated a revision of the national guidelines and established two committees: a Scientific Review Committee (SRC) responsible for reviewing recent scientific evidence from a public health perspective and a Communications/Implementation Committee (CIC) responsible for developing consumer advice and implementation strategies that would embody the revised nutrition recommendations. The SRC adopted as the Nutrition Recommendations for Canadians[6] the key statements presented in box 2.4.

The CIC identified many gaps between estimated current consumption patterns and those recommended by the SRC. These gaps indicate nutrition problems for many Canadians, whose dietary practices place them at greater risk of diet-related chronic disease. To make the

BOX 2.4

NUTRITION RECOMMENDATIONS FOR CANADIANS

- The Canadian diet should provide energy consistent with the maintenance of body weight within the recommended range.
- The Canadian diet should include essential nutrients in amounts recommended.
- The Canadian diet should include no more than 30% of energy as fat (33 g/1,000 kcal or 39 g/5,000 kJ) and no more than 10 percent as saturated fat (11 g/1,000 kcal or 13 g/5,000 kJ).
- The Canadian diet should provide 55 percent of energy as carbohydrate (138 g/1,000 kcal or 165 g/5,000 kJ) from a variety of sources.
- The sodium content of the Canadian diet should be reduced.
- The Canadian diet should include no more than 5 percent of total energy as alcohol, or two drinks or less daily.
- The Canadian diet should contain no more caffeine than the equivalent of four cups of regular coffee per day.
- Community water supplies containing less than 1 mg/L of fluoride should be fluoridated to that level.

BOX 2.5

CANADA'S GUIDELINES FOR HEALTHY EATING

- Enjoy a variety of foods.
  - Emphasize cereals, breads, other grain products, vegetables, and fruits.
  - Choose low-fat dairy products, lean meats, and foods prepared with little or no fat.
  - Achieve and maintain a healthy body weight by enjoying regular physical exercise and healthy eating.
- Limit salt, alcohol, and caffeine.

guidelines more accessible to the public, translation of the science was based on focus group research at the consumer level and advice from nutrition educators. Box 2.5 shows the Guidelines for Healthy Eating, which were developed in 1990.

PUTTING U.S. DIETARY GUIDELINES INTO PRACTICE

The Food Guide Pyramid and the Nutrition Facts label found on most processed foods in the grocery store are educational tools that put the Dietary Guidelines for Americans into practice.[8,23,34] The pyramid translates the RDAs and the Dietary Guidelines into the kinds and amounts of food to eat each day. The Nutrition Facts label is designed to help consumers select foods for a diet that will meet the Dietary Guidelines.[8,23]

The Food Guide Pyramid

The Pyramid is the official guide for the United States and the only one recognized by federal agencies[34] (figure 2.6). The Pyramid teaches the total diet instead of the foundation diet represented by the basic four food groups (see box 2.6). Based on health concerns that may result from nutritional excesses, the Pyramid addresses overnutrition as well as undernutrition. Achterberg has indicated that educators should appreciate this change because they now have a guide that allows them to offer advice to consumers about the total diet, not just about parts of it.[1] Consumers may also find this approach less confusing. The Pyramid was based on consumer research. Contrary to the food guides and illustrations created in the past, a great deal of research effort was spent identifying an image that was both measurable and understandable to a variety of audiences.[34] The result is an easily recognizable figure that presents both opportunities and challenges for nutrition professionals and consumers.

The Pyramid illustrates the three principal concepts that are the key teaching objectives of the Dietary Guidelines: variety, moderation, and proportionality.

Variety is defined as eating a wide selection of foods within and among the major food groups. It is also important to eat a variety of foods within each food group. No one major food group is more or less important than any other food group.

Food Guide Pyramid
A Guide to Daily Food Choices

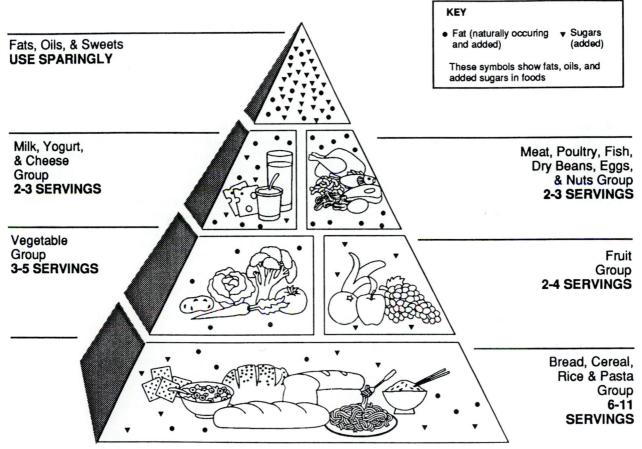

KEY

● Fat (naturally occuring and added) ▼ Sugars (added)

These symbols show fats, oils, and added sugars in foods

Fats, Oils, & Sweets
USE SPARINGLY

Milk, Yogurt,
& Cheese
Group
2-3 SERVINGS

Meat, Poultry, Fish,
Dry Beans, Eggs,
& Nuts Group
2-3 SERVINGS

Vegetable
Group
3-5 SERVINGS

Fruit
Group
2-4 SERVINGS

Bread, Cereal,
Rice & Pasta
Group
**6-11
SERVINGS**

FIGURE 2.6   Food Guide Pyramid
(*Source:* USDA, Food Guide Pyramid, April 28, 1992, Washington, DC.)

Moderation is defined by two components:

- Eating food portions, especially those high in fat and in added sugar, in recommended serving sizes.
- Eating fats, oils, and sweets sparingly.

Proportionality is defined as eating relatively more foods from the larger food groups at the bottom of the pyramid and fewer foods from the smaller food groups at the top of the pyramid.[20]

Achterberg indicates that when using the Food Pyramid, the most important consideration in working with audiences is to have compassion and respect for clients—respect for their belief system, their food preferences, their ethnic heritage, and their lifestyle.[1] The process must begin by acknowledging and using the ethnic foods that clients eat. With the input of representative foods from different cultures, the Food Guide Pyramid can be developed to illustrate the foods of these cultures.

FOOD LABELING

The passage by the U.S. Congress of the Nutrition Labeling and Education Act of 1990 (NLEA) has led to the most sweeping set of food labeling reforms in U.S. history. The new food labeling regulations are destined to dramatically alter food packaging, advertising, product

MAJOR CHANGES IN THE FOOD GUIDE PYRAMID COMPARED TO THE BASIC FOUR FOOD GROUPS[34,1]

- Dietary advice has shifted from a foundation diet to the total diet.
- The number of food groups has changed to five food groups. Each group provides some but not all of the nutrients needed for good health, and no one group is more important than another. The tip of the Pyramid (the fats, oils, and sweets group) does not count as a major food group, therefore, no foods are depicted schematically. Foods in the tip provide energy and little else nutritionally.
- The names of the food groups have changed (see figure 2.6) but their purpose is to clarify the complete composition of each food group.
- Fruits are now separated from vegetables. The vegetable group—on the left side of the Food Guide Pyramid—is now bigger than the fruit group to the right. The bigger size of the vegetable group means that people should consume more servings from this group. The left-hand placement emphasizes the change from previous food guides.
- The number of servings per group have changed. The recommended number of servings for each food group will make sense only if they are matched to the recommended serving size. Also, the term "use sparingly" has been introduced, although many people, especially youngsters, have no idea what the word sparingly means.
- The tip of the Pyramid is now called the fats, oils, and sweets group. Community nutritional professionals tend to put more items in the tip than actually belong there. For example, alcohol, hot dogs, potato chips, and french fries are not included in this group. The rationale for what does or does not go in the tip is based on the function or use of the food. Most items in the tip are condiments and/or contribute no other important nutrients besides sugar or fat. Some items in the tip of the Pyramid are butter, jelly, margarine, and honey.
- Serving sizes have changed for some foods and food groups. The suggested serving sizes on the Pyramid do not correspond to the serving sizes on the new food label. The Pyramid's serving sizes are the recommended amounts; the label's standardized serving sizes are the amounts that most Americans currently consume.[34] A comparison of the serving sizes for the label, ADA Exchange List and the Food Guide Pyramid are shown in the "Expert Speaks" by C. Geiger on page 50.
- Protein equivalents have changed. For example, an egg, 2 T peanut butter, or 1/2 cup cooked beans now count as 1 oz lean meat.
- Symbols for fat and sugar have been added. The circles on the Pyramid signify added or naturally occurring fat; the inverted triangles signify added, but not naturally occurring sugar. The purpose of the symbols is to teach that fat and sugar are found in all of the food groups, not just in the tip.

research, composition of food, and ultimately, consumer eating habits (see box 2.7). The changes mark the first extensive renovation of the food label since 1974 when the FDA and USDA established voluntary nutrition labeling. The new food label is mandated for most packaged foods affecting over 400,000 food products. In May 1994, food regulated by FDA, which includes almost all packaged processed foods, were required to have new labels. In 1994, foods regulated by the Food Safety and Inspection Service (FSIS), a division of USDA, were required to be labeled.

Serving Sizes

Whatever the format, the serving size remains the basis for reporting nutrient amounts. The FDA and FSIS define serving size as the amount of food "customarily consumed per eating occasion." Reference Amounts are determined by national food consumption surveys. Only the "serving size" will appear on the label.

Required Nutrients

The nutrients required on the "Nutrition Facts" panel have been changed in response to consumer concerns and the new public health emphasis on preventing chronic disease. The nutrients required, in order of appearance on the label are:[20]

Calories

Calories from Fat (new)

Total Fat

Saturated Fat (new)

Cholesterol (new)

BOX 2.7

KEY CHANGES IN FOOD LABELING[10,24]

There are six key changes in the food label (see figure 2.7) and these include:

- A new standard format. Bold graphics emphasize important information.
- Serving sizes are derived from reference amounts. These reference amounts are based on amounts people customarily eat at one time. Serving size information is provided in household and metric units.
- A new list of required nutrients based on major health concerns.[24] The emphasis is now on the prevention of chronic disease instead of the prevention of deficiency diseases. Calories from fat and saturated fat, amounts of cholesterol, dietary fiber, and sugar have been added to the label. Thiamin, riboflavin, and niacin have been deleted.
- New label standards for nutrients, known as Daily Values, are based on current health and nutrition information.

For example, the cholesterol Daily Value is 300 mg. The Daily Values consist of two sets of dietary standards, which are discussed later. The Percent Daily Values are based on the Daily Value standards. The Percent Daily Values show how a food fits into a total daily diet. They show at a glance how much or how little of a nutrient is contained in a food product.

- Nutrient content descriptors that are more rigidly confined and consistent for all food products such as "fat-free" and "high" in fiber.
- Approved health claims that describe the relations between food, nutrient, or substance in a food and a disease. For example, calcium and osteoporosis, and fat and coronary heart disease.

Sodium

Total Carbohydrate

Dietary Fiber (new)

Sugars (new)

Protein

Vitamin A, vitamin C, calcium, and iron are the only micronutrients required on the label unless a nutrient content or health claim is made.

Voluntary Nutrients

As before, additional nutrients may be listed on a voluntary basis:

Calories from unsaturated fat

Polyunsaturated fat

Other carbohydrate

Soluble fiber

Insoluble fiber

Sugar alcohol such as xylitol/sorbitol

Monounsaturated fat

Potassium

Beta-carotene as % of vitamin A

Other vitamins and minerals

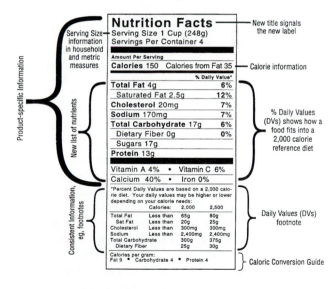

FIGURE 2.7   The New Food Label
© 1994, The American Dietetic Association. *Learning the New Food Labels: An Education Slide Kit.* Used by permission.

TABLE 2.5
Daily Values

The following is a list of the daily values for the nutrients that may appear on the food label.

Food components	Daily value*	Food components	Daily value*
Daily Reference Values (DRVs)			
Total Fat	65 g+	Potassium	3,500 mg
Saturated Fat	20 g+	Total carbohydrate	300 g+
Cholesterol	300 mg	Dietary fiber	25 g+≠
Sodium	2,400 mg	Protein	50 g+
Reference Daily Intakes (RDIs)			
Vitamin A	5,000 IU	Folate	400 mcg
Vitamin C	60 mg	Vitamin B_{12}	6.0 mcg
Calcium	1 g	Biotin	0.3 mg
Iron	18 mg	Pantothenic acid	10 mg
Vitamin D	400 IU	Phosphorus	1 g
Vitamin E	30 IU	Iodine	150 mcg
Thiamin	1.5 mg	Magnesium	400 mg
Riboflavin	1.7 mg	Zinc	15 mg
Niacin	20 mg	Copper	2.0 mg
Vitamin B_6	2.0 mg		

* Daily Value for adults and children four years of age or older.
+ Daily Value based on a 2,000-calorie reference diet.
≠ Daily Value based on 11.5 g per 1,000 calories.
© 1994, The American Dietetic Association. *Learning the New Food Labels: An Education Slide Kit.* Used by permission.

Daily Values

Arriving at a way to help consumers use food labels to plan an overall healthy diet was no small task. To meet this need, a new dietary reference value was developed called Daily Values (DVs). The term "Daily Values" replaces the previously used term "US Recommended Dietary Allowance" (USRDA). The USRDA, based on the 1968 RDAs were the highest level of that nutrient established for any age group. Daily Values actually comprise two sets of reference values for nutrients: **Daily Reference Values** (DRV) and **Reference Daily Intakes** (RDIs) (see table 2.5). But these two sets are behind the scenes in food labeling; to make label-reading less confusing, only the DVs appear on the label.

DVs are not required levels of nutrients. They are just reference points to help people get some perspective on what their overall diet needs should be. DVs appear as 2,000 calorie and 2,500 calorie nutrient recommendations in the DV footnote on many labels.

Percent Daily Values

The Percent Daily Values show how an individual food fits into a 2,000-calorie reference diet. It also shows how a serving of the food contributes to the total daily value for each nutrient for the day. For example, a one-cup serving of yogurt provides 40 percent of the DV for calcium. The consumer would need to obtain the remaining 60 percent of calcium needs in other foods consumed the rest of the day. The Percent Daily Value also allows consumers to determine at a glance if a food is high or low in a certain nutrient. For example, if a food contains 20 percent or more of the DV for calcium, it is considered high in calcium.

Daily Reference Values

DRVs are the standards for nutrients that have a significant impact on health and disease, but do not have established RDAs. DRVs for the energy-producing nutri-

EXAMPLES OF THE APPROVED USE OF DESCRIPTOR WORDS FOR SPECIFIC NUTRIENTS

"Fat-free" claims are allowed on a label if one serving of the product contains:

- Less than half a gram (0.5 g) fat, and
- No added ingredient that is a fat or is generally understood to contain fat. "Low fat" claims are allowed if the product contains no more than:
- Three grams of fat and no more than 30 percent of calories from fat. "Light" or "lite" is also stringently defined.
- The term "light" can refer to calories, fat, sodium, color, or texture. Each of these characteristics has a definition. To be called "light" the product must be nutritionally altered to contain 1/3 fewer calories or 1/2 the fat of the reference food. If food derives 50 percent or more of its calories

from fat, the fat reduction must be 50 percent to qualify for a "light" claim. "Light" also can be used to describe a sodium reduction in a "low-calorie," "low-fat" food. "Light" may also describe the characteristics of a product if qualifying information is given (e.g., "light in color").

These are just some examples of descriptors that have been regulated. Even the term "healthy" is now regulated. The term "healthy" can be used if the food is low in fat and saturated fat and a serving does not contain more than 480 mg sodium or more than 60 mg cholesterol and as well contains at least 10 percent of RDA for vitamin A, vitamin C, calcium, protein, or fiber.

---

ents (fat, saturated fat, carbohydrate, protein, and fiber) are based on the number of calories consumed per day. For labeling purposes, 2,000 calories has been established as the reference for calculating Percent DV. It is a rounded number that is easy to use for calculating individual nutrient needs.

DRVs for cholesterol, sodium, and potassium are not based on calorie intake, but are recommendations for all adults based on the NAS/NRC's Diet and Health Report.[24] The DRV for fat, saturated fat, cholesterol and sodium represent the uppermost limit that is currently recommended because of their association with certain diseases (table 2.5).

Reference Daily Intakes

Reference Daily Intakes are a set of dietary references based on the 1989 RDAs for essential vitamins, minerals, and protein (table 2.5). Unlike DRVs, the RDIs are established estimated values for intakes of vitamins, minerals, and proteins.

Nutrient Content Claims or Descriptors

Consumers were bombarded with all kinds of nutrition messages before the new food label was put into place. Many claims were nothing more than advertising hype and added to consumer's confusion. The public was misled with products like "light" vegetable oil that was just light in color and "lite" cheesecake that was just

light in texture. Now, food-labeling regulations, define terms and spell out which nutrient content claims are allowed and under what circumstances they can be used.

There are eleven core terms. A nutrient content claim or descriptor is any direct statement about the level of a nutrient in a food (e.g., low-fat, lite/light, no cholesterol). A food package cannot carry these terms unless the product meets government guidelines. No matter where they appear, the words mean the same thing. The absolute terms or descriptors describe the amount of a nutrient in a food (see box 2.8). These terms include free, low, good source, high, lean, and extra lean.

Comparative claims (e.g., reduced, less, light, and more) are allowed between a regular product and a nutritionally altered product.[10,11]

Health Claims for Foods

A health claim describes the relation between a food, a nutrient, or other substance in a food, and the risk of a health-related disease or condition. The world of food is changing rapidly, not only in scientific and technical areas, but also in the area of policy. International organizations such as the World Health Organization and the Food and Agriculture Organization (FAO) are shifting their attention to diseases related to overconsumption of food. This new worldwide emphasis on preventing chronic diseases is awakening policy interest in the use of health claims as a way of encouraging consumers to make healthy food choices.

Further, in areas of the world where trade harmonization efforts are paramount—for example, in the European Community (EC)—labeling is gaining acceptance as the best policy to afford the consumer protection and to allow for free circulation of food. Claims can be divided into various categories, but from the standpoint of liberalizing their use, two categories seem most useful—nutrient content claims and food-disease relationship claims. The latter category is strictly prohibited by Codex (a Joint FAO/WHO food standard program to protect the health of consumers and to ensure fair practices in the food trade), the EC, Canada, and Australia. Nutrient claims are permitted in Canada and are being considered by Codex, the EC, and Australia.[11]

U.S. Experience with Health Claims

Even after voluntary nutrition labeling was introduced in the United States in 1975, the prohibition against health claims remained. The rationale has been that the consumer is easily misled by such claims and the regulatory agency has a duty to protect the consumer. However, the Nutrition Labeling and Education Act 1990 does permit health claims. The NLEA assigned authority to regulate health claims on food to FDA.

Health Claim Requirements

For a food product to carry a health claim, it must meet specific requirements. The food carrying the health claim must be a "good source" containing 10 to 19 percent of the DV of at least one of these six nutrients without fortification—fiber, protein, vitamin A, vitamin C, calcium, or iron. The food must meet specific nutrient criteria for each of the health claims. For example, to carry a health claim regarding fat and cancer, the food product must contain 3 g or less of fat per serving.

One of the new developments in the health claims area was the proposal by FDA to develop the first food-specific health claim. In January 1997, the FDA determined that there is enough scientific evidence to support the claim that a diet high in oatmeal and low in saturated fat and cholesterol may reduce the risk of heart disease.[30] The first food-specific health claim is as follows:

> Soluble fiber from oatmeal, as part of a low saturated fat, low cholesterol diet, may reduce the risk of heart disease.

The FDA is also allowing food labels to have a health claim that use of sugar alcohol does not promote dental caries and may reduce the risk of tooth decay.[12]

Approved Health Claims

Approved health claims are allowed if there is significant scientific agreement among qualified scientific reports. The food labeling rules allow health claims about seven relationships (see table 2.6). The FDA provided model language for health claims. Some health claims emphasize decreasing certain nutrients (fat, saturated fat, cholesterol, sodium) and some emphasize increasing certain nutrients (calcium, fiber). Another emphasizes diets rich in fruits and vegetables. Health claims cover nutrients that are linked to the prevention of diseases such as cancer, heart disease, hypertension, and osteoporosis.

Together, the Dietary Guidelines for Americans, the Food Guide Pyramid, and the Nutrition Facts label represent a carefully designed and coordinated approach to dietary guidance for American consumers. These tools can help consumers make wise food choices that promote health and prevent disease. The scientific basis of these tools makes them important in the work of community nutrition professionals.

IMPLICATIONS FOR COMMUNITY NUTRITION PROFESSIONALS

The goal of public health is to create an environment to promote and protect the health of all people in the community. Public health agencies have three core functions including assessment, policy development, and assurance. The Health Promotion and Disease Prevention Objectives (Healthy People 2000) act as a template for public health. Public health nutrition is a key component of public health. Community nutrition professionals and public health nutritionists focus primarily on health promotion and disease prevention to improve the nutritional status of the population.

Dietary recommendations are the tools used by the community nutrition professional to develop effective interventions. Current dietary guidance tools for all Americans include Dietary Guidelines for Americans, the Food Guide Pyramid, and the Nutrition Facts label.

COMMUNITY NUTRITION PROFESSIONALS IN ACTION

1. Public health services protect and promote health and prevent disease. List the ways in which you personally have benefited from public health efforts.
2. Interview a public health nutritionist in your community. Identify the key functions that this person

TABLE 2.6
Health Claim Requirements

Disease	Health claim	Requirements*	Model health claim
Cancer	1. Fruits and vegetables— cancer	• Food must be or must contain a fruit or vegetable • Food is "low fat," 3 g or less • Food is a "good source" of at least one of the following: vitamin A, vitamin C, or fiber	Development of cancer depends on many factors. Eating a diet low in fat and high in fruits and vegetables, such as oranges, which are fat free and high in vitamin C, vitamin A, and fiber, may reduce the risk of some cancers.
	2. Fiber-containing grain products, fruits, and vegetables— cancer	• Food must be or must contain a grain product, fruit, or vegetable • Food is (prior to fortification) a "good source of dietary fiber," 2.5 g to 4.9 g • Food is "low fat," 3 g or less	Low-fat diets rich in fiber-containing grain products, fruits, and vegetables may reduce the risk of some types of cancer, a disease associated with many risk factors.
	3. Fat—cancer	• Food is "low fat" or • Fish and game meats are "extra lean"	Development of cancer depends on many factors. A diet low in total fat may reduce the risk for some cancers.
Coronary heart disease	1. Saturated fat and cholesterol— coronary heart disease	• Food is "low saturated fat," "low cholesterol," and "low fat" or • Fish and game meats must be "extra lean"	Diets low in saturated fat, cholesterol, and total fat may reduce the risk of heart disease. Heart disease is dependent on many risk factors, including diet, a family history of the disease, elevated blood LDL-cholesterol levels, and physical inactivity.
	2. Fruits, vegetables, and grain products that contain fiber—coronary heart disease	• Food must be or must contain a fruit, vegetable, or grain product • Food is "low saturated fat," "low cholesterol," and "low fat" • Food contains (prior to fortification) at least 0.6 g soluble fiber per Reference Amount; soluble fiber content is listed on Nutrition Facts Panel	Diets low in saturated fats and cholesterol and rich in fruits, vegetables, and grain products that contain some types of dietary fiber, particularly soluble fiber, may reduce the risk of heart disease, a disease associated with many risk factors.
Hypertension	1. Sodium— hypertension	• Food is "low sodium," 140 mg or less	Diets low in sodium may reduce the risk for high blood pressure, a disease associated with many risk factors.
Osteoporosis	1. Calcium— osteoporosis	• Food is "high calcium," 200 mg or more • Calcium source is easily absorbed • Food contains no more phosphorus than calcium per Reference Amount	Regular exercise and a healthy diet with enough calcium helps teen and young adult White and Asian women maintain good bone health and may reduce the risk of osteoporosis later in life.

*All foods that carry health claims must also contain, prior to fortification, at least 10 percent DV of one of the mandatory nutrients (fiber, protein, vitamin A, vitamin C, iron, or calcium) per Reference Amount, and must not contain any nutrients above the disqualifying levels established by the FDA. See the Code of Federal Regulations for more information.

© 1994, The American Dietetic Association. *Learning the New Food Labels: An Education Slide Kit.* Used by permission.

provides and compare the list to the core functions of public health and the definition of public health nutrition.

3. What are the key competencies that a public health nutritionist must have to function effectively in the community?

4. The evolution of the Dietary Guidelines from the 1980 edition to the 1995 edition reveals many subtle changes. Discuss the impact of these changes on the public's understanding and acceptance of the Dietary Guidelines message.

5. How do you use the Dietary Guidelines, the Food Guide Pyramid, and the Nutrition Facts label to help a targeted group in your community make wise food choices?

6. Search the grocery store for ten food products that make health claims.

7. What are the accepted health claims in the United States today? What agency is in charge of monitoring health claims?

GOING ONE STEP FURTHER

1. Make an appointment with a community nutrition professional in your community. Select a clinic or site of a nutrition intervention program and observe the activity occurring. Identify the target audiences and the goals and objectives of the intervention. Determine the type of intervention provided—individual-, community-, or system-based—and the level of prevention—primary, secondary, and tertiary. Present your findings to the class and have a discussion as to the merits of this and other intervention approaches for accommodating the goals and objectives.

2. Referring to a copy of *Healthy People 2000,* select one of the nutrition objectives to explore in detail. Compare the current status of your community to the national data and objectives for the year 2000. Determine the range of intervention programs that are now in place to work on this particular problem and identify all the organizations and agencies in the public, private, and voluntary sectors who are involved.

3. Select a group of people (coworkers, classmates, family members, or a church group) of ten people to follow the Food Guide Pyramid for three days. Then, interview them to determine if they understand the concepts involved in the Pyramid. Summarize the results for the group and how it affected their food choices including a comparison of how they are meeting the food groups listed on the Pyramid.

ADDITIONAL INFORMATION

Professional societies develop statements, scientific status summaries, commentaries, and position papers to clarify an issue in which the particular society has expertise. The American Dietetic Association Position Statement and the Surgeon General's Report relevant to chapter 2 are listed below:

ADA Position Statement

Nutrition Education for the Public: Nutrition education for the public—*J Am Diet Assoc* 96:1183, 1996 and Nutrition education of health professionals—*J Am Diet Assoc* 91:611, 1991.

Surgeon General Report

Physical Activity and Health: A Report of the Surgeon General. USDHHS, Centers for Disease Control and Prevention, 1996. Superintendent of Documents, P.O. Box 371954, Pittsburgh, PA 15250-7954 (S/N 017-023-00196–5).

REFERENCES

1. Achterberg C, McDonnell E, Bagly R: How to put the Food Guide Pyramid into practice, *J Am Diet Assoc* 94:1030–1035, 1994.
2. *Basic document,* ed 15, Geneva, 1964, World Health Organization.
3. Beaton, GH: Uses and limits of the use of the RDA for evaluating dietary intake data, *Am J Clin Nutr* 41:155–64, 1985.
4. Dever AGE: *Community health analysis: global awareness at the local level,* ed 2, Gaithersburg, MD, 1991, Aspen Publishers, 23.
5. Dietary Guidelines Advisory Committee: *Report of the Dietary Guidelines Advisory Committee on Dietary Guidelines for Americans 1995 to the Secretary of HHS and the Secretary of USDA,* Beltsville, MD, 1995, USDA/ARS.
6. Dodds JM, Kaufman M., editors: *Personnel in public health nutrition for the late 1990s: a comprehensive guide,* Washington, DC, 1991, The Public Health Foundation.
7. Egan MC: Public health nutrition: an historical perspective, *J Am Diet Assoc* 1994;94:298–304.
8. *FDA Consumer* (Special Issue), *Focus on food labeling: read the label, set a healthy table,* Washington, DC, 1993, FDA/HHS.
9. Federal, Provincial, and Territorial Advisory Committee on Population Health: Centers for Disease Control & Prevention: *Strategies for population health: investing in*

Canadians' health, Ontario, Canada, 1994, Health and Welfare Canada.

10. Geiger CJ, Harper PH: *Learning the new food labels: an education slide kit,* Chicago, IL, 1994, The American Dietetic Associaton.

11. Harris SS: Health claims for food in the international marketplace, *Food Technology* 46:92, 1992.

12. Health claims: Sugar alcohols and Dental Caries: *Federal Register:* Aug 23, 1996 (Vol 61, No 165) Rules & Regulations Pg 43433–43447.

13. Hess NA, Haughton B: Continuing education needs for public health nutritionists, *J Am Diet Assoc* 96:641–736, 1996.

14. Institute of Medicine: *The future of public health,* Washington, DC, 1988, National Academy of Sciences, National Academy Press.

15. Kaufman M: *Nutrition in Public health: a handbook for developing programs and services,* Gaithersberg, MD, 1990, Aspen Publishers.

16. Kennedy E, Myers L, Layden M: The 1995 dietary guidelines for Americans: an overview, *J Am Diet Assoc* 96:234–237, 1996.

17. Mason M, Wenberg BG, Welch PK: *The dynamics of clinical dietetics,* New York, 1977, John Wiley & Son, p. 49.

18. Monsen ER: New Dietary Reference Intakes proposed to replace the Recommended Dietary Allowances, *J Am Diet Assoc* 96:754–755, 1996.

19. National Academy of Sciences/National Research Council: *Recommended dietary allowances,* ed 10, Washington, DC, 1989, National Academy Press.

20. National Research Council: *Diet and health: implications for reducing chronic disease risk,* Washington, DC, 1989, National Academy Press.

21. *The Nation's Health,* Washington, DC, 1997. American Public Health Association, p. 6.

22. Nielsen H: Achieving health for all: a framework for nutrition in health promotion, *Journal of the Canadian Dietetic Association* 50:77–80, 1989.

23. Nutrition and your health: *Dietary Guidelines for Americans,* ed 4, USDA & HHS. Home and Garden Bulletin no. 232, 1995.

24. Nutrition Labeling Education Act. Publication No. 101-535 Stat. 2353.

25. Nutrition Reviews 55(9): 327, 1997.

26. O'Donnell MP: Definition of health promotion: Part II: Levels of programs, *American Journal of Health Promotion* 1(Fall): p. 6, 1986.

27. Olmstead-Schaefer M, Story M, Haughton B: Future training needs in public health nutrition: results of a national Delphi survey, *J Am Diet Assoc,* 96:282–283, 1996.

28. Owen GM, Kram KM, Garry PJ, et al: A study of nutritional status of preschool children in the United States, 1968–1970, *Pediatrics* 53:(Part II): 597–646, 1974.

29. Pickett G, Hanlon JJ: *Public health administration and practice,* ed 9, St. Louis, 1990, Mosby–Year Book.

30. The Quaker Oats Company: Petition for Health Claims: Form Labeling: health claims; soluble fiber from whole oats and risk of coronary heart disease. Federal Register. Formal Rule Volume 62, number 61. Pp. 15343–15344. March 31, 1997.

31. Sims LS: Uses of the Recommended Dietary Allowances, *J Am Diet Assoc* 96:659–662, 1996.

32. *Surgeon General's report on physical activity and health,* Atlanta, GA, 1996, Centers for Disease Control & Prevention.

33. *Ten-state nutrition survey, 1968–1970,* DHEW Publication No. (HSM) 72-8130–8134, Volumes I–V, Centers for Disease Control and Prevention. Atlanta, GA.

34. U.S. Department of Agriculture and US Department of Health and Human Services: *Food Guide Pyramid: a guide to daily food choices,* Home and Garden Bulletin no. 252, 1992, The Human Nutrition Information Service, US Dept of Agriculture, Hyattsville, Md.

35. U.S. Department of Health, Education and Welfare (HEW), *Healthy people: the Surgeon General's report on health promotion and disease prevention,* Washington, DC, 1979, Superintendent of Documents.

36. U.S. Department of Health and Human Services, *Healthy people 2000: national health promotion and disease prevention objectives,* Washington, DC, 1990, U.S. Government Printing Office.

37. U.S. Department of Health and Human Services (PHS): *Healthy people 2000: national health promotion and disease prevention objectives. Mid-course review,* Washington, DC, 1995, U.S. Government Printing Office.

38. U.S. Department of Health and Human Services, Public Health Service: *Promoting health/preventing disease: objectives for the nation,* Washington, DC, 1980, Government Printing Office.

39. U.S. Senate Select Committee on Nutrition and Human Needs: *Dietary Guidelines for the US,* ed 2, Washington, DC, 1977, U.S. Government Printing Office.

40. Winslow C-EA: The untilled field of public health, *Mod Med* 2:183, 1920.

USING PUBLIC POLICY EDUCATION TOOLS FOR NUTRITION COMMUNICATIONS THAT WORK: INTEGRATING THE FOOD LABEL, THE FOOD GUIDE PYRAMID AND THE DIETARY GUIDELINES

CONSTANCE J. GEIGER, PHD, RD, PRESIDENT

GEIGER AND ASSOCIATES, SALT LAKE CITY, UT

How can you as a community nutrition professional create an effective positive environment for consumer education? Learning to use and to integrate the principles of the *Dietary Guidelines* with the Food Label and the Food Guide Pyramid makes it easier to be a more effective educator of the American consumer. Americans need to learn how to make wise food choices as part of a healthy lifestyle. Making available accurate, consistent information on processed and fresh food labels and in educational materials, advertising and marketing allows the consumer to make informed judgments about food selections to build a healthy eating pattern.

The key changes that facilitate wise food choices for consumers and that make educating people easier for community nutrition professionals include:

- Expanded nutrition information on most foods in a revised format
- A changed and reordered required list of nutrients, including saturated fat, cholesterol, fiber, and other nutrients that are of public health concern and that reflect the emphasis on preventing chronic disease
- More uniformity in serving sizes, including consumer-friendly measurements, to help consumers compare similar products
- New standards, Daily Values, which replaced the USRDA for almost all nutrients that appear on the label
- Listing of the percent Daily Value (Percent DV) for nutrients, which allows you to teach people how a particular food product fits into a 2,000 calorie reference diet
- List of the DV for key nutrients is a boxed footnote in which *Dietary Guideline* recommendations are supported
- Consistent definitions for nutrient content claims that describe a food's nutrient content (e.g., low-fat, light and calorie-free)

- Defined permissible health claims about the relationship between a food or nutrient and disease, or health-related condition, such as "diets adequate in calcium may reduce the risk of osteoporosis"

INTEGRATION OF THE *DIETARY GUIDELINES* WITH THE FOOD LABEL AND THE FOOD GUIDE PYRAMID

There are many interrelationships between the *Dietary Guidelines,* the Food Guide Pyramid, and the Food Label. Table 2.A illustrates how closely they are integrated. Most of the *Dietary Guidelines* are supported by mandatory listing of key nutrients on the Nutrition Facts Panel and the nutrients' percent DV, nutrient content claims, and health claims as well as recommended servings from each of the five food groups on the Pyramid (figure 2.A).

The Food Guide Pyramid provides an overall plan that shows what types and how much food should be eaten on a daily basis for a healthy diet. The percent DVs on the Nutrition Facts Label can help people make wise food choices among the foods in a food group to balance their intake of certain nutrients or to choose foods highest or lowest in certain nutrients. The percent DV also allow people to compare foods in different groups.

You can relate the serving size information on the Nutrition Facts Label to the Food Guide Pyramid. Estimate the number of servings from each major food groups of the Food Guide Pyramid using a daily menu. Relate the total amount for one food to the serving size on the food label.

Be aware that the serving sizes for the Food Guide Pyramid and the Nutrition Facts panel do not match up (table 2.B). This discrepancy confuses people and

TABLE 2.A

Interrelationships between the Dietary Guidelines, the Food Label and the Food Guide Pyramid

Dietary Guideline	Food Label tie-in	Food Guide Pyramid tie-in
Eat a variety of foods	Mandatory labeling on almost all processed foods; voluntary labeling on fresh fruits, vegetables, meat, fish, and poultry helps consumers build a healthy diet. The percent Daily Value allows you to show clients how to balance the variety of foods choices to achieve a healthy diet. The percent DV allows consumers to choose foods that meet their individual needs (e.g., foods high in iron for pregnant women); foods high in calcium for adolescent females and women.	The Food Guide Pyramid illustrates the importance of balance among food groups in a daily eating pattern. Encourage clients to choose from each of the five food groups to build a healthy diet. Tell clients to choose different foods within and across food groups.

Balance the food you eat with physical activity—maintain or improve your weight	Calories must be listed on the label, as well as calories from fat, to allow consumers to make informed choices to meet their caloric requirements.
	The Daily Value set for calories is lower than the national average (e.g., 2,000).
	Nutrient content claims:
	    "low" or "reduced calories"
	    "calorie-free"
	    "light"
	(Note: fat-free does not mean calorie-free.)
		The Pyramid provides a range of servings depending on your clients' caloric requirements; symbols for sugar and fat illustrate the importance of choosing lower fat and sugar choices for persons with lower caloric needs.

Choose a diet with plenty of grain products, fruits, and vegetables	Required information on the Nutrition Facts Panel supports the guidelines: • absolute amounts and percent DV for fiber • percent DVs for vitamins A and C Daily Values for • fiber–25 g • vitamin A–5000 IU • vitamin C–50 mg Specific nutrient content claims are cues for consumers: • "good source of" and "high" fiber • "good source of" and "high" vitamin A or C • healthy. Specific health claims reinforce this guideline: 1. Diets low in saturated fat and cholesterol and high in fruits, vegetables, and grain products that contain fiber, especially soluble fiber, and a reduced risk of coronary heart disease. 2. Diets low in fat and high in fiber-containing grain products, fruits, and vegetables and a reduced risk of cancer.	The Pyramid shape relates to the number of servings from each group needed to achieve a healthy diet. It emphasizes building the diet from the base of the Pyramid using plenty of grain products, fruits, and vegetables.

TABLE 2.A—CONTINUED

Dietary Guideline	Food Label tie-in	Food Guide Pyramid tie-in
Choose a diet low in fat, saturated fat and cholesterol	Mandatory listing of certain nutrients as well as their percent DV helps consumers identify these nutrients in foods: • fat • saturated fat • and cholesterol Daily Values are set for these nutrients: • fat–30% of 2,000 calories (e.g., 65 g) • saturated fat–10% of 2,000 calories, 20 g • cholesterol–300 mg. Specific health claims reinforce this guideline: 1. Diets low in saturated fat and cholesterol and a reduced risk of coronary heart disease 2. Diets low in saturated fat and cholesterol and high in fruits, vegetables, and grain products that contain fiber, especially soluble fiber, and a reduced risk of coronary heart disease 3. Diets low in fat and high in fiber-containing grain products, fruits, vegetables and a reduced risk of cancer. 4. Diets low in fat and a reduced risk of cancer. Specific nutrient content claims are cues for consumers: • "low" and "reduced" fat, saturated fat and cholesterol • fat-, saturated fat- and cholesterol-"free" • "healthy" and "light." Strict standards for health claims and nutrition content claims protect consumers from taking in large quantities of nutrients that are of public health concern: • disqualifying levels for health claims (e.g., a health claim cannot be made if a food contains more than 13 g fat, 1g saturated fat, 60 mg cholesterol, and 480 mg of sodium) • disclosure levels for nutrient content claims (e.g., same levels as above). If a nutrient content claim is made and the food exceeds any of these levels, a disclosure statement must be made (e.g., high in fiber); see side panel for information about fat.	Fat is located at the top of the Pyramid, which indicates using sparingly. Symbols show fat added in foods.

Dietary Guideline	Food Label tie-in	Food Guide Pyramid tie-in
Choose a diet moderate in sugars	For the first time sugars are a mandatory component of the Nutrition Facts Panel. Consumers can identify foods containing sugars. Be aware no differentiation occurs between natural and added sugars as they have the same metabolic fate. No Daily Value (Daily Reference Value) is set for sugar, as no national guideline has been set. It is not a concern in the American diet at current levels of consumption. Therefore the label does not strongly support the Dietary Guidelines on this one.	Sugars are located at the top of the Pyramid, which indicates using sparingly. Symbols show sugars added in foods.
Choose a diet moderate in salt and sodium	Required information on the Nutrition Facts Panel supports the guideline: • sodium and • percent DV of sodium. A Daily Value is set for sodium: • 2,400 mg. Specific nutrient content claims are cues for consumers: • "low," "light" and "reduced" sodium • "sodium-free." A specific health claim reinforces this guideline: • Diets low in sodium may reduce the risk of hypertension.	The Food Guide Pyramid food groups contain foods with a wide range of sodium. Have your clients check the Nutrition Facts Panel for the amount of sodium in foods they eat.
If you drink alcoholic beverages, do so in moderation	Not labeled on the Nutrition Facts Panel Alcohol's calories are reflected in total calories on wine cooler Nutrition Facts Panel. However, alcohol is not listed on the label.	Not mentioned in the Food Guide Pyramid.

Developed by Geiger & Associates, Salt Lake City, UT 1996.

makes integration of these two educational tools difficult. Remember, the serving sizes on the label reflect on average what people consume during one eating occasion. Derivation of serving sizes in this manner was mandated by the NLEA. The Food Guide Pyramid serving sizes are based on the amounts needed to obtain certain key nutrients. Furthermore, if you use the American Dietetic Association/American Diabetes Association Exchange list, be aware their recommended serving sizes are also different. Table 2.B compares the recommended serving sizes for the ADA/ADA exchange list *versus* the Nutrition Facts Panel. The best advice is to personalize the serving size on the label to the amount your client consumes (e.g., if the label serving size is 1 cup of orange juice and your client drinks 1/2 cup, halve the nutrient amounts).

For your clients who do not need 2,000 calories per day, adjust the percent DVs to their caloric intake (e.g., 2,000 calories = 100 percent, 1,500 calories = 75 percent, and 3,000 calories = 200 percent. The percent DVs for fat, saturated fat, carbohydrate, dietary fiber and protein (when listed) should add to the adjusted level. All other nutrients still should total 100 percent of the DV.

By integrating the *Dietary Guidelines,* the Food Label, and the Food Guide Pyramid, you will successfully educate your clients to maximize their food choices to build a healthy diet.

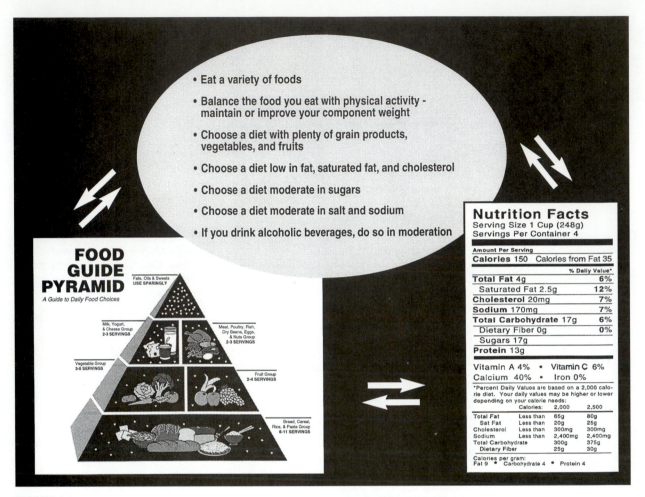

FIGURE 2.A
There are many interrelationships between the Dietary Guidelines, the Food Guide Pyramid, and the Food Label.
Developed by Geiger and Associates, Salt Lake City, UT 1996.

TABLE 2.B
Comparison of Serving Sizes for Various Nutrition Education Tools

Food group	USDA Food Guide Pyramid	Food label serving size (Reference amount customarily consumed)	ADA/ADA exchange list
Breads	1 slice (1 oz)	1–2 slices (50 g)	1 slice (1 oz)
Cereals, cooked	½ cup prepared	1 cup prepared	½ cup prepared
Cereal, ready-to-eat	1 oz	Cups vary (15 g to 55 g)	¾ cup
Vegetables, cooked	½ cup	½ cup (85 g for fresh or frozen, 96 g for vacuum canned, 130 g for canned)	½ cup
Juices	¾ cup	1 cup (240 ml)	½ cup standard
Cheeses	1 ½–2 oz	1 oz (30 g)	1 oz
Meats, luncheon	2 ½–3 oz	2 oz (55 g)	1 oz
Meats, cooked	2 ½–3 oz	85 g	1 oz
Fat (margarine, butter, oils)	Limit	1 tbsp (15 g)(15 ml)	1 tsp

Developed by Geiger and Associates, Salt Lake City, Utah, 1996.

CHAPTER THREE

ASSESSMENT OF NUTRITIONAL STATUS
AN EPIDEMIOLOGIC APPROACH

*If we are to move forward in our understanding of the role
of diet in both the etiology and treatment of disease,
improved methods for estimating food and nutrient
intake are urgently needed.*

—MARILYN BUZZARD

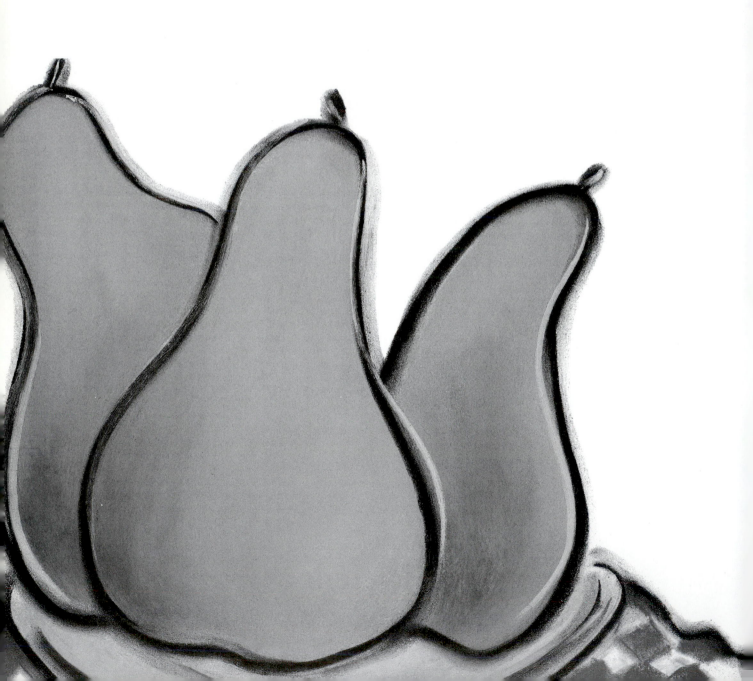

Core Concepts

Assessment is a core function of public health. Community nutrition professionals routinely use individual and community nutrition assessment methods to identify and prioritize problems and then track progress over time in reducing the problems. Nutrition assessment methods include anthropometric, biochemical, clinical, and dietary intake measurements. Each of the dietary intake methods has its strengths and limitations and consideration must be given to selecting and using these methods properly. Data on individuals is aggregated to give a picture of the nutritional status of the population. This information is supplemented with findings from descriptive and analytical epidemiologic studies and sociodemographic information, lifestyle and environmental factors, and information on the availability and appropriateness of health and nutrition services. Extensive activities of the federal government to assess and monitor the nutritional status of the population are coordinated through the National Nutrition Monitoring and Related Research program.

Objectives

When you finish chapter three, you should be able to:

~ Define concepts and terminology related to epidemiology.

~ Describe epidemiologic methods used by community nutrition professionals.

~ Recognize commonly used anthropometric, biochemical, clinical, and dietary measures of nutritional status.

~ Discuss the strengths and weakness of dietary assessment methods and give examples of their appropriate use.

~ Describe the major components of the National Nutrition Monitoring and Related Research Program.

Key Words

Word	Page Mentioned
Risk factor	58
Modifiable factors	58
Epidemiology	58
Determinants	58
Incidence	58
Prevalence	58
Population at risk	58
Odds ratio	60
Relative risk	60
Screening test	61
Valid	61
Reproducible	61
Sensitivity	61
Specificity	61
Descriptive or ecologic study	61
Analytic etiologic study	61
Experimental study or intervention trial	61
Case-control study	61
Cohort study	61
Bradford Hill criteria	66
Nutritional status	66
Anthropometric	67
Biochemical	67
Clinical	67
Dietary	67
Epidemiologic	67
Food records	67
Twenty-four-hour recall	69
Food frequency questionnaire	71
National nutrition monitoring	76

The planning and management of community nutrition services requires knowledge of the distribution and determinants of nutrition-related health problems within the community and feasible opportunities for intervention. Many of the recommended tools for acquiring knowledge of diet and determinants of problems are found within the specialty of epidemiology. Unlike the clinician, who focuses on the diagnosis of problems in the individual patient and that patient's health, the epidemiologist focuses on diagnosing problems of population groups in the community and identifies the variation of risk factors of disease and health status among the individuals within the group. The objectives are to identify the determinants related to risk and occurrence of disease so that intervention methods can be planned for the primary and secondary prevention of disease and the promotion of health.

The nutrition professional in the community uses procedures similar to those of the epidemiologist to identify the determinants associated with nutrition-related health problems. Individual data on dietary intakes, biochemical and anthropometric measurements, and other indicators of health status, along with demographic data on age, sex, ethnicity, education, and socioeconomic level, are collected and aggregated together to describe the population and to identify subgroups of the community who have or who are at high risk of developing nutrition-related health problems. With these descriptive data and analytical data about the community, the nutrition professional selects target groups and plans appropriate interventions to prevent disease and promote health (see figure 3.1).

The objectives of the nutrition professional are to estimate the rates of occurrence of nutrition-related health problems, **risk factors,** especially **modifiable factors,** and to use this information to plan and conduct community or public health nutrition programs for their control and prevention. We want to know the probability that people who are without a disease but exposed to certain risk factors will acquire the disease at some point in their lives. Risk factors can be inherited, although for nutrition-related health problems, the factors are more likely to be environmental. The nutrition professional is the key member of the health team responsible for identifying the dietary risk factors associated with various diseases. Thus, although the rates of occurrence of diseases are of major concern, it is equally important to identify the nutritional determinants of these diseases and the associated risk factors.

EPIDEMIOLOGY

Epidemiology can be defined as the study of the distribution and determinants of health-related diseases and conditions in particular populations and the application of this study to the control and prevention of health problems. "Distribution" refers to the subjects affected, the place of the event, and the time period of the occurrence. "Subjects" includes descriptive factors such as age, sex, race or ethnicity, occupation, socioeconomic status, and education. "Place" refers to country, state, or urban or rural area, or a particular subsection of a city or country. **"Determinants"** are the causes or agents responsible for the disease or condition. A classic example of a nutritional epidemiologic study that included particular subjects, place, and time is the historical study of James Lind in the mid-1700s.[38] The subjects were British sailors who were at sea for long periods of time. Their diet included staples, but there was no adequate refrigeration for fresh fruits and vegetables. Many sailors became ill and died. Doctor Lind, a Scottish surgeon, conducted a series of clinical controlled trials and found that the feeding of two oranges and one lemon a day had a sudden and beneficial effect on the course of the disease. Later, the beneficial substance in these foods was found to be ascorbic acid, and the cause of the disease, known as scurvy, was due to vitamin C deficiency. The significance of this report is relevant because epidemiologists are often able to recommend methods of preventing a particular disease before the specific cause has been identified.

Several epidemiologic concepts have application for nutrition practice. Disease frequency is a measure of the amount of disease or morbidity in a population group and is stated as **incidence** or **prevalence.**[33] These measures are usually expressed as "rates." The incidence rate is the number of new cases in a **population at risk** during a particular time period, such as one year. The "population at risk" refers to the target population; that is, all persons who are initially free of the particular disease or condition. The incidence rate is defined as

$$\frac{\text{Incidence}}{\text{rate}} = \frac{\text{No. of new cases}}{\text{No. in population at risk}} \times \frac{\text{Time}}{\text{period}}$$

Prevalence, on the other hand, is the proportion of the group or the population that is affected with a particular disease or condition at a given time and includes both new and existing cases; thus, it represents the total number affected, including individuals with long duration and newly identified cases. The prevalence rate is defined as

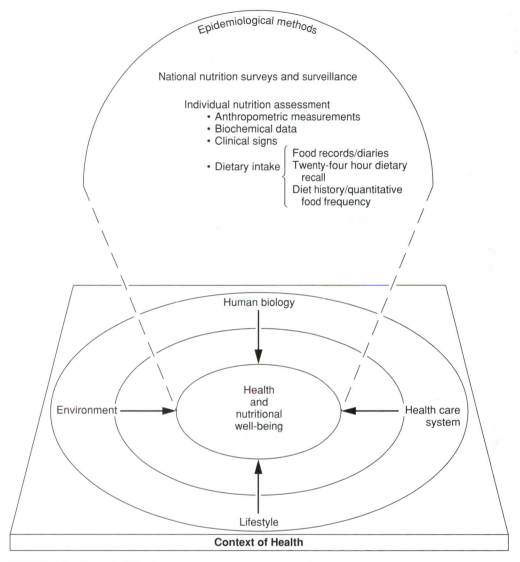

FIGURE 3.1   Context of Health
Epidemiologic Approach to the Assessment of Nutritional Status.

$$\text{Prevalence rate} = \frac{\text{No. of new and existing cases}}{\text{No. in population at risk}} \times \text{Time period}$$

For both of these rates, the numerator is part of the denominator. For many diseases or conditions, incidence data may not be available. For example, it may not be possible to obtain the frequency of new cases of obesity, whereas a survey within a population could provide the estimated prevalence of obesity in which both new and existing cases are identified. On the other hand, registries for some reportable diseases, such as cancer or birth defects, can provide numbers of new cases of specific cancers or birth defects within a particular interval of time, so that incidence rates can be estimated.

Mortality rates, which are measures of the number of deaths due to particular diseases, the number of deaths within particular age or sex groups, or total mortality, are actually incidence rates. They represent new cases—that is, new cases of deaths—occurring in a particular population during a specified time interval. There are several different standardized indices used for computing death rates, depending on the age group, cause, or total mortality.

These vital statistics are useful for understanding problems or conditions within the population and for identifying high-risk groups in particular geographic areas. Table 3.1 lists some of the commonly used vital statistics available from public health agencies.[33]

The comparison of defined rates among different subgroups of persons often yields clues regarding the existence of a health problem and related environmental conditions. In using these data, we need to understand that a rate is a proportion involving a numerator and a denominator, both of which must be clearly defined. Also, as noted above, in the case of a rate, the numerator is a subset of the denominator, whereas in the case of a *ratio,* the numerator refers to a different group than the denominator. For instance, as seen in table 3.1, the fetal death ratio is the number of fetal deaths during the year divided by the number of live births during the year. This information would be useful for planning prenatal nutrition and health programs in particular high-risk groups of the population.

In conducting analytical research, epidemiologists seek to assess whether there is an *association* between particular exposures and a disease and to assess the

strength of the association.[34] We want to know the probability of developing a disease when exposed, compared with the probability of developing a disease when not exposed. These associations are defined according to relative risk or odds ratio, the choice of their use is dependent on the research design. The **odds ratio** is an estimate of the relative risk derived from case-control studies. For **relative risk,** a comparison is made using the following equation:

$$\frac{\text{Relative}}{\text{Risk (RR)}} = \frac{\text{Incidence of disease in the exposed}}{\text{Incidence of disease in the unexposed}}$$

For example, a surveillance study among a multiethnic cohort in Hawaii found that breast cancer occurred in 3.4 percent of women who ever drank alcohol, compared to 2.0 percent of women who never drank alcohol (unpublished data). The RR is the ratio of 3.4 to 2.0, or 1.7. This implies that female drinkers are 70 percent more likely to develop breast cancer than nondrinkers.

Another important concept in conducting epidemiologic studies is risk of disease. *Risk* refers to the probability that people who are without a particular disease or condition, but who are exposed to certain risk fac-

TABLE 3.1
Commonly Used Indices of Vital Statistics

Crude birth rate (per 1,000 population)	=	No. of live births during year / Average (midyear) population
Infant mortality rate (per 1,000 live births)	=	No. of deaths of children < one year of age during year / No. of live births in same year
Neonatal mortality rate (per 1,000 live births)	=	No. of deaths of children < twenty-eight days of age during year / No. of live births in same year
Fetal death ratio (per 1,000 live births)	=	No. of fetal deaths* during year / No. of live births in same year
Fetal death rate (per 1,000 live births and fetal deaths)	=	No. of fetal deaths during year / No. of live births and fetal deaths in same year
Maternal (puerperal) mortality rate (per 100,000 or 10,000 live births)	=	No. of deaths from puerperal causes during year / No. of live births in same year
Crude death rate (per 1,000 population)	=	No. of deaths during year / Average (midyear) population
Age-specific death rate (per 1,000 population)	=	No. of deaths among persons of a given age group during year / Average (midyear) population in specified age group
Cause-specific death rate (per 100,000 population)	=	No. of deaths from a stated cause during year / Average (midyear) population

> 20 weeks' gestation

From Sherry B: Descriptive epidemiologic research. In Monson ER, editor: *Research: successful approaches,* Chicago, 1991, American Dietetic Association.

tors, will acquire the disease at some point in their lives. This concept has led to the aggregation of certain characteristics associated with particular diseases. For example, risk factors associated with coronary heart disease are high blood pressure, hypercholesterolemia, cigarette smoking, and obesity. Risk factors are often referred to as determinants, and may include dietary and other environmental factors as well as genetic characteristics. Thus, individuals who are currently healthy but possess the risk factors of high blood pressure, hypercholesterolemia, cigarette smoking, and obesity are more likely to develop coronary heart disease than persons without these risk factors.

To identify persons who are at high risk for a disease or at early stages of disease, researchers have developed **screening tests** that can be applied to large groups of persons.[33] For instance, nutrition and other health professionals use screening tests to identify children with anemia for iron supplementation. They also use serum cholesterol measurements to identify adults with hypercholesterolemia who may benefit from an American Heart Association Step I diet. Tests used for screening must be **valid** and **reproducible.** A reproducible test gives the same results when repeated on the same person several times. A valid test is one that measures what it is designed to measure.

Epidemiologists use two parameters to assess the validity of a test. **Sensitivity** is the proportion of persons with the disease or condition who test positive on a test. In other words, the person who is found to have high serum cholesterol is truly hypercholesterolemic. **Specificity** is the proportion of persons without the disease or condition who test negative on a test. The greater the specificity, the less likely it is that a positive result will misclassify the person. The goal with any diagnostic test is to maximize both sensitivity and specificity.

Types of Epidemiologic Studies

Epidemiologists use several different methods for studying the distribution of health and disease and the factors that influence this distribution in population groups. These studies progress along a continuum of complexity from **descriptive or ecological studies,** to **analytical etiologic studies,** in which persons with a disease are compared to persons without the disease to identify potential causal factors, to **experimental studies** in which **intervention trials** are conducted to test hypotheses.

Descriptive Studies Descriptive or ecologic studies provide data on the pattern of diseases among different population groups. For example, investigators have analyzed food consumption data in different countries and correlated the intake data with rates of particular diseases, such as cancer. The dietary information in these international studies is based on food disappearance data, which are computed from the national figures of food produced plus imported minus the food exported, fed to animals, or otherwise not available for humans. The total amounts of food available are divided by the estimated total population to yield the per capita dietary intakes for each country. The per capita intakes of individual foods, food groups, and nutrients are published by the Food and Agriculture Organization (FAO) of the United Nations.[6] For example, figure 3.2 compares the average daily per capita fat intakes with the breast cancer incidence rates of several countries.[31] The findings revealed strong correlations between the per capita dietary fat intakes and breast cancer incidence rates. However, these data are weak because they represent only the foods and nutrients *available* per person and not the amounts consumed. Nor is there information on the distribution of food and nutrient intakes by age and sex. It also is not known whether the persons with higher fat intakes are the ones who will develop cancer.

In some descriptive studies, such as one conducted in Hawaii a few years ago, dietary histories were obtained among random samples of various ethnic groups of women.[18] Analysis of the dietary intakes by ethnic group revealed strong correlations with dietary fat and the ethnicity-specific breast cancer incidence rates. Although findings such as these are suggestive, the major values of ecologic studies are to provide hypotheses that can be tested in epidemiologic analytical studies and intervention trials with groups of individuals.

Analytical Studies Analytical studies are more rigorous than descriptive studies. They are conducted to develop as well as to test hypotheses regarding the associations of diet and other factors and diseases among individuals in population groups. The two major types of analytical studies are retrospective or **case-control studies** and prospective or **cohort studies.** Both terms can be used for each type of study. In case-control studies, the subjects are selected according to whether they have a particular disease. These are the cases. Controls are randomly selected individuals of the same sex, age,

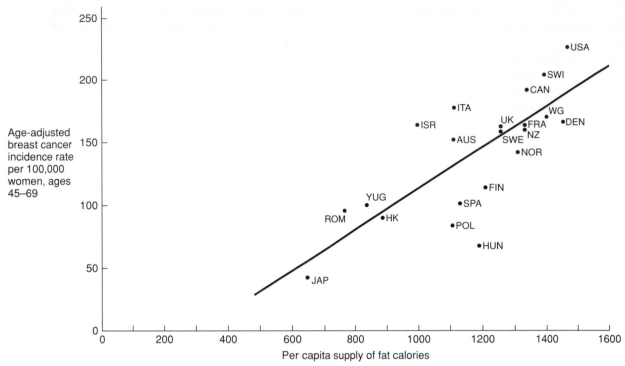

FIGURE 3.2   Association of Breast Cancer Incidence Rates and Per Capita Intakes of Fat Calories in Twenty-One Countries
From Prentice RL, Kakar F, Hursting S, et al.: Aspects of the rationale for the women's health trial, *J Natl Cancer Institute;* 80:802, 1988.
Reprinted with permission.

ethnicity, and other matching variables who do not have the disease. Generally, the investigator develops a questionnaire that includes a number of potential exposure factors. Trained interviewers collect the same information in the same way from both cases and controls. The data are analyzed, and the investigator compares the various exposure factors in the cases and controls to determine their association with the particular disease. The aim is to identify those risk factors that are found more commonly in the cases than the controls.

Risk factors are usually variables that are suspected to increase the likelihood of developing a disease. For example, excess dietary fat intake is a risk factor for some diseases. In addition, the lack of some dietary components, such as dietary iron or calcium, is a risk factor for various health problems. During recent years, several case-control studies on the relationship of diet and various cancers have been conducted. Most of these studies have used diet history or food frequency questionnaires to estimate the usual past dietary intakes among cases and matched controls. For instance, several investigators have postulated an association of dietary fat and breast cancer. However, the findings from case-

control studies, as well as cohort studies, of diet and breast cancer have been equivocal, with some studies suggesting a modest positive association with total fat or saturated fat and others suggesting no association.[12,16] On the other hand, case-control studies of diet and prostate cancer have generally been supportive of a positive association with some component of dietary fat.[17] It is important to note that studies such as these do *not* provide evidence of cause and effect. Confirmatory information is necessary, and this is possible only through experimental studies or intervention trials.

Several limitations to the dietary information in case-control studies result from the potential bias in responding to questionnaires about a person's recall of past diet. In studies of cancer, epidemiologists seek knowledge on the usual diet before diagnosis of disease. Chronic diseases, such as cancer, coronary heart disease, and osteoporosis, are likely to have their origin several years before diagnosis. However, most persons are not able to recall their diets of several years in the past. Consequently, in case-control studies, the cases are usually asked to recall their dietary intakes the year prior to diagnosis of disease, whereas the controls are asked to recall

TABLE 3.2

Comparison of Strengths and Limitations of Retrospective (Case-control) and Prospective (Cohort) Studies

Retrospective study	
Strengths	**Limitations**
Relatively inexpensive	Recall possibly biased
Smaller number of subjects	Biological data antedating disease not obtainable
Relatively quick results	Potential bias in selection of controls
Practical for rare diseases	Only odds ratio rather than relative risk obtainable
Prospective study	
Strengths	**Limitations**
No bias for exposure factors	Very expensive
Relative risk and incidence rates obtainable	Large number of subjects required
Study of exposure variables with many diseases enabled	Many years to get results
	Potential loss of subjects over time
Biologic data antedating disease obtainable	Possible bias in ascertaining disease
	Rare disease study not possible

their diets during the year prior to the interview. Several investigators believe that people who are diagnosed with a potential diet-related disease may unconsciously alter their responses about their past diet. If this occurs, their dietary data would be biased and any *differences* between cases and controls would most likely be underestimated.

For this reason, epidemiologists prefer to begin with a healthy group of individual participants in a cohort or prospective study. In cohort or prospective studies, the baseline diets of a large number of healthy persons are assessed, and the diets of persons who subsequently develop a disease are then compared with persons of the same sex, age, and ethnicity who remain healthy. Recall bias should be minimized because the dietary data are collected from all participants before disease occurred.

A number of large cohort studies have been established by epidemiologists in the United States as well as in other countries. These studies consist of large population groups (up to 200,000 persons or more), selected on the basis of particular criteria, such as belonging to the same profession or being members of particular ethnic groups. Various data are collected from each person, including biographical information, estimates of usual dietary intakes, history of diseases, smoking and drinking habits, anthropometric measurements, physical activity, and other health indices and practices. In some studies, blood and urine samples are also obtained for laboratory analyses of biochemical and genetic parameters. Then, all individuals who are initially healthy or free of known

diseases are followed periodically for several years to obtain data on the incidence of particular diseases or conditions. The epidemiologist compares the baseline characteristics of persons developing the disease (new cases) with comparable persons who remain disease free (controls). These data are used to compute incidence rates and to identify the risk factors associated with particular diseases or conditions. Table 3.2 compares the strengths and limitations of the retrospective or case-control and the prospective or cohort studies.

Experimental Studies Investigators may review the findings from several analytical studies (both case-control and cohort) and propose particular hypotheses that can be tested in experimental studies or intervention trials. For example, the Women's Health Initiative is a large multi-center study of chronic disease in postmenopausal women.[35] The major health outcomes are coronary heart disease, breast and colorectal cancers, and osteoporosis. One component of the study is testing the hypothesis that a low-fat dietary pattern with increased fruits, vegetables, and grains will reduce the risk of breast and colorectal cancers and coronary heart disease. About 48,000 women in forty clinical centers in the United States are participating in this component of the study, with 40 percent randomized to a 20 percent fat diet, and with 60 percent consuming their usual diet. This ten-year intervention trial will provide evidence of the role of dietary fat in the etiology of these cancers and of heart disease.

Findings from analytical studies may also lead to different types of intervention trials. For instance, a case-control study on lung cancer conducted in Hawaii revealed that a high intake of dark green vegetables and of all vegetables was negatively associated with lung cancer.[20] The negative or inverse condition with vegetables was greater than with any nutrient, such as beta-carotene, or other dietary component. These findings formed the basis for the development of an intervention trial among successfully treated lung cancer and head and neck cancer patients who are at high risk of developing a recurrence or a second cancer in five years. The feasibility of testing this hypothesis was demonstrated in a preliminary pilot study.[19] The hypothesis that a diet of nine servings of specific vegetable and fruit groups each day will prevent the development of a new cancer or recurrence of lung cancer is being tested scientifically in an intervention trial. Qualified patients who meet the study criteria are randomized either to the experimental diet or to their usual diet. The intervention is being monitored through repeated dietary recalls and measured food records and through periodic measurements of serum carotenoids and ascorbic acid.

EPIDEMIOLOGIC METHODS USED BY THE COMMUNITY NUTRITION PROFESSIONAL

Defining the Population and Sampling

Review of the demographic and health statistics of the population may suggest a need for conducting a nutritional status survey among the particular high-risk subgroup. This population group will comprise the denominator for analyzing the data. In collecting the dietary and health data of this population, it is important to consider the methods of selecting the sample for the nutritional assessment. The sample will be biased if the participants are volunteers or are self-selected. This is avoided by selecting a random sample of the population for the particular survey. As noted later, the various surveys conducted by the U.S. Departments of Agriculture (USDA) and Health and Human Services (HHS) are based on randomly selected subjects who meet particular criteria in the U.S. population. The nutrition professional should consult with an epidemiologist or biostatistician to develop a method of random sampling for assessing the nutritional status of the community. This is the only objective procedure for identifying the risk for developing nutrition-related health problems by members of the population.

A further epidemiologic concept is to ensure that the measuring techniques are performed accurately and consistently in the same way among all persons in the sample. Thus, all personnel need to be trained to ensure that the information is not biased by inaccuracy or inconsistency among the data collectors. For instance, if a diet history or quantitative food frequency questionnaire has been developed or selected for estimating dietary intakes, then all interviewers need to be trained so that each of them is following the same protocol. It also is important to obtain data from all of the randomly selected persons. If there are too many refusals among the selected persons, the findings will be biased. The refusals could be made by individuals with particular nutrition problems or with atypical eating patterns. Preplanning and staff training should be done to maximize the participation of all persons, possibly by interviewing or examining them at their most convenient days and times. If necessary, interviewers may need to alter their working hours to accommodate the survey participants. In addition, the participants need assurance that the purpose of the survey is to identify possible health problems and to develop programs and materials that will benefit them and their families. They need assurance that the information they provide is confidential, that individual names are not included in reports, and that they are not being judged!

The epidemiologist and the nutrition professional weigh the information obtained from a representative sample of the population to identify the importance of findings related to the health status of various subgroups in the population and rank the findings for follow-up action. For example, suppose you are concerned about obesity as a risk factor for coronary heart disease in males. A random sample of middle-aged men reveals that the body mass index is greater than 30 among 30 percent of the men who are currently free of coronary heart disease (CHD). Since obesity is a risk factor for CHD and other health problems, the nutrition professional may decide to develop a nutrition education/intervention program that includes both dietary and physical activity components.

Criteria for Selecting Methods and Tools

Standardized methods should be selected for any nutritional/health status assessment. It is particularly useful to select methods that will provide comparable data with other population surveys, such as the National

Health and Nutrition Examination Surveys (NHANES). Dependent on the health statistics, available trained personnel, and financial resources, the nutrition professional may select a variety of anthropometric, biochemical, clinical, and dietary assessment procedures that are indicative of nutrition/health status of the particular at-risk population. The particular methods should have been tested for validity and reproducibility and reported in published manuals or studies. However, it is essential that methods used and reported in the medical and nutrition literature from other studies be critiqued before their use is adopted. An excellent comprehensive reference is the *Plan and Operation of the Third National Health and Nutrition Examination Survey, 1988–1994*.[26] This manual includes well-tested assessment methods and provides guidance for use among various age groups of the population. Also, the anthropometric procedures used in NHANES III have been published as a video and provide an excellent description and illustration of all measuring procedures followed by the National Center of Health Statistics (NCHS).[25] Standardized procedures for the following measurements are included: body weight, standing and sitting heights; upper leg and upper arm lengths; knee height; arm, waist, buttocks, thigh, and head circumferences; thigh, triceps, subscapular, and supriliac skinfolds; and wrist, biacromial, biiliac and elbow breadths. By following procedures used by the NCHS, the findings can be compared to nationally representative reference data.

Careful review is also essential in the selection or development of a dietary assessment method for use in the survey. In selecting the dietary method for assessing the nutritional status or health status of a population, it is important to test its validity and reproducibility. Although it may appear easier to use a survey instrument developed for another population, that instrument may not necessarily be appropriate for your population. Before use, the instrument should be pretested in a sample of the population to determine if the survey instrument includes a majority of the usual foods consumed in your geographic area and racial or ethnic population. For example, a questionnaire developed for Caucasians living in the New England states would most likely not include the usual food items consumed by Asians, Hispanics, or African-Americans living in southern California. The particular method should also be tested for validity and reproducibility within your population before use.

Validity is the ability of the dietary assessment instrument to measure what it is expected to measure, that is, the individual's dietary intake over a period of time, which could be a day, week, month, or year. Validity requires that the truth be known, which is most likely impossible to obtain among free-living persons for extended periods. However, in congregate eating facilities, it has been possible to validate one-day recalls by weighing the portions served to individuals and weighing what was left on plates, and then asking the subjects to recall their diets the next day. This procedure was followed by Madden and associates[21] and Gersovitz and associates[8] among subjects sixty or more years old eating at congregate meal sites. Recalls the following day revealed that the mean intakes between the observed and recalled diets were not significantly different. However, there was a tendency for participants with lower observed intakes to overreport, and for those with higher observed intakes to underreport their previous day's intake.

The quantitative photographic diet history designed for the multiethnic population of Hawaii, was validated among persons who completed four weekly food records during a one-year period.[14] The study indicated that the questionnaire gave reasonably accurate estimates of the usual dietary intakes of the population. Validity has also been assessed for various food frequency questionnaires and is reported in the *Dietary Assessment Resource Manual*, a supplement published by the *Journal of Nutrition*.[37]

Biomarkers have also been used for validation of dietary questionnaires.[37] Although correlations between serum levels of carotenoids and ascorbic acid and dietary intakes of fruits and vegetables may be imperfect, they are useful for monitoring changes in intakes of these food items through corresponding changes in serum levels.[19] This is an important monitoring procedure for intervention trials in which subjects are asked to increase their intakes of fruits and vegetables.

Reproducibility (also called *reliability*) is the ability of the instrument to produce the same dietary estimates on two or more separate occasions, assuming that there was no change in diet during the time interval. A number of nutritionists and epidemiologists have tested the reproducibility of their food frequency or diet history questionnaires by repeated administration to subjects after intervals of a few months or years.[10,37] In general, reproducibility was higher for nutrients than for foods, for shorter intervals of a few months than for longer time spans of several years, and for standard size portions than for variable size servings.

Interpreting Epidemiologic Findings on Nutritional Status

The nutrition professional must use care in interpreting epidemiologic findings concerning the relationship between diet and nutritional/health status. Although the link between these variables may suggest *cause and effect,* we need to remember that both parameters are measured with considerable uncertainty. Nonetheless, public or community health problems often demand some action despite our imperfect knowledge. Some thirty years ago Bradford Hill proposed a set of standards known as the **Bradford Hill criteria** for causal inference.[32] Before assuming a causal relationship between a dietary finding and health status, all of the following conditions should be satisfied:

1. *Strength of association.* The evidence must show a correlation (association) between the dietary finding and the outcome. The greater the correlation when the causal dietary factor is present, the greater the likelihood of a causal relationship.
2. *Consistency.* Similar studies in other populations and environments should reveal similar findings. In other words, the findings should be replicated in other situations.
3. *Specificity.* The disease or health outcome must be associated only with the potential causal factor under study. However, this condition may be difficult to satisfy because there may be several determinants of the particular disease, and a particular determinant may have an effect on more than one health outcome, as seen in figure 3.3.
4. *Temporality.* The causal factor must be present before the occurrence of the disease or health problem. In other words, coronary heart disease does not cause a high fat diet, whereas years of a high fat diet may contribute to the development of CHD.
5. *Plausibility.* Plausibility refers to the biological rationale of the evidence. For example, it is biologically plausible that a child consuming a diet low in protein and iron will develop iron-deficiency anemia.
6. *Coherence.* Coherence implies that the cause-and-effect associaton does not conflict with what is known scientificaly.

These criteria are not necessarily "hard and fast rules" to be followed for inferring cause and effect, according to Hill.[15] Causal inference is tentative and is a somewhat subjective process. Nonetheless, these criteria should be considered before concluding that a particular dietary or nutritional status finding is the "cause"

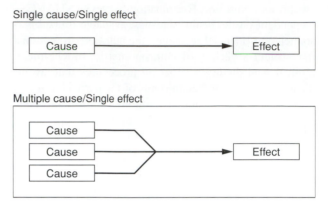

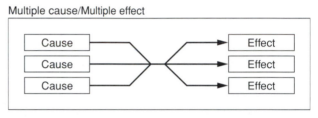

FIGURE 3.3   Relationship of Determinants to Health Effects in Epidemiologic Studies

of a particular condition. It also is necessary to review relevant published scientific reports in the literature and to confer with epidemiologists and other nutrition and health professionals in the community before drawing a conclusion. Finally, for nutrition-related health problems, there will seldom be only one particular cause. Generally, there will be multiple environmental as well as genetic determinants related to the etiology of the problem. Thus, the nutrition professional needs to identify all potential determinants of disease, use the skills and knowledge of other health professionals, plan and implement an intervention program to alleviate the health problems, and use appropriate measures to evaluate the effectiveness of the program.

DEFINING NUTRITIONAL STATUS

The Joint Nutrition Monitoring Evaluation Committee describes "the **nutritional status** of an individual as the condition of his or her health as influenced by the intake and utilization of nutrients."[4] The committee points out that nutritional status cannot be measured directly by a single test; rather assessment is dependent on the collective interpretation of relevant dietary and health data. There are five major types of data needed to identify nutrition-related health problems or risks of related diseases:

1. **Anthropometric** measurements, such as weight, height, body mass index (BMI), waist and hip circumferences, height for weight ratio, and waist/hip ratio. Norms for various age-sex groups are published in the *Third Report on Nutrition Monitoring in the United States.*[5]

2. **Biochemical** data, including concentrations of substances in body fluids or tissues, such as red blood cell fatty acids, plasma cholesterol, urinary creatinine, serum iron, and glucose tolerance levels. Norms for the U.S. population are also found in the *Third Report.*[5]

3. **Clinical** signs, such as characteristics of the skin and hair associated with nutritional deficiency or excess, should be identified.

4. **Dietary** intake data, including assessment of intakes of individual food items, mixed dishes, dietary supplements, and food preparation methods. Although the recommended dietary allowances (RDAs) have been the only quantitative guidelines available for estimating nutrient needs, they were not designed to be applied to any one individual.[29] The RDAs are intended for planning diets and food supplies for groups of individuals; setting public policy for food stamp allowances; and designing school food services, congregate meals for the elderly, and the like. However, in practice, researchers and practitioners compare the dietary intakes of particular age-sex subgroups with the RDAs. This practice may change as new reference values for nutrient intake are released by the National Research Council of the National Academy of Sciences. Different nutrients are important in different conditions and different subgroups of the population, and are described in the various life cycle chapters.

5. **Epidemiologic** data on the incidence or prevalence of nutrition-related health problems are also needed. All of these parameters can be thought of as the ABCs of nutrition assessment. In addition, nutritional status is affected by socioeconomic factors, behavioral patterns, physical activity, medical care, and genetics.

As shown in figure 3.4, each piece of information identifies a different level of nutritional and health status. Dietary data alone are insufficient for indicating if the individual is at risk for poor health. The whole picture is essential for the assessment of nutritional/health status. In addition to measuring nutritional/health status per se, as noted previously, the nutrition professional is concerned with the identification of risk factors for diseases with nutritional components, such as coronary heart disease, hypertension, and several cancers. Biochemical, anthropometric, clinical, and dietary measurements are used to assess such risks. Information on the prevalence of risk factors is particularly useful for planning primary prevention programs because the initiation of many chronic diseases most likely begins at an early age.

DIETARY INTAKE METHODS AND THEIR USE IN SURVEYS

For more than sixty years, diet has been increasingly recognized as a major determinant of health and disease throughout the life cycle. In addition to individual assessment and dietary counseling, nutrition professionals play a major role in selecting the appropriate dietary method for nutrition assessment studies of populations as well as for epidemiologic investigations of diet and disease. The various types of dietary assessment tools have different functions; yield different kinds of information; and vary in method of administration, complexity, and cost. Nutrition professionals need to understand each major method, its purpose, and its strengths and weaknesses. In addition, it is most helpful to be familiar with reported studies that have utilized various methods as well as potential formats that can be modified for your own situation. This chapter includes a brief description of each dietary assessment method, along with its strengths and weaknesses and illustrations of a few questionnaires or formats in use today. Further details can be found in two major publications: the *Dietary Assessment Resource Manual,* published by the *Journal of Nutrition,*[37] and *Research: Successful Approaches,* published by the American Dietetic Association.[10]

Food Records or Diaries

Food records or food diaries require the subject or proxy to record all foods and beverages and amounts consumed over several days, usually three to seven consecutive days, and possibly at multiple times during the year.[10,37] Amounts consumed may be weighed; measured with household utensils; or estimated from models, pictures, package labels, or no particular aids. The respondent must be trained to describe adequately the foods and amounts consumed, including preparation methods, recipes for mixed dishes, and portion sizes. In addition, dietary supplements are generally recorded in detail. The quality may be enhanced by a personal review of the record after the first day; and it is essential that a trained interviewer review the data at the end of

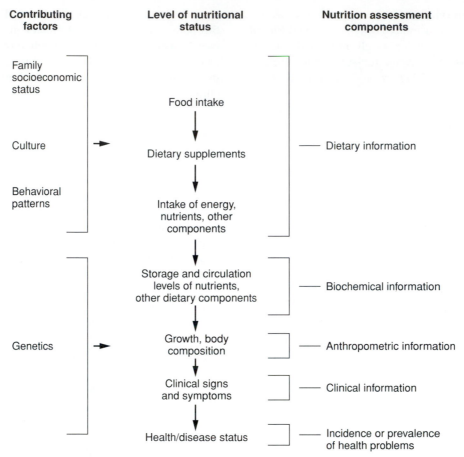

FIGURE 3.4   Relationship between Levels of Nutritional Status and Components of Nutritional Assessment

the recording period to clarify all entries and to probe for missing information. Usually the format is open-ended, permitting the subject to record the time and place of each meal or snack, the name of the food item, the components of mixed dishes, and the quantity consumed. Table 3.3 is an example of the format for a food record using household measurements. This example shows written instructions as well as a sample so the subject knows how to complete the food record.

Strengths   The food record has the potential of providing quantitatively accurate information on food consumed during the recording period. Consequently, it has often been considered to be the "gold standard" for use in validating other dietary methods based on long-term dietary recall. If foods are recorded as consumed, the problem of omission is lessened and the measurement of amounts should be more accurate than is likely with past recalls.

Weaknesses   Bias may occur in the sample selection and the choice of foods during the recording period. Record keeping requires motivated and literate subjects, which can limit its use in some population groups, such as recent migrants, children, and very elderly persons. Thus, the information may not be representative of the general population. Also, the demanding task of measuring and recording foods as consumed can affect the types of foods selected and the amounts consumed. For example, it is far easier to consume a frozen entree with a label that lists the ingredients and amounts than to prepare a similar mixed dish in which all of the ingredients need to be measured and recorded. Some studies have also found that dietary intakes from food records tend to be underestimated.[37] This could be due to incomplete recording or an actual dietary change during the recording period. Finally, food record data are burdensome to code and can lead to high personnel costs.

T A B L E   3 . 3
Food Record Form

GENERAL INSTRUCTIONS FOR KEEPING RECORD

1. Write LEGIBLY. Use BLACK INK.
2. Record each meal/snack IMMEDIATELY after it is eaten.
3. Complete the TIME EATEN and PREPARED sections for each meal or snack.
4. In the PREPARED column, use 1 for foods prepared in a HOME, 2 for foods prepared in a RESTAURANT, and 3 for foods prepared in an OTHER location.
5. Record each food on a SEPARATE LINE.
6. Leave 1 BLANK LINE after each meal or snack.
7. Start EACH NEW DAY on a NEW PAGE.
8. If additional space is required for the same day, CONTINUE on the NEXT PAGE.

INSTRUCTIONS FOR RECORDING OF FOODS

The study interviewer has discussed the information that must be recorded about the foods you eat. Keep the following major points in mind.

1. Record BRAND NAMES if known.
2. Specify METHODS OF PREPARATION. Example: whether meat is fried, broiled, baked, breaded, etc.
3. For foods PREPARED WITH FAT, specify fat used. Example: fried in margarine (with brand name).
4. Record NAMES OF RESTAURANTS in the Foods and Beverages column.
5. FULLY DESCRIBE all foods, beverages, condiments, spreads, etc. Example: chicken thigh, skin not eaten; decaffeinated coffee; low calorie French dressing.
6. LIST INGREDIENTS for sandwiches and mixed dishes.
7. Record EXACT AMOUNTS. Specify weight, volume (example: cup, tsp, Tb, fl oz), or dimensions in inches.
8. Include ADDITIONS AT THE TABLE. Example: baked potato with 1 TB butter; coffee with 1 tsp sugar. Record each addition on a separate line.
9. Describe all VITAMINS, MINERALS and other SUPPLEMENTS.

If you have any questions call your study contact person.

SAMPLE

LINE	PREP	DAY Monday / DATE 0 7 - 0 1 - 9 1 / PAGE ☐ OF ☐	WAS SALT ADDED IN PREPARATION? 1=NO 2=YES 3=UNKNOWN / WAS FAT ADDED IN PREPARATION? 1=NO 2=YES 3=UNKNOWN		

LINE	Hour	Min.	A=a.m. P=p.m.	PREPARED	FOODS AND BEVERAGES	AMOUNT		
01	0 7	4 5	A	1	Orange Juice	1/2 cup		
02					Buttermilk pancakes	3 cakes	2	2
03					from scratch with			
04					brand x oil, 5" diam			
05					Margarine, unkn	1 tsp		
06					brand, stick			
07								
08	1 0	0 0	A	1	Apple with peel	1 med		
09								
10	1 2	3 0	P	1	Tomato soup	1 cup		
11					diluted with water			
12					Lettuce salad	1 cup		
13					Lo-cal Italian dressing	1 Tb		
14					Ginger Ale	12 oz		
15					Chocolate pudding from	1/2 cup		
16					mix with skim milk			
17								
18	0 5	3 0	P	2	Ham, baked, trimmed	3 1/2 oz		
19					Baked potato, skin eaten	1 med		
20					Butter	1 tsp		
21					Carrots, ckd	1/2 cup	1	2
22					Rye roll	1 avg		
23					Skim milk	1/2 cup		
24				☐	* IF PAGE CONTINUES			

Form provided by the Nutrition Coordinating Center, Division of Epidemiology, University of Minnesota, 1300 S. 2nd St, Suite 300, Minneapolis, MN, 55454-1015.

Twenty-four-Hour Dietary Recalls

In the **twenty-four-hour dietary recall,** the well-trained interviewer (usually a dietitian or a non-nutritionist trained in the use of the method) obtains information on all food items consumed during the past twenty-four hours or the previous day. It may be computer assisted[37] or recorded directly on paper forms. This method requires interviewers to have knowledge about available local foods and preparation practices and experience in probing for all necessary details. The recall can be administered in person or by telephone. A quality control system is needed to minimize errors and increase reliabil-ity of interviewing. Training and retraining sessions for interviewers are essential. For example, periodic conference calls to discuss problems among the interviewers and taping of telephone interviews have increased quality control in a large multiethnic population study that uses twenty-four-hour recalls for calibration of a structured diet history (personal information). Table 3.4 is an example of a twenty-four-hour recall form. It includes columns to assure consistent probes about fat and salt.

Strengths   There are many advantages of the twenty-four-hour recall. Because the information is obtained by an interviewer, literacy of the respondent is not required.

TABLE 3.4
Dietary Intake Form Used for Twenty-four-Hour Recall

STUDY ID

DIETARY INTAKE Collection Method 1-Record 2-Recall

DATE OF VISIT — MONTH — DAY — YEAR VISIT NO.

PARTICIPANT ID

INITIALS Interviewer ID

INTERVIEWER'S OPINION OF INFORMATION
1 = RELIABLE
2* = UNABLE TO RECALL ONE OR MORE MEALS
3* = UNRELIABLE FOR OTHER REASONS

INTAKE WAS
1 = TYPICAL
2 = CONSIDERABLY LESS THAN USUAL
3 = CONSIDERABLY MORE THAN USUAL

INTAKE DAY
1=SUN 2=MON 3=TUE 4=WED 5=THU 6=FRI 7=SAT

DID YOU TAKE ANY SUPPLEMENTS ON DAY OF INTAKE?
1=NO 2=YES
IF YES, DESCRIBE UNDER "FOODS AND BEVERAGES"

FOR NCC USE
BATCH NO:

Explain starred (*) items in the comments space below

Page ___ Of ___

Amount of Salt Product Added at Table
1 = light 2 = medium 3 = heavy 9 = unknown
Kind of Salt Product Added at Table
1 = none 2 = salt 3* = salt substitute 9 = unknown
Kind of Salt Product Added in Preparation
1 = none 2 = salt 3* = salt substitute 9 = unknown

1 – Home 2 – Restaurant 3 – Other
PREPARED
Was Fat Added In Preparation?
1 = no 2 = yes 9 = unknown

LINE NO.	TIME A=a.m P=p.m. Hour Min.		FOODS AND BEVERAGES	AMOUNT		COMPLETE DESCRIPTION		
01								
02								
03								
04								
05								
06								
07								
08								
09								
10								
11								
12								

*IF CONTINUATION PAGE FOLLOWS

COMMENTS: (Give Line No. if appropriate)

Review using Documentation Checklist by: Initials: Date:

Nutrition Coordinating Center

NCC Form No.100-1B Rev. 4/91

Form provided by the Nutrition Coordinating Center, Division of Epidemiology, University of Minnesota, 1300 S. 2nd St, Suite 300, Minneapolis, MN, 55454–1015.

Also, the respondents are usually able to recall what they have eaten fairly well due to the recency of the recall period. Furthermore, because of the low burden, the participants are likely to be more representative of the population, and refusals occur far less often than in food record studies. Another strength is that the information is collected after the food was consumed, and thus the recall is less likely to affect the eating practices.

Direct coding of the foods reported during the interview is now possible, using automated software that specifies the information needed for coding each response. This is being done in several studies in the United States, including the National Health and Nutrition Examination Surveys,[37] as well as in some international studies. However, this procedure does have a potential problem due to the loss of the respondent's verbal description, which would be available in the written recall conducted by the interviewer. In addition, the automated procedures may be difficult if interviews are being conducted in a variety of ethnic populations who prepare and consume foods unfamiliar to the interviewer and that may not be available in the food composition database.

Multiple twenty-four-hour recalls from the same individuals on randomly selected days can be used for the validation or calibration of a diet history or a quantitative food frequency questionnaire.[39]

Weaknesses   A single twenty-four-hour recall cannot be used to characterize the individual's usual diet because most people's diets vary greatly from day to day. In addition, most persons do have atypical eating patterns on occasional days due to sickness, travel, or many other reasons. It also is not appropriate to use single twenty-four-hour recalls to estimate the proportion of the population that has adequate or inadequate diets. The principal use of a single twenty-four-hour recall is to describe the average dietary intakes of a group. For example, the method has been used to characterize the average dietary patterns of groups of Pacific Islanders according to the degree of Westernization[13] and in epidemiologic studies comparing diet and coronary heart disease among Japanese males living in California, Hawaii, and Japan.[36]

Diet Histories or Quantitative Food Frequencies

The first diet history was developed by Burke about fifty years ago.[2,10,37] This was a subjective method that included a detailed interview (usually a twenty-four-hour recall with questions about typical variations), a

food list with frequencies and amounts eaten, and a three-day food record. The frequency and food record data were used as cross-checks of the history. From these data, dietitians calculated the average daily intakes of energy and nutrients. This method was used in diet and child growth studies[1] and for epidemiologic studies of diet and heart disease in Framingham, Massachusetts.[22] The Burke method was the forerunner of the more structured diet histories in current use.

The collection of information on past dietary intakes can be thought of in the same way as past clinical information on health and disease. In both cases, the information refers to the past and may be thought of as "histories." To simplify the collection of past dietary intakes, investigators who wish to obtain data on individuals' usual diets develop a list of selected food items and food groups with similar nutrient values used interchangeably in the diet for use in large epidemiologic or nutritional status studies.[10,37] The instruments can be described as *diet histories* or *quantitative food frequencies*. Respondents are asked to indicate their usual frequencies of eating each listed item and to choose one of the listed serving units. Usual intakes of foods are obtained by multiplying the frequency or midpoint of the frequency interval (e.g., the midpoint of three to five times a week is "4") by the weight of the serving size of each item. Usual intakes of nutrients and other dietary components are computed in the same way, using the amount of nutrients in the particular size serving times the reported frequency.

Some investigators solicit frequency data only,[9,40] although a convenient serving size can be listed with each item. This approach is often called a *food frequency* or *semiquantitative* **food frequency questionnaire.** Figure 3.5 is a section from a self-administered semiquantitative food frequency questionnaire being used in the Male Health Professionals' Cohort Study.[9] The assumption is made that frequency is the more important component in a person's diet, and food and nutrient intakes are estimated by multiplying the frequency by the listed or assumed portion size. This assumption may be true or appropriate among some populations. However, in other populations that include a variety of ethnic groups, such as Asians and Polynesians, portion size may be as important as frequency of consumption in assessing usual individual intakes.

To develop a meaningful diet history (or quantitative food frequency) questionnaire, preliminary information is needed on the population's usual eating practices. General guidelines are to choose foods consumed by a

BREADS, CEREALS, STARCHES	Never, or less than once per month	1–3 per month	1 per week	2–4 per week	5–6 per week	1 per day	2–3 per day	4–5 per day	6+ per day	P
Cold breakfast cereal (1 cup)	○	○	Ⓦ	○	○	Ⓓ	○	○	○	○
Cooked oatmeal/cooked oat bran (1 cup)	○	○	Ⓦ	○	○	Ⓓ	○	○	○	○
Other cooked breakfast cereal (1 cup)	○	○	Ⓦ	○	○	Ⓓ	○	○	○	○
White bread (slice), including pita bread	○	○	Ⓦ	○	○	Ⓓ	○	○	○	○
Dark bread (slice), including wheat pita bread	○	○	Ⓦ	○	○	Ⓓ	○	○	○	○
Bagels, English muffins, or rolls (1)	○	○	Ⓦ	○	○	Ⓓ	○	○	○	○
Muffins or biscuits (1)	○	○	Ⓦ	○	○	Ⓓ	○	○	○	○
Brown rice (1 cup)	○	○	Ⓦ	○	○	Ⓓ	○	○	○	○
White rice (1 cup)	○	○	Ⓦ	○	○	Ⓓ	○	○	○	○
Pasta, e.g., spaghetti, noodles, etc. (1 cup)	○	○	Ⓦ	○	○	Ⓓ	○	○	○	○
Tortillas (1)	○	○	Ⓦ	○	○	Ⓓ	○	○	○	○
Other grains, e.g., bulgar, kasha, couscous, etc. (1 cup)	○	○	Ⓦ	○	○	Ⓓ	○	○	○	○
Pancakes or waffles (serving)	○	○	Ⓦ	○	○	Ⓓ	○	○	○	○
French fried potatoes (4 oz.)	○	○	Ⓦ	○	○	Ⓓ	○	○	○	○
Potatoes, baked, boiled (1) or mashed (1 cup)	○	○	Ⓦ	○	○	Ⓓ	○	○	○	○
Potato chips or corn chips (small bag or 1 oz.)	○	○	Ⓦ	○	○	Ⓓ	○	○	○	○
Crackers, Triscuits, Wheat Thins (1)	○	○	Ⓦ	○	○	Ⓓ	○	○	○	○
Pizza (2 slices)	○	○	Ⓦ	○	○	Ⓓ	○	○	○	○

FIGURE 3.5   Sample Page from a Semi-Quantitative Food Frequency Questionnaire Used in the Male Health Professionals' Cohort Study

Harvard University food frequency questionnaire used with permission of Walter Willett.

sizable number of persons and to include those items that will provide 85 to 90 percent of the estimated intakes of energy, nutrients, and other dietary components of interest. Various procedures can be used for selecting the items, such as food records or recalls of a representative sample of the population. For example, Hankin and Wilkens collected three-day measured food records from representative samples of the five major ethnic groups in Hawaii, grouped the items into meaningful categories, and developed a diet history questionnaire for use in epidemiologic studies in the population.[11] The food record data were also used to select the distribution of three serving sizes for each listed food item or group. Colored photographs of the serving sizes of each food item or food group were prepared, and interviewers used these aids to obtain frequency and quantitative data from each participant in the studies. This technique was modified and adapted for use in a multiethnic cohort study being conducted in Hawaii and Los Angeles, California. The self-administered questionnaire includes photographs of three portions of several food groups and allows the participant to select the usual frequencies and amounts consumed during the previous twelve months. Figure 3.6 illustrates a page of the diet history questionnaire used in the multiethnic cohort study.

Strengths   The diet history or quantitative food frequency questionnaire has the advantage of collecting estimates of the usual diet during a previous time period, usually the past year. It may include food preparation data, such as the usual methods of preparing meat, poultry, and fish; the kinds of fats and oils used in cooking; and the degree of browning and doneness of meat items. Information on condiments, alcohol consumption, and particular kinds of fats added to bread items and of kinds of milk used may be included. With data such as these, epidemiologists and nutrition professionals derive estimates of the dietary intakes and eating practices of the respondents and use the information for intervention studies to test associations of diet and disease and for public health nutrition programs.

With optical scanning of the questionnaire data, processing time and labor have been reduced considerably. If the food items are representative of the dietary patterns of the particular population, the questionnaire is an efficient way of collecting usual dietary intake data in a large cohort study.

Limitations   There are potential weaknesses of this method. Although investigators strive to include 85 to 90 percent of foods consumed by the study population,

For **EACH FOOD GROUP**, fill in the circle ◯ that best describes **HOW OFTEN** you ate those items during the last year. Then fill in the circle ◯ that best describes your **USUAL SERVING SIZE**.

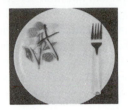
A

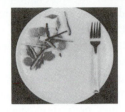
B

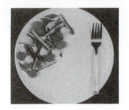
C

RAW OR COOKED VEGETABLES (NOT IN SOUPS OR MIXED DISHES)	AVERAGE USE DURING LAST YEAR								YOUR USUAL SERVING SIZE
	Never or hardly ever	Once a month	2 to 3 times a month	Once a week	2 to 3 times a week	4 to 6 times a week	Once a day	2 or more times a day	
Broccoli (raw or cooked)	◯	◯	◯	◯	◯	◯	◯	◯	**CHOOSE ONE** ◯ Photo A (1/4 cup or less) **OR** ◯ Photo B (about 1/2 cup) **OR** ◯ Photo C (1 cup or more)
Cabbage (such as head, Chinese or Napa cabbage, Brussels sprouts)	◯	◯	◯	◯	◯	◯	◯	◯	**CHOOSE ONE** ◯ Photo A (1/4 cup or less) **OR** ◯ Photo B (about 1/2 cup) **OR** ◯ Photo C (1 cup or more)
Dark Leafy Greens (such as spinach, collard, mustard or turnip greens, bok choy, watercress, chard)	◯	◯	◯	◯	◯	◯	◯	◯	**CHOOSE ONE** ◯ Photo A (1/4 cup or less) **OR** ◯ Photo B (about 1/2 cup) **OR** ◯ Photo C (1 cup or more)
Green Beans or Peas	◯	◯	◯	◯	◯	◯	◯	◯	**CHOOSE ONE** ◯ Photo A (1/4 cup or less) **OR** ◯ Photo B (about 1/2 cup) **OR** ◯ Photo C (1 cup or more)
Other Green Vegetables (such as zucchini, celery, asparagus, green pepper, okra)	◯	◯	◯	◯	◯	◯	◯	◯	**CHOOSE ONE** ◯ Photo A (1/4 cup or less) **OR** ◯ Photo B (about 1/2 cup) **OR** ◯ Photo C (1 cup or more)
Cauliflower	◯	◯	◯	◯	◯	◯	◯	◯	**CHOOSE ONE** ◯ Photo A (1/4 cup or less) **OR** ◯ Photo B (about 1/2 cup) **OR** ◯ Photo C (1 cup or more)
Carrots (raw or cooked)	◯	◯	◯	◯	◯	◯	◯	◯	**CHOOSE ONE** ◯ Photo A (or 4-5 sticks or less) **OR** ◯ Photo B (1/2 cup or 1 med.) **OR** ◯ Photo C (1 cup or more)
Corn (fresh, frozen, or canned)	◯	◯	◯	◯	◯	◯	◯	◯	**CHOOSE ONE** ◯ Photo A (1/4 cup or less) **OR** ◯ Photo B (1/2 cup or 1 cob) **OR** ◯ Photo C (1 cup or more)
Pumpkin or Yellow-Orange Winter Squash	◯	◯	◯	◯	◯	◯	◯	◯	**CHOOSE ONE** ◯ Photo A (1/4 cup or less) **OR** ◯ Photo B (about 1/2 cup) **OR** ◯ Photo C (1 cup or more)
Other Vegetables (such as white or summer squash, beets, eggplant)	◯	◯	◯	◯	◯	◯	◯	◯	**CHOOSE ONE** ◯ Photo A (1/4 cup or less) **OR** ◯ Photo B (about 1/2 cup) **OR** ◯ Photo C (1 cup or more)

FIGURE 3.6   Sample Page from the Diet History Questionnaire for the Multiethnic Cohort Study in Hawaii and Los Angeles
Self-administered diet history questionnaire used with permission of the Epidemiology Program, Cancer Research Center of Hawaii.

the list may be incomplete for some persons. The quantification will not have the details of a food record, and due to the problems of recalling past diet it may not be as accurate as a twenty-four-hour recall. Some recall errors are expected in the estimation of frequencies and serving sizes. This can be partially corrected by conducting a calibration study (similar to a validation study) among a random sample of the ethnic-sex groups in the population. For instance, representative participants can be interviewed at various times in the year to obtain three or four twenty-four-hour recalls. This is generally followed with a second diet history or food frequency questionnaire to ensure a similar reference period. For each subgroup, the twenty-four-hour recall data are used to derive equations that predict the dietary intakes from the second questionnaire. These equations are then applied to the data from the first questionnaire of all persons in that specific subgroup to correct for measurement error.[39]

As noted above, the development of the food list for the questionnaire is critical.[37] Obtaining accurate information on foods eaten alone or in mixtures is a problem. Some questionnaires ask respondents to average all the ways they eat a particular food; for example, a question may pertain to ground beef, such as in fast food hamburgers, tacos, meat balls, and meat loaf. The respondent then needs to summarize the average frequency of eating these items. This method results in a shorter questionnaire, but may be cognitively difficult for many individuals. The alternative method is to ask about various mixed dishes separately, such as stews, stir-fried meats, spaghetti, and so on. These questions are followed with a listing of separate questions that are not part of mixed dishes, such as beef steak or roast, pork chops, and the like. This procedure results in a longer questionnaire but tends to be easier for subjects to complete.

NUTRITIONAL ASSESSMENT COMPARED TO COMMUNITY ASSESSMENT

The goal of comprehensive community nutrition assessment is to develop a picture of the pressing nutrition-related needs in the community along with the discovery of opportunities for intervention. To do this one needs data on the problems and their determinants. Nutrition assessment of the community uses nutritional status measures, drawing from anthropometric, biochemical, clinical, and dietary intake data as well as epidemiological information. However, in addition to these biological determinants of health and nutritional status, a community nutrition assessment includes information about the other determinants of health. As illustrated in figure 3.1, these include the health care system and the availability of appropriate health and nutrition services; lifestyle factors that influence food access, food selection, preparation, and consumption and other behavioral factors related to health risk; and environmental factors including social and physical aspects of the environment. These topics are incorporated into comprehensive community nutrition needs assessment as it relates to planning which is expanded in chapter 13.

NATIONAL NUTRITION SURVEYS AND SURVEILLANCE SYSTEMS

National Nutrition Surveys

As noted earlier, measurement of dietary intake is only one of the components in nutritional status assessment. The assessment includes taking anthropometric body measurements, collecting results of biochemical and laboratory tests, and assessing clinical signs of nutritional deficiencies or excesses as well as estimating dietary intakes. The United States has developed a highly sophisticated system of monitoring the nutritional status of the population, following the comprehensive nutrition surveys which had their beginnings almost thirty years ago.

The Ten-State Nutrition Survey, conducted from 1968 to 1970, was the first survey that evaluated the nutritional status of a large segment of the population.[7] In each of the selected states from various regions of the country, families with incomes below the poverty level of 1960 were randomly selected to participate in the survey. The objectives were to identify the prevalence and location of serious hunger, malnutrition, and related health problems in low-income populations. Nutritional status was assessed on the basis of dietary intakes, dental examinations, clinical and anthropometric examinations, biochemical assessment, and demographic information among all family members. This survey documented a high prevalence of undernutrition and malnutrition among the 24,000 families surveyed.

Also, during the 1960s, George Owen, a pediatrician and researcher, conducted the Preschool Nutrition Survey among 3,400 children one to six years of age in thirty-six states and the District of Columbia.[30] Clinical and dental examinations, anthropometric and laboratory measurements, and dietary intake data were obtained. Similar to the Ten-State Survey, this study demonstrated that poor diet was associated with clinical signs of malnutrition, poor health, and low economic status and revealed that these conditions were not rare in the United States.

The importance of a comprehensive assessment of nutritional status of the U.S. population was documented at the 1969 White House Conference on Food, Nutrition, and Health. This was followed by the U.S. Department of Health and Human Services' inclusion of nutritional status assessments into its ongoing Health Examination Survey.[7] Three national Health and Nutrition Examination Surveys have been conducted (NHANES I in 1971 to 1975, NHANES II in 1976 to 1980, and NHANES III in 1988 to 1991),[23,27,28] along with a special survey of Hispanic Americans (HHANES in 1982 to 1984).[24] The HHANES survey included representative samples of Mexican-Americans, Cubans, and Puerto Ricans in the United States. The NHANES samples were randomly selected from the fifty states or the forty-eight conterminous states and included information on health histories; sociodemographic characteristics; dietary intakes based on a twenty-four-hour recall and food frequency; biochemical levels; and clinical, anthropometric, and dental examinations.[41]

Since 1936, the USDA has conducted periodic Household Food Consumption Surveys on a stratified probability sample of the forty-eight conterminous states.[41] Information was obtained from the person in the household who was most responsible for food purchasing and preparation about the quantity, source, and cost of food used during the previous seven days. Since 1965, information has also been collected from individual household members about their food intakes. The interviewer obtains a twenty-four-hour recall and instructs the individual on measuring and recording their food intakes for the following two days. The major aim of these individual intake surveys has been to describe food consumption behavior and assess the adequacy of food and nutrient intakes and to establish national nutrition policies related to food production, marketing, food safety, food assistance, and nutrition education.

During the 1980s, food and nutrition professionals and Congress recognized that the Food Consumption Surveys should be conducted more frequently due to large changes in food availability and in eating behavior within ten-year periods. Consequently, smaller surveys known as the Continuing Survey of Food Intakes by Individuals (CSFII) have been conducted on a continual basis since 1985.[5,41] The survey samples represent only selected segments of the population. For example, during 1985 to 1986 and 1989 to 1991, data were obtained from women nineteen to fifty years old and their children one to five years old. Representative samples of these groups from the general population and from low-income individuals were included, and twenty-four-hour recalls were obtained every two months during the year from each person. A one-day recall was also obtained from a national sample of nineteen- to fifty-year-old men in 1985. In addition, from 1989 to 1996, twenty-four-hour dietary recalls and two-day diaries have been collected from all household members in about 1,500 households from the general population and about 750 low-income households within the forty-eight conterminous states. Beginning in 1989 the CSFII has included all persons in the household, including infants. These USDA surveys have been useful for determining the effects of family income and other demographic characteristics on food expenditures, estimating the allowances for food stamps to needy families, and following the trends in Americans' diets by region of the country, race, and income.

National Surveillance Systems

The national surveillance systems, which are coordinated by the Centers for Disease Control and Prevention (CDC), are statistical service programs that provide data to state health agencies concerning low-income populations of children and pregnant women who obtain services in publicly funded food assistance, nutrition, and health programs.[5,41] Nutrition surveillance data are analyzed by the CDC and returned to the states periodically for their use in making programmatic decisions. The Pediatric Nutrition Surveillance System (PedNSS) began in 1974 and is active in more than forty states, territories, and Indian tribes. Simple indicators of nutritional status, such as short stature, underweight, overweight, anemia, and low birthweight, are monitored, compared with data from reference populations to estimate prevalence rates, and returned to the states for use in program planning.

The Pregnancy Nutrition Surveillance System (PNSS) began in 1979.[5,41] Using clinic information, the PNSS monitors pregravid underweight and overweight, prenatal weight gain, and anemia. Since 1987, self-reported data on smoking and alcohol consumption have been used to examine the dose effect of these practices on infants' birthweights.

Although these surveillance statistics are valuable for program planning among these particular populations, it is important to consider their limitations as well.[5] These populations are self-selected, based on their participation in existing federal programs, and are not representative of the nutritional status of all children and pregnant women in the community. Participants differ in socioeconomic status, nutrition or health risk and are generally overrepresented by racial or ethnic minority groups as compared with the general population. Further information on the use of these data for program planning is available from the Nutrition Division of the Centers for Disease Control and Prevention, HHS, Atlanta, Georgia.

A third surveillance activity useful for the nutrition professional is the Behavioral Risk Factor Surveillance System (BRFSS).[5,41] The objectives of this system are to monitor personal risk factors for the ten leading causes of premature death in the United States. The CDC assists participating states in the use of random-digit dialing telephone methods. In each household, one adult, aged eighteen years or older, is selected randomly for the telephone interview. A core questionnaire is administered with information on such items as alcohol consumption, cigarette smoking, hypertension, exercise, dietary fat intake, fruit and vegetable consumption, and self-reported weight and height. Participating states use results from the BRFSS to plan public education and intervention programs on nutrition and health.

National Nutrition Monitoring

During the 1980s, coordination of the nationwide USDA and HHS surveys and surveillance activities increased, and in 1990, Congress passed the **National Nutrition Monitoring** and Related Research Act (NNMRR). The act directed the HHS and USDA to share responsibility for implementing the program and to contract with the National Academy of Sciences (NAS) or the Federation of American Societies for Experimental Biology (FASEB) to interpret the data and publish a report on the dietary, nutritional, and health-related status of the American people at appropriate intervals.

The major components of the **National Nutrition Monitoring** and Related Research Program are:

  Nutritional status and nutrition-related health measurements

  Food and nutrient consumption

  Knowledge, attitudes, and behavior assessments

  Food composition and nutrient databases

  Food supply determinations

These five components are illustrated in figure 3.7, which depicts the interrelationships between food and

health.[5] Descriptions of studies, surveys, and databases used in each component of the NNMRRP are summarized in table 3.5. The national surveys and surveillance systems participating in the **national nutrition monitoring** system, such as NHANES III and CSFII, target the noninstitutionalized population residing in households in the entire United States or in the forty-eight conterminous states. A fixed address for mailings or personal interviews is required for inclusion. Thus, persons with no fixed address, such as migrants, military personnel living on U.S. bases, and American Indians living on reservations are often not included. Analysis of nutritional data at the national level generally includes non-Hispanic Whites, non-Hispanic Blacks, and Hispanics. Although ethnic subgroups such as Asian-Americans and Pacific Islanders are included in national surveys and surveillance systems, the numbers of individuals in these subgroups are usually insufficient for analysis by subgroup at the national level. However, the nutrition professional working in a community with ethnic subgroups such as these should include random samples in nutritional status surveys.

The *Third Report on Nutrition Monitoring in the United States,* prepared by FASEB, was published in 1995.[5] The findings and implications are particularly useful for nutrition professionals. They provide clues to problems and risk factors at the national level and serve as references for planning the nutritional status components to be included in the community assessment as well as for comparing community findings on nutritional status with national reference values or norms.

Limitations of the National Monitoring System and Findings

The epidemiologic data in the Third Report are cross-sectional, and it is likely that the participants selected for each cycle will not be the same persons.[5] Although these data provide accurate information about a target population at a particular point in time, caution is needed in inferring changes of nutritional status over time.

Variations in nutritional status methods among the various reported surveys limit the ability to make direct comparisons of the findings. Differences due to sampling strategies, interviewing methods, dietary questionnaires, and analytical laboratory methods reduce the comparability. As noted previously, the target populations in the pregnancy and pediatric nutritional surveillance systems represent high-risk groups and are not useful for charac-

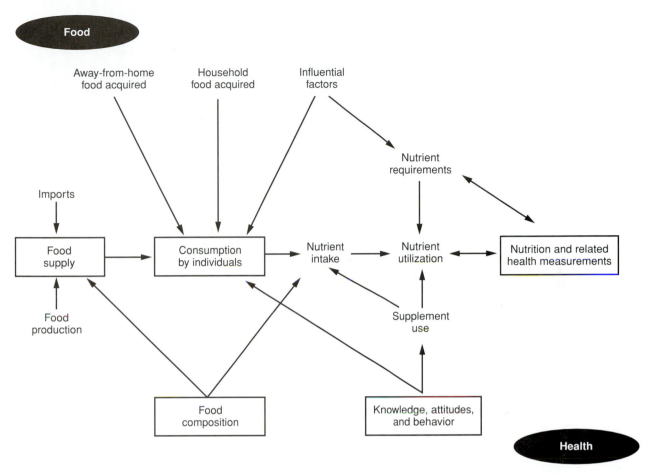

FIGURE 3.7   Relationship of Food to Health, Highlighting the Five Major Components of the National Nutrition Monitoring and Related Research Program
(*Source:* From Third Report on Nutrition Monitoring in the United States, Vol. 1, 1995.)

terizing the status of all pregnant women, infants, and children. However, these data are extremely helpful for identifying nutrition-related risk factors, such as anemia, in these populations participating in government-sponsored programs. The nutrition professional needs to understand the various biochemical methods used for different surveys to determine their comparability. For instance, prevalence values for some health risks, such as iron-deficiency anemia, based on hemoglobin and hematocrit data collected in the pregnancy and pediatric surveillance systems differ from prevalence values of iron-deficiency anemia in NHANES, which are based on multiple measures of iron status. Consequently, the estimates of iron-deficiency anemia are likely to differ due to differences in definition of anemia, methodological differences, and population differences.

Furthermore, as stated in the report, these data "may be used to provide assessments of dietary status, nutritional status, and nutrition-related health status of *populations* and of the roles of factors associated with these conditions at the points in time when the data were collected. But, the dietary, nutritional, and nutrition-related health status of *individuals* cannot be determined from data collected for nutrition monitoring purposes."[5] However, individual assessment is covered in the life cycle chapters of Section II of this text.

There is an important caveat concerning the nutrient intakes in the National Nutrition Monitoring report. The estimated nutrient intakes described in this report represent only partial estimates because they do not include nutrient intakes from dietary supplements, drinking water, discretionary salt use, or medications.[5] There

Sources of Data from the Five Component Areas of NNMRRP Considered in the *Third Report on Nutrition Monitoring*

Component area and survey or study	Sponsoring[1] agency (department)	Date	Population	Data collected
1. Nutritional status and nutrition-related health measurements				
Third National Health and Nutrition Examination Survey (NHANES III)	NCHS, CDC (HHS)	1988–1991	Civilian, noninstitutionalized population two months of age and older; oversampling of non-Hispanic Blacks and Mexican Americans, children < six years of age, and adults aged ≥ sixty years	Dietary intake (twenty-four-hour recall and food frequency), socioeconomic and demographic data, biochemical analyses of blood and urine, physical examination, body measurements, blood pressure, bone densitometry, dietary and health behaviors, health conditions; two additional twenty-four-hour recalls for participants ≥ fifty years of age
Hispanic Health and Nutrition Examination demographic Survey (HHANES)	NCHS (HHS)	1982–1984	Civilian, noninstitutionalized Mexican Americans in five Southwestern States, Cuban Americans in Dade County, Florida, and Puerto Ricans in metropolitan New York City; six months to seventy-four years of age	Dietary intake (twenty-four-hour recall and food frequency), socioeconomic and demographic data, dietary and health behaviors, biochemical analysis of blood and urine, physical examination, body measurements, health conditions
Pregnancy Nutrition Surveillance System (PNSS)	NCCDPHP, CDC (HHS)	1992	Convenience population of low-income, high-risk pregnant women	Demographic data, pregravid-weight, maternal weight gain during pregnancy, anemia (hemoglobin, hematocrit), behavioral risk factors (smoking and drinking), birthweight, breast-feeding and formula-feeding
Pediatric Nutrition Surveillance System (PedNSS)	NCCDPHP CDC (HHS)	1973–1992	Low-income, high-risk children, birth to seventeen years of age, with emphasis on birth to five years of age	Demographic data, anthropometry (height and weight), birthweight, hematology (hemoglobin, hematocrit), breast-feeding
Maternal Longitudinal Followup to the 1988 National Maternal and Infant Health Survey (NMIHS)	NCHS, CDC (HHS)	1991	Mothers of three-year-olds who participated in the 1988 NMIHS, pediatricians, and hospitals	Use of vitamin and mineral supplements, WIC participation, and growth and hematological measurements from birth to three years
2. Food and nutrient consumption				
Continuing Survey of Food Intakes by Individuals (CSFII)	HNIS (USDA)	1989–1991	Individuals in households in the forty-eight conterminous states; survey composed of two samples: households with incomes at any level (basic sample) and households with incomes ≤ 130% of the poverty thresholds	One-day and three-day food and nutrient intakes by individuals of all ages, names and times of eating occasions, and sources of food eaten away from home; data for three consecutive days using a one-day recall and two-day record; intakes available for twenty-eight nutrients and food components

Survey	Agency	Year	Population	Content
Continuing Survey of Food Intakes by Individuals (CSFII)	HNIS (USDA)	1985–1986	Individuals in households in the forty-eight conterminous states; survey composed of two samples: households with incomes at any level and households with incomes ≤ 130% of the poverty threshold, including in 1985, women nineteen to fifty years of age and their children one to five years and men nineteen to fifty years of age, and in 1986, women nineteen to fifty years of age and their children one to five years	Six one-day food and nutrient intakes by individuals; names and times of eating occasions, and sources of food obtained and eaten away from home; data collected at about two-month intervals over a one-year period
Nationwide Food Consumption Survey (NCFS)	HNIS (USDA)	1987–1988	Households in the forty-eight conterminous states and individuals residing in those households; survey composed of two samples: a basic sample of all households and a low-income sample of households with income ≤ 130% of the poverty threshold	For households: quantity and money value and nutritive value of food used; for individuals: one-day and three-day food and nutrient intakes by individuals of all ages, names and times of eating occasions, and sources of food obtained and eaten away from home; data collected over three consecutive days using a one-day recall and a two-day record; intakes of twenty-eight nutrients and food components
National Health Interview Survey on Vitamin and Mineral Supplements	NCHS and FDA (HHS)	1986	Civilian, noninstitutionalized children two to six years of age and adults eighteen years of age and older	Prevalence of use; sociodemographic characteristics of users; intakes of twenty-four nutrients from supplements; potency, form, and units used to declare potency; specific chemical compounds for mineral supplements; number of supplements taken, duration of use, and whether supplement was prescribed
Total Diet Study (TDS)	FDA (HHS)	1982–1989	NA	Chemical analysis of nutrients and contaminants in U.S. food supply; food composition data merged with food consumption data to estimate daily intake of nutrients and contamination

3. Knowledge, attitudes, and behavior assessments

Survey	Agency	Year	Population	Content
Behavioral Risk Factor Surveillance System (BRFSS)	NCCDPHP CDC (HHS)	1992	Adults eighteen years of age and older in households with telephones in participating states	Demographic data; height, weight, smoking, alcohol use, weight-control practices, diabetes, preventable health problems, mammography, pregnancy, cholesterol-screening, modified food frequencies for fat, fruit, and vegetable consumption by telephone interview
Diet and Health Knowledge Survey (DHKS)	HNIS (USDA)	1989–1991	Main meal planner and preparer in households in the forty-eight conterminous states who participated in CSFII 1989–1991	Self-perceptions of relative intake levels, awareness of diet-health relationships, use of food labels, perceived importance of following dietary guidance for specific food components, beliefs about food safety, and knowledge about food sources of nutrients: these variables can be linked to individuals' food and nutrient intakes from CSFII 1989–1991

continued

TABLE 3.5—CONTINUED

Component area and survey or study	Sponsoring[1] agency (department)	Date	Population	Data collected
4. Food composition and nutrient data bases				
National Nutrient Data Bank	ARS (USDA)	NA	NA	Nutrient content of foods used in USDA Survey Nutrient Data Base for analysis of national dietary intake surveys. Also available in published tables of food composition and as computerized data bases. Periodic updates available on Nutrient Data Bank Electronic Bulletin Board.
USDA Nutrient Data Base for Standard Reference	ARS (USDA)	NA	NA	A computer file for *Agricultural Handbook* No. 8 (USDA, 1992) produced from National Data Bank and main source for USDA Survey Nutrient Data Base. Includes data on food energy, 28 food components and 18 amino acids for 5,200 food items.
USDA Survey Nutrient Data Base	ARS (USDA)	NA	NA	The data base is used for analysis of nationwide dietary intake surveys. It is updated continuously and includes data on food energy and 28 food components for >7,100 food items. The data base used for CSFII 1989–91 and NHANES III 1988–91 contained approximately 6,700 items.
Food Label and Package Survey (FLAPS)	FDA (HHS)	Biannually 1977–90	NA	Use of nutrition labeling; declaration of selected nutrients and ingredients; nutrition claims; other label statements and descriptors; nutrient analysis of representative sample of packaged foods.
5. Food-supply determinations				
U.S. Food Supply Series	CNPP and ERS (USDA)	1970–92	U.S. total population	Quantities of foods available for consumption on a per capita basis; quantities of food energy, nutrients, and food components provided by these foods (calculated).

[1]Sponsoring agency and department: NCHS, National Center for Health Statistics; CDC, Centers for Disease Control and Prevention; HHS, Department of Health and Human Services; NCCD-PHP, National Center for Chronic Disease Prevention and Health Promotion; HNIS, Human Nutrition Information Service; USDA, U.S. Department of Agriculture; FDA, Food and Drug Administration; ARS, Agricultural Research Service; CNPP, Center for Nutrition Policy and Promotion; ERS, Economic Research Service.
Source: Federation of American Societies for Experimental Biology, Life Sciences Research Office: Third report on nutrition monitoring in the United States, vols. 1 and 2, Washington, DC, 1995, U.S. Government Printing Office.

also may have been some underreporting by the participants. Although estimates of energy and food and nutrient intakes may appear less than recommended levels, these estimates do serve an important role in assessing the dietary consumption and nutrition-related status among representative population groups.

COLLECTING AND INTERPRETING NUTRITION ASSESSMENT DATA

Community nutrition professionals gather and use information specific to the community or selected populations within the community. They plan and conduct nutrition surveys and assessments. Relevant data are also abstracted from reports and files of nutrition monitoring and surveillance systems and studies conducted by others on similar population groups. Together this range of data helps to build a more complete picture of nutrition-related problems and their determinants. The data are summarized and used as a benchmark to monitor trends in nutrition-related problems over time and to measure progress toward goals for improvement of nutritional status or reduction of risk factors.

IMPLICATIONS FOR COMMUNITY NUTRITION PROFESSIONALS

The community nutrition professional must be informed about the distribution and determinants of nutrition-related health problems in his or her country, state, and community. This is the knowledge base for decision making about community nutrition programs and services. Nutrition assessment data guide program development and serve as benchmarks for evaluating the impact of programs and services. The use of epidemiologic methods for identifying nutrition-related health problems of a particular population was emphasized in this chapter. However, in addition to epidemiologic methods, nutrition professionals also need to use methods of behavioral scientists and market researchers to diagnose the community, its needs, and acceptable ways to intervene. Comprehensive community nutrition assessment incorporates multiple methods to identify problem areas. These topics are addressed in later chapters.

This chapter points out the rigors of high-quality assessment methods that produce valid and reproducible data. Since crucial decisions are based on assessment data, the community nutrition professional must know which methods are appropriate for which purposes and be able to conduct nutrition assessments with care and skill.

COMMUNITY NUTRITION PROFESSIONALS IN ACTION

- Request a report of "vital health statistics" from a local or state health department. Which rates listed in table 3.1 are included in the report? What are the top causes of death for the population? Which causes of death could be related to dietary factors?
- The local Head Start program is required to complete a nutrition assessment of each child in the fall. The director contacts you for guidance on what should be included. Identify one method for each of the "ABC's of nutrition assessment" that could be used with young children in the Head Start setting.
- Use two or more methods of dietary assessment to assess your dietary intake. Compare and contrast the ease of use and your findings from the methods.
- Contact nutrition professionals in a number of settings (i.e., prenatal clinic, WIC program, Meals on Wheels program, university research program) and collect tools and procedures used for dietary assessment. What are the strengths and weaknesses of the tools and methods being used for specific purposes in different population groups?
- Review the range of nutrition surveys and studies conducted by the federal government (see table 3.5). Discuss the kind of information produced by each study or survey. What value does this information have to you as a community nutrition professional? Who else would find this information useful?
- Do you think tracking the health, nutritional status, behavior, food consumption, and such information concerning Americans is an appropriate role for the federal government? Why or why not?

GOING ONE STEP FURTHER

- Design a nutrition survey to be conducted in a specific population group. Provide a rationale for the methods and tools selected. Identify steps that must be taken to assure the data collected are valid and reproducible.
- Review the scientific literature for a pressing health problem in the community. Identify the chain of causes (risk factors and determinants) that lead to the health problem. Use the Bradford Hill criteria to critique the level of confidence one should have in concluding a cause-and-effect relationship for nutrition factors identified. According to the literature, what points in the chain of causes may be modifiable with a known intervention?

• Review one of the latest reports from surveys and studies under the jurisdiction of the National Nutrition Monitoring and Related Research Program (see table 3.5). What conclusion can be drawn about the current nutritional well-being of the American population based on this report?

REFERENCES

1. Beal VA: The nutritional history in longitudinal research, *J Am Diet Assoc* 51:426, 1967.
2. Burke BS: The dietary history as a tool in research, *J Am Diet Assoc* 23:1041, 1947.
3. Centers for Disease Control and Prevention (CDC): *CDC Wonder/PC,* Atlanta, Department of Health and Human Services, CDC.
4. Department of Health and Human Services, Public Health Service, and U.S. Department of Agriculture, Food and Consumer Services: *Nutrition monitoring in the United States,* DHHS Pub (PHS) 89–1255, Washington, DC, 1989, U.S. Government Printing Office.
5. Federation of American Societies for Experimental Biology, Life Sciences Research Office: *Third report on nutrition monitoring in the United States,* vols. 1 and 2, Washington, DC, 1995, U.S. Government Printing Office.
6. Food and Agriculture Organization of the United Nations: *Food balance sheets, 1975–77 average,* Rome, 1980, FAO.
7. Frankle RT, Owen AY: *Nutrition in the community. The art of delivering services,* St. Louis, 1978, Mosby.
8. Gersovitz M, Madden JP, Smickilas-Wright H: Validity of the 24-hr dietary recall and seven-day record for group comparisons, *J Am Diet Assoc* 73:48, 1978.
9. Giovannucci E, Rimm EB, Stampfer MJ, and others: Intake of fat, meat and fiber in relation to colon cancer risk in men, *Cancer Res* 54:2390, 1994.
10. Hankin J: *Dietary intake methodology.* In Monsen ER, editor: *Research: successful approaches,* Chicago, 1991, American Dietetic Association.
11. Hankin J, Wilkens LR: Development and validation of dietary methods for culturally diverse populations, *Am J Clin Nutr* 59(Suppl):198S, 1994.
12. Hankin JH: Role of nutrition in women's health: diet and breast cancer, *J Am Diet Assoc* 93:994, 1993.
13. Hankin JH, Reeds S, Labarthe S, Nichaman M, and others: A survey of dietary and disease patterns among Micronesians, *Am J Clin Nutr* 23:346, 1970.
14. Hankin JH, Wilkins LR, Kolonel LN, Yoshizawa CN: Validation of a quantitative diet history method in Hawaii, *Am J Epidemiol* 133:616, 1991.
15. Hill AB: The environment and disease: association or causation? *Proc R Soc Med* 58:295, 1965.
16. Hunter DJ, Willett WC: Nutrition and breast cancer, *Cancer Causes Control* 7:56, 1996.
17. Kolonel LN: Nutrition and prostate cancer, *Cancer Causes Control* 7:83, 1996.
18. Kolonel LN, Hankin JH, Nomura AMY, Chu SY: Dietary fat intake and cancer incidence among five ethnic groups in Hawaii, *Cancer Res* 41:3727, 1981.
19. Le Marchand L, Hankin JH, Carter FS, Essling C, and others: A pilot study on the use of plasma carotenoids and ascorbic acid as markers of compliance to a high fruit and vegetable dietary intervention, *Cancer Epidemiol Biomarkers Prev* 3:245, 1994.
20. Le Marchand L, Yoshizawa CN, Kolonel LN, Hankin JH, and others: Vegetable consumption and lung cancer risk: a population-based case-control study in Hawaii, *J Natl Cancer Inst* 81:1158, 1989.
21. Madden JP, Goodman SJ, Guthrie HA: Validity of the 24-hr recall, *J Am Diet Assoc* 68:143, 1976.
22. Mann GV, Pearson G, Gordon T, and others: Diet and cardiovascular disease in the Framingham study. I. Measurement of dietary intake, *Am J Clin Nutr* 11:200, 1962.
23. National Center for Health Statistics (NCHS): *First National Health and Nutrition Examination Survey (NHANES I), 1971–1974,* Hyattsville, MD, 1976, Department of Health and Human Services, NCHS.
24. National Center for Health Statistics (NCHS): *Hispanic Health and Nutrition Examination Survey (HHANES), 1982–1984,* Hyattsville, MD, 1987, Department of Health and Human Services, NCHS.
25. National Center for Health Statistics: *NHANES III anthropometric procedures video,* Hyattsville, MD, 1996, Department of Health and Human Services, NCHS.
26. National Center for Health Statistics (NCHS): *Plan and operation of the Third National Health and Nutrition Examination Survey, 1988–1994. Vital and health statistics series 1, No. 32,* Hyattsville, MD, 1994, Department of Health and Human Services, NCHS.
27. National Center for Health Statistics (NCHS): *Second National Health and Nutrition Examination Survey (NHANES II), 1976–1980,* Hyattsville, MD, 1982, Department of Health and Human Services, NCHS.
28. National Center for Health Statistics (NCHS): *Third National Health and Nutrition Examination Survey (NHANES III), 1988–1991,* Hyattsville, MD, 1994, Department of Health and Human Services, NCHS.
29. National Research Council (U.S.), Committee on Dietary Allowances: *Recommended dietary allowances,* ed 10, Washington, DC, 1989, National Academy Press.
30. Owen GM, Kram KM, Garry PJ, and others: A study of nutritional status of preschool children in the United States, 1968–1970, *Pediatrics* 53(Suppl):597, 1974.
31. Prentice RL, Kakar F, Hursting S, and others: Aspects of the rationale for the women's health trial, *J Natl Cancer Inst* 80:802, 1988.
32. Rothman KJ: *Modern epidemiology,* Boston, 1986, Little, Brown & Company.

33. Sherry B: *Descriptive epidemiologic research.* In Monsen ER, editor: *Research: successful approaches,* Chicago, 1991, American Dietetic Association.

34. Sherry, B: *Epidemiologic analytical research.* In Monsen ER, editor: *Research: successful approaches,* Chicago, 1991, American Dietetic Association.

35. Tinker LP, Burrows ER, Henry H, Patterson RE, and others: The *Women's health initiative: overview of the nutrition components.* In Krummel DA, Kris-Etherton PM, editors: *Nutrition in women's health,* Gaithersberg, MD, 1996, Aspen.

36. Tillotson JL, Kato H, Nichaman MZ, and others: Epidemiologic studies of CHD and stroke in Japanese men living in Japan, Hawaii, and California: methodology for comparison of diet, *Am J Clin Nutr* 26:177, 1973.

37. Thompson FE, Byers T: *Dietary assessment resource manual, J Nutr* 124(Suppl):2245S, 1994.

38. Wardlaw GM, Insel PM: *Perspectives in nutrition,* ed 3, St. Louis, 1996, Mosby.

39. Willett W: *Nutritional epidemiology,* New York, 1990, Oxford University Press.

40. Willett WC, Sampson I, Stampfer MJ, and others: Reproducibility and validity of a semiquantitative food frequency questionnaire, *Am J Epidemiol* 122:51, 1985.

41. Woteki CD, Wong FL: *Interpretation and utilization of data from the National Nutrition Monitoring System.* In Monsen ER, editor: *Research: successful approaches,* Chicago, 1991, American Dietetic Association.

CASE STUDY

NUTRITION ASSESSMENT FOR PRIMARY CANCER PREVENTION

DESCRIPTION

This case presents a realistic situation faced by many community nutrition professionals—deciding what to do and how to do it. The newly employed nutrition professional systematically applies needs assessment methods and tools to develop an understanding of the problem and its determinants as well as opportunities for addressing the problem. In this situation, the population is persons living in a city who may be at risk of cancer. The case also illustrates how a voluntary health agency (American Cancer Society is one of dozens of such agencies) directs resources to identify problems and work with community groups to develop and evaluate intervention strategies to reduce risk factors or determinants related to the problem.

TEACHING/LEARNING OBJECTIVES

By reading the case study and discussing the questions, students should gain an understanding of how assessment methods are selected and applied in real community situations. Important lessons of this case study include:

- A nutrition professional accesses information from many sources to determine needs and identify opportunities for intervention.

- Existing data play a significant role in prioritizing problems.
- Program planning decisions follow from the needs assessment information.
- Nutrition assessment methodologies are also used to evaluate the progress and success of intervention programs.

Students should read the case and answer the questions as a homework assignment. Then during class, divide into groups to discuss the questions.

CASE STUDY

You are the first nutrition professional employed by the American Cancer Society affiliate in a large metropolitan city of California and have been requested to develop and implement an educational program concerning primary prevention of cancer among potential high-risk population groups. You begin by examining a very important piece of information—the incidence and distribution of various cancers in the state, which are usually available from the Cancer Registry in the city or state or the local Cancer Society. It is clear that breast cancer is the leading cancer among women, and prostate cancer is the leading cancer among men. Breast cancer is highest among the Caucasian women followed by the African-American women, and then the Asian women; whereas the African-American men have the highest prostate cancer rates, followed by the Caucasian men, with the Asian men having the lowest rates. Cancer is more prevalent in the lower socioeconomic status groups. The incidence rates of both of these cancers are increasing about 1 percent per year. Next, you review the census data to determine the demographic profile of the state, paying attention to age, ethnicity, income, and other factors associated with cancer risk.

To have comparative data on other populations, you utilize a relatively new data source, namely, the Centers for Disease Control and Prevention (CDC) WONDER/PC.[3] This is an electronic link, allowing health professionals to access, analyze, and exchange health information. It is a software program for microcomputers that is available free of charge. By request, you can quickly obtain information on cancer incidence rates in various areas. You may also speak to persons at the CDC regarding nutrition intervention programs conducted in various communities that are aimed at primary prevention of cancer in children as well as adults. In fact, you are able to obtain e-mail addresses of nutrition professionals who may assist you in program planning at the community level.

It is also helpful to meet with public health nutritionists at local and state health departments and other voluntary health agencies to learn about their recent nutrition education programs and their involvement in cancer prevention.

You do a literature search and read published scientific articles and reports of intervention studies to understand the risk factors for and antecedents of breast and prostate cancer. You find that epidemiological studies from different countries suggest a positive association between prostate cancer and high fat intake; but the relationship with fat intake is inconclusive for breast cancer. Other possible risk factors for breast cancer include alcohol intake, excess weight, and level of exercise. Recent studies suggest that isoflavones, a component of soy beans and products derived from them, explain the lower the incidence of breast and prostate cancer among Asian women and Asian men, respectively. Intervention studies are emphasizing a plant-based diet, including five to nine servings of fruit and vegetables per day.

After considering all this information, you propose to conduct a nutrition education and physical activity intervention trial among preadolescent girls and boys

(aged ten to eleven years). Epidemiologists have suggested that this age period may be crucial for the development of breast cancer; and it is an age where both boys and girls are learning to make more independent decisions about food and activity. Furthermore, it is known that lifestyle habits are formed during the preadolescent and adolescent years. Thus you decide to include both sexes in this primary prevention program.

This proposal is discussed with the Cancer Society professionals who concur with your suggestion and arrange meetings with public and private school administrators in the city. Since this is a "first" for this community, the educational leaders suggest that a pilot study be conducted in three schools: a private school in a high-socioeconomic area, a public school in another high-socioeconomic area, and a public school in a relatively low-socioeconomic area. Working with the epidemiologist of the public health agency, you randomly select three schools meeting these criteria. Contacts are made with the administrative directors and the relevant teachers in each school; subsequently these core individuals will be asked to participate in the development and demonstration of the intervention programs.

Your plan is to select two to three classrooms at each school and to involve both girls and boys in the program. You have several aims: (1) to decrease total fat intake, (2) to increase physical activity among all students, and (3) to promote normal body weight and growth while preventing obesity. Because of your interest in promoting good lifestyle dietary practices, you also will promote increased vegetables, fruits, and grains in the diet, which is also a goal of the American Cancer Society and public health officials.

To measure the success of the program, you plan to do nutritional assessments at the beginning of the program and at regular intervals throughout the pilot study. The nutritional assessments will include: weight and height measurements, dietary recalls, physical activity diaries (checked by the teacher), health histories (completed by the school nurse and possibly the parent), and food frequency questionnaires completed by the mothers. Additional clinical or biochemical measurements are unnecessary for this particular intervention program. The assessments will be repeated at six-month intervals and monitored to ensure that the program is proceeding satisfactorily. Prior to the beginning of the study, meetings will be arranged with the parents and with the school food service personnel to ensure that the school lunch menus and the meals consumed at home are planned to meet the goals of the program. Consequently, this particular program should have beneficial effects for other students at these schools as well as family members. You plan to use educational materials available from the American Cancer Society, the National Cancer Institute, and the Department of Health and to work with the classroom teachers, school nurses, and physical education teachers in implementing the program. The project is expected to continue among the same children for a minimum of three years.

For the evaluation, you may wish to consult with an epidemiologist or a biostatistician to determine differences by school, sex, ethnicity, and socioeconomic status along with other parameters that may explain variations in the findings. A report of your nutrition intervention program should be prepared, and the findings presented to the Cancer Society, public health agency, schools, and parent groups. If the results of this intervention program are successful, the program may be modified and expanded to other schools in the city and state.

CASE STUDY QUESTIONS

1. What *community* is the setting for the project?
2. What is/are the *health problem* or problems to be reduced?
3. What are the *causes/risk factors/determinants* for the health problem?
4. What *assessment methods and tools* were used to understand the problem and opportunities for addressing the problem?
5. Who is the *target audience* for intervention?
6. What are the known *characteristics* of the target audience? Be clear about the "facts" versus assumptions. Consider what else you may need to know about the target audience and its needs, wants, attributes, and behaviors before you can design a program that can achieve the stated aims of the program.
7. What *nutrition assessment and dietary methods* will you use to measure the success of the program? What issues should you be concerned with when using these methods?

CHAPTER FOUR

THE SEAMLESS HEALTH CARE SYSTEM
IDEAL OR REALITY?

*Only 10% of the morbidity of any population can be traced to
the presence or absence of a medical care system. 90% of
morbidity is affected by nutrition, sanitation, lifestyle, education
and income. Unless the 10% cooperates with the 90%, we will
not improve the health status of communities.*

—LELAND KAISER

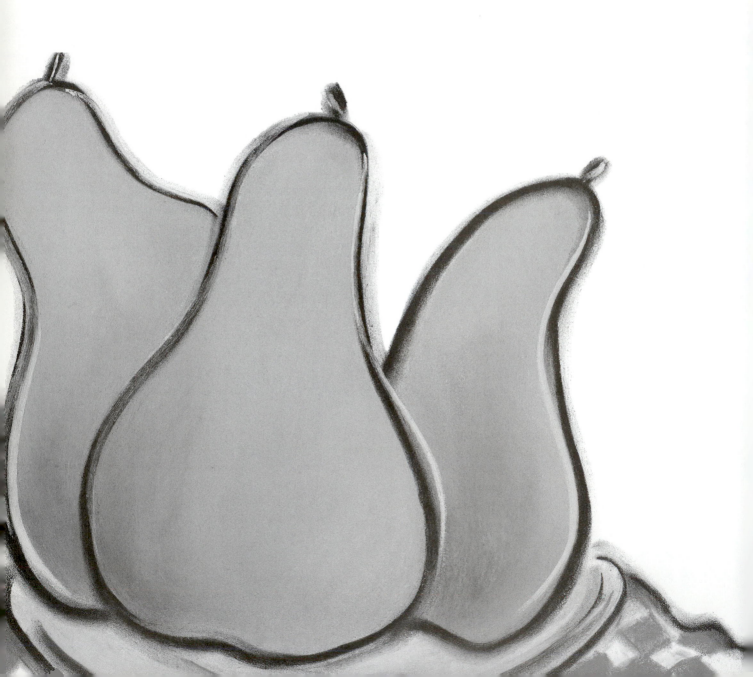

Core Concepts

Driven by cost, access, and quality concerns, health care is undergoing a major paradigm shift—from a treatment-oriented, biotechnological medical model to a managed health care system. The emerging system emphasizes prevention and cost-effective disease management in a seamless, coordinated, integrated network of providers in a wide range of settings. Within this system the role of public health will be to monitor the health of the population and assure health services are available to meet the needs of special populations. Because nutrition screening, assessment, intervention, and follow-up are integral to clinical preventive services and disease management, nutrition is an essential service in all health settings. Practice guidelines, outcomes assessment, and performance improvement will be used extensively by community nutrition professionals in managed care systems.

Objectives

When you finish chapter four, you should be able to:

~ Discuss critically the forces leading to reform of the health care system.

~ Contrast the traditional medical system with the emerging managed health care system.

~ Recognize terminology and acronyms related to the organization and financing of health care in the United States.

~ Diagram the network of health care settings in an integrated delivery system.

~ Identify government agencies responsible for delivery of health services to vulnerable population groups.

~ Explain the role of public health in the emerging managed health care system.

~ Describe the role of nutrition services in clinical prevention services and disease management.

Key Words

Word	Page Mentioned
Medicare	88
Medicaid	88
Access	88
Fee-for-service	88
Appropriate care	89
Managed care	90
AHCPR	90
Indemnity	90
Health maintenance organization	90
Integrated delivery systems	93
Primary care	93
Capitation	93
Vulnerable populations	98
CDC	101
HCFA	101
Report cards	102
Medical nutrition therapy	102
Outcomes assessment	103
Practice guidelines	103

FORCES DRIVING HEALTH CARE REFORM: COST, ACCESS, AND QUALITY

Almost a decade ago in "The Public's Health Care Paradigm is Shifting," Freymann said that Americans are undergoing a paradigm shift in attitudes and beliefs about health care and that the health care system itself is undergoing a transition from centralized biomedical and technologic care to a more decentralized ecological system of care.[16] Under the biomedical model, the health care delivery system has placed greater emphasis on disease treatment in specialty centers than on community-based primary and preventive health care. The disease-oriented system is no longer viewed by policy makers and the American public as the ideal model for organizing and providing health care services.

In contrast, public policy makers and providers are beginning to see the benefits of a more ecological model that views health as a natural state that is affected by several interrelated factors: (1) access to health care services, (2) human biology, (3) social and physical environments, and (4) personal lifestyle and behavior,[12] as illustrated in the foundation of figure 4.1, in this chapter and in every chapter.

The catalyst behind this paradigm shift is dissatisfaction with the traditional health care system and its inherent problems of cost, access to care, and quality. Another aspect of this shift is the changing patterns of disease and the advent of "new morbidities," such as chronic diseases, violence, and HIV/AIDS.

Health Care Costs

National health care expenditures have been growing significantly faster than the rest of the economy for thirty years. As shown in figure 4.2, the proportion of our economy consumed by the health care sector has zoomed from just under 6 percent in 1965—the year government-funded **Medicare** and **Medicaid** were born—to a projection of 16 percent by 2005.[12] The Medicare and Medicaid programs (described later) cost a great deal more now than originally expected for a number of reasons. People are living longer and the biotechnological advances have led to more costly care. In addition, defensive medicine is practiced to avoid malpractice litigation and "extraordinary measures" are often used at the end of life.

Cost reduction and realignment of services to reduce costs while providing medically necessary care in the most cost-effective setting is becoming a key strategy in health care organizations. Traditionally, health care was provided almost exclusively in **fee-for-service,** acute care settings (hospitals and physician clinics). According to American Hospital Association statistics published in 1995, community hospital admissions dropped almost 13 percent—from about 35 million to almost 31 million. During the same period, outpatient visits rose almost 81 percent—from about 212 million to almost 383 million.[4] As care shifts to less expensive points along the health care continuum, hospitals are eliminating services judged to be redundant or nonessential. Curative medical care continues to dominate, however, and less than 5 percent of health care expenditures are used for preventive services and only 1 percent is spent on population-based prevention.

Health Care Access

Access to health care is more strongly determined by income and health insurance than by health needs and health status. The escalating costs of health care and the lack of health insurance has made health care services unaffordable and, thus, inaccessible to millions of Americans. It is now estimated that 37 to 40 million Americans do not have health insurance and an equal number are thought to have inadequate insurance. The uninsured are disproportionately young, minority, employed in small businesses, and poor.[54] Lack of health insurance, which discourages the use of primary and preventive care, often shifts the pattern of care to more costly urgent and emergency services provided in hospitals and emergency departments. A study by the Robert Wood Johnson Foundation revealed that the uninsured were less likely to be immunized, to receive early prenatal care, to have a blood pressure check, and to seek medical care for serious symptoms.[54] There are many other factors preventing access to care including acceptability as it relates to patient satisfaction and accessibility as it relates to geographic, cultural, and language barriers. Baker[6] and many others have indicated that the only clear means of reestablishing equitable access to essential health care services is to provide universal and compulsory coverage for all Americans.

One step to keeping American families covered by health insurance was the passage of the Health Insurance Portability and Accountability Act of 1996. This legislation was designed to prevent insurance companies from discontinuing a person's coverage if he or she changes jobs and a family member has a preexisting condition (e.g., diabetes or a birth defect).

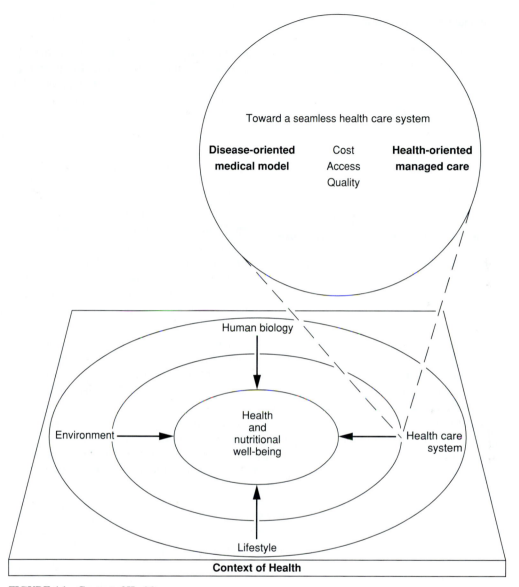

FIGURE 4.1   Context of Health
The development of a seamless health care system.

Quality of Care

Infant mortality rates in some urban areas of the United States exceed rates in many developing countries; unacceptable numbers of poor and minority children remain unimmunized; many women do not have access to adequate prenatal care, and the needs of the aging population have, to a large extent, gone unattended. This picture of the ineffectiveness of the American health care system is one of the reasons why the traditional medical system is rapidly losing the public's trust. The traditional

system has been serving a shrinking population of fully insured individuals who often receive the bulk of care in a high-cost, technologically oriented environment.

Appropriateness, effectiveness, and quality care are criteria of a sound health care system. **Appropriate care** is defined as the care that best matches the health needs of an individual or group of individuals and that is the most cost-effective intervention for preventing or resolving health problems. Effectiveness means the procedure or therapy produces a positive result for most patients when used under usual circumstances. While effectiveness is a

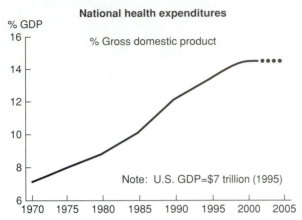

National health expenditures

% GDP

% Gross domestic product

Note: U.S. GDP=$7 trillion (1995)

FIGURE 4.2   Growth of Health Care Spending in the United States
(*Source:* HCFA/Health Care Financing Review/Fall 1996: Vol. 18, No. 1, p. 199. STRATEGIC GRAND ROUNDS® © 1997 Abbott HealthSystem Division.)

criterion, only 20 percent of commonly used medical interventions have been proven to be effective.[43] To address this gap, the U.S. Agency for Health Care Policy and Research (**AHCPR**) and other organizations and agencies have directed extensive resources toward the medical effectiveness research or outcomes research (discussed later in this chapter). Quality care is the combined perception of providers and patients that health care and its results have a positive value in terms of the time and resources invested. The definition of quality is expanded in box 4.1.[26]

To balance cost, access, and quality, a new system based on managed care is evolving. After an overview of the financing of health care in the United States, **managed care** is discussed. Refer to the glossary of terms used in managed care to understand and learn terminology used in this new system (Appendix A).

Health Care Financing in the United States

Before the end of World War II, most people paid for physician visits, hospitalization, and other medical care out-of-pocket from family resources on a fee-for-service basis. County hospitals and charity organizations covered care for the indigent. After World War II and into the 1960s, medical insurance became popular in the form of fee-for-service **indemnity** plans, which were initiated as a fringe benefit to employed workers. These plans were predominately "hospital insurance" and protected beneficiaries from financial loss due to large medical bills.

During the 1970s and 1980s, the second era in health care financing saw the rise of new organizational and payment mechanisms to contain costs. These mechanisms include **health maintenance organizations** (HMOs), preferred provider organizations (PPOs), and government-initiated payment systems such as the diagnosis-related groups (DRGs), which set standard rates for hospital services. The reimbursement rate is determined by the primary diagnosis of the patient.

BOX 4.1

QUALITY OF CARE DEFINED

Quality of care can be defined as the degree to which health services for individuals and populations increase the likelihood of desired health outcomes and the degree to which health services are consistent with current professional knowledge.

The term *health services* refers to a wide array of services that affect health, including those for physical and mental illness. The definition applies to many types of health care practitioners (physicians, nurses, dentists, dietitians, therapists, and other health professionals) and to all settings of care (from hospitals and long-term care facilities to physicians' offices, community clinics, and private homes).

Individuals and populations draws attention to the different perspectives that need to be addressed: the quality of care that health plans and clinicians deliver to individuals, and the quality of care across the entire system.

The phrase *desired health outcomes* highlights the crucial link between how care is provided and its effects on health. It underscores the importance of being mindful of people's well-being and welfare and of keeping patients and their families well informed about alternative health care interventions and their expected outcomes.

Current professional knowledge emphasizes that health professionals must stay abreast of the dynamic knowledge base in their profession and take responsibility for explaining to their patients the processes and expected outcomes of care.

Adapted from Institute of Medicine: *Focusing on quality in a changing health care system,* Washington, DC, 1997, National Academy of Sciences.

In 1988, traditional insurance, the indemnity plans, accounted for almost 72 percent of the private health insurance market. By 1993, it had shrunk to a third due to the expansion of HMOs. By 1994 one in five Americans was enrolled in an HMO.[52] The American Association of Health Plans (formerly the Group Health Association of America) reported that by the end of 1995, 56 million Americans were enrolled in HMOs.[1]

The current wave of health care reform is ushering in a third era of health care financing that takes a broader approach to the challenge of providing high-quality health care while containing overall costs. This broader vision of managed care includes not only personal episodic health services in physicians' clinics and hospitals but also community-focused services that, over a period of time, protect and promote health as well as prevent illness.[35]

Throughout these eras of health care financing, it has been a challenge to secure payment for nutrition services (see box 4.2). Community nutrition professionals with their knowledge of food, nutrition, and health are in a prime position to provide essential nutrition-related services in hospitals and clinics, as well as health promotion and disease prevention education and services through other community-based set-tings. In this chapter, the terms "registered dietitian" and "dietitian" are used when the topic refers to clinical activities that specifically require the expertise of a nutrition professional who has education in dietetics or nutrition and approved clinical training and who has passed a written exam. In many states, these persons are licensed as or have the protected title of "dietitian." Otherwise, as in the rest of the text, the term community nutrition professional is used to refer to a broader range of persons who are involved in promoting the nutritional well-being of people through services delivered in a managed care system or through other community organizations.

Medicare and Medicaid: The Background

No discussion of the evolving health care system can proceed without considering the nation's two largest health care programs—Medicare and Medicaid. The priority for both of these government-funded programs is to control costs and integrate themselves into the changing paradigm of health care delivery. Federal spending on the Medicare and Medicaid programs totaled $267 billion in 1995. These programs accounted for over 16 percent of the entire federal budget for that year. Unless there is

BOX 4.2

PAYMENT FOR NUTRITION SERVICES

MEDICARE

Medicare Part B covers services and supplies furnished "incident to a physician's professional services." For nutrition services to be reimbursed the following must all be true:

- The community nutrition professional must be employed by the physician.
- The service must be rendered under the direct, personal supervision of the physician.
- The service must be medically necessary.

Medical nutrition therapy legislation has been introduced to modify these requirements and enable payment to registered dietitians for nutrition services rendered.

MEDICAID

Coverage policies for nutrition services differ by state. All states are required to include nutrition assessment as part of Early and Periodic Screening and Diagnosis and Treatment Services (EPSDT) to low income children. If the screening identifies a problem, the state Medicaid program must pay for health services to treat identified conditions, including nutrition needs. Thus, follow-up services must be provided to treat identified nutrition-related problems.

MANAGED CARE ORGANIZATIONS

Managed care organizations vary greatly in their inclusion of nutrition services. Many health maintenance organizations have dietitians on staff, other types of organizations include dietitians as preferred providers.

MAJOR INDEMNITY PLANS

Insurance companies provide payment for ambulatory nutrition services when they are preapproved or when they are within coverage benefits defined in insurance contracts.

reform, Medicare and Medicaid spending are projected to double every five to seven years.[5]

Medicare: How It Works

Medicare is a federal program that pays for many of the medical services received by the elderly and the disabled. The Medicare program became law in 1965 as Title XVIII of the Social Security Act. Today, Medicare covers 95 percent of the nation's elderly in addition to many disabled persons who are on social security. Medicare covers most medically necessary and reasonable services delivered as inpatient hospital care, short-term skilled nursing facility care, home health care, doctor's services, diagnostic and laboratory tests, hospital outpatient services, home dialysis, and ambulance services. However, it does not provide for all health care services. Standards for Medicare include requirements for medical and nursing staff, nutrition services and staff, the physical environment in which care is provided, and the maintenance of records and overall quality of care. State agencies—usually health departments—implement the standards and provide consultative services.

Services are provided under two separate but coordinated programs: the compulsory Part A or Hospital Insurance and the voluntary Part B or Supplementary Medical Insurance. Part A beneficiaries are eligible to receive inpatient hospital care, inpatient care in a skilled nursing facility following a hospital stay, home health care, and hospice care. This portion of the program is financed by a federal tax paid by employers and employees.

Medicare's Part B covers various "medical and other health services," such as physician services, emergency room and outpatient services, laboratory tests and x rays, and rehabilitation services. Medicare beneficiaries are responsible for an annual deductible and a cost-sharing contribution (co-payment) for services, usually 20 percent of charges. Beneficiaries also must pay any

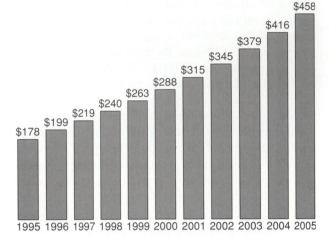

FIGURE 4.3   Projected Growth of Medicare Spending
(*Source:* Congressional Budget Office: *Social state of the nation,* Washington DC, 1995, Fiscal Year 1996 Budget of US Government.)

charges above the Medicare allowed charge and are totally responsible for any services not covered by Medicare. Many elderly carry private supplementary (Medi-Gap) insurance to cover these costs.

In 1994, 36 million persons were enrolled in Medicare Part A at a cost of $104.5 billion, and 35.1 million persons enrolled in Medicare Part B at a cost of $60.3 billion.[8,21,45] Figure 4.3 shows the projected growth in Medicare spending from 1995 through 2005.[9]

Medicaid: How It Works

Medicaid was also established in 1965 as an amendment (Title XIX) to the Social Security Act. It provides access to health care for eligible low-income Americans. The data in box 4.3 illustrate the role Medicaid plays in providing health services. Unlike Medicare, Medicaid is jointly paid by federal and state governments. States are responsible for administering the

BOX 4.3

MEDICAID STATISTICS

- One out of every ten Americans, or 35 million people, rely on Medicaid for some form of health care.
- One out of every four American children depends on Medicaid for basic health care. Children comprise nearly 50 percent of all Medicaid recipients; however, children only use 15 percent of Medicaid costs.
- One third of all births in the United States are paid for by Medicaid.
- The disabled and the elderly use the majority of Medicaid funds—39 percent and 28 percent, respectively.[5]

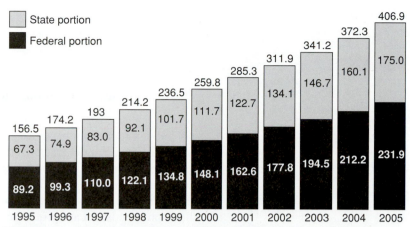

FIGURE 4.4   Projected Growth of Medicaid Spending (in Billions of Dollars)
(*Source:* Congressional Budget Office: *Social state of the nation,* Washington DC, 1995, Fiscal Year 1996 Budget of US Government.)

Medicaid program, but the federal government has paid the majority of the cost (57 percent in 1995).[5]

Medicaid coverage and eligibility varies from state to state and within each state over time. Each state establishes its own Medicaid eligibility standards, but must cover certain individuals to receive federal funds. Each state also determines the type, amount, and scope of its Medicaid services, but must include certain basic services that are similar to a basic private insurance plan.

Total outlay for Medicaid in 1995 reached $156.6 billion ($89.2 billion in federal and $67.3 billion in state funds).[5,8,21,45] Medicaid is funded through general tax revenues of the federal government and general and special taxes at the state level. Figure 4.4 shows the projected growth in Medicaid spending from 1995 through 2005.[9]

THE NEW WORLD OF MANAGED CARE: CREATING INTEGRATED DELIVERY SYSTEMS

Health care organizations are changing rapidly in response to the paradigm shift in health care and the push of cost, access, and quality concerns. The nation's hospitals are merging, consolidating, and aligning with other health care organizations at a dizzying pace. The majority of physicians are now practicing in groups and existing physician groups are consolidating. Physicians and hospitals are forming new strategic alliances. Region by region across the United States, health care organizations are reorganizing and reinventing themselves as broad-based, vertically and horizontally **integrated delivery systems** that embrace **primary care,** wellness, home health, long-term care, and hospice care as well as hospital care and specialty clinics. The organizational model that incorporates the new paradigm is known as integrated delivery systems (IDSs) or managed care (see appendix A for a definition of terms used in managed care). The IDS is illustrated in figure 4.5. Managed care entities combine the organization, financing, and delivery of health care in ways that respond to the demographics and economics that prevail in different regions of the country. The expected outcome of this new system is the capacity to provide appropriate care in a seamless continuum that uses limited resources most effectively.[44]

The Integrated Delivery System Model

The integrated delivery system shown in figure 4.5 depicts a defined or enrolled population that has insurance coverage for a predetermined set of benefits. These persons receive care from an integrated system of providers that encompasses primary care providers, public health specialists, ambulatory care centers, home health care agencies, hospitals, and so on. Payments could come from a variety of arrangements, ranging from fee-for-service to **capitation** (fixed rate per member).

Shortell and associates define an integrated delivery system or managed care as a network of organizations that provides or arranges to provide a coordinated continuum of services to a defined population

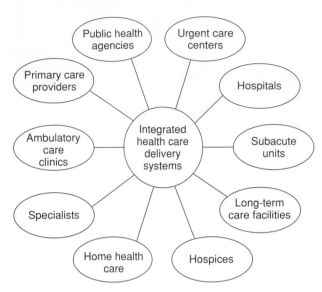

FIGURE 4.5   Model of Integrated Delivery Systems
(*Source:* Adapted from Shortell SM, Gillies RR, Anderson DA: The new world of managed care: creating organized delivery systems, *Health Affairs*; 13(5):46–64, 1994. Adapted with permisison.)

and is willing to be held clinically and fiscally accountable for the outcomes and the health status of the population served.[44] What ties the system together is its clinical and fiscal accountability for a defined population. Within integrated delivery systems, care is managed to encourage cost containment and selective

and appropriate use of providers and to review the performance of health care services to maximize outcome and quality.[33]

Evolution of Managed Care

As managed care is introduced in a region, it typically goes through four evolutionary stages.[40] The early stage (premanaged care) is characterized by many independent hospitals and physicians paid on a fee-for-services basis, and some small HMOs and community health centers. Hospital use is high. The goal of providers is to fill hospital beds; create profit (revenue) centers; reward managers for financial performance; secure more referral sources; and build high-technology, specialist-oriented "centers of excellence."

In the second stage, a loose framework of providers begin to emerge. Managed care organizations (MCOs) (including HMOs, independent practice associations, and preferred provider organizations—see box 4.4) grow and begin to penetrate the market with 20 to 25 percent of the population covered. Excess bed capacity in hospitals develops as care shifts to ambulatory settings, which leads to offers of discounts to fill hospital beds. Health care providers begin to maximize fee-for-service business by cost shifting and managing contractual allowances to maximize net revenue. The emphasis is on payer mix (the combination of indemnity fee-for-

B O X   4 . 4

TYPES OF MANAGED CARE ORGANIZATIONS

HMO. Health maintenance organizations are responsible for the financing and delivery of comprehensive health care services to an enrolled membership. Under an HMO plan, the purchaser (an employer, an insurance company, Medicaid, Medicare, or an individual) buys a health care service package from the HMO for a prepaid, monthly fee. Only the capitated fee is paid regardless of the amount and type of services provided. HMO members must obtain services from participating providers and may be responsible for minimal co-payments for various services. Members usually are not subject to meeting deductibles.

PPO. Preferred provider organizations are a variation of indemnity insurance. In a PPO, a purchaser (e.g., an insurance company, an employer, or an employees' union) arranges contracts with groups of independent health care providers

who agree to provide services to plan members for discounted fees. A PPO may consist of hundreds of physicians and other providers and hospitals throughout a state or region.

Managed fee-for-service. Some traditional fee-for-service (FFS) or indemnity insurance plans have become part of the managed care industry. The objective of managed FFS programs is to control costs while allowing patients free choice of providers and coverage for out-of-plan specialty services. As in traditional indemnity plans, providers receive payment after the patient receives care.

Physician-hospital organization. A legal entity formed by hospitals and physicians to negotiate contracts with payers to provide services under managed care. These organizations may also be involved in the management and oversight of the facilities.

service, Medicare, Medicaid, and discounted contracts with HMOs) and case management.

In the third stage of evolution, leading HMOs, physician groups, and hospital systems begin to align into a small number of integrated delivery systems or networks through affiliation, consolidations, mergers, and acquisitions. Unnecessary, duplicative tests and procedures are eliminated and evidence of outcome and cost-effectiveness is gathered. Greater emphasis is placed on keeping people well and out of the hospital. The focus at stage three is developing comprehensive coordinated networks, measuring value, and controlling use. The elements of the continuum of care are put in place.

In the final stage of the evolution to managed care, purchasers contract with HMOs, IDSs, PPOs, and physician-hospital organizations. MCOs provide health care to over 50 percent of the population. Capitation (a set monthly rate per enrollee) is the prevailing model of payment with primary care providers assuming greater service risk. Hospitals operate as cost centers, not as revenue sources. Hospital use is reduced as much as 50 percent. Redundant systems and fragmentation are eliminated. The system eventually uses a comprehensive medical record and a single information management format.[40]

In the new paradigm of managed care, MCOs are risk-based organizations with a strong focus on the provision of primary care. As capitation payment systems and IDSs develop in managed care, delivery of care will become more proactive and prevention-oriented instead of request and acute care driven. The focus will be on keeping clients well. Prevention and health promotion will be an important inroad for community nutrition professionals. The paradigm shift from hospital-centered to community-centered care requires a complete shift in the organizational culture. Box 4.5, adapted from Shortell,[44,45,5] outlines the shift in capabilities and focus as the traditional medical system makes the transition to managed care.

The shift to managed care has tremendous implications for nutrition services and the role of nutrition professionals. Box 4.6 describes nutrition professionals in each stage of the evolution.

As we have seen, a managed care health plan can take many forms. Plans vary according to the amount of choice a patient has and the level of control of services exerted by the provider. In general, managed care plans have the following attributes in common:[17]

- Arrangements with selected providers for comprehensive health services for members
- Explicit standards for selection of providers
- Formal quality assurance programs
- Significant financial incentives for plan members to use plan services (e.g., must pay out-of-pocket for nonplan services or providers)

Common types of managed care organizations in existence are described in box 4.4. The three most prominent types are HMOs, PPOs, and managed fee-for-service plans; however, the distinctions among types is becoming blurred and many managed care organizations are now hybrids.

BOX 4.5

CHANGING ORGANIZATIONAL CULTURE UNDER MANAGED CARE

Old Capability		*New Capability*
Provide for acute inpatient care	→	Provide a continuum of care
Treat illness	→	Maintain and promote wellness
Care for individual patients	→	Be accountable for health status of a defined population
Provide products and services based on biotechnology	→	Provide value-added services—emphasis on primary care, health promotion, ongoing management of chronic conditions
Fill beds	→	Provide care in appropriate setting
Manage an organization	→	Manage a network of services
Manage a department	→	Manage a regional market
Coordinate services	→	Actively manage and improve quality
Document services	→	Measure outcome

BOX 4.6

IMPLICATIONS FOR NUTRITION PROFESSIONALS AND NUTRITION CARE SERVICES AT EACH STAGE OF EVOLUTION TOWARD MANAGED CARE

STAGE ONE: TRADITIONAL MEDICAL MODEL

- Dietitians and dietetic technicians fill traditional clinical positions in hospitals and outpatient clinics.
- Many hospitals have nutrition support teams.
- Hospital patients and long-term care residents are screened for nutritional risk at admission.
- Consultant dietitians and food service managers provide for nutrition needs of long-term care residents.
- Community nutrition professionals in community-based agencies focus on food and nutrition programs.
- Access to nutrition care is often inconsistent from setting to setting and is tied to physician referrals and accreditation requirement.

STAGE TWO: COST-DRIVEN CONSOLIDATION; SHIFT TO AMBULATORY CARE

- Nutrition services and nutrition positions are scrutinized for revenue-generating potential.
- Nutrition professionals and organizations give attention to billing and reimbursement for nutrition services.
- Closing of hospital beds results in cuts of nutrition personnel.
- Some nutrition counseling shifts to outpatient clinics.
- Dietitians explore new opportunities with physician groups and home health care agencies.
- Hospital patients are sicker and have shorter stays.
- Nutrition professionals in long-term care must be prepared to provide nutrition support for more complex conditions and seriously ill residents.
- Costly nutrition support and visits for nutrition counseling are scrutinized by payers.
- Essential role of nutrition in disease management and the cost-effectiveness of nutrition services must be defended.

STAGE THREE: NETWORKS DEVELOP

- Priority is given to services with known effectiveness and the most cost-effective setting for care.
- Lines of authority and communication shift; improved linkages develop across components of the continuum of care.
- Dietitians and other community nutrition professionals exert greater flexibility and draw on a broader knowledge base to work effectively across a range of providers and patients in multiple settings.

- Nutrition practice guidelines and protocols become important.
- Nutrition professionals become involved in outcome assessment, cost-effectiveness analysis, and continuous quality improvement.
- Using information from these evaluation processes, nutrition professionals contain costs while advocating for the availability of appropriate nutrition care to patients in all settings.

STAGE FOUR: MATURE MANAGED CARE ENVIRONMENT

- Integrated delivery systems, coordination, and communication develop across a seamless continuum of care.
- Dietitians and other nutrition professionals are no longer organized primarily in nutrition service departments.
- Some nutrition professionals become preferred providers with networks, others are integrated into teams of clinical specialists (e.g., diabetes center or cardiovascular center) or work out of health plan-sponsored patient education and health promotion departments.
- Expanded roles for nutrition professionals develop in hospices and home care agencies.
- Continuity of nutrition care across time and settings is a priority; this is facilitated by open communication and electronic information and data systems using common terminology and general and disease-specific indicators of care processes and outcomes.
- An emphasis of nutrition care is an early identification of nutrition risk and appropriate intervention to prevent disease advancement and complications. Nutrition services with a health promotion focus expand. The role of nutrition in rehabilitation and palliation is recognized.
- Nutrition professionals develop and adopt new models of intervention to improve effectiveness and expand availability and access to nutrition care.
- Nutrition professionals break away from dependence on one-to-one nutrition counseling and printed education materials and use information technology including telephone, fax, e-mail, and computer-based education and counseling programs.

Managed Care and the Community

Mature managed care organizations recognize that promoting the health of the community; offering timely, effective diagnostic and treatment services; and managing chronic disease and rehabilitation, all in the most accessible and cost-efficient setting, is the ultimate way to control health care costs and assure quality.

To achieve this requires true integration and coordination throughout all parts of the system shown in figure 4.5 using a comprehensive community care management system.[44] The development of a community care management system begins with assessing population needs, developing resource requirements based on those needs, and then engaging in a continuous cycle of what is called community-based management. This cycle includes knowledge of the current state-of-the-science and -art of medical practice and health care, which requires staying attuned to the latest research regarding outcomes and clinically effective practices. This, in turn, becomes input for the design of the system's own clinical care protocols and guidelines, which leads to development of the system's overall continuous improvement processes. Performance data and assessment of outcomes are combined with evidence from other sites nationally to monitor performance. All of this is facilitated by an information management system, at the center of figure 4.5.

TOWARD A SEAMLESS HEALTH CARE SYSTEM

The goal for delivery of health care in the future is a seamless system. The ideal is an integrated health system that provides all persons with access to a continuum of services needed for health promotion and disease management in a highly coordinated manner. It allows the individual patient to move to different settings and services across the system with a strong continuity of care. To arrive at a seamless system, as managed care promises, regions go through the four evolutionary stages already described. (See box 4.6)

The movement toward a seamless, coordinated, integrated system has resulted in dramatic growth in long-term care, home care, and hospice care with the primary care provider serving as gatekeeper to these components of the system. A description of these important components follows.

Primary Care

Primary care, including preventive care, stands at the cornerstone of the new health care paradigm and integrated delivery systems. Primary care includes the first contact or the basic level of medical care for ambulatory patients who receive care in physician's offices, community neighborhood or managed health centers, health maintenance organizations, or public health departments.[27] Primary care had traditionally been provided by physicians, including family practitioners, general practitioners, pediatricians, obstetricians/gynecologists, and internists. Now, in many settings, primary care is being provided by physicians assistants or nurse practitioners with backup by a physician. Other practitioners such as dentists, dietitians, and other community nutrition professionals, social workers, health educators, and pharmacists also provide service in primary care settings. The primary care physician is designated as a gatekeeper for referral to specialized services. An excellent resource on primary care was developed by the U.S. Preventive Services Task Force. The second edition, called the *Guide to Clinical Preventive Services*,[42] provides recommendations for clinical practice in preventive intervention. The *Guide* identifies nutrition risk screening and counseling priorities for each stage of the life cycle.

Long-Term Care

In 1994, 1.5 million people lived in the nation's more than 16,300 skilled nursing facilities. Almost 90 percent are over age 65. Medicaid is this segment's primary payer source. The Congressional Budget Office estimates that the number of nursing facility residents will rise steadily until 2020 and then increase sharply for the next 20 years, doubling the 1994 level. By the year 2050, the nursing facility population will triple. As more Medicaid recipients are channeled into HMOs, long-term care should become even more integrated into the continuum of health care.[50]

Home Care

Home care is also growing significantly, reflecting the increasing number of older people and the advances in technology that make medical care in the home possible. Home care is less expensive than hospital care and thus more attractive to managed care providers. At an average 1995 cost of $86 per day, home care is a bargain when compared to acute care ($1,810) and long-term care

($293).[7] According to the Bureau of Labor Statistics, home care is the fastest growing segment of the health services industry. More than 17,000 providers deliver home care services to approximately 7 million individuals. Medicare is the largest single payer for home care services. In 1995, about 3.5 million Medicare enrollees received home care, twice the number of 1990 recipients.[7]

An emerging specialty within home care is home-based nutrition support. This a cost-effective means to serve individuals who must receive their nutritional needs through specialized medical foods taken orally as supplements, enterally by feeding tube, or parenterally by the intravenous route.

Hospice Care

The American hospice movement began in the 1960s and the first hospice began offering services in 1974. There are approximately 2,000 organizations providing compassionate, appropriate care for the terminally ill and their families. Over the past decade, hospice care has become an important aspect of the total continuum of care. Hospice care is palliative rather than curative and may occur in a number of settings, including the home. It involves a multidisciplinary team of physicians, nurses, social workers, community nutrition professionals, and counselors as well as family members and community volunteers. Hospice care treats the person, not the disease, focuses on the family, not the individual; and emphasizes the quality of life, not its duration.[24]

Nontraditional Health Care Services

In the seamless health care system, it is important to be aware of other providers, programs, and organizations outside the "traditional" health care system that provide useful health care services in certain situations. These range from the services of traditional healers (e.g., medicine man or woman or Shaman) to weight loss programs to chiropractic and acupuncture services. Under managed care, services such as these may be utilized when indicated by patients' needs and cultural beliefs. Nontraditional health services must be considered in the new health care system because they can be a route to appropriate and cost-effective care when used selectively.

PUBLIC HEALTH IN THE MANAGED CARE ENVIRONMENT

The rapid changes occurring within the U.S. health care system are creating an opportunity to reassess and reori-ent the relationships between the public and private sectors. The long history of separation between public health and private medicine has not been conducive to maximizing the health of the U.S. population.[49]

The medical care system has traditionally provided services directed at the diagnosis and management of the ailments of people who seek the services. In many regions, public health agencies have undertaken this role as a provider of last resort for the socially disadvantaged. On the other hand, public health has assumed the primary responsibility for organizing programs directed at population-based prevention and disease control. Clinical preventive services (e.g., immunizations and cancer screening) have been divided between the two, largely through opportunity rather than design.

Designed primarily to contain costs and serve those already insured, the managed care system has little experience meeting the special needs of populations traditionally served by public health. Providers, policy makers, and advocates are working to ensure managed care systems, in collaboration with public health, maintain a safety net designed to offer at least basic health care to every American.[49]

Health Services to Vulnerable Populations

A variety of public health agencies at federal, state, and local levels provide health care for **vulnerable populations,** those considered to be at risk. These services must continue to be provided for vulnerable groups by either the public or private sectors or by a combination of the two. In these populations, nutrition factors are recognized as significantly contributing to medical risks. Thus, most of these programs include nutrition services as part of screening, assessment, clinical preventive services, and disease management. Some major programs include community or neighborhood health centers, migrant health services, Indian health services, school health, maternal and child health programs, family planning, and the military health care system.

Community or Neighborhood Health Centers   Begun in 1964, neighborhood health centers were created to deliver comprehensive, responsive care to low-income populations, the uninsured, and minority groups. Services include medical care and preventive health services such as well-child care, adult physical examinations, prenatal care, and chronic disease treatment and follow-up. The health clinics are located in medically underserved (rural and inner city) communities. Most have strong links to other health programs (such as Medicaid), social services, financial assistance programs, and food assistance programs such as food stamps programs and the Special Supplemental Nutrition Program for Women, Infants and Children (WIC). Many employ nutritionists to plan and provide education, counseling, and programs to address nutrition-related health problems. Nutrition assistants, who are often recruited from the community to match the age and ethnic background of the service area, are trained to extend nutrition services. They provide nutrition information in the clients' primary languages and are culturally sensitive to their food preferences, health beliefs, and lifestyles.

Migrant Health Services   Migrant health centers provide primary health services similar to those offered by community or neighborhood health centers. In addition, migrant health services offer environmental health services, infections and parasitic disease screening and control, accident prevention, and prevention of excessive pesticide exposure. These services directly reflect the needs of the people who are responsible for planting, cultivating, and harvesting the nation's produce and take into account the factors of poverty, inadequate housing, and the stress common among migrant communities.

A challenge in migrant health services is to provide continuity of care as families move from one location to the next. The National Migrant Referral Project enables exchange of medical information between migrant health centers. Many migrant families also carry personal health cards summarizing major health problems, medications, and immunizations and including clinic phone numbers of previous providers.[10] Nutrition services, including screening, counseling, and education, must be based on clients' traditional food ways, what they can afford to buy, and the type of cooking facilities available.

Indian Health Service   Health services to Indian and Alaskan natives became the responsibility of the Public Health Service in 1954. The mandated role of the Indian Health Service (IHS) is to provide Indians and Alaskan natives with access to comprehensive health care including preventive, curative, rehabilitative, and environmental services. The Indian Health Service provides medical care, emergency medical services, preventive health services, environmental health services, and professional training. Health conditions commonly addressed include pregnancy, child health, accidents and injuries, aging, alcoholism, mental health, diabetes, and otitis media. IHS hospitals and clinics generally in-clude services of dentists, dietitians and nutrition assistants, health educators, and social workers. Nutrition priorities for community nutrition professionals in the Indian Health Service are diabetes, maternal and child nutrition, and weight control. Nutrition and other services must take into account environmental conditions leading to nutrition and health problems such as poverty, unemployment, substandard housing, educational deficits, alcohol abuse, and social stress.

School Health   School nurses have had a presence in schools for more than eighty years. Nurses may be employees of the school district or supplied by the local health department. A new trend is to place primary care clinics in school buildings. Clinics staffed by a physician, a nurse practitioner, a nurse's aid, and a dietitian are in place in many inner city middle schools and high schools. Generally, health services are available for health screening, sport physicals, minor infections and complaints, and sexually transmitted disease testing, and many sites offer prenatal care. The unique and challenging aspect of school-based health services is the collaboration with principals, teachers, parents, and the students to determine what health services are needed, desired, appropriate, acceptable, and feasible. Supportive services available at schools such as guidance, counseling, psychological testing, and the assistance of social workers are utilized to support health aims.

Rural Health Care   Rural health care facilities have been recognized as being patient-centered and cost-effective, but low funding and lack of trained personnel are serious constraints to access and quality in rural areas. Shared staff arrangements are common since physician specialists, therapists, nurse practitioners, and community nutrition professionals are in short supply in rural areas. Linkages are necessary to provide specialized diagnostic and treatment procedures and to coordinate care delivered in separate parts of the system. To meet the needs of rural populations, rural providers must redefine their roles and relationships to include a more integrated approach to health care delivery.[23]

Maternal and Child Health   In 1935, Title V of the Social Security Act provided grants to the states for maternal and child health and crippled children's services. The current Maternal and Child Health (MCH) block grant program enables states to foster family-centered, community-based, coordinated services for mothers, children, and families. Services focus on preventive and primary care services for children, specialized services for children with special health care needs, and prenatal care for disadvantaged women. Community nutrition professionals serve as core team members in MCH programs. MCH services are often coordinated with other family support and financial assistance programs such as Medicaid, WIC, and Food Stamps in "one-stop" service centers. MCH funds also help provide for the development of standards of practice and guidance materials, technical assistance to providers, support for special projects, and professional training and research.

Family Planning Clinics   Federally supported family planning clinics are mandated to "offer medically-accepted methods of family planning, education and counseling, outreach and public information services." The population served includes girls and women twelve to forty-four years of age. Women who use the clinics are low income, uninsured, or underinsured. Government funding (Title X) at one point provided nutrition counseling with family planning, but continuation of these services today varies by state and among clinics within a state. While family planning clinics offer a logical opportunity to reach women with nutrition information, critics feel nutrition assessment and counseling can be a deterrent to using family planning services by some women. Family planning clinics are staffed by nurse practitioners; medical assistants; health educators; and, in some cases, dietitians or other community nutrition professionals.

Military Health Care System   The military health care system ensures the health of members of the armed services so they are physically and mentally ready to carry out their worldwide defense mission.[46] Active duty members are covered along with their dependents. The military health care system has been generally much more successful in health promotion than the civilian system. The evidence is clear in the benefits derived from smoking cessation, reduced alcohol consumption, weight control, and other "lifestyle" programs.[46]

Vital Role for Public Health in the "New" System

In addition to providing a safety net for vulnerable populations, there are many opportunities for the public and private sectors to work in an integrated, coordinated fashion.

Public health is likely to have an enhanced monitoring function consistent with its role as an agent for assessment, policy development, and quality assurance

(see chapter 2). Ensuring the accountability of managed care requires systems to document the adequacy of such care in meeting health needs. Maintenance of vital statistics data and conducting of surveys have always been part of the public health role; the expansion of such activities into monitoring medical care services is a natural extension of that role.[37]

If integrated delivery systems are to be held responsible for the health status of populations, they will need to do a better job of assessing the needs, demands, and preferences of their populations. This will involve using existing data but also collecting primary data on population segments—such as the poor and near-poor, minorities, and others for whom adequate health care data are lacking. Conducting such assessments will require closer linkages among managed care organizations, public health, and social agencies in the community. Results of these assessments can reveal areas in which organizations and agencies can forge cooperative programs and agreements to assure health care and related services for certain populations.

It is particularly important that such assessments focus on community wellness and health promotion and not exclusively on diagnosed or perceived illness. With this focus, it may be possible to use appropriate secondary prevention programs to forestall the need for acute care or to minimize the cost of managing long-term chronic illness. Community nutrition professionals, with their knowledge of food, nutrition, and epidemiology can play a major role in providing nutrition and health assessment to properly diagnose community nutrition and appropriate interventions.

Within the assurance function, public health agencies either encourage necessary action by other entities in the private or public sectors or provide services directly. Public health agencies could contract with managed care entities to offer services that are more efficiently provided by public health agencies (e.g., preventive health campaigns and immunizations). As part of the assurance function, public health also fosters equity. Public health can develop mechanisms to assess the equity of services provided by subpopulations within the community.

According to a policy paper of the American Public Health Association, essential roles to be played by public health agencies include environmental health protection and health promotion/disease prevention, the assurance of a community infrastructure for health services for the uninsured, and the mechanism for assuring accountability of managed care organizations.[33] Thus, public health should be viewed as an integral component of the integrated health system, as shown in figure 4.5.

Models for Public and Private Partnerships

There are several models of effective collaboration. The Missouri Department of Health, concerned that the period of confusion that marks the transition to managed care for their Medicaid population could pose a risk to public health, decided to carve out as their perview immunizations; services for HIV/AIDS, sexually-transmitted diseases, communicable diseases, and tuberculosis; and lead environmental assessment. Managed care plans may directly provide these services to their own members. But if members obtain the services from local health departments, managed care plans will reimburse the local health agencies on a fee-for-service basis.[29]

In Minnesota, where managed care has reached the fourth stage of evolution, managed care organizations are making a commitment to promote the health of the community. In 1994, the "Partners for Better Health" program was announced by HealthPartners, a large, not-for-profit health care organization. This program established a set of measurable goals for the organization and its members[23] (see box 4.7).

HealthPartners see themselves as a "health improvement" organization as opposed to a "health maintenance" organization. Their mission is to improve the health of members of their community. The basic philosophy underriding the Partners for Better Health goals is a disease prevention model.[36] It divides the population into people who are at no or low risk, at risk, at high risk, have early symptoms, or have active disease (see figure 4.6). The aim of services is to keep members at the lowest risk level possible. Health messages and educational tools are targeted to members at the appropriate point in the spectrum. Several major successes have been achieved through this prevention initiative.

Other Government Agencies Foster Quality

The many government agencies within the Department of Health and Human Services play major roles in funding research and demonstration projects to develop and improve health care delivery systems. The Centers for Disease Control and Prevention (**CDC**), the Health Care Financing Administration (**HCFA**), the Agency for Health Care Policy and Research, and many other government agencies are involved in fostering effective and efficient systems for delivering health services to Americans.

The CDC has several programs that support research and demonstration projects; these include cancer control, diabetes control, hypertension control, pediatric and pregnancy surveillance of low-income populations, and immunization programs. To address the issue of managed care, the CDC created its Office of Managed

BOX 4.7

"PARTNERS FOR BETTER HEALTH" GOALS

1. Increase from 75 to 95 percent the proportion of children who are fully immunized by age two years.
2. Reduce by 30 percent infant and maternal complications among members, including preterm deliveries, the number of infants affected by substance abuse, and repeated teen pregnancies.
3. Decrease by 25 percent the number of childhood injuries severe enough to require medical care and reduce by 10 percent the number of injuries so severe that hospitalization is necessary.
4. Help identify members who may be victims of abuse and continually link them with appropriate services and preventive resources at HealthPartners and within the community.

5. Improve early detection of diabetes by screening 90 percent of high-risk members; reduce by 25 percent the progression from a high-risk state to active disease; and reduce by 30 percent the onset and progression of eye, kidney, and nerve damage resulting from diabetes.
6. Improve early detection of breast cancer, reducing by 50 percent the cases that reach an advanced stage before being detected.
7. Reduce by 50 percent new dental caries in all age groups.
8. Reduce the number of heart disease events among members by 25 percent. This includes myocardial infarction, angioplasty, coronary artery bypass, and congestive heart failure.

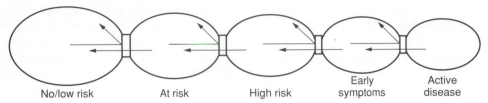

FIGURE 4.6   HealthPartner's Health Improvement Model
(Reprinted with permission of HealthPartners, Inc., Minneapolis, MN.)

Care in late 1995 to track managed care trends and determine the impact of managed care on Medicaid recipients, provide research guidance and recommend essential services for such health plans to adequately serve the public. The CDC will concentrate on prevention effectiveness and guidelines, Medicaid, managed care, and quality assurance.

The HCFA is involved in developing and evaluating innovations in the care of the elderly Medicare population such as community-based care. The HCFA Office on Managed Care is actively involved in identifying ways to measure quality and has developed disease-specific indicators of quality. The AHCPR was created by Congress in 1989 to stimulate the evaluation of medical effectiveness and the development and dissemination of guidelines evolving from outcomes research. The Bureau of Maternal and Child Health has funded projects to assure access to and quality of health care for high-risk pregnant women and children and to track outcomes for the MCH population.

MEASURING PERFORMANCE AND OUTCOME OF HEALTH CARE

Within the health care system, organizations are examining their performance and using data to improve the system. This has taken many forms over the years including peer review, quality assurance, total quality management, continuous quality improvement, and more recently, outcomes measurement, and performance improvement. Most organizations have mechanisms for internal monitoring to track key indicators of performance and management procedures to introduce adjustments in operations and clinical practices to foster effectiveness and patient satisfaction along with cost controls. External groups are also exerting pressure to foster quality through standardized comparisons applied across organizations and performance measurement required as a condition of accreditation.

Health Plan "Report Cards"— Measuring Performance

One type of assessment that is becoming widely used is health plan **"report cards"** to enable comparison of standard performance measures across managed care organizations and health plans. Published summaries of health plan performance can be used by individual consumers and employers to select a health plan on the basis of cost and quality.[51] Developing a universal system for assessing and reporting health plan quality began as an effort by a coalition of employers and health plan administrators. This coalition worked to standardize quality reporting process and to develop a manageable set of data elements that document certain characteristics of a health plan. Thus, the development of the Health Plan Employers Data and Information Set (HEDIS) came to fruition.[34] The National Committee for Quality Assurance (NCQA), a group that also evaluates health plans through an accreditation process, has taken the lead on this initiative.

HEDIS includes an evolving set of health plan performance measures, standardized definitions, and methods for data collection. HEDIS is used as the basis for many report cards initiatives and is the preferred tool of the managed care industry for measuring health plan performance. Examples of the health plan performance evaluation in HEDIS version 3.0 are listed in table 4.1. They include indicators relevant to Medicaid and Medicare.[34]

The current list of HEDIS performance measures omits many health services including nutrition. Nutrition measures have the potential for wide appeal among health care stakeholders (i.e., payers, consumers, and providers). Turner and Dwyer proposed four measures related to **medical nutrition therapy** for managed care report cards: staffing for nutrition services and medical nutrition therapy for high cholesterol levels, gestational diabetes, and cardiovascular disease.[51] Barriers to adding nutrition measures in HEDIS include competition from other potential measures and the need to resolve technical issues related to measurement and documentation before

TABLE 4.1
HEDIS® 3.0 Selected Reporting Measures

Use of services
- Well-child visits in the first fifteen months of life
- Well-child visits in the third, fourth, fifth, and sixth years of life
- Adolescent well-care visit
- Frequency of selected procedures
- Inpatient utilization—nonacute care
- Inpatient utilization—general hospital/acute care
- Ambulatory care
- Cesarean section and vaginal birth after cesarean rate (VBAC-rate)
- Discharge and average length of stay for females in maternity care
- Births and average length of stay, newborns
- Frequency of ongoing prenatal care
- Mental health utilization—percentage of members receiving inpatient day/night and ambulatory services
- Readmission for specified mental health disorders
- Chemical dependency utilization—inpatient discharges and average length of stay
- Chemical dependency utilization—percentage of members receiving inpatient, day/night care, and ambulatory services
- Mental health utilization—inpatient discharges and average length of stay
- Readmission for chemical dependency
- Outpatient drug utilization

Cost of care
- High-occurrence/high-cost DRGs
- Rate trends

Informed health care choices
- Language translation services
- New member orientation/education

Health plan descriptive information
- Board certification/residency completion
- Provider compensation
- Physicians under capitation
- Recredentialing of physicians
- Pediatric mental health network
- Chemical dependency services
- Arrangements with public health, educational, and social service entities
- Weeks of pregnancy at time of enrollment
- Family planning
- Preventive care and health promotion
- Quality assessment and improvement
- Case management
- Utilization management
- Risk management
- Diversity of Medicaid membership
- Unduplicated count of Medicaid members
- Enrollment by payer (member years/months)
- Total enrollment

Reprinted with permission from the National Committee for Quality Assurance; *HEDIS® 3.0, Volume I: Narrative—What's In It and Why It Matters;* pgs. 30–34 © 1997. HEDIS® is a trademark of the National Committee for Quality Assurance.

considering new measures. The involvement of community nutrition professionals in the development of performance measures and outcome indicators is equally important for positioning nutrition services in managed care.

Outcomes Assessment and Management

The outcomes movement is having a strong impact on health care systems. Outcomes management uses data collected within the system or studies conducted by others to determine "What works best for whom and at what cost?"[47] **Outcomes assessment,** also called outcomes research, is used to evaluate the effectiveness of current clinical diagnostic procedures and treatments, considering multiple consequences of concern to patients, medical experts, health care administrators, payers/buyers, and policy makers. Carefully selected evaluation and research methods are applied to determine whether the procedure or care process does, in fact, produce the desired results (this topic is expanded in chapter 15). Based on

the results of outcomes assessment, guidelines for care delivery such as protocols or **practice guidelines** are developed and implemented to foster use of the best practices across the system.

The three outcome categories generally assessed are clinical outcomes, patient outcomes, and cost outcomes. These outcomes are illustrated in the following section.

NUTRITION CARE AND SERVICES IN THE HEALTH CARE SYSTEM

Nutrition Care and Its Outcomes

Nutrition care is an essential service in all health care settings, including acute care, hospitals, subacute care, outpatient clinics, long-term care facilities, home health, and other community-based services (figure 4.5). The prevalence of nutrition risk and severity of these risks vary according to the setting. In acute care hospitals, nutrition risks on admission have been reported in up to 46 percent of patients.[47] Rates as high as 59 percent have been reported among patients admitted to long-term care facilities.[47] As many as 85 percent of home health clients have nutrition risk factors.[52] Nutrition services includes screening, assessment, selection and implementation of the appropriate nutrition care intervention, referral when necessary, and follow-up. Refer to appendix B for definitions of nutrition care terms.[2,38]

In all settings, nutrition screening can be used to identify patients who require special nutrition intervention. When indicated, the initial screening can be followed by in-depth nutrition risk assessment and nutrition intervention planning. Many specific diseases and diagnoses require nutrition intervention for successful clinical outcomes. Once a patient is designated for nutrition intervention, nutrition care is initiated based on practice guidelines, if they exist, and on the best judgment of the practitioner. Optimal nutrition intervention may be complicated by several factors, including:

- Variation in patients' acceptance and compliance with the nutrition intervention
- Staffing patterns and other organizational limitations that hinder implementing nutrition care according to practice guidelines or protocols
- Interruption of specialized nutrition support for other medical procedures

Consequently, to provide high-quality nutrition care it is essential to monitor and compensate for impeding factors. The nutrition intervention should be adjusted, if necessary, to match patients' needs with the capacity for specialized nutrition care in the specific delivery setting.

Nutrition in Clinical Preventive Services

Good nutritional status is an integral part of health promotion and disease prevention and enhances growth and development. Adequate maternal nutrition, for example, is important for a healthy pregnancy and a healthy newborn. Children with good nutritional status are healthier and recover from intercurrent illnesses more quickly than do malnourished children. Well-nourished individuals are better able to tolerate and recover from acute illnesses and trauma. Poor nutritional status can precipitate disease or increase its severity. The association of nutrition and dietary practices with chronic disease risk is well established.[39] Certain dietary patterns have been associated with increased risk for five of the ten leading causes of death in the United States, particularly heart disease, diabetes, and cancer.

Many diseases can harm the nutritional status of patients unless steps are taken to provide adequate nourishment and treat malnutrition if it exists. Early detection and nutrition intervention has been demonstrated to be effective prevention for secondary diseases.[39] Based on this information, nutrition screening, assessment, and intervention when indicated should be incorporated into clinical preventive services and primary care, including prenatal care; infant, child, and adolescent health; wellness programs; adult health maintenance; and geriatric health visits. The goals of nutrition in preventive care are to keep people healthy and active in their communities, to reduce the incidence and severity of preventable diseases, to improve health and quality of life, and to reduce total medical costs, particularly costs for drug therapy, surgery, hospitalization, and extended care.[38]

A national objective has been established to "Increase to at least 75 percent the proportion of primary care providers who provide nutrition assessment and counseling and/or referral to qualified community nutrition professionals by the year 2000."[22] The U.S. Preventive Services Task Force recommends that clinicians who lack time or skills to obtain a complete dietary history, understand barriers to changes in eating habits, or offer individualized guidance on food selection and preparation should refer patients to a registered dietitian or qualified nutritionist for appropriate counseling.[42]

Nutrition in Disease Management

Patients with nutrition-related diseases are seen in all settings from primary care in outpatient clinics to acute care in hospitals, home care, hospice care, and long-term care. Nutrition screening, assessment and medical nutrition therapy (MNT) are essential in the management of many diseases.[14] After nutrition screening identifies those at risk, assessment and appropriate MNT can lead to improved clinical outcomes and improved quality of life for patients and economic benefits for the organization. The goals of nutrition in disease management are to:

- Restore and maintain optimal nutritional status
- Modify dietary and nutrient intake as required by the altered metabolic or physiologic state
- Empower the patient (or caretaker) to manage the nutritional aspects of the person's disease or condition
- Monitor and adjust the nutrition intervention over the course of the disease or condition as necessary to achieve the above goals

CLINICAL, COST, AND PATIENT OUTCOMES OF NUTRITION SERVICES

Clinical Outcomes

With sufficient exposure to the appropriate nutrition intervention, patients should experience improved dietary or nutrient intakes, which lead to changes in intermediate outcomes of biochemical or physiological indicators. These changes help improve or stabilize the disease state or condition and help improve adverse events. This cascade of outcomes is illustrated in figure 4.7.

The nutrition intervention is judged effective when this cascade of outcomes is observed and when the degree of change is clinically meaningful. The major clinical outcome is the impact of nutrition intervention on the disease state. Intermediate outcomes are also important, however, because they measure and demonstrate the nutrition intervention's value. For example,

• Improved food or nutrient intakes provide health care providers feedback about the success of nutrition counseling and dietary modification.

• Changes in biochemical and physiological indicators provide physicians and patients with evidence of the nutritional intervention's impact. These changes also provide the other members of the health care team with information about the effectiveness of the specific nutrition intervention or the need for adjustment. The results also allow for predictions of future outcomes, including the effect of the nutrition intervention on the disease state, on potential adverse effects, and on the associated health care costs.

Clinical "effectiveness" is achieved when the preventive or therapeutic nutrition intervention has the desired impact on the disease state or condition. Documented effectiveness provides important evidence of the value of nutrition intervention to a wide range of players in the health care arena, including physicians and medical directors, administrators in the health care organization, decision makers in managed care organizations, benefits managers for employee groups, and payers. Adequate nutritional support in trauma patients, for example, is associated with earlier stabilization and fewer infection-related

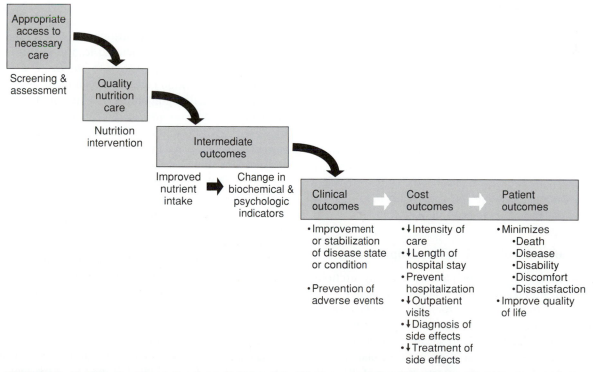

FIGURE 4.7 The Cascade of Events Leading to Evidence of the Effectiveness and Cost-Effectiveness of Nutrition Interventions (Reprinted with permission of Mead Johnson & Company, © 1996.)

complications. These and other positive clinical outcomes translate into cost savings for the health care organization and the payer.

Cost Outcomes and Economic Benefits

Numerous studies have shown that effective MNT can save money as an alternative to most costly therapies (e.g., pharmaceutical intervention), by preventing the need for more specialized technologies and hospitalization, and by reducing the length of hospital stay.[15,18,31,38,40,48] Better nutritional status is also related to fewer outpatient visits. Patients are less likely to experience complications as their nutritional status improves and their nutritional risk is reduced. As a result, they minimize their utilization of health care resources.

Benefits of MNT in Diabetes Mellitus

Recent studies have established the need for MNT in management of diabetes, a disease that had a total economic cost, including costs for diabetes as a secondary diagnosis, of $91.8 billion in 1992.[40] Although 40.5 percent of this cost was attributable to inpatient hospital costs, less than 0.03 percent ($31.9 million) was spent on MNT and diet counseling.[40] MNT costs, although small, appear to offer considerable opportunity for a positive health and economic impact.

In a study of MNT in the outpatient management on non-insulin-dependent diabetes mellitus, Johnson and Valera[28] found that in 44 percent of the patients evaluated, medication (oral hypoglycemic agents) could be reduced or stopped after an average of four counseling sessions over the course of four to six months. In the management of insulin-dependent diabetes mellitus (type I diabetes), the Diabetes Control and Complications Trial clearly demonstrated that MNT is needed in the management of patients to optimize glycemia control.[11,15]

Benefits of MNT in Hyperlipidemia

The benefits of MNT for patients with hypercholesterolemia were reported in a study conducted by the Massachusetts Dietetics Association.[31] In this evaluation, 285 patients were treated with diet alone for cholesterol reduction. Mean serum cholesterol reduction was 8.6 percent, resulting in an estimated reduction of risk for coronary artery disease of 17.2 percent. The researchers concluded that MNT should be utilized as an initial, effective and low-cost approach in the management of patients with mild to moderate hypercholesterolemia.[31]

Patient Outcomes

Assessment of patients' perceptions of nutrition care services and the effect of nutrition on quality of life is a relatively new area in nutrition research and outcomes assessment. One study identified a range of health and nonhealth benefits that patients gained from nutrition counseling including reassurance, sense of control, and relief of symptoms.[20] Nutritional status has been shown to be related to patients' functional status including psychological and cognitive performance, psychosocial status, and activities of daily living.

Patient outcomes are also related to the willingness of individuals and society in general to pay for health care. If it is perceived that improved health outcomes result from nutrition intervention, then individuals and society demand and are willing to pay for these interventions. Demand and willingness to pay diminish, however, if care is perceived to be of poor quality, have little effect, and be of high cost.[47]

PRACTICE GUIDELINES FOR NUTRITION

Necessary and appropriate nutrition care that is available and consistently delivered should lead to positive outcomes for most patients. A way to improve and assure the quality of nutrition care is through the development and use of practice guidelines. Practice guidelines are systematically developed statements or specifications designed to help practitioners and/or patients choose appropriate health care. Practice guidelines define appropriate care under specific situations (e.g., setting and diagnosis). They are based on the best available research and professional judgment and are validated through field testing[15] (see figure 4.8). Practice guidelines are not new to the profession of dietetics. They have been known in the past as quality assurance standards, protocols, or standards of care.[19] In other fields, they are also called clinical practice parameters, and in some settings, they are being applied as critical care maps or clinical pathways.[25] The term "guidelines" reflects their purpose, which is to guide the practitioner rather than to replace professional judgment.

Dietitians and other community nutrition professionals working in MCOs or IDSs will need to increasingly use practice guidelines in delivery of MNT. They can develop practice guidelines specific for their organization or

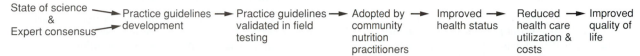

FIGURE 4.8   Process and Potential Result of Developing Practice Guidelines

adapt nationally recognized guidelines such as the practice guidelines for diabetes mellitus[30] or the recommendations of the National Cholesterol Education Program.[32]

The advantages of practice guidelines are as follows:[19]

- They define appropriate care for patients within a specific diagnosis or condition.
- They provide a common language for practitioners to use in providing care and evaluating the patient's response.
- They ensure consistency and thoroughness among providers within a system or within a profession by specifying the type and amount of care and defining data elements (or indicators) necessary for complete assessment of care and its outcomes.
- They identify key information needed in documentation and may lead to the formation of documentation forms or computerized documentation systems.
- They facilitate measurement of outcomes.
- They establish more uniform expectations for payers and primary care physicians so they know what to expect when referred for a particular diagnosis.

In addition, documented use of practice guidelines may be a prerequisite for payment in some settings or managed care plans.

Various dietetic practice groups of the American Dietetic Association (ADA) and other organizations have developed standards of practice or practice guidelines. Some are shown in table 4.2.

ROLE AND RESPONSIBILITY OF COMMUNITY NUTRITION PROFESSIONALS

In all settings, dietitians and other nutrition professionals must develop and deliver interventions and services that are effective, cost-efficient, and accessible. Although many health plan representatives recognize the benefits of MNT, not all are actively seeking to incorporate nutrition screening, assessment, and MNT in their current mix of services. As capitated systems develop, primary care gatekeepers (e.g., physicians and nurse practitioners) are likely to control access to nutrition services; thus, they need tools for screening, guides

for referral, reasonable expectations for the content and outcome of nutrition services, and knowledge of the cost-effectiveness of MNT.[40] Community nutrition professionals must play an active role in developing screening tools and procedures and referral guidelines that can be routinely used by primary care gatekeepers. Further, community nutrition professionals must be available and accessible when needs are identified. To be judged as high quality by physicians, nutrition service must be timely, relevant to the patient's needs, and effective; and the primary provider must be informed as to the progress of the nutrition intervention.[41]

As discussed above, MCOs are beginning to rely on outcomes assessment as a method of evaluating care and making decisions about services offered. Community nutrition professionals must actively assess outcomes among the patient population served and use data to maintain and improve the quality of nutrition care processes.[3]

FUTURE DIRECTIONS FOR COMMUNITY NUTRITION PROFESSIONALS

As the health care system in the United States continues to evolve into a seamless system of managed care, dietitians and other community nutrition professionals must initiate the following actions to ensure the availability of necessary and appropriate nutrition services to patient groups across the continuum of care:

1. Develop, implement, and evaluate practice guidelines for nutrition in all settings.
2. Work as members of multidisciplinary teams to develop critical pathways that define nutrition as an integral step in patient care for persons with specific diagnoses or conditions.
3. Develop relationships with primary physicians and case managers and help them recognize the essential role of nutrition screening, assessment, intervention, and follow-up in clinical preventive services and disease management.
4. Continue to educate health care consumers on the essential nature of nutrition services across the continuum of health care.

TABLE 4.2
Practice Guidelines for Nutrition Care

Standards of Practice

Standards of Practice: Statements of dietetic practitioner's responsibility for providing quality nutrition care. (Standards of Practice for the Profession of Dietetics *J Am Diet Assn.* **1985; 85(6):723–726.)**

Standards of Practice for Gerontological Nutritionists: A Mandate for Action, Gerontological Nutritionists DPG [*J Am Diet Assoc.* 1995; 95(12):1433–1438]

National Standards for Diabetes Self-Management Education, Diabetes Task Force. [*Diabetes Care,* 1995; 95(18): Supplement 1: 94–96]

Standards of Practice Criteria for Clinical Nutrition Managers, Clinical Nutrition Management DPG [*J Am Diet Assoc.,* 1997; 97(6):673–678]

Standards of Practice for the Consultant Dietitian, Consultant Dietitians in Health Care Facilities DPG [*J Am Diet Assoc.,* 1993; 93(3):305–308]

Standards of Practice for the Nutrition Support Dietitian, Dietitians in Nutrition Support DPG (Joint Project with A.S.P.E.N.). [*J Am Diet Assoc.,* 1993; 93(1):1113–1116]

Standards of Practice for the Profession of Dietetics. [*J Am Diet Assoc.,* 1985; 85(6):723–726]. Revision approved 1996; to be submitted to the *J Am Diet Assoc.,* 1998]

Practice Guidelines

Practice Guidelines: Systematically developed statements or specifications designed to help practitioners and/or patients/clients choose appropriate health care in "typical" clinical or foodservice systems circumstances. ADA (adapted from the Agency for Health Care Policy and Research)

Nutrition Practice Guidelines for Dysphagia Dietetics in Physical Medicine & Rehabilitation DPG [ADA © 1996]*

Nutrition Practice Guidelines for Gestational Diabetes Mellitus Diabetes Care & Education and Perinatal Nutrition DPGs. [Approved March 1997, expected publication January 1999].

Professional Performance Standards for Gerontological Dietitians Practicing in Specific Settings, project alliance with the Administration on Aging. [Approved June 1996; in progress]

Practice Guidelines for the Care of Renal Patients (Third Edition), Renal Dietitians DPG [Approved June 1996, in progress].*

Guidelines of Practice for Dysphagia in Rehabilitation. Dietetics in Physical Medicine and Rehabilitation DPG [ADA, © 1996].*

Nutrition Practice Guidelines for Type I & Type II Diabetes Mellitus, Diabetes Care & Education DPG [ADA © 1996].*

Practice Guidelines for Medical Nutrition Therapy Provided by Dietitians for Persons with Non-Insulin-Dependent Diabetes Mellitus (Joint Project with IDC), Diabetes Care & Education DPG [*J Am Diet Assoc.,* 1995; 95(9):999–1006].

Suggested Guidelines for Nutrition and Metabolic Management of Adult Patients Receiving Nutrition Support, Dietitians in Nutrition Support DPG [ADA, © 1993].*

Suggested Guidelines for Nutrition Care of Renal Patients (Second Edition), Renal Dietitians DPG [ADA, © 1992]*

Indicators, Protocols & Other QI Projects

Medical Nutrition Therapy Protocols: Protocols clearly define the level, content, and frequency of nutrition care that is appropriate for the disease or condition. Reimbursement and Insurance Coverage for Nutrition Services © 1991 ADA. Indicators: A quantitative measure used to measure and improve performance of functions, processes, and outcomes. *LEXIKON, Dictionary of Health Care Terms, Organizations, and Acronyms for the Era of Reform JCAHO © 1994.*

Patient Acuity Clinical Staffing Study, Clinical Nutrition Management DPG [Approved April 1997, *J Am Diet Assoc.,* 1997].

Clinical Benchmarking Survey, Clinical Nutrition Management DPG. [Approved April 1997; (in progress).

Documenting Nutrition Care: Are We Prepared for our Future Practice? Clinical Nutrition Management DPG and Dietitians in Nutrition Support DPG. [Approved December 1994, expected publication *J Am Diet Assoc.,* 1997].

Enteral Practitioner Cards, Dietitians in General Clinical Practice DPG. [Approved 1996; in progress].

Parenteral Practitioners Cards, Dietitians in General Clinical Practice DPG [ADA & Mead Johnson 1997].*

Medical Nutrition Therapy Across the Continuum of Care. (Joint Project with Morrison Health Care Inc.), Diabetes Care and Education, Oncology Nutrition, Perinatal Nutrition, Renal Nutrition and HIV/AIDS [ADA © 1996]. Includes 12 adult ambulatory based MNT protocols:

Cancer (medical, radiation oncology), Chronic Obstructive Pulmonary Disease, High-risk Prenatal Care, Hypertension, Pre-End-Stage Renal Disease, Diabetes Mellitus (gestational, insulin-dependent, non-insulin dependent) Hyperlipidemia, Irritable Bowel Syndrome, HIV/AIDS.

Supplement to Medical Nutrition Therapy Across the Continuum of Care, (Joint Project with Morrison Health Care Inc.), Consultant Dietitians in Health Care Facilities DPG, Pediatric Nutrition DPG, Perinatal Nutrition DPG, and Dietitians in Nutrition Support DPG. [ADA October 1997].* Includes 9 additional MNT protocols for various age groups and settings: Anorexia and Bulimia Nervosa/Adolescent and Adult, Congestive Heart Failure/Adults, Enteral Feeding Support/Adults, Hyperemesis Gravidarum/Adults, Parenteral (PEN) Feeding Support/Adults, Pediatric Failure to Thrive (0–7 years), Pressure Ulcer/Older Adults, Prevention of Unintentional Weight Loss/Older Adults, Weight Management/Adults.

Clinical Indicators Associated with Unintentional Weight Loss and Pressure Ulcers in Elderly Residents of Nursing Facilities, Consultant Dietitians in Health Care Facilities DPG and Dietitians in Nutrition Support DPG [*J Am Diet Assoc.,* 1995; 95(9):984–992].

Clinical Indicator Workbook for Nutrition Care Systems, The Quality Management Committee [ADA © 1994].*

Clinical Indicators for Oncology, Cardiovascular and Surgical Patients, [*J Am Diet Assoc.,* 1993; 93(3):338–344].

Quality Assurance Criteria Sets for Pediatric Nutrition Conditions (Includes supplements), Pediatric Nutrition Practice Group [ADA © 1988, 1990, 1993].*

Guidelines for a Standard Documentation System for Clinical Dietitians, Dietitians in Nutrition Support and Clinical Nutrition Management DPGs [Approved 1994; in progress].

From *Current ADA and DPG quality improvement projects,* Chicago, 1997, The American Dietetic Association.

5. Implement internal outcomes assessment and performance improvement programs for all nutrition services.
6. Use clinical outcomes assessment data to evaluate and report the effectiveness of MNT.
7. Determine the cost-effectiveness of MNT.
8. Communicate the importance of MNT as a cost-effective intervention to MCOs and IDSs.
9. Influence decision makers to include nutrition screening, assessment, and MNT in managed care plans.
10. Establish nutrition services and nutrition indicators as a component of utilization review and performance improvement efforts.

IMPLICATIONS FOR COMMUNITY NUTRITION PROFESSIONALS

The health care delivery system traditionally placed greater emphasis on the medical model and disease treatment rather than on community-based primary and preventive health care. The disease-oriented system is no longer considered by policy makers and the American public to be the ideal model for organizing and providing health care services. The catalyst behind the shift is the dissatisfaction with the traditional system and the problems of cost, access to care, and quality. To control costs, Medicare and Medicaid, the two largest health care programs, must be integrated into the changing paradigm of health care delivery. The lack of health insurance and the cost of health care has made health care services inaccessible to millions of Americans. Appropriateness, effectiveness, and quality care are criteria for a sound health care system.

To balance cost, access, and quality, a new system based on managed care has evolved. Throughout the United States, health care organizations are restructuring and reinventing themselves as broad-based integrated delivery systems. These systems include primary care, wellness, home health, long-term care, and hospice care as well as hospital care and specialty clinics. The changes occurring within the health care system provide an opportunity to reassess and reorient the relationship between the public and private sectors. The history of separation between public health and private medicine has not maximized the health of U.S. citizens. Public health has provided health care to vulnerable populations through community and neighborhood health centers, migrant health services, Indian health services, school health, rural health, maternal and child health, family planning clinics, and the military health care system. In the new system, there are many opportunities for the public and private sectors to work in an integrated and coordinated system.

Nutrition care is an essential service in all health care settings. Nutrition services include screening, assessment, selection and implementation of appropriate nutrition care interventions, referrals, and follow-up. With appropriate intervention, patients should experience improved nutrient intakes, which lead to changes in intermediate outcomes of biochemical or physiological indicators. Clinical effectiveness is achieved when the preventive or the therapeutic nutrition intervention has the desired impact on the disease state or condition. Practice guidelines have been developed for the profession of dietetics. They define appropriate care under specific conditions. In all settings, community nutrition professionals must develop and deliver intervention services that are effective, cost-effective, and accessible.

COMMUNITY NUTRITION PROFESSIONALS IN ACTION

Questions for investigation and discussion.

- If you had a need for health services for yourself where would you go? What choices do you have? Are the services you need conveniently located? How easy is it to access specialized help for a specific problem? How would the costs be paid? Are you uninsured, covered by an indemnity plan, or covered by a capitated health plan? Are you required to pay a deductible or co-payment?
- What kind of health insurance policy does your family have? How has that changed over the years?
- How satisfied were you with your last experience in the health care system as a patient or as a visitor? How do you judge quality as a patient? If you were director of a managed care organization, how would you measure quality?

Projects.

- Collect information about the major health care delivery systems in your area. Are comprehensive services available across the continuum of care? What components of the continuum of care are part of a network or integrated delivery system? What is the level of evolution toward managed care in your area?

- Interview dietitians in each of the major health care systems in your area to explore issues related to the cost, access, and quality of nutrition services. Are essential nutrition services available for disease management and clinical preventive services? To what degree are hospital and clinic nutrition services linked with other components of the continuum of care? Is there continuity of nutrition care from the hospital to home health care, for example? What protocols or practice guidelines for nutrition care are in use?
- Contact your state or local dietetic association to identify the nutrition services payment system contact person. Meet with this person to explore avenues for payment of nutrition services in your state.
- Select one of the following (child with cystic fibrosis, high-risk pregnancy, elderly person with advanced rheumatoid arthritis, adult with angina and eventual myocardial infarction, failure-to-thrive infant, person with HIV/AIDS, healthy adult interested in staying well) and track a person with that disease or condition through the health care system across settings and over time. Find out where nutrition-related needs are identified and addressed over the course of the disease or condition.

GOING ONE STEP FURTHER

- Outline basic nutrition services that should be available in clinical preventive services and disease management. Prepare this as a protocol that could guide the actions of primary care gatekeepers.
- Design the plans for an ideal, seamless system to assure essential and appropriate nutrition services are available to all persons in a health care system.
- Prepare a presentation to introduce the plan to the top leadership of a managed care organization.
- Review the literature on the scientific bases for clinical outcomes of nutrition services in a specific disease or condition. Summarize your findings to be submitted to decision makers in the HCFA, which sets policy for Medicare, or your state Medicaid agency.
- Critique an existing set of practice guidelines for nutrition care. Do the guidelines identify when a primary care provider should refer the patient to a dietitian or community nutrition professional? Do the guidelines foster continuity of nutrition care across settings and over time? Revise the guidelines, as necessary, to assure access and quality in a managed care environment.

- Investigate the success of available health care systems in meeting the needs of vulnerable populations in your area. What changes would you propose to assure that all people have access to appropriate and affordable health and nutrition care?

ADDITIONAL INFORMATION

Professional societies develop statements, scientific status summaries, commentaries, and position papers to clarify an issue in which the particular society has expertise.

The American Dietetic Association position statements relevant to chapter 4 are as follows:

1. Cost-effectiveness of medical nutrition therapy (*J Am Diet Assoc* 95:88, 1995)
2. Nutrition services in managed care (*J Am Diet Assoc* 96:391, 1996)
3. Management of health care food and nutrition services (J *Am Diet Assoc* 93:914, 1993)
4. Nutrition monitoring of the home parenteral and enteral patient (*J Am Diet Assoc* 94:664, 1994)

REFERENCES

1. American Association of Health Plans HMO Fact Sheet: Washington DC, 1995.
2. The American Dietetic Association Council on Practice Quality Management Committee: ADA's definitions for nutrition screening and nutrition assessment, *J Am Diet Assoc* 94:838–839, 1994.
3. The American Dietetic Association and Ross Products Division of Abbott Laboratories: *Nutrition intervention and patient outcomes: a self-study manual,* Columbus, OH, 1995, Ross Products Division of Abbott Laboratories.
4. American Hospital Association, *1994 annual survey,* Chicago, 1995, American Hospital Association.
5. Bagby M: *Annual report of the USA: Social state of the union,* New York, 1996, Harpers Business.
6. Baker EL, Melton RJ, Stange PL, Fields ML, Koplan JP, Guerra FA, Satcher, D. Health reform and the health of the public: forging community health partnerships, JAMA 272:16, 1994.
7. *Basic statistics about home care 1995,* Washington DC, 1995, National Association for Home Care.
8. Brief summaries of Title XVIII and Title XIX of the Social Security Act, Washington DC, 1995, Health Care Financing Administration.
9. Congressional Budget Office 1995 Social State of the Nation: Fiscal Year 1996 Budget of U.S. Government, Washington DC.

10. COSSMHO: *Delivering preventive health care to Hispanics: a manual for providers,* Washington DC, 1990, National Coalition of Hispanic Health and Human Service Organizations.

11. DCCT Research Group: Expanded role of the dietitian in the Diabetes Control and Complications Trial: implications for clinical practice, *J Am Diet Assoc* 93:758–764, 1993.

12. Dwyer WM: National health care outlook: strategic grand rounds, Abbott Park, IL, 1995, Abbott Laboratories.

13. Escott-Stump, S: *Nutrition and diagnosis-related care,* 4th ed. Williams and Wilkins, 1997.

14. Finn SC: President's page. Standards, guidelines and indications position dietitians for competitive advantage, *J Am Diet Assoc* 93:1173–1174, 1993.

15. Franz M, Splett PL, Monk A: Cost-effectiveness of medical nutrition therapy provided by dietitians for persons with non-insulin dependent diabetes mellitus, *J Am Diet Assoc* 95:1018–1024, 1995.

16. Freymann JG: The public's health care paradigm is shifting: medicine must swing with it, *J Gen Intern Med* 4:313–319, 1989.

17. *The fundamentals of managed care,* Washington, DC, 1991, Health Insurance Association of America.

18. Gallagher-Allred CR, Voss AC, Finn SC, McCamish MA: Malnutrition and clinical outcomes: the case for medical nutrition therapy, *J Am Diet Assoc* 96:361–369, 1996.

19. Harritz MR, Johnson EQ: Devaluation in the 21st century: the impact of health care reform, *Clin Nutr* 11:27–32, 1996.

20. Hauchecorne CM, Barr SI, Sork TJ: Evaluation of nutrition counseling in clinical settings: do we make a difference? *J Am Diet Assoc* 95:437–440, 1994.

21. Health care, *Social Security Bulletin* 57(Suppl):83–102, 1994.

22. *Healthy people 2000: national health promotion and disease prevention objectives,* DHHS (PHS) publication no. 91–50213, Washington, DC, 1990, U.S. Department of Health and Human Services.

23. Hicks LL, Bopp KD: Integrated pathways for managing rural health services, *Health Care Manage Rev* 21:65–72, 1996.

24. *Hospice facts and statistics,* Washington, DC, 1996, Hospice Association of America.

25. Incorporating nutrition care into critical pathways for improved outcomes, Gaithersburg, Md., 1994, Ross Products Division, Abbott Laboratories.

26. Institute of Medicine: *Focusing on quality in a changing health care system,* Washington, DC, 1997, National Academy of Sciences.

27. Institute of Medicine: *Primary care: America's health in a new era,* Washington, DC, 1997, National Academy Press.

28. Johnson EQ, Valera S: Medical nutrition therapy in non-insulin dependent diabetes mellitus improves clinical outcomes, *J Am Diet Assoc* 95:700–701, 1995.

29. Kivlahan C: Missouri carves out public health to safeguard Medicaid population during shift to managed care, *State Health Watch* 2:12, 1995.

30. Kulkarni K, Castle G, Gregory R, Holmes A, Leontos C, Powers M, Snetselaar L, Splett P, Wylie-Rosett J: Nutrition Practice Guidelines for Type I Diabetes Mellitus positively affect dietitian practices and patient outcomes. *J Am Diet Assoc* 98:62–70, 1998.

31. McGee M, Johnson EQ, Rasmussen HM, Sahyoun N, Lynch MM, Carey H and Mass. Dietetic Assoc: Massachusetts Dietetic Association. Benefits and costs of medical nutrition therapy by registered dietitians for patients with hypercholesterolemia, *J Am Diet Assoc* 95:1040–1043, 1995.

32. MHLBI. Second report of the Expert Panel on Detection, Evaluation, and Treatment of High Blood Cholesterol in Adults (Adult Treatment Panel II) Public Health Service, NIH Pub. No. 93–3095, Washington, DC, 1993.

33. The national health. APHA policy paper: public health services and managed care. In *The Nation's Health,* Washington, DC, 1996, American Public Health Association.

34. HEDIS 3.0 Reporting Measures National Committee for Quality Assurance (NC2A) Washington DC, 1996.

35. Oswald JW: Quality assurance and epidemiology in the third era of managed health care, *Learning Resources Journal* (February)11: 1995.

36. Partners for Better Health: "HealthPartners" Report of a conference "Americans simply can't go on living like this." Health Futures Institute, *Minn MN* Vol 2. No 12 pg 5&6.

37. Pew Health Professions Commission: *Critical challenges: revitalizing the health care professions for the twenty-first century,* San Francisco, CA, 1995, UCSF Center for the Health Professions.

38. Position of the American Dietetic Association. Cost-effectiveness of medical nutrition therapy, *J Am Diet Assoc* 95:88–91, 1995.

39. Position of the American Dietetic Association. The role of nutrition in health promotion and disease prevention programs, *J Am Diet Assoc* 98:205–208, 1998.

40. Position of the American Dietetic Association: Nutrition services in managed care, *J Am Diet Assoc* 96:391–395, 1996.

41. Reinhardt M. Splett PL: Physician's expectations for quality nutrition expertise and services, *J Am Diet Assoc* 94:1375–1380, 1994.

42. Report of the US Preventive Services Task Force: *Guide to clinical preventive services,* ed 2, Baltimore, MD, 1996, Williams & Wilkins, pp. 625–634.

43. Roos NP, Shapiro E, Tate R: Does a small minority of elderly account for a majority of health care expenditures? A sixteen year perspective, *Milbank* 68:347–369, 1990.

44. Shortell SM, Gillies RR, Anderson DA: The new world of managed care: Creating organized delivery systems, *Health Affairs* 13:46–64, 1994.

45. Social Security programs in the US, *Social Security Bulletin* 56:3–82, 1993.
46. Southby RF: Military health care in the 21st century, *Mil Med* 158:637–640, 1993.
47. Splett PL: *Cost outcomes of nutrition intervention. Outcome research* (Part 1 of 3-part monograph), Evansville, IN, 1996, Mead Johnson.
48. Splett PL: Effectiveness and cost-effectiveness of nutrition care: a critical analysis with recommendations, *J Am Diet Assoc* 91(Suppl):S7–S50, 1991.
49. Starfield B: Public health and primary care: a framework for proposed linkages, *Am J Public Health* 86:1365–1369, 1996.
50. *Today's nursing homes and the people they serve: facts and trends: 1994,* Washington, DC, 1994, American Health Care Association.
51. Turner MA, Dwyer JT: Nutrition measures for managed care report cards, *J Am Diet Assoc* 96:374–380, 1996.
52. Webber CB, Splett PL. Nutrition risk factors in a home health population. *Home Health Care Service Quarterly* 1995, 15(3):97–110.
53. Weiss B: Managed care: there's no stopping it now, *Medical Economics* 13:26–28, 31–34, 36, 43, 1995.
54. Wright, RA: Community-oriented primary care: the cornerstone of health care reform, *JAMA* 269:2544–2547, 1993.

CASE STUDY

QUALITY AND CONTINUITY OF NUTRITION CARE

SUSAN FINN, PHD, RD, DIRECTOR OF NUTRITION SERVICES, ROSS LABORATORIES, COLUMBUS OHIO

This case illustrates the importance of establishing nutrition practice guidelines that transcend acute care and community-based components of the health care system. When hospital patients are discharged, steps should be taken to assure continuity of care. A smooth transition is possible when providers in separate parts of the health care delivery system have similar guidelines. This is important whether the providers are operating under the traditional model of medical care or are part of an integrated delivery system within a mature managed care environment.

The main question in this case study concerns assurance of quality nutrition care when patients on specialized nutrition support are discharged from the hospital to community-based care. The case study can be used for general class discussion or as the basis for a student project (individual or team). It illustrates principles of quality improvement, outcomes assessment, and practice guidelines.

SCENARIO

Mary Beth Hart is a registered dietitian working as coordinator of a hospital nutrition support team. The hospital's nutrition services, including nutrition screening, assessment, therapy plans, and selective use of enteral and parenteral nutrition support, have a reputation of being successful in identifying patients at nutritional risk and intervening early to reduce complications and shorten length of hospital stay.

After two weeks of home enteral nutrition support, one of the nutrition support team's patients, Mr. James, was readmitted with weight loss and dehydration. Mr. James was not the first patient on home enteral feeding to return to the hospital with these problems. Mary Beth suspected that something was going wrong after stabilized enterally fed patients were discharged to home care. Since she has been following developments in home care over the past year, Mary Beth knows this is a growing component of the health care system and an emerging area of nutrition practice. Clarifying and correcting the problem now could prevent more extensive problems and associated costs in the future.

The home care agency to which the hospital refers is a part of the managed care organization's network of providers. The agency includes nutrition in its services and is accredited by the Joint Commission on Accreditation of Healthcare Organizations (JCAHO). Consequently, even though the home care agency does not employ any nutrition professionals at this time, to be accredited it must meet certain nutrition care standards such as conducting nutrition screening to identify individuals at high risk and developing a multidisciplinary care plan for those individuals, including measurable goals, interventions, and time frames.

To assure quality nutrition care for patients, Mary Beth believes it is desirable to strengthen the link between the hospital's nutrition support team and the home care agency. This could help assure patients' nutritional needs continue to be met when they are discharged to other components of the health care network. This approach is supported by the hospital's mission and that of the managed care organization, which both reflect commitment to quality, cost-effective services, and continuity of care for patients.

All members of the nutrition support team were concerned about Mr. James and were interested in the outcomes of other patients who were discharged with enteral or parenteral feedings. In the course of their discussion, some inconsistencies in the team's understanding of home nutrition support emerged. The team decided to initiate an outcomes assessment to look at clinical outcomes, readmission rates, and patient satisfaction.

They planned an audit of medical records of all nutrition support patients discharged to home-based enteral or parenteral feeding in the last year, and conducted a telephone survey to determine their current status. The results of the medical record review are pending. However, in the telephone survey, patients and their caretakers told about their anxiety at home and how it took several days before they understood how to operate the equipment and use the formula.

Mary Beth wanted to know more about the experience of other nutrition professionals in home nutrition support. She posed a question about guidelines and practices used in home nutrition support to her colleagues using a nutrition support bulletin board she subscribes to. She was not surprised to uncover a wide range of recommendations and guidelines for home enteral and parenteral feeding. One problem emphasized by many bulletin board respondents was a gap in appropriate education materials and guidelines suitable for patient and caretaker use. Another problem was the lack of community nutrition professionals with expertise in nutrition support.

Based on this information Mary Beth recommended a formal review of the hospital's guidelines for discharge of patients on enteral and parenteral feedings. In planning for this home care project she invited representatives from the home care agencies and other hospitals in the network.

When the group met, Mary Beth shared the data she had gathered. The group decided to divide the task of searching for and reviewing information on nutrition support in community-based settings. They planned to specifically look at procedures necessary for successful transition to home-based nutrition support including recommendations and instructions for patients and caretakers. This new home care project group set goals and outlined a plan of work.

QUESTIONS

1. What are the goals of the new group?
2. As the group leader, what steps should Mary Beth expect in the process of developing practice guidelines that assure conformity of care from hospital to home for patients on nutrition support?
3. How could an outcomes assessment be helpful to the deliberations of the group? What other information do they need? Where should they look for information?
4. What actions might be taken among all parties to assure quality nutrition care?
5. What performance measures could be used to track quality of nutrition support in hospitals and home care agencies?
6. In a time of lean operations and tight budgets, how can the nutrition support team use the home care project to enhance its image and keep its visibility in the managed care organization high?
7. How can the home care project experience be used to build and integrate other essential nutrition services into the continuum of care?

CHAPTER FIVE

THE DYNAMICS OF PUBLIC POLICY

*If it is true that knowledge culminates in politics, it is rarely
good that scholars end up as politicians.*
—Jacques deGoff

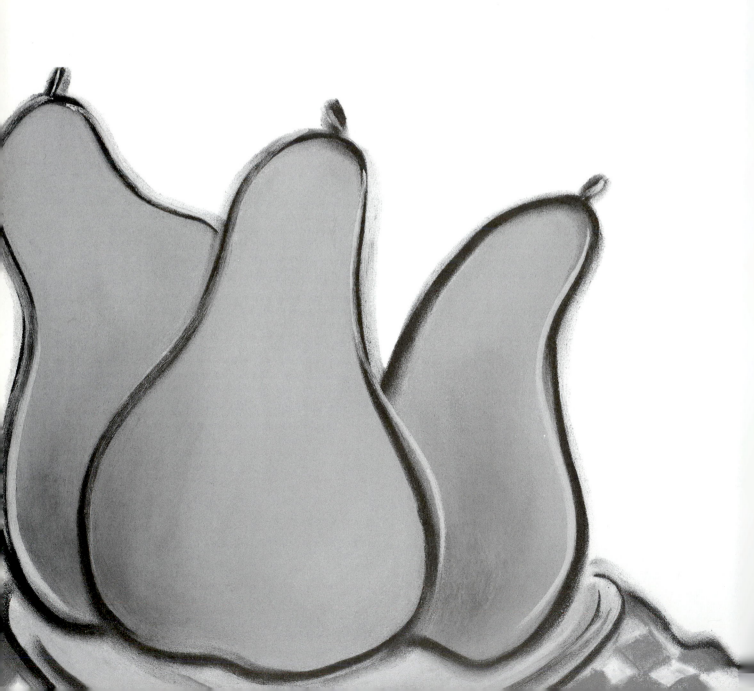

Core Concepts

Nutrition policy influences nearly all programs and services offered by nutrition professionals who practice in the community. Therefore, community nutrition professionals must be familiar with the issues and the public policy process to provide leadership and direction to both the types of nutrition programs that are funded and to the nature of professional practice and services offered in those programs.

Objectives

When you finish chapter five, you should be able to:

~ Define public policy and discuss its importance in the field of community nutrition.

~ Describe the policymaking process and steps at which informed advocacy on the part of community nutrition professionals can be effective.

~ Compare and contrast the functions of the legislative, executive, and judicial branches of government in the policymaking process.

~ Describe the major elements in nutrition, the programs now in existence, and the political and economic forces that may cause them to change in the future.

~ Develop advocacy skills needed to shape public policy dealing with nutrition issues.

Key Words

Word	Page Mentioned
Public policy	116
Policy	116
Nutrition policy	116
Problem recognition	116
Agenda setting	116
Policy formulation	118
Policy implementation	118
Policy evaluation	119
Bills	119
Law	119
Rules	119
Legislative process	119
Hearings	121
Budget process	122
Entitlement	122
Regulatory process	123
Food security	125

UNDERSTANDING PUBLIC
AND NUTRITION POLICY

Community nutrition professionals often ask why they need to know about **public policy** and how they can influence it. After all, they say, we practice in a clinic setting where we provide patient counseling and talk to groups about changing their diets in a more healthful way. What does this have to do with public policy? *Absolutely everything*! The nature of the nutrition message, how services are delivered, and the types of programs and services with which community nutrition professionals are involved are all shaped by public policy decisions.

Policy statements set the general tone for how an agency, group, or even government operates. Policies provide guidelines for setting priorities among competing goals, the allocation of funds, selection of personnel, standards for program operation, and future direction. *Public policy is simply what government does.*

Nutrition policy is commonly assumed to be synonymous with food and agricultural policy. This conceptual pairing was fostered in the language of the 1977 Farm Bill, which gave "lead agency" responsibility for nutrition research to U.S. Department of Agriculture (USDA). The view that "nutrition policy is food policy" is changing. Indeed, events outside the policy arena, such as in the media, advertising, and the public's demand for certain food products, have influenced the nutrition policy agenda. Health policy, especially that portion that addresses disease prevention and health promotion, regards dietary guidance as an essential component of its programs. Also in the late 1970s, there was a push to develop and implement a comprehensive, coordinated national nutrition policy; however, none has yet evolved. Thus, at present, nutrition policy can be regarded as a collective set of government actions in a number of separate arenas resulting in a number of distinct food, health, and social programs. Nutrition policy exists as a nexus among other policies—agricultural, health, medical, social, economic, educational, and environmental—each of which is the product of its own set of external influences, directives, actors, and infrastructures.[35]

The Public Policy Process

The policy process has been described as *how* public problems are acted on by government. The process of policymaking is actually a very dynamic one in which a number of participants—including influential organizations, interest groups, and legislators—work toward attaining mutually satisfactory goals by compromise and consensus.

The policy process can be viewed as a series of stages, as illustrated in Figure 5.1. The following discussion identifies each of these stages in terms of the actors involved and the nature of the policy process at each stage. Further, how government institutions interact with forces outside the government (such as interest groups and influential parties) at each stage as they formulate or change policy is described. This process influences the context of health and affects the health and nutritional well-being of the population.

Stage I: Problem Recognition   The development of a public policy begins with **problem recognition,** that is, with public realization that a problem exists. This situation exists when some undesirable social condition exists but has not yet captured much public attention, even though some experts or interest groups may already be alarmed by it. Ethical and ideological perspectives play an important role during this first stage, because groups with different perspectives will see and define problems differently. The media have often been instrumental in bringing public attention to problems defined by professionals and are useful at this stage for galvanizing public interest in the problem. If the public becomes convinced that a problem exists, it will more often generate attention from public officials. To put all views in the proper context, specific information should be gathered: data or results drawn from scientific research studies, social indicators such as demographic changes and trends, and results of program evaluations or demonstration projects. A sound knowledge base is important at this stage to document the nature and the extent of the problem.

But what if the evidence gathered is less than complete? When do we know *enough* to proceed? Chapter 19 reviews the criteria to guide ethical decisions related to policymaking.

Stage II: Agenda Setting   The process by which issues successfully compete for governmental attention is called **agenda setting.** Even if it is recognized a problem exists, this is not enough to ensure it will be placed on the policy agenda. At least two other conditions must be met: the political circumstances must be right, and significant political actors must back placement of the issue on the policy agenda. A supportive political climate is necessary to convince officials to take ownership of the problem and share in the goals for setting policy.

In the process of agenda setting, the policymakers act as gatekeepers, deciding which items go into the

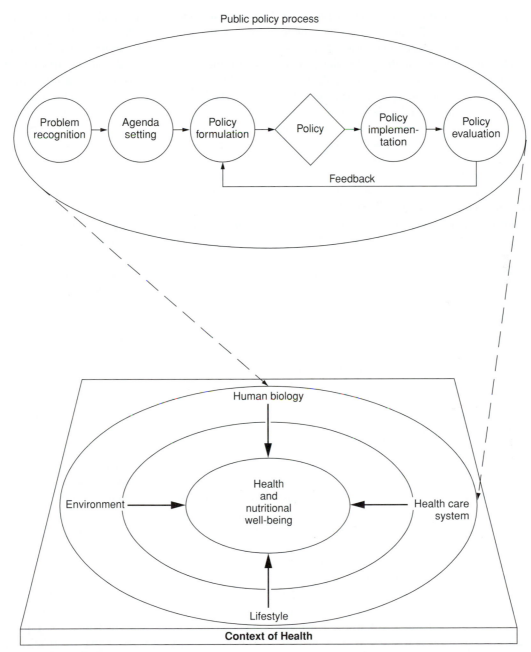

FIGURE 5.1   Context of Health
How the policy process affects nutrition and health policy.

agenda and which do not. Moving an issue onto the public agenda may be the most difficult aspect of achieving policy change. An issue may be so sensitive that policymakers or public attitudes work to keep it from reaching the agenda setting stage. In other situations, an issue may be perceived as a problem by only a small number of people who lack the political influence to get the issue onto the institutional agenda. Yet in other circumstances, the process may take place quickly. For example, major catastrophes such as an earthquake, riot, famine, or an unusual human event may trigger public outcry to such an extent that the issue is pushed almost effortlessly onto the policy agenda.

Stage III: Policy Formulation   To reach the point of stating the preferred choice of action surrounding public interest, an issue is further defined, additional information about the problem is collected and discussed, and alternative solutions are considered throughout the **policy formulation** stage of the policymaking. With the input of interest groups, policy experts, and constituents, decision makers debate alternative policy formulations, select an alternative or a combination of alternatives, and respond to the problem.

Unmistakably, public policy is shaped by groups who attempt to influence the form, pace, or direction of policymaking for their own interests. The business of policymaking often involves an ongoing struggle among conflicting values, vested interests, and ambitious personalities. Even when interested parties share the same lofty goals, effective negotiation and trade-off skills are needed to construct functional policy. A complex balancing act is required to satisfy consumers' concerns, industry interests, scientific principles, and budget realities.[5] Members of the nutrition community must be prepared to work with other professional organizations and interest groups with related agendas that, together with policy makers, can develop a set of workable, coordinated policy guidelines.

The political atmosphere must be receptive to a cause before it can gain approval from legislators. Nutrition rarely appears as a separate issue. Improved nutrition and other food issues are often linked with other political concerns such as health care reform, welfare reform, the economic security of farmers, or even national defense. Further, the voting public must view the issue as important. Politicians must perceive that there is sufficient public sentiment in favor of a cause before they will support it.

A good example of this dynamic occurred in 1995 when the Republicans gained leadership in both houses of Congress for the first time in forty years. One of the first actions taken in the House of Representatives was introduction of the Personal Responsibility Act, which targeted food assistance programs for massive budget cuts. Federal funding was to be replaced by a system of discretionary block grants to the states.

Many considered block granting of the Food Stamp Program a sure thing. After all, proponents explained, those closest to the problem could better identify how to administer it and design it to serve the truly needy. As discussions wore on, the advocacy community used the media to help spread the notion that block grants were nothing more than "a mean-spirited, hard-hearted policy to take food from children and poor families."[21]

Public sentiment waned, and block grants faded as an option for dealing with the Food Stamp Program.

The block grant concept never gained momentum because the states and local communities recognized the benefits they received from existing programs. They already had management control, and did not need block grants for that purpose. Instead, state and local government leaders began to see that if they were recipients of block grants, they would then be blamed for cutting food programs among their own constituencies. State and local governments said "no thanks" to congressional leaders, and many state and local political leaders quietly urged Congress to keep the programs as currently structured.

In summary, the policy formulation stage results in *policy*. This can come in the form of legislation (usually), regulations, executive orders, or policy statements. Although policy can assume any number of forms, it must be publicly exhibited, and articulated to be valid.

Stage IV: Policy Implementation   At this stage, decisions arrived at by policy makers must be acted on. The implementation process involves writing regulations, spending money, enforcing laws, hiring employees, and formulating plans of action. The implementers of public policy in the United States include employees of federal, state, and local governments who work with private organizations, interest groups, volunteers, and other parties to carry out government policy.

What happens at this stage is affected by numerous elements. Even seemingly simple programs can be difficult to implement if there are too many participants with differing perspectives, and if numerous decisions have to be made before the policy is fully implemented. One example involves the wording of public laws or decisions. Laws enacted by Congress and signed by the president are often vaguely worded as a result of the bargaining and negotiation that may have been necessary to get a majority to support the bill. This results in a document with unclear guidelines for implementation. Other problems may also exist. Insufficient resources may have been appropriated for program implementation; two or more agencies may have been given authority for implementation; or an agency charged with implementing a given policy may be hostile to it, and end up undermining implementation of the program.

Policy implementation includes outputs and impacts. *Policy outputs* are what governments do in a particular policy area. The policy outputs of the Food Stamp Program include the moneys spent, coupons printed, poor persons served, and personnel hired. *Policy impacts* (also called policy outcomes) are the effects that policy outputs have on society. For the Food Stamp Program, major impacts include the total amount of money spent by a family on food, or changes in recipients' diets.

Stage V: Policy Evaluation We usually equate policy success or failure with the observed performance and consequences of that policy. Evaluation attempts to assess how policy effects society compared to intended goals. It asks whether the goals have or have not been met, with what costs, and with what unintended consequences. It considers whether policy is equitable and efficient, and whether it has satisfied the interests of those who demanded action in the first place.

Because evaluation is part of the policymaking cycle, it can be viewed both politically and technically. Evaluation is political because those people who support a policy or program are likely to believe it has succeeded, whereas those who are ideologically opposed are likely to conclude that the program has failed. Evaluation also has a technical component because it involves a formal, institutionalized process that draws on scientific principles and both qualitative and quantitative methods to help policy makers make good decisions about what has and what has not worked. It is important, however, that understanding the facts empirically must precede judgment about whether or not a program will continue. **Policy evaluation** therefore must be accompanied by empirical analysis of policy content. Such data (and conclusions reached from such analyses) are often used by congressional committees as they exercise their charge to perform program oversight and provide feedback for those who seek to change or modify existing policy.

The Special Supplemental Nutrition Program for Women, Infants and Children (WIC), for example, has been evaluated thoroughly for both program efficiency and effectiveness. Written into enabling legislation were requirements for substantive data collection, such as heights, weights, infants' head circumferences, and measures of iron status, which were not only a means for assessing recipients' eligibility but were useful indicators to evaluate cost-benefits of the program. The General Accounting Office (GAO) used these measures as well as infant birth weights to conclude that WIC was a very cost-effective program; for every federal dollar spent, between $2.89 and $3.50 was saved throughout the child's first 18 years of life.[12]

This is the rational, "ideal" model for policymaking. All too often, however, policymaking depends on the raw emotions of policy makers and those who seek to influence the process. Policymaking is about bringing together individuals and groups (including the media) who want to work together to change the status quo. For the nutrition community, it means bringing together forces that have the time, resources, expertise, and intensity to work on public issues that will improve the nutritional status of the American population.

THE WORK OF GOVERNMENT

Congress, the president, and the judiciary perform most of the policy functions of formulation, implementation, and interpretation. Laws that initiate, modify, authorize, and appropriate funds for all programs and services administered by the federal government are passed by Congress, the principal arm of the legislative branch. Congress is composed of 100 senators and 435 representatives who have been elected in their own geographic district. Each member of the House represents an average of 500,000 people. Two senators are elected from each state for six-year terms.

Legislatures often assume three roles: a law-making role, a representative role, and a constituency service role. In the United States, these sometimes conflicting roles are all the responsibility of members of Congress.

Making Laws

Of the several thousand **bills** introduced during the two years of a Congress, only a small handful ever become **law.** For example, during the 103rd Congress from January 1993 to December 1994, only 577 of the 9,822 bills introduced actually were passed by Congress, and signed into law by the president.[7]

Because of the volume of work, and the potential for chaos in such a large legislative body, certain rules and procedures influence the process. Political party leadership, the committee structure, and procedural **rules** all greatly affect legislative affairs. Thus, the chances of any particular piece of legislation being passed do not depend solely on the number of members who support it. The ability of a bill's sponsors to propel it through complicated committee and floor procedures and their expertise in the topic of the bill are both important in ensuring passage.[1]

The general sequence of stages or steps through which a bill passes on its way to becoming a law are shown in figure 5.2.[8] Actually, all steps can be recombined into six major phases as indicated below.[6] Concerned professionals can take appropriate actions if they know the steps in the **legislative process,** as well as the

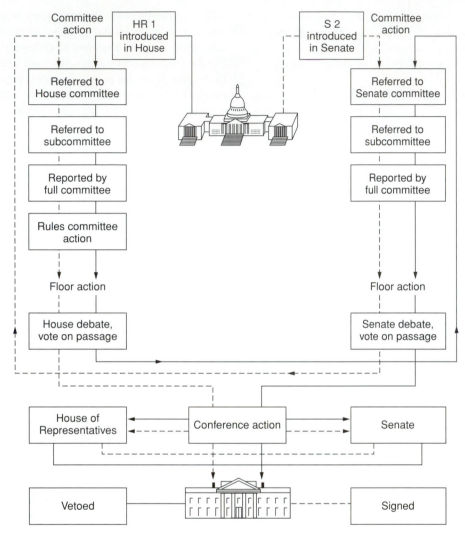

FIGURE 5.2   How a Bill Becomes a Law
(*Source:* From Wormser MD, editor, *CQ's guide to congress,* ed 4, Washington, DC, 1996,
Congressional Quarterly, Inc.)

key decision makers and their responsibilities at each
step of the process. Appendix C identifies Internet sites
of Congress and important legislative resources to assist the community nutrition professional.

Introduction   The bill is introduced in either the
House or Senate. (In practice, most bills begin as similar proposals and are introduced in both houses.) Unless
enacted into law, bills die at the end of the Congress in
which it was introduced. However, a bill not enacted
into law during the two years of the current Congress
can be reintroduced at the start of the next one.

Committee Action   Once introduced, the bill is assigned a number and then referred to the appropriate
committee for action. The predominant role of the
committee system is the most distinguishing characteristic of the legislative branch. Committees have their
own operating rules with the authority to draft, amend,
and vote on legislation. To make workloads more
manageable, each committee is given responsibility for
a specific area of public policy. The speaker of the
house decides which committee has jurisdiction and he
or she can also issue joint or sequential referral to
committees.

Once assigned to committee, the bill may be referred to one of that body's subcommittees. Subcommittees are assigned responsibility for specific portions of the legislative jurisdiction of the full committees. Subcommittees also exercise oversight power over the federal agencies, boards, and departments that regulate matters within their subject areas.

Committees and subcommittees have the ability to control, change, stall, or even eliminate a proposed piece of legislation. Most substantive work on proposed legislation is done at the committee and subcommittee level. If a major committee decides against taking action on a particular bill, it is difficult to bring it to the floor of the House or Senate for vote. This is especially true in the House. While committee bills may be amended on the floor, the committees themselves usually are responsible for most of the details of any legislation that passes. The House Rules Committee may also limit the number or type of amendments of any bill that reaches the floor. To make workloads more manageable, each committee is given responsibility for a specific area of public policy. The speaker of the house decides which committee has jurisdiction and can also issue joint or sequential referral to committees. The importance of legislative committees cannot be overemphasized.

There are forty-four standing (or permanent) committees in the House and Senate but only a few have jurisdiction for issues dealing with food, nutrition, and health. In the Senate, the two most prominent committees are the Committee on Agriculture, Nutrition and Forestry (with its subcommittee on Research, Nutrition and General Legislation) and the Committee on Labor and Human Resources (with its subcommittees on Aging; Children and Families; Education, Arts and Humanities; and, Disability Policy). In the House, most bills dealing with food and nutrition issues are referred to Agriculture (with its subcommittees on Department Operations, Nutrition and Foreign Agriculture), Economic and Educational Opportunities (and its subcommittee on Early Childhood, Youth and Families), or Science. Committee chairmanships are held by members of the majority party. These are extremely powerful positions. The committee chair decides which matters the committee will act on during the course of a congressional session. This person may also be important in guiding the bill through passage by the full chamber.

When needed, temporary committees may be created for limited and specific purposes. Although helpful for calling public attention to an issue or for information gathering, these special or select committees have no authority to authorize or appropriate funds for programs.

Hearings   The committee chair determines what action, if any, will be taken on bills referred there. Committees and subcommittees can choose to take no action, thus killing a bill, or they can take action through such procedures as **hearings** and markup sessions (see below). Usually, the first step in any committee action is a public hearing to solicit views of members of Congress, experts in the field, and the general public. Hearings are called by the committee chair to gather public and expert testimony on whether legislation is needed and, if so, what form should it take. Hearings are also used to establish a public record of the history and controversy surrounding a particular piece of legislation. They may be used to form or affect public opinion, especially when testimony is presented by celebrities. Hearings may be held to delay action on the legislation or to pacify a particular interest group. The committee to draft new legislation, amend the legislation already before it, or decide that no final legislative action is necessary uses the information gathered during hearings.

Markup Sessions   If a hearing shows support for the bill, the next step is a meeting of subcommittee members to make any necessary or desired changes to the bill in what is called a "markup" session. In these sessions, the subcommittee goes over the bill line by line and rewrites it to reflect the subcommittee's views. If the subcommittee determines that the bill needs considerable revision, it may be completely redrafted, given a new number, and responsored by the full committee. Once a subcommittee approves a bill, it is sent to the full committee, which can make more changes. However, if the subcommittee approves the bill by a substantial margin, the full committee generally agrees to support the bill with few if any further changes.

Report   When the committee has taken a final vote on the legislation and all its recommended amendments, the committee staff writes a report that explains the reasons for approving the bill, and the legislation is "ordered reported." This step directs the committee staff to compile various drafts of the legislation and recommended amendments into the bill format.

Scheduling for Vote   Once a bill is approved, the committee chair asks that it be scheduled for floor debate. In the House this request goes to the Rules Committee; in the Senate it goes to the Majority Leader. In the House the rules of debate are often restricted so that only a few specified amendments can be considered by the full membership. As a result, it is usually the subcommittees and committee that give final shape to any legislation passed in the House. In the Senate bills are open to any amendment. However, there are unanimous agreements to limit both debate and votes.[7]

Decision   The bill is debated (and perhaps amended) on the floor of the chamber. The debate over the bill includes time allotted to supporters and opponents. If an open rule is in effect, amendments may be adopted by a majority vote. Finally, the bill is voted up (approved) or down (rejected). The bill is passed in the first chamber (either House or Senate).

Conference   A bill must be passed by both the House and Senate. When the two chambers pass similar but not identical bills, a joint conference committee composed of equal numbers of senators and representatives works out the differences. As a rule, the conferees are members of the committees that had original jurisdiction over the bill(s). Once the conferees agree on identical language, it is sent back to both the House and Senate for approval. Only when both chambers pass the bill with identical language can it be sent to the president for signature.

Executive Action   The bill, now an Act of Congress, goes to the president for signature. If the president signs the bill, it becomes law. However, if the president disapproves of the bill, he can veto it. When that happens, the only way for the bill to become law is for both the House and the Senate to vote by a two-thirds majority to override the veto. Also, if the president refuses to sign the bill within ten days after Congress has adjourned at the end of its two-year life span, the bill dies; this is called a "pocket veto."

Federal Budget Process

Fiscal power—the power to raise revenues through taxes and to spend money through appropriations—is a fundamental power of the legislative branch. However, budgetary debate and decision making on Capitol Hill is shaped by what the president emphasizes in his budget message to Congress each year. A strong case can be made that the **budget process** makes the president

the main initiator of policy—not only of fiscal policy, but also of policy in every area requiring expenditure of public funds. By approving, modifying, or disapproving proposed legislation, Congress can change the level of program funding, eliminate programs, or add programs not requested by the president. It can also enact legislation to raise or lower various types of federal taxes or generate other sources of revenue.

The federal budget process is complex. A number of stages and considerable delays take place from legislative approval of spending to when the agencies actually provide the services and the bills are paid. The massive growth in federal government activity in this century is another complication, as is the number of congressional committees with responsibility at various stages of the budget process. One set of committees—Ways and Means in the House, and Finance in the Senate—determine revenue policy, whereas another set—the two appropriations committees—determines spending policy.[6]

In 1990, Congress made far-reaching changes in its 1974 budget process law. The law continued to provide for congressional approval of budget resolutions and reconciliation bills, but discarded provisions that automatically cut federal spending in certain areas when predetermined targets were exceeded. Two funding categories were created—*discretionary funds* (a minor proportion of the total budget) are limited by spending caps set by the appropriations committees, and *mandatory funds* cover all **entitlement** programs. Under rules set by the 1990 budget summit, pay-as-you-go restrictions (the so-called PAYGO rules) cover tax cuts and mandatory spending chiefly for entitlement programs such as Medicare, Medicaid, and food stamps. Any changes must be "revenue neutral"; that is, any tax cut, new entitlement program, or change that increases spending in an entitlement program must be offset by a tax increase or cutbacks in entitlement spending.[8]

Entitlement programs—those for which persons qualify because they meet certain income or other eligibility requirements—are funded out of the *mandatory* portion of the budget. Medicare, Medicaid, and food stamps and most other food assistance programs are all entitlement programs. (Food assistance programs were first included under the 1977 Farm Bill in an effort to garner support from urban legislators for agricultural programs. This action essentially ties funding for food assistance to funding earmarked for price supports and other agricultural and food production programs.) An example of a program that competes for funds in the *discretionary* category is the WIC program. Only about 65 percent of people eligible to participate in WIC receive services because when appropriated funds are exhausted, none are left for program expansion.

Policy Implementation and Regulations: Roles of the Executive Branch

Once the legislation is passed and signed into law, implementation and enforcement of the law become the responsibility of the agency in the executive branch to which it is assigned. The executive branch is headed by the president. His fourteen cabinet secretaries are political appointees, and many are "first line" administrators of these agencies. Most of the laws enacted that affect nutrition, food, and health are passed to the U.S. Department of Agriculture or the Department of Health and Human Services (DHHS) for implementation.

Some agencies, but not all, are considered to be regulatory agencies. The two types of regulatory agencies are independent agencies and executive department agencies. *Independent agencies* include the Federal Trade Commission (FTC), which has regulatory responsibility for food advertising and truth-in-labeling laws; the Consumer Product Safety Commission; and the Federal Commerce Commission. Examples of *executive department agencies* are the Food and Drug Administration (FDA) in the DHHS, and the Food Safety Inspection Service (FSIS) and the Animal and Plant Health Inspection Service (APHIS) in the USDA.

Regulations are written by each agency to carry out the intent of Congress. The statements issued by agencies in the executive branch carry the power of law and can be legally enforced with fines for noncompliance. How closely the regulations carry out the legislative intent may depend on whether the philosophy and policies of Congress and the agency officials coincide.

Rulemaking Regulatory tools include *rule making, informal methods,* and *adjudication.* Rulemaking is a process of setting the rules or regulations that define the requirements for implementing the law.[24] In rulemaking, the **regulatory process** follows a stipulated course of action, and agencies must adhere to certain procedures in issuing new regulations. Rules are detailed restrictions and guidelines that agencies establish to implement congressional statutes. The enabling regulatory statute typically defines the scope of agency authority and describes

any specific rulemaking procedures the agency must follow. The interpretation of the intent and nature of the statute by the administrative agency (through administrative rules that the agency established) gives the statutory law some life and determines the extent and scope of impact. The rule may apply to products (e.g., food labels or medical devices) or to procedures to be followed by the regulated industry or the agency. In the case of complicated legislation, such as Medicaid, the administratively developed regulations are usually much longer and more detailed than the enabling legislation. Congress has also sought to control and expedite agency rulemaking by imposing statutory deadlines for completing rulemaking actions. This has been particularly true for laws pertaining to public health and the environment.

To begin the process, the agency can issue a public statement of general or particular applicability and future effect. The agency may publish an "advance notice of proposed rulemaking" in the *Federal Register.* In the *Federal Register,* the "notice of proposed rulemaking" (NPRM) describes the planned regulation and provides background on the issue. It also gives the address for submitting written comments, a contact for more information, and the deadline for public comments. There is no special form to fill out for comments, nor do submitters have to follow a certain style. However, comments *must* be on paper, either handwritten or typed. No phone calls will be processed.

By law, anyone can participate in the rulemaking process by commenting in writing on rules the FDA proposes. Comments can be written in response to both the NPRM and the proposed rules. The agency has the discretion to set the length of the "comment period" depending on the complexity of the proposed rule. Nonetheless, the public must be given an opportunity to comment on a proposed rule (usually, thirty, sixty, or ninety days) and must be given adequate notice that a rule has been adopted before it becomes effective.

After public comment period has ended and the agency has had sufficient time to review comments and revise wording, the final rule is published in *Federal Register.* The final rule is sent to the Office of Management and Budget (OMB) for determination of costs and benefits of new regulations and then the final rule is printed in *Code of Federal Regulations* (CFR); also known as codified. The CFR is a compilation of all general and permanent agency rules and is revised annually.

Besides accepting public comments and petitions, the FDA also schedules public meetings and hearings to discuss and explain its proposals. These are usually held with industry representatives or consumer groups, but anyone interested may attend, and, with advance notice, may comment on a proposal. Meetings for the public to present views are announced in the *Federal Register*.

Petitions are also published in the *Federal Register*. A petition is a formal request made to an agency by an individual, firm, or organization that a certain action be taken or not taken or that a regulation or order be established, revoked, or revised. Contact the FDA Dockets Management Branch (301–443–7542) if you have any questions about the comment, petition, or hearing process.[14]

When FDA receives a comment it is logged in, numbered, and placed in a file for that docket. It then becomes a public record and is available for anyone to examine in the FDA's reading room. Under the Freedom of Information Act (FOIA), visitors to the reading room can receive free copies of comments up to fifty pages.

After the comment period has closed, the agency then has the responsibility for reviewing the comments received, seriously considering alternatives, revising when appropriate, and issuing a final rule, which must undergo approval at both the agency and the administration level by the OMB. The final rule carries an effective date that can range from immediately to several years in the future. Corrections are issued to rectify problems with the content of regulations; generally, these are technical corrections such as dates, rates, and program formulas. Final rules are published as regulations for federal programs; the compilation of regulations is revised and published annually in the CFR.

One example of this process of interest to most community nutrition professionals was the action taken by the FDA after passage of the Nutrition Labeling and Education Act (NLEA) in November 1990. The statute specified that rules for its implementation had to be proposed by the agency within one year after its enactment. They were published in the *Federal Register* by FDA in November 1991 with a ninety-day comment period allowed. During that time, the FDA received more than 40,000 comments, 8,000 on the last day alone! Implementation of the final rules were effective May 8, 1994. This example emphasizes how important it is for community nutrition professionals interested in public policy to comment on proposals or other items of interest published in the *Federal Register* as well as communicating with Congress about pending legislation.

Advice on how to comment on the FDA regulations are available.[14] Petitions and comments need to clearly indicate if you are for or against the proposed rule or some part of it and why. The comments should be accurately indexed to the regulatory citations (dockets) specified in the *Federal Register*. Comments should be stated succinctly; and where appropriate, references from the scientific literature should be cited and included. The expertise of the respondent should also be identified. If an article or reference is in a foreign language, you must submit a copy of the original document and an English translation verified by a qualified translator to be accurate. To promulgate the fairest rules, regulatory agencies must receive comments from individuals informed about the issues by the last day of the comment period. FDA regulatory decisions are based largely on law and science, and agency reviewers look for reasoning, logic, and good science in public comments.

Interim final rules fall somewhere between a proposed rule and a final rule. An agency usually adopts interim final rules when it is rushed to issue a regulation, but because of Congressional time mandates, public crisis, and the like, does not have time to go through the proposed stage process. Interim final rules do provide the public with an opportunity to comment, but an agency is likely to make only minor changes.

Another process used when the regulations proposed are particularly contentious to all parties is called "negotiated rulemaking," or "reg-neg."[37] This procedure is growing in use and involves bringing all the parties together to hammer out a new rule with a skilled neutral such as the Federal Mediation and Conciliation Service. Unlike traditional rulemaking, in which the agency takes the lead, proposes the rule, and asks for written comment, reg-neg is done face to face. It is usually a short-term process and results in rules that seldom, if ever, are challenged in court. Proponents of the method say it avoids some of the biggest pitfalls of rulemaking in the more traditional manner— lengthy delay, impasse, vicious bickering, or endless proposals that no one can agree on. This procedure was recently brought to the attention of the food and nutrition community. School food service administrators dissatisfied with USDA proposed rules for changing the school program threatened to invoke "reg-neg" to arrive at a mutually satisfactory agreement. Negotiations were successful, however, and this approach was not used.

Informal Action and Adjudication In addition to rulemaking, significant agency policy decisions also result from either informal actions or adjudication. Informal actions include inspections, meetings, recalls, and advisory opinions. The term informal may be misleading because these actions are informal only in a legal sense. To the agency and to the regulated industry, they can have the same impact as any formal action. An adjudication is basically a decision issued by the judicial system for how the law is to be carried out. The outcome of the adjudication or the court decision is called an "order," similar to the "rule" that results from the rulemaking process. In addition to these mechanisms of action, administrative agencies use a variety of informal means to articulate policy under a statute; these may include press releases, speeches, statements, letters, advisory opinions, and other types of communications.

Role of the Judicial Branch

The judicial branch has responsibility for legal oversight of the activities of the other branches of government. The judicial role also applies to all the rulings or court actions taken by the FDA to condemn unsafe food or reduce fraudulent sale of supplements. Each issue of the *FDA Consumer* has a section entitled "Summaries of Court Actions" that describe seizure proceedings, criminal proceedings, and injunction proceedings. Seizure proceedings are civil actions taken against goods alleged to be in violation of federal regulations, while criminal and injunction proceedings are against firms and individuals charged to be responsible for violations. These cases generally involve food, drugs, devices, or cosmetics alleged to be adulterated or misbranded or otherwise violating the law when introduced into and while in interstate commerce or while held for sale after shipment in interstate commerce.[40]

A SYSTEMS MODEL SURROUNDING NUTRITION POLICY

A "systems" model shows the role of each component of the nutrition policy picture. Figure 5.3 demonstrates both the simplicity and the complexity of nutrition policy. "Input" to the system is in the form of those sets of policies (mainly agricultural) that affect the quantity and quality of food available. "Process" is best conceptualized as all those events and situations that affect how the food supply is used. The major process in this

scenario is food consumption, which in turn affects the output of the food system. The output of the system can be shown as a range of outcomes, including those related to health outcomes of individuals and to "healthy" sustainable environments.[22]

Agricultural policy sets the stage for nutrition policy by influencing the quantity and quality of the food supply. We rely on the food production system to provide ample quantities of food at reasonable prices for consumers, a basic tenet of food policy. The types and amounts of food that are produced are directly affected by agricultural; that is, farm policy, which, in turn, affects the types, supply, and costs of foods from which the public can choose.

While agricultural policy directly affects the food supply, both health and medical policy and environmental policy influence food consumption practices by means of a vast array of programs and services. Health policy, especially that segment that deals with health promotion and disease prevention, has embraced nutrition as a vital component of its strategies. Because food consumption patterns are now seen as having a major role in the prevention of chronic degenerative diseases, nutrition has been described as "an ideal area in which to demonstrate the principles of health promotion and healthy public policy."[38]

Science policy affects agricultural, health, and environmental policies because of its role in setting funding priorities for research and new product development. Socioeconomic policy is influential in its capacity as a delivery system for the economically disadvantaged in society and is also of major importance in this context by setting eligibility standards for participation in food assistance programs. Educational policy, in addition to its use as a delivery system for many nutrition education programs, influences students' literacy and numerical abilities, thus affecting consumers' ability to make informed food choices.

ELEMENTS OF NUTRITION POLICY

To understand the complexity of nutrition policy, we must examine the components that together make up the whole. Examples of elements found within nutrition policy include the availability of safe, wholesome food as well as the provision of **food security.** Governmental involvement in nutrition policy has traditionally focused on providing food-related information and educational programs; maintaining price supports

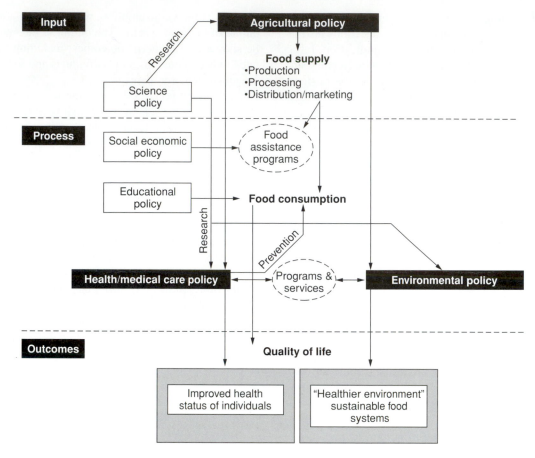

FIGURE 5.3   Nutrition Policy Overview
(*Source:* From Sims, LS. Public policy in nutrition: a framework for action, *Nutrition Today;* 28(5):14, 1993.)

on commodities (such as milk, sugar, grain products, and animal foods); and regulating the quality and safety of the food supply.[27] Providing food and income assistance to the economically disadvantaged has also been encompassed in food and nutrition policy activities.

In summary, six elements can be considered within the realm of food and nutrition policy. Table 5.1 identifies these six elements and then connects these elements to the array of structures and groups that initiate, influence, and implement nutrition policy. For example, this table links the six primary policy elements in food and nutrition with government structures in the legislative branch (those that have authority for initiating policy), units in the executive branch (those that have responsibility for implementing policy), and with groups outside of government (such as advocacy organizations, professional associations, interest groups). All converge to in-

fluence both initiation and implementation of policy. A visualization provided by table 5.1 is only a snapshot of a very complex and dynamic process. It does, however, illustrate the diverse nature of the units and groups (both inside and outside of government) involved with the process of nutrition policymaking and the intended nutrition policy element. As each element is discussed, please refer to this table as a reference.

Policy Element 1: Providing an Adequate Food Supply at Reasonable Cost

One of the basic tenets of nutrition policy is that adequate quantities of food must be produced and made available to consumers at reasonable cost. Farm policy basically determines the quantity of agricultural products produced, which, in turn, influences the kinds of food available and the prices of those foods for the consumer.

TABLE 5.1

Elements of Nutrition Policy and How They Relate to Selected Government and Private Sector Groups that Initiate, Implement, and Influence Public Policy

Policy element	Legislative branch (congressional committees) — House	Legislative branch (congressional committees) — Senate	Executive branch— Administrative (regulatory agencies)	Nongovernment branches— private sector groups (examples)
I. Providing adequate food at reasonable cost	Agriculture (SC on "Production and Price Competitiveness")	Agriculture, Nutrition and Forestry (SC on "General Farm Commodities")	U.S. Department of Agriculture (USDA)	American Farm Bureau Federation, National Farmers Union; Farm Credit Council
II. Ensuring quality, safety, and wholesomeness of food supply	Commerce (SC on "Health and Environment") Agriculture	Labor and Human Resources	USDA (Food Safety and Inspection Services) (Animal and Plant Health Inspection. Services [APHIS]) Environmental Protection Agency (EPA) Department of Health and Human Services (DHHS) (Food and Drug Administration)	Public Voice for Food and Health Policy Food Marketing Institute; Center for Science and Public Interest
III. Ensuring food access and availability	Agriculture Economic and Education Opportunities	Agriculture, Nutrition, and Forestry (Special Committee on Aging; Indian Affairs)	USDA (Food and Consumer Services [FCS]) DHHS (Administration on Aging)	Center for Budget and Policy Priorities; Bread for the World; American School Food Service Assoc.; Food, Research and Action Center
IV. Providing research-based information and education programs	Agriculture (Economic and Education Opportunities)	Agriculture, Nutrition, and Forestry (SC Research, Nutrition, and General Legislation) Labor and Human Resources (SC Education)	USDA (Food and Consumer Services) (Food Safety and Inspection Services) (National Center for Nutrition Policy and Promotion) (Food and Nutrition Information Center) DHHS (National Heart, Lung, and Blood Institute) (Food and Drug Administration) (National Cancer Institute)	Society for Nutrition Education; American Dietetic Association
V. Supporting an optimal science research base in food and nutrition	Agriculture Science	Agriculture, Nutrition and Forestry Commerce (Science and Transportation) Labor and Human Resources	USDA (Agricultural Research Service) (Human Nutrition and Research Center) (Cooperative Research, Education & Extension Services [CREES]) DHHS (National Institutes of Health [NIH]) (Food and Drug Administration [FDA]) (National Center for Health Statistics [NCHS])	National Academy of Sciences; Institute of Medicine; Food and Nutrition Board; Institute of Food Technology
VI. Integrating nutrition into the health care system	Commerce Ways and Means	Labor and Human Resources Finance	DHHS (Health Care and Financing Admin.) (Public Health Service) (National Institutes of Health)	American Dietetic Association; American Public Health Association; ASCN; American Society for Parenteral and Enteral Nutrition

Note: SC stands for subcommittee.

The goal of agricultural policy, simply stated, is to provide relatively inexpensive food for consumers while protecting farm income.

In Congress, food production issues are under the jurisdiction of the Agriculture Committee in the House, and the Agriculture, Nutrition and Forestry Committee in the Senate. Implementation is primarily in the domain of the USDA in the executive branch. A variety of farm, environmental and consumer groups exercise a direct role in influencing policy directions in this arena. Outside interest groups include the American Farm Bureau Federation, the National Farmers Union, and the Farm Credit councils.

Policy Element 2: Ensuring a Safe and Wholesome Food Supply

Food Safety   Food safety includes issues as varied as environmental contaminants, pesticide residues, product tampering, nutritional imbalances, and microbial contamination. The FDA is responsible for the safety and labeling of foods, as well as a broad range of important nutrition-related food issues, such as fortification, infant formula, medical foods, and dietary supplements. In recent years, consumers have developed a growing concern about safety of their food and its impact on their health. Consumer advocates, the food industry, and even some government regulators have widely divergent views on the food safety issue. Given these often conflicting perspectives, it is not surprising that some food safety concerns have become highly charged public policy issues.[31]

Congressional responsibility for food safety is handled by the Commerce Committee in the House and the Labor and Human Resources Committee in the Senate. Inspection and regulation duties for food and water safety are shared among several regulatory agencies within the U.S. Department of Agriculture, the Department of Health and Human Services, and the Environmental Protection Agency. Food safety issues that have emerged as topics of recent concern include the safety of pesticide residues, food additives, microbiological contamination, and seafood inspection.

The existing food safety policy presents unique challenges. Current laws and regulations must be revised to adequately address long-standing issues such as uniformity of standards for food additives versus pesticides, and contemporary concerns about detection of the complete range of emerging chemical and microbiological hazards. In addition, food safety regulations now must extend to those actions needed to implement current diet and health recommendations. These new duties include controlling microbiological contamination of food, assessing the range of significant chemical hazards, and communicating the relative risks from various food products to the public. Also involved is the regulation of new genetically engineered or formulated food products, such as "fat substitutes."[28]

Food Fortification and Enrichment   Between 1906 and 1930, the science of nutrition was born with the discovery of vitamins and their roles in human health. This precipitated what Hutt has called "one of the most difficult regulatory problems that FDA has had to confront."[15]

One of the first examples of fortification (adding a nutrient not originally contained is a food) was in 1924 when the Michigan Department of Health and the Michigan Medical Society convinced all salt manufacturers that goiters were such a problem that they should add iodine to table salt at no additional cost to the consumer. Thus, the first fortification policy was to correct a recognized deficiency of a nutrient in the diets of a significant number of individuals.[27] Fortification of flour and bread with vitamins and minerals dates back to the 1920s, when some millers added vitamin D to flour. In the early 1930s to prevent rickets, the federal government mandated that vitamin D be added to milk, and the fortification of low-fat milk and margarine with vitamin A followed in 1939. In 1943, the enrichment (replacing nutrients lost during processing) of flour and bread with thiamin, niacin, riboflavin, and iron was mandated by War Food Order No. 1. The addition of calcium and vitamin D was optional. Soon after, similar standards were set for corn meal, grits, macaroni, and rice. In 1973, the FDA amended its enrichment standards to allow for the increase in the level of the three B vitamins in bread and cereal products by at least 50 percent and an increase in the level of iron by 300 percent.[41]

As the nation moved from an agricultural base to one focused on an industrial-urban locale, the food supply needed to be transported from where it was produced to where it was consumed. Various preservatives had to be added to retain the nutritional quality and integrity of the food product. Thus, as dietary habits changed, the second principle of fortification policy became the maintenance of the nutritional quality of the food supply.[27]

As science continues to underscore the importance of individual nutrients in preventing disease and achieving optimal health, many have called for the FDA to reevaluate its fortification policy taking this knowledge into account. The agency may be moving in that direction. The FDA has issued a new fortification rule for the first time in over fifty years. Beginning in 1998, all food manufacturers are required to fortify specific grain products with folic acid in an effort to reduce the incidence of certain birth defects. Manufacturers currently add a wider array of nutrients, such as calcium, beta-carotene, and vitamin E, to a diet that already includes a myriad of superfortified foods. Unlike the rules for fortification of grain products, dairy products, butter, and salt, there are no regulations or even guidelines that address how much of a certain nutrient may be added to other foods. The FDA recognizes the need to reevaluate its current food fortification policy.[41]

Policy Element 3: Providing Food Access and Availability, Regardless of Income

Hunger and Food Security Issues   Policy options to meet the needs of the "hungry" depend, in part, on the public perception of hunger and how it is defined. Hunger is frequently defined in two ways. The first is in terms of measurable forms of malnutrition, such as anemia, low birthweight, or infant mortality. The second way, which is more useful for policymakers, is hunger as a lack of **"food security."** This definition focuses on "food purchasing power and food availability to families in their community, thus making it possible to detect and measure the extent of hunger, develop strategies to alleviate the problem, and monitor progress in its elimination."[2] Food security has been defined as "access by all people at all times to enough food for an active, healthy life, and at a minimum includes the following: 1) the ready availability of nutritionally adequate and safe foods, and 2) the assured ability to acquire personally acceptable foods in a socially acceptable way."[4] It follows that potential consequences of food insecurity include hunger, malnutrition, and negative effects on health and quality of life caused either directly or indirectly by the lack of adequate food.

Government has addressed the issue of food insecurity by providing economic assistance to individuals and households in the form of a variety of programs. More than any other aspect of food and nutrition policy, food assistance programs are a form of government action directly tied to the nation's economic well-being. Food assistance programs employ a variety of strategies, but the two main ones involve transferring resources or providing supplemental foods. In some programs, nutrition education and health referrals are provided. The fundamental challenge facing food assistance policy makers in the 1990s is the need to hold down food program costs but continue to provide needed nutritional assistance. In light of increasing recognition that nutrition is an essential component of preventive health care, implementation of a more effective federal initiative will require closer linkages between local, state, and federal activities; consumer and advocacy groups; and those supported by industry, foundations, or other funding sources.

History of Food Assistance   Federal food assistance programs evolved as an outgrowth of farm support laws enacted during the Great Depression of the 1930s. A commodity distribution program was established that distributed surplus agricultural commodities directly to the needy and in 1939, some 13 million Americans received such food assistance. In large measure, today's food programs have retained their original goals—to improve the nutrition of low-income people and other groups, while providing an outlet for surplus agricultural commodities from the farm programs.

Two forces helped to place the hunger and malnutrition issues in the public policy agenda during the late 1960s.[26] In 1968, the Senate Select Committee on Nutrition and Human Needs was formed, and in early 1969, President Nixon committed his administration to "putting an end to hunger in America itself for all time."[50] An outgrowth of this vow was the White House Conference on Food, Nutrition and Health held in December 1969, and chaired by Dr. Jean Mayer, a renowned nutritional scientist. A number of recommendations from that conference have helped shape nutrition policy in the ensuing twenty-five years.

During the 1970s, cash subsidies and vouchers increasingly replaced agricultural commodities in federal food programs as the means by which the purchasing power of the poor would be improved. This strategy was employed to create the Supplemental Nutrition Program for Women, Infants and Children in 1972, expand the Food Stamp Program, and develop the Nutrition Program for Older Americans. From 1969 to 1977, annual federal expenditures for food assistance increased nearly sixfold, and donated farm products declined to less than 10 percent of the total value of federal expenditures.[32] By the late 1970s, the positive effects of these efforts were evident. Representatives of the Field Foundation who had toured the south ten years earlier returned in 1979 to report that nutrition programs were working, and evidence of hunger and malnutrition had declined considerably.

With the onset of the 1980s and the election of a Republican president, responsibility for nutrition policies shifted notably from the federal government to states and the private sector. One of the hallmarks of the Reagan administration was a mandate to reduce government spending, and offer services only to the "truly needy," that is, those who met the objective criteria for program participation.[34] From 1980 to 1982, Congress reduced expenditures on food assistance programs by one third as part of the effort to trim the federal budget.[5]

The consequences of these cutbacks soon became evident. Concomitant with a reduction in benefits was the economic downturn of 1981, which caused a significant rise in unemployment, and consequently increased the rolls of food assistance program participants, especially the numbers applying for food stamp benefits. Emergency food and shelter providers (such as food banks, homeless shelters, and "soup kitchens") began to report an increasing demand for their services by what they termed the "new poor": children, unskilled and unemployed youth, underemployed families with insufficient resources, and the deinstitutionalized mentally ill.[26]

In recent years, both the White House and Congress have taken steps to improve access to and benefits from food assistance programs. The Food Security Act of 1985 reinstated lost nutritional benefits for low-income households through changes in the Food Stamp Act and the Temporary Emergency Food Assistance Program (TEFAP). In 1986, Congress passed the School Lunch and Child Nutrition Program amendments that included increased funds for WIC and the School Breakfast Program and reauthorized the expiring Child Nutrition Programs. Congress began to focus attention on the homeless by holding hearings and adopting legislation to extend food program benefits to this group.[5] The Hunger Prevention Act of 1988 provided federal matching funds to states to conduct outreach to households potentially eligible for the Food Stamp Program. In 1993, additional legislation (the Leland Bill) became law. This is viewed as one of the most important pieces of anti-hunger legislation since 1974.

In January 1995, the 104th Congress gave the Republicans leadership of Congress for the first time in forty years. Part of the Republican House members' "Contract with America," was a promise to reform the welfare system. Under these proposals major nutrition programs would have been repealed; federal funding for nutrition programs would have been reduced and combined into a single discretionary "block grant" to the states. Such a block grant would have provided a set amount of funding to each state based on a national formula and would have permitted states to spend the funds with little federal direction or constraint.[19] Proponents of block grants claim that this approach will save money, and allow states to better target assistance to those in need by giving states increasing flexibility to tailor their programs to their own populations. Those who oppose block grants feel that such an approach undermines the four key functions of federal nutrition programs that have contributed to their proven success: health-based nutrition standards, economic responsiveness (automatic funding adjustments built into current law would be eliminated by block-granting funds to states), national eligibility (and benefits) standards, and adequate funding.[23,48]

In summary, food assistance programs are designed to enhance participants' buying power by issuing vouchers or stamps for the purchase of food, or to provide food directly.[39] The effectiveness of each program must be judged by how well it meets its specific stated objectives. Government officials point out that these programs are not intended to meet all needs. Categories of food assistance are family nutrition programs, child nutrition programs, supplemental food programs, and food distribution programs.

Food Stamp Program   The family nutrition programs include the Food Stamp Program (FSP), the Nutrition Assistance Program for Puerto Rico, and the Food Distribution Program on Indian Reservations (needy Family Program). The FSP, the largest food assistance program, was established in its present form in 1964 and is described as the "nation's single most important program in the fight against hunger."[11] The program is designed to improve the diets of people with low incomes by providing coupons (food stamps) to cover part or all of their household's food budget.[49] The food stamps provided to eligible recipients are a form of currency that can be used only to purchase food at participating grocery stores.

The FSP is the only entitlement food program available to all who meet eligibility standards, regardless of their age or family composition. Eligibility is determined on the basis of both financial (income and resources) and nonfinancial (citizenship, work requirements, etc.) factors. To qualify, households must have gross incomes below 130 percent of the official poverty level; households with elderly and disabled members must have "net incomes" (all the household's income minus the deductions for which it qualifies) below 100 percent of the poverty line. Most households may have up to $2,000 in assets. Fully 98 percent of food stamps go to households with incomes equal to or below the poverty line. Over half of all food stamp recipients are children, and 87 percent are children, the elderly, or women.[43]

The FSP is administered at the federal level by USDA Food and Consumer Services, and at the state and local levels by welfare, social service, or human service agencies. The federal government pays the full cost of food stamps and at least half of the program's administrative costs, with states and local governments paying the remainder. An Electronic Benefit Transfer (EBT) system, the use of a "credit-card-like" mechanism in place of paper coupons, is being tested as a means to enhance recipients' security and to discourage trafficking of food stamp benefits.

The FSP is over thirty years old, yet surprisingly few studies have documented program impact. The basic premise underlying the program is that use of food stamps increases family food expenditures, which in turn improves dietary intake and ultimately improves health. The FSP functions well as an income maintenance program, and has been demonstrated to provide basic support during times of economic hardship. However, because nutrient consumption in the United States is not highly responsive to changes in income, the magnitude of the effect of the FSP is likely to be small. Strengthening the nutrition education component may enable participants to make better-informed food choices.[36]

Child Nutrition Programs   Five child nutrition programs are offered: the National School Lunch Program, the School Breakfast Program, the Child and Adult Care Food Program, the Special Milk Program, and the Summer Food Service Program. The largest and oldest of these is the School Lunch Program. The National School Lunch Program (NSLP) is administered at the federal level by Food, Nutrition and Consumer Services, the largest agency in the USDA; at the state level by one of a variety of state agencies (usually the department of education); and at the local level by school district administrators.[11]

The NSLP is an entitlement program, which means federal funds must be provided to all schools that

apply and meet the program's eligibility criteria. A three-tiered reimbursement system is used to calculate benefits: children from households with incomes at or below 130 percent of poverty receive free meals; those between 130 and 185 percent receive reduced-price meals; and those above 185 percent of poverty pay "full-price," for which the school districts receive a small federal subsidy. In 1996, more than 26 million children were served lunch each school day in over 90,000 schools. Despite the fact that the NSLP is available to 92 percent of all students in the United States, however, only 56 percent participate on a typical day.[3]

Meals served in the NSLP must meet specific requirements if participating institutions are to qualify for federal funds. Lunch must include 1/2 pint fluid milk (whole milk must be one of the options offered); 2 ounces protein; 3/4-cup servings of two or more vegetables or fruits or both (juice can meet half of this requirement); and eight servings of bread, pasta, or grain per week.

How effective is the NSLP? Surveys have documented that the food consumed makes an important dietary contribution to children's diets. The *School Nutrition Dietary Assessment Study* found that lunches provided one third or more of the RDAs for energy; protein; vitamins A, C, B_6; calcium; iron; and zinc but higher than recommended amounts of fat, saturated fat, and sodium.[3]

The School Breakfast Program (SBP) provides assistance to schools and residential child care institutions that operate nonprofit breakfast programs. In 1975, amendments to the Child Nutrition Act of 1966 permanently authorized the SBP. The meal pattern requirements of school breakfasts are intended to provide one fourth of the RDAs. The SBP is available to slightly more than half of the nation's school children, but only about 20 percent participate.[3] Of those who do take part in the SBP, 87 percent are considered to be "at-risk" children.[30]

Evaluations of school meals have indicated that they contained higher than recommended amounts of fat, saturated fat, and sodium. In response, the USDA developed the "School Meals Initiative for Healthy Children," to deal with this problem. It is a comprehensive integrated plan to ensure that children are offered healthful meals at school. In June 1994, the USDA promulgated regulations to make critical improvements in the nutritional quality of school meals and bring them into compliance with the Dietary Guidelines for Americans. That same year, the Healthy Meals for Healthy Americans Act of 1994 (PL 103-448) mandated that school meals comply with the Dietary Guidelines for Americans by school year 1996 to 1997, and directed the USDA to offer schools a choice of menu-planning options, including a food-based menu system.

To implement the initiative, the USDA developed "Team Nutrition," an integrated network of public/private partnerships intended to improve the health and education of children by promoting food choices for a healthful diet through the media, schools, the community, and families. The two main components to the USDA's Team Nutrition are nutrition education and training and technical assistance. Nutrition education efforts have been enhanced with a number of partnerships with the private sector, including a subsidiary of the Walt Disney Company to use two movie characters in nutrition education promotions; with Scholastic, Inc., an educational publisher to develop teaching kits for use in schools, and with home economist in the Cooperative State Research, Education, and Extension Services (CREES) to implement community nutrition action kits. Training and technical assistance will be provided to school food service personnel by partnering with chefs to develop new recipes for use in the updated school meals program, by changing the specifications for foods offered in school meals, and by funding training grants to assist states in developing a sustainable training infrastructure for local school districts.[44]

The Child and Adult Care Food Program (CACFP), which began in 1968, is designed to assure nutritious meals for children to age 12, the elderly, and certain handicapped individuals who participate in a nonprofit, licensed, or approved day-care program. Centers receive federal funds for two meals and one snack per participant per day, plus one additional meal or snack if the recipient is in attendance for eight hours or longer. All meals in participating organizations are subsidized with federal funds. This program currently serves 1.5 million participants daily, only 1 percent of whom are elderly. Because more women are in the workforce, and more nonworking mothers are using supplemental child care, larger numbers of children are spending more time in child care settings, which makes it imperative that we continue to monitor the quality of food served to children in these settings.[47]

The Special Milk Program provides milk in schools not participating in the NSLP. The Summer Food Service Program provides funds and commodities for breakfast, lunch, and snacks free to all children under age eighteen who attend the meal site of a sponsor organization, usually schools, residential camps, state or local government units, or private nonprofit organization locations.

Supplemental Feeding Program   The most notable program in this category is officially named the Special Supplemental Nutrition Program for Women, Infants and Children, but it is better known as WIC. This program was created as a pilot program in 1972 and then authorized as a national program in 1974. The program grew quickly in the 1980s and now includes special provisions under the Hunger Prevention Act of 1988 to reach the homeless.

Currently authorized through fiscal year 1997, WIC is not an entitlement program like most of the other food assistance programs. Instead, there is a cap on the amount of federal money allocated, which limits the number of participants who can be served. In 1996, nearly 7 million individuals participated in the WIC program at a cost of $3.6 billion. However, it is estimated that the program serves only about two thirds of those eligible. Because insufficient funds have been appropriated to provide services to all who have been determined to be eligible and in need of the program, coverage is provided on a priority basis. Local agencies maintain priority levels for eligible persons based on national guidelines. Many government officials believe that if eligibility for WIC were to cap for children at age three or four, the percentage of "coverage" for the total population served nationwide would improve dramatically.[12]

For pregnant, postpartum, and lactating women, and infants and children up to age five who qualify, WIC offers supplemental nutritious foods, nutrition education, and access to health care. Participants must meet economic eligibility criteria (between 100 and 185 percent of the poverty level), must be certified by a qualified health professional to be at nutritional risk (which includes such medical problems as abnormal prenatal weight gain, history of high-risk pregnancies, anemia, or inadequate dietary pattern), and must meet state eligibility requirements. In addition, any individual who receives benefits from FSP, Aid to Families with Dependent Children (AFDC), or Medicaid is automatically deemed to meet the WIC income eligibility requirement. (See chapters 8 and 9 for further discussion of the WIC program.)

The WIC program is administered at the federal level by the Food, Nutrition and Consumer Services agency within the USDA, which grants funds to state health departments and Indian tribal agencies. The state agencies, in turn, fund local sponsors such as health agencies, social service agencies, or other nonprofit agencies that are capable of providing nutrition and health services. Currently, more than 8,000 local WIC clinics are in operation throughout the nation.

WIC is generally regarded as one of the most effective nutrition programs.[12] Regardless of the type of research design employed, studies conducted since the mid-1970s consistently show increased prenatal weight gain, increased mean birthweight, decreased prematurity rate, decreased neonatal mortality, and decreased prevalence of anemia in children. Most of the more positive results associated with program participation have been reported for pregnant women and infants.

Food Distribution Programs   Several commodity distribution programs also assist households with food insufficiency. The Commodity Assistance Program (CAP) (PL 104–37) was created by consolidating funding for the Emergency Food Assistance Program (TEFAP), the Soup Kitchens and Food Banks Program (SK/FB), and the Commodity Supplemental Food Program (CSFP), into a single account. TEFAP provides administrative expenses and certain commodities to the network of food banks and other programs that assist households in need of immediate, short-term food assistance. The SK/FB provides commodities to soup kitchens and food banks, primarily to benefit the homeless; and in a number of states, the CSFP provides commodities to low-income elderly and women, infants, and children not enrolled in the WIC program.[42]

Nutrition Programs for Seniors   Nutrition programs for the elderly are designed to provide older Americans with low-cost nutritious meals, nutrition education, and an opportunity for social interaction. The Older Americans Act of 1965 authorized the Congregate Meals Program and the Home-Delivered Meals Program both of which are still in existence today. The USDA contributes to the senior nutrition programs through the Elderly Nutrition Program (ENP), which provides cash and commodities to local elderly nutrition centers for use in both programs. In 1995, ENP served approximately 230 million meals at 14,000 sites at a cost estimated to be $152 million.[42] In coordination with the DHHS, the ENP subsidizes meal service to persons sixty or older at low-income elderly centers or in the Meals On Wheels program. In 1997, the funding and administration of this program was transferred from the USDA to the Administration on Aging (AOA) of the DHHS.

Anyone sixty years or older can participate in the congregate meals program and their spouse, regardless of age, can also participate. Congregate meals are usually served once a day, Monday through Friday, at a local site, such as a senior center, community center, or neighborhood church. Program participants enjoy a nutritious meal and have the opportunity to socialize. Many centers also provide other services, including transportation to and from the center, information and referral for health and social services counseling, nutrition education, shopping assistance, and recreation. Participants in the home-delivered meals program must be older than sixty years of age, live in the program's service area, and be unable to prepare meals for themselves. This program delivers nutritious meals to the homes of disabled elderly persons. This type of program provides invaluable assistance to the frail elderly who wish to remain in their community and avoid institutionalization.

Policy Element 4: Providing Research-Based Information and Educational Programs to Encourage Informed Food Choices

In large measure, dietary guidance policies have followed closely behind related scientific discoveries in nutrition. Food guides such as the Basic Four Food groups and its precursor were based on the concept of selecting a recommended number of servings from a number of different food groups and maintaining a balance between the proportion of micronutrient-dense foods and energy-yielding foods.

In the past twenty-five years, the type of dietary guidance provided to consumers has shifted in focus. Early food guides had emphasized the quantity of foods to be selected from specific food groups, not on the quality of those food choices. This changed when groups such as the Senate Select Committee on Nutrition and Human Needs and noteworthy events such as the 1969 White House Conference on Food, Nutrition and Health began to call public attention to the links between diet and chronic disease. In 1977, the Senate Select Committee on Nutrition and Human Needs released a report, *Dietary Goals for the United States.*"[47] This document was among the first publications to link certain food components (such as fat, saturated fat, sodium, and dietary cholesterol) to the prevalence of debilitating chronic diseases, such as coronary heart disease and certain forms of cancer. Dietary recommendations now reflect general concern about excessive consumption of certain dietary components, such as saturated fat and cholesterol, because these substances have been shown to be associated with the risk of certain chronic diseases. Thus, the nature of the general message is changing to become more specific. Consumers are now advised not only to make *quantitative* judgments to consume certain types of foods but also to make *qualitative* distinctions among foods.[33]

The debate about content of dietary guidance messages has largely subsided with the publication of the *Surgeon General's Report on Nutrition and Health*[45] and the National Research Council report, *Diet and Health.*[25] Both reports proposed similar modifications in the U.S. diet to reduce the risk of chronic disease. Issues that remain regarding dietary guidance include:

• How will the message be presented—will guidelines remain qualitative in nature or will quantitative targets (such as 30 percent of calories as fat) be recommended?
• How can the same dietary guidance message be geared to individuals with different genetic profiles?
• How can dietary guidance be made more effective in actually changing dietary behavior?
• How best to implement the dietary recommendations?[28]

Government-Supported Programs in Nutrition Education

Extension Homemakers Programs and the Expanded Food and Nutrition Education

Program (EFNEP)   USDA assigned responsibility to the Extension System (ES) to administer a general food and nutrition education program for the public. Based on the extension delivery system, the program is designed to deliver research-based information through specialists at land grant universities to agents located in each county throughout the country. Recently, a national assessment of extension food and nutrition programs found that health and wellness was one of the three most frequently covered topics in the program.[18]

Also administered at the federal level by the USDA's ES is the Expanded Food and Nutrition Education Program, which is designed to teach low-income families, especially those with small children, the skills needed to choose and prepare an adequate, varied and balanced diet.

Recently, new initiatives have strengthened the relationship between the ES and food assistance programs. A WIC-ES initiative has received special funding that has enabled the ES to develop nutrition education programs in some states for WIC families. Some states have developed breast-feeding promotion programs for WIC mothers, often using EFNEP aides as lactation counselors. In addition, a number of ES programs are using funds reserved in the Food Stamp Program for

nutrition education to help food stamp families make wiser use of their limited food resources.[16]

Nutrition Education and Training Program (NET)   Since its inception in 1977, the NET has been integrally linked to school food programs. The goal of the program is to "provide nutrition education training to teachers and food service personnel so they, in turn, can teach children the relationship between food and health and encourage good eating habits.[17] The NET is not only designed to teach children the concepts of food and nutrition, but it also puts these concepts into practice in the lunchroom.

Federally Supported Educational Campaigns   As evidence linking diet and risk of chronic disease has increased, several groups have initiated communication campaigns to encourage the consumption of more healthful diets. Two of these federally supported educational campaigns are the National Cholesterol Education Program (NCEP), sponsored by the National Heart, Lung, Blood Institute (NHLBI), and the 5-a-Day for Better Health program, initiated by the National Cancer Institute (NCI), both units within the National Institutes of Health (NIH).

The NCEP was introduced in 1985 with the objective of "reducing coronary heart disease morbidity and mortality related to elevated blood cholesterol by developing a national education effort and by stimulating extensive cooperation and coordination among responsible government agencies and interested public organizations."[20] Based on research linking fruit and vegetable consumption to cancer prevention, and a tested state-based campaign prototype, the NCI launched the national "5-a-day" program in 1991.[13] The program is a collaborative effort between the NCI and the Produce for Better Health (PBH) using retail, media, and health channels to encourage Americans to improve their eating habits. The goal of the national 5-a-day program is to increase the per capita consumption of fruit and vegetables in the United States from the current 3.5 servings per day to 5 servings a day by the year 2000. The objectives include increasing public awareness of the importance of eating more fruits and vegetables for better health and providing specific information about how to turn these recommendations into dietary practices. It is anticipated that the program will run through the year 2000 and will consist of an ongoing media program, retail grocery involvement, and community interventions.[29]

Nutrition Labeling Although not identified specifically as a nutrition education program, providing information on food labels is a powerful tool for helping consumers make informed food choices. The Nutrition Labeling and Education Act (NLEA) of 1990 (PL 101-535) replaced the voluntary system of labeling established by the FDA regulations in 1973. The new food labels provide consumers with accurate and useful information about the nutrient content of products.

Policy Element 5: Providing for an Adequate Science and Research Base in Food and Nutrition

Research-based information needed for policymaking include data on human nutrition requirements throughout the life cycle, food consumption patterns, and the nutrient composition of food. Such information forms the scientific basis for policy decisions on food assistance programs, food labeling, and dietary guidance. Other research results, particularly those derived from epidemiological studies, clinical trials, and animal experiments, which delineate the nature of substantive relationships between diet and chronic diseases, have been used to justify requests for increased public funding for nutrition research.[5]

Recommended Dietary Allowances An example of the linkage between nutrition research and policy are the recommended dietary allowances (RDAs).[10] The scientific evidence on which the RDAs are formulated include nutrient balance studies; biochemical measurements of tissue saturation; nutrient intake studies of apparently healthy people; epidemiological observations; and in some cases, extrapolation of data from animal experiments. The RDAs have served as a basis for a variety of government and private activities and programs, such as a starting point for determining desirable nutrient intakes on which federal food assistance programs are based, or as the starting point for establishing comparison standards commonly referred to as "daily values."[29]

Research Activities and Support The USDA has traditionally been responsible for supporting research in the agricultural and food production system, up to and including food consumption and normal human nutrition needs. This role was strengthened by the 1977 Food and Agriculture Act (also called the 1977 Farm Bill), in which the USDA was identified as the lead agency in the federal government for food and agricultural sciences, including human nutrition.

Within the USDA, a number of agencies conduct or support human nutrition research. The Agricultural Research Service (ARS) supports a program that is primarily conducted by scientists or staff rather than by providing grants to outside scientists. A newly merged agency, the USDA's Cooperative Research Education and Extension Service, supports research at state land grant universities, oversees the federal funds (the so-called Hatch Grants) that go to state agricultural experiment stations, and provides assistance and technical support to extension staff at state and local levels. This agency also administers the Competitive Research Grants Program in human nutrition.

Other USDA agencies have more limited research programs. The Food and Nutrition Service (FNS) supports research projects related to the evaluation of service delivery issues in the food assistance programs. The FSIS conducts research primarily related to the safety and inspection systems for meat and poultry. The Economic Research Service (ERS) conducts intramural research on economic issues related to food consumption and food assistance programs.

At the DHHS, human nutrition research dealing with the metabolic effects of dietary consumption patterns, particularly as related to chronic diseases, has largely been in the domain of the NIH. The research program at the NIH consists mainly of extramural support provided to researchers at universities and medical school research facilities. The FDA, also an agency in the DHHS, conducts research related to food labeling and food safety issues.

The level and sources of federal support for nutrition research are of concern to most nutrition professionals because this indicates the commitment of the government to food and nutrition. Before 1950, the principal funding of human nutrition research was provided by three sources: the private sector, appropriated state funds, and the USDA formula grants to Agricultural Experiment Stations in land grant colleges and universities. Today, support for nutrition research has followed public and congressional interests in issues primarily related to the relationship between nutrition and health and disease. However, as Ostenso has reminded us, "regardless of the source of funding, the federal contribution to nutrition research has kept pace neither with the rate of inflation nor with the percentage increase allocated by the government to basic research in most other disciplines."[27]

Nutrition Monitoring   Nutrition monitoring is vital to policymaking and research.[46] Timely, complete, and accurate data are essential for developing nutrition policies and programs to meet the changing health needs of the nation. Monitoring activities can contribute to a database for public policy decisions related to food assistance programs; federally supported food service programs; nutrition education; public health nutrition programs; the regulation of fortification, safety, and labeling of the food supply; and food production and marketing. It also provides a database on which to establish research priorities. Figure 5.4 shows how nutrition monitoring and nutrition research affect policymaking.

On October 22, 1990, the National Nutrition Monitoring and Related Research Act of 1990 (PL 101-445), was passed. In accordance with the requirements of the act, a ten-year comprehensive plan was developed to "establish a comprehensive nutrition monitoring and related research program by collecting quality data that are continuous, coordinated, timely, and reliable; using comparable methods for data collection and reporting of results; conducting relevant research; and efficiently and effectively disseminating and exchanging information with data users."[46]

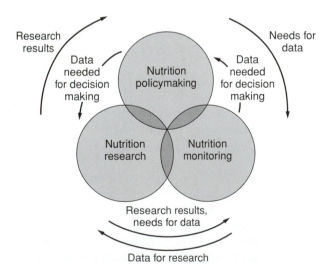

FIGURE 5.4   Relationship between Nutrition Policymaking, Nutrition Research, and Nutrition Monitoring
(*Source:* From US Department of Health and Human Services and US Department of Agriculture: *Ten-year comprehensive plan for the national nutrition monitoring and related research program,* 1992.)

Policy Element 6: Integrating Support for Nutrition Services as Part of the Health System

Issues such as health care financing, credentialing of health service providers, and standards of practice for nutrition professionals have attracted attention from policymakers over the past few years. Nothing has challenged the American system more seriously or proved more daunting to policymakers in recent years than ensuring that every citizen has access to good and affordable health care.

Nutrition in Health Care Reform   Shortly after taking office in early 1993, President Clinton announced the formation of a task force to conduct a serious study of the health care system and make recommendations for widespread reform. Sweeping changes and numerous plans were vociferously debated. The nutrition community, as well as every other health profession, rose to the occasion. The American Dietetic Association (ADA) developed a platform entitled, "The Economic Benefit of Nutrition Services," which focused on prevention as well as acute, long-term, outpatient, and home care. The platform also addressed maternal and child health and the nutrition needs of the elderly.[9] Like those of the Clinton administration and most groups promoting health care reform, the ADA backed the position that quality health care should be available, accessible, affordable, and reimbursable for all Americans. Further, the ADA maintained that government-mandated benefits must include nutrition services.[51] Other health associations and consumer groups joined the battle to include nutrition services in the health care reform debate. The resulting paper, "Rx: Good Nutrition, Putting 'Health' into Health Care Reform," presented a detailed analysis of the cost-benefits of nutrition services and was used extensively in talks with legislators.[51] The elections of November 1994 put the Republican Party in control of Congress, dramatically changing the political agenda. House Republicans do not refer to health care reform in their "Contract with America," and the issue seems to have been replaced by welfare reform, which is now a law.

THE COMMUNITY NUTRITION PROFESSIONAL'S ROLE THROUGHOUT THE POLICYMAKING PROCESS

So often we hear community nutrition professionals complain that they don't wish to become involved in the public policy process for a number of reasons—the problems are so great and their abilities to make a difference too weak; they don't know how or are scared to approach policy makers; or they think others should do this part of the job. The truth is that community nutrition professionals must be concerned about public policy and the process by which it can be changed because their very positions often depend on it.

Community nutrition professionals can successfully influence the policymaking process if they develop a positive working relationship with public officials, are savvy and sensitive about the political environment, and provide knowledgeable input (both support and criticism) for a policy maker's efforts. This section of the chapter highlights the roles of community nutrition professional as the issue moves through the public policy process (see figure 5.5).

Problem Recognition

Community nutrition professionals come in contact every day with a myriad of problems that could—and should—be solved by public policy actions. It is at this stage that community nutrition professionals may make important contributions by providing scientific evidence or data to strengthen the case for the issue. Without scientific backing, any cause will likely fall on "deaf ears" in Congress. Antihunger advocates and nutrition experts have found that documenting the prevalence of hunger and the benefits of good nutrition for human health has been helpful in securing support for new or expanded programs. The following sources of information are suggested as useful references to review key policy issues and build a strong case using scientific information:

- *Scientific bodies*—An example includes the Food and Nutrition Board of the Institute of Medicine, which provides impartial, comprehensive reviews of key policy issues.
- *Government publications and databases*—Examples include the National Nutrition Monitoring System, which provides an ongoing repository of data from various federally sponsored surveys. Their databases are the National Health and Nutrition Examination Surveys (NHANES), the Continuing Survey of Food Intakes of Individuals (CSF110) and the Diet-Health-Knowledge (DHK) survey.

The Centers for Disease Control and Prevention operate an on-line database (CDC Wonder), which contains U.S. Census, mortality and morbidity data useful in documenting nutrition-related health concerns.

State and local health departments also collect health and program data that is available to health professionals for program-planning purposes.

- *Consumer groups*—An example is The Food Research and Action Center (FRAC), which has prepared *How to Document Hunger in Your Community*, and Bread for the World publishes *Hunger Watch*.
- *Evaluation reports*—Examples include the School Nutrition Dietary Assessment Study conducted by the Mathematica Policy Research Group and the National WIC Evaluation Study.

Community nutrition professionals must be warned that grim statistics alone do not motivate policy makers to act. Providing examples of local program successes, anecdotal stories (especially those involving children), or sharing personal experiences that support the statistics will put a human face on all the numbers. In this changing political climate, Dr. M. R. C. Greenwood, former associate director of the Office of Science Technology Policy at the White House, advises

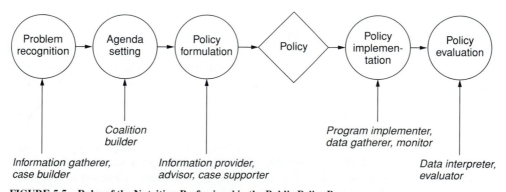

FIGURE 5.5   Roles of the Nutrition Professional in the Public Policy Process

that nutrition and health issues must be positioned to show how the proposed solutions will specifically benefit the interests of the nation as well as a disadvantaged group of people. Specific descriptions of how to effectively present nutrition program outcomes are found in chapter 15.

Agenda Setting

Community nutrition professionals must work with policy makers to get their issue onto the agenda and progress through the public policy process. Tips for getting policy makers to listen and common methods of reaching government officials are summarized in box 5.1.

The agenda-setting stage of the public policy process calls for the community nutritional professional to excel as coalition builder. Forming active coalitions among diverse groups such as researchers, health professionals, educators, farmers, and consumer groups as well as influential citizens, friends of decision makers, and respected community groups is the key to success. Such coalitions, often representing diverse points of interest on the issue, usually have greater political clout than individuals or organizations working alone.

Every coalition must have effective leadership or nothing will happen. Among the coalitions of groups focusing their attention on specific food and nutrition policies are the following:

- *Child Nutrition Forum:* Organized to express a unified voice about support for child nutrition programs, its members include the Society for Nutrition and Education (SNE), the American Dietetic Association, the American School Food Service Association (ASFSA), the Food Research and Action Center, the National Parent Teacher Association (PTA), and the Community Nutrition Institute (CNI).
- *End Childhood Hunger:* More than 100 different public health organizations, church groups, and trade associations joined the FRAC in a national campaign to end childhood hunger.
- *The Food and Nutrition Labeling Group:* Formed originally in 1988 by the Center for Science in the Public Interest (CSPI) to support and lobby for nutrition labeling reform, this group represents more than twenty different groups.
- *Task Force on Aging:* Comprised of sixty member organizations that support legislative initiatives on health care, food assistance, and transportation for senior citizens.

Appendix C provides addresses and telephone numbers of organizations involved in domestic food and nutrition policies.

Policy Formation

The process of formulating public policy is actually within the purview of the legislative or regulatory body. It is the job of various stakeholders on the issue under debate to influence the policy makers about the content of the policy as well as the process it will follow. It is the role of the community nutrition professional to be an advisor, supporter, and communicator.

Community nutrition professionals working in community programs have two positions of access and influence: first, they are tax-paying voters who are constituents of a particular congressional district; second, they have information to assist the legislator in supporting worthwhile legislation, the goal of all policy makers. Constituent support greatly facilitates an issue's chances of moving quickly and smoothly through the policy process. It is important to be patient and not get discouraged. Many legislative initiatives require several sessions of Congress before they get passed. The Nutrition Monitoring bill, which eventually passed in 1990, took more than six years before the proposed legislation actually became law.

Policy Implementation

Once a policy has been enacted, the programs it created must be carried out. At this stage of the policy process, the community nutrition professional assumes the role of program planner, implementer, and data gatherer to document and monitor program outcomes.

Policy Evaluator

Once program data have been collected, the community nutrition professional becomes a program evaluator. It is important to document program outcomes and impacts. In addition, the role of data interpreter becomes important. One so closely identified with the program and how it works should be able to "feed back" these data to policy makers to inform them how well the program is working. These feedback data are crucial to continuing program success; often changes in regulations or legislation is needed to improve how well the program functions. Community nutrition professionals are able and prepared to undertake this responsibility.

BOX 5.1

VOICING EFFECTIVE MESSAGES

TO POLICYMAKERS

- *Know what to say:* Before voicing messages, one must define the purpose and desired outcome. Do you want a member of Congress to introduce a bill to educate the public on safe food handling or to reform meat inspection completely?
- *Research the audience you want to reach:* The target audience determines what to say and how to deliver the message. An analysis of the target audience includes learning the values, concerns, and existing opinions of the group. What language do they speak? About what do they care? Who do they believe? From what sources do they get information?
- *Make a persuasive message:* To make your voice heard, you need to develop a clear, concise, and consistent message. Convey your passion toward the issue and the urgency of finding a solution.
- *Select the best communication channel:* Citizens communicate with government officials through many channels. The best way to voice your opinion depends on your target audience, your goals, and your circumstances.
- *Repeat the message, repeat the message!*

TO GOVERNMENT OFFICIALS

Letter Writing: A handwritten letter with a personal touch sends a powerful message to the Hill.

Phone Call: Congressional staff who are responsible for an issue answer most phone calls and relay your concerns to the official. Follow-up a letter with a call.

Town Meetings: If your representative participates in a town meeting, come prepared with a specific question that addresses your concerns.

Personal Visit: You can visit elected officials when they return to the local office or when you visit the state or federal capital.

Visits to Your Program: If you invite an elected official to visit your program, show how it benefits the community and what really goes on in your program.

Testify at a Hearing: Whether you testify at a public hearing or simply submit written comments on an issue, timing can make or break your cause. The first five lines of your testimony make the strongest impression, so state your name, organization, background on the issue, and legislative concerns immediately and concisely.

Gimmicks: For years, advocates have relied on gimmicks to communicate their messages. Bread for the World, a Christian antihunger group, mobilized members to send a single birthday candle to their congressional members with a letter noting the impact WIC had in getting poor kids through the first year of life.

TO COLLEAGUES

Telephone or Fax Tree: Organizations can generate immediate action by establishing a telephone or fax tree whereby a member will receive a call and then contact two additional appointed members until everyone in an organization is reached.

E-mail: Many groups sign on to the information superhighway to transfer information to members through the Internet.

TO THE PUBLIC

Direct Mail: Some groups send mailings that describe the issue and often ask for funding to support reform.

Newsletters: Some advocacy groups use their newsletters that reach the public to encourage mailing post cards on specific issues to local or national political leaders.

Mass Media: The most successful policy campaigns depend on mass media to raise public awareness and even consumer outrage. Powerful ideas and emotions can move voters to contact legislators, and in turn, force legislators to respond through the media. The media informs the public about current issues to give legislators a gauge of public sentiment on key issues.

Source: From Chapman N, Kehoe R: *Let your voice be heard: how to shape food policy,* Washington, DC, 1995, N. Chapman Associates, Inc. Used with permission of Nancy Chapman, N. Chapman Associates, Inc.

IMPLICATIONS FOR COMMUNITY NUTRITION PROFESSIONALS

Public policy governs the actions of governmental units. In the absence of a clearly defined nutrition policy in the United States, policy is set de facto by a number of programs, advisory groups, legislative actions, partnerships, and publications. Six elements of nutrition policy are identified. These elements are crucial in understanding how the actors, structures, and groups contribute toward the public policy process. Appendices C and D list specific resources as well as sources of information that will be helpful to those who wish to be actively involved in the nutrition policy process. Since much public policy has shifted away from the federal government to actions at the state and local levels in the past few years, community nutrition professionals need to recognize and address problems close to home by applying advocacy skills throughout the five stages of the public policy process. Community nutrition professionals can change policy when they are knowledgeable about the process, adopt a proactive stance, and advocate change based on sound science that benefits populations.

COMMUNITY NUTRITION PROFESSIONALS IN ACTION

- Do research on your representatives in Congress— your local member of the House of Representatives and the two Senators representing your state. What are their interests, their "pet projects"? How can you contribute to their understanding of food and nutrition issues that may appear as proposed legislation?
- Select a food- or nutrition-related issue of interest. Using Appendix D, identify the organizations that are interested in this food- or nutrition-related issue. Contact one of the organizations to request any related publications. Locate other documented research or monitoring data to support your position. Review ways of "voicing effective messages" and generate a postcard mailing for the public to raise awareness about your issue of interest.
- Attend a hearing at your state legislature. Prepare a report, noting who the speakers were, what their positions were, and how these hearings are likely to impact the outcome of the proposed bill.
- Review the efforts in the development of food assistance programs. Do current food assistance programs resolve the policy element of "providing adequate food at reasonable cost"? Why or Why not? If not, what is needed to strengthen these programs. Prepare a convincing statement that could be mailed to your congressperson.

GOING ONE STEP FURTHER

Select one nutrition-related legislative or regulatory issue. Using current resources, track the following:

- The science base on which the proposal is based.
- The "political climate" under which it was proposed. Who favored it? Who opposed it? On what grounds?
- To which committee was it referred? Do you think this was an appropriate assignment? Why or why not?
- Were hearings held? Who testified? What were their positions? Were they effective in conveying their positions? What made for a "convincing" testimony?
- Describe the course of the legislative process for this issue. Was it passed? Vetoed by the president? What are the next steps?
- If bill was passed and signed into law, to which agency was it referred for implementation? Describe the process for writing regulations for this bill. What were the particularly contentious issues? Write a comment on proposed regulations. Compare the proposed with the final regulations. How do they differ?
- Write a concise overview of the legislative and regulatory processes, and outcomes that occurred for this particular nutrition-related issue.

ADDITIONAL INFORMATION

Professional societies develop and publish statements, scientific status summaries, commentaries, and position papers to clarify an issue in which the particular society has expertise.

The American Dietetic Association position statement relevant to chapter 5 is as follows:

1. Cost-effectiveness of medical nutrition therapy (*J Am Diet Assoc* 95:88, 1995)

REFERENCES

1. Blumer P: How a bill becomes a law, Paper presented at the legislative symposium of the American Dietetic Association, Washington, DC, 1992.
2. Boisvert-Walsh C, Kallio J: *Reaching out for those at highest risk.* In Kaufman M, editor: *Nutrition in public health,* Rockville, MD, 1990, Aspen.
3. Burghardt J, Devaney B: *The School Nutrition Dietary Assessment Study,* Princeton, NJ, 1993, Mathematica Policy Research Institute.
4. Campbell, CA: Food security: a nutritional outcome or predictor variable? *J Nutr* 121:408, 1991.
5. Chapman N: Consensus and coalitions: key to nutrition policy development, *Nutr Today* 22:22, 1987.
6. Clem, AL: *Congress: powers, processes, and politics,* Pacific Grove, CA, 1989, Brooks/Cole.
7. *Congressional Directory for the 104th Congress,* Washington, DC, 1995, National Committee to Preserve Social Security and Medicare.
8. *CQ guide to current American government,* Washington, DC, 1996, Congressional Quarterly Inc.
9. Finn SC, Gallagher A, Blumer P: President's page: health care reform—making nutrition part of the package, *J Am Diet Assoc* 93:337, 1993.
10. Food and Nutrition Board, National Research Council, National Academy of Sciences: *Recommended dietary allowances,* ed 10, Washington, DC, 1989, National Academy Press.

11. Food Research and Action Center (FRAC): *Fact sheets on the federal food programs,* Washington, DC, 1991, FRAC.

12. General Accounting Office: *Early interventions: federal investments like WIC can produce savings, Food assistance programs,* GAO/HRD–92–18, Washington, DC, 1992, General Accounting Office.

13. Heimendinger J, VanDuyn MA, Chapelsky D, Foerster S, Stables G: The national 5-a-day for better health program: a large-scale nutrition intervention, 1996, Unpublished.

14. Henkel J: How to comment on proposals and submit petitions, *FDA Consumer* 30:6, 1996.

15. Hutt PB: National nutrition policy and the role of the Food and Drug Administration, *Currents* 2:2, 1986.

16. Joy AB, Doisy C: Food stamp nutrition education program: assisting food stamp recipients to become self-sufficient, *J Nutr Educ* 28:123, 1996.

17. Kalina BB, Phillips CA, Minns HV: The NET program: a ten-year perspective, *J Nutr Educ* 21:38, 1989.

18. Kaltreider DL, Sims LS, Brown JL: Extension food and nutrition programs: a national assessment, *Extension Review* 58:46, 1987.

19. Kennedy E, Morris PM, Lucas R: Welfare reform and nutrition programs: contemporary budget and policy realities, *J Nutr Educ* 29:67, 1996.

20. Lenfant C: A new challenge for America: the National Cholesterol Education program, *Circulation* 73:855, 1986.

21. Leonard RE: Block grants fading as food program option, *CNI Nutrition Week* (August 18):4–5, 1995.

22. McNutt K: Integrating nutrition and environmental objectives, *Nutr Today* 25:40, 1990.

23. McNutt K: Pros and cons of block grants, *J Nutr Educ* 28:76, 1996.

24. Mintz BW, Miller NG: *A guide to federal agency rulemaking,* ed 2, Washington, DC, 1991, Administrative Conference of the United States.

25. National Research Council: *Diet and health: implications for reducing chronic disease risk,* Washington, DC, 1989, National Academy Press.

26. Nestle M, Guttmacher S: Hunger in the United States: rationale, methods, and policy implications of state hunger surveys, *J Nutr Educ* 24:18S, 1992.

27. Ostenso GL: Nutrition, policies and politics, *J Am Diet Assoc* 88:909, 1988.

28. Palmer S: Food and nutrition policy: challenges for the 1990s, *Health Affairs* (Millwood) 9:94, 1990.

29. Porter DV: Food assistance programs: nutrition standards, *Nutr Today* 30:177, 1995.

30. Robinson D: *Federal programs for children and families,* CRS Report for Congress No. 03-50 EPW, Washington, DC, 1992, Congressional Research Office, The Library of Congress.

31. Senauer B, Asp E, Kinsey J: *Food trends and the changing consumer,* St. Paul, MN, 1991, Eagan Press.

32. Sims, LS: The ebb and flow of nutrition as a public policy issue, *J Nutr Educ* 15:4, 1983.

33. Sims, LS: Government involvement in nutrition education: panacea or Pandora's box? *Health Educ Res,* 5:517, 1990.

34. Sims LS: *Nutrition policy through the Reagan era: feast or famine?* Pew/Cornell lecture series on food and nutrition policy, Ithaca, NY, 1988, Cornell Food and Nutrition Policy Program.

35. Sims LS: Public policy in nutrition: a framework for action, *Nutr Today* 28:10, 1993.

36. Sims LS, Voichick J: Our perspective: nutrition education enhances food assistance programs, *J Nutr Educ* 28:83, 1996.

37. Skrzycki C: The rise of "reg-neg": finding common ground in the middle of the table, 23 February 1996, *Washington Post.*

38. Spasoff RA: The role of nutrition in health public policy, *Rapport* 4:6, 1989.

39. Splett PL: Federal food assistance programs: a step to food security for many, *Nutr Today* 29:6, 1994.

40. Summaries of court actions, *FDA Consumer* 30:35, 1996.

41. Ternus M: Food fortification: it can be a lifesaver, but are we going too far in creating "no-brain" super foods? *Environ Nutr* April(Spec. Suppl):9–12, 1996.

42. U.S. Department of Agriculture, Food and Consumer Service: *USDA's 1997 budget summary,* Washington, DC, 1996, USDA.

43. U.S. Department of Agriculture/Food and Nutrition Service, Office of Analysis and Evaluation: *Characteristics of food stamp households: Summer 1993,* Washington, DC, 1994, USDA.

44. U.S. Department of Agriculture: *Team nutrition: program summary,* Washington, DC, 1995, USDA.

45. U.S. Department of Health and Human Services: *The Surgeon General's report on nutrition and health,* U.S. Public Health Service Pub. No. 88–50201, Washington, DC, 1988, U.S. Public Health Service.

46. Department of Health and Human Services and Department of Agriculture: Ten-year comprehensive plan for the national nutrition monitoring and related research program; notice, *Federal Register* 56:55716, 1991.

47. U.S. Senate Select Committee on Nutrition and Human Needs: *Dietary goals for the United States,* ed 2, Washington, DC, 1977, U.S. Government Printing Office.

48. Wagner PA: Proposed changes in the nation's system of food assistance, *Hunger & Food Security Issues* 4:1, 1995.

49. Wagner PA, Gaumer A: Food stamps: a nutrition resource in times of economic hardship, *Hunger & Food Security Issues* 4:1, 1995.

50. White House Conference on Food Nutrition and Health: *Summary of actions on food nutrition and health,* Washington, DC, 1970, U.S. Government Printing Office.

51. Wootan M and others: *Rx: good nutrition: putting "health" into health care reform,* Washington, DC, 1994, National Coalition for Nutrition in Health Care Reform.

CASE STUDY

A POLICY-BASED APPROACH TO PREVENTING HUNGER IN WISCONSIN*

LAURA S. SIMS, PHD, MPH
PROFESSOR OF NUTRITION
DEPARTMENT OF NUTRITION AND FOOD SCIENCE
UNIVERSITY OF MARYLAND

INTRODUCTION

This case study illustrates the process by which a recognized problem is transformed by the public policy process into actionable programs. This case demonstrates an actual event, an example of how the dedicated work of a relatively small number of people who were focused on a single, galvanizing topic resulted in the passage of hunger prevention legislation in Wisconsin in 1994.

THE CASE

The Setting

Although state legislatures may vary in details of organization, they have similar functions: lawmaking, representation, and administrative oversight. In their structure, state legislatures reflect the structure of Congress. For the most part, they adhere to the same traditions of seniority and legislative norms, such as legislative work, specialization, reciprocity, party loyalty, institutional loyalty and interpersonal courtesy as does Congress.[1]

The Wisconsin legislature is a two-chamber body consisting of a thirty-three-member senate and a ninety-nine-member assembly. Each senate district is made up of three assembly districts. Senators serve four-year terms and representatives to the assembly serve two-year terms. A new legislature is sworn into office in January of each odd-numbered year to meet a two-year period called a "biennium."

During the biennium, the legislature is in continuous session with a schedule of alternating floor periods and committee work periods. The session schedule, which sets the dates for these, is adopted by joint resolution of both houses at the beginning of the session. Standing committees are the "workhorses" of the Wisconsin legislature. They are established by the rules of each house. The senate president and assembly speaker are responsible for referring newly introduced bills or resolutions to the appropriate standing committee.[3] This, then, is the body with which those who seek to influence Wisconsin legislature must work.

THE POLICYMAKING PROCESS

Problem Recognition

In Wisconsin, as in many other states, a number of advocacy groups that began in the 1970s have been continuously committed to bringing public attention to the issues of hunger and food security. Two such organizations—the Hunger Task Force of Milwaukee (HTFW) and the Wisconsin Nutrition Project (WNP)—were instrumental in formulating the initial case for policy solutions to the hunger problem in Wisconsin and have worked closely with local community action agencies to promote WIC, school nutrition programs, and the like over the years. The HTFW, which started in 1974 to focus attention on the problems in Milwaukee and the urban southeast corner of Wisconsin, now works statewide; it comprises an emergency food bank as well as a policy advocacy component. The WNP began in 1978 as a pilot program of the National Children's Project and became an independent, private, nonprofit organization in 1979. These groups have also had successful networking experiences with the faith community, including the Archdiocese of Milwaukee and the Evangelical Lutheran Church of America, and were joined in their efforts by a former member of the Wisconsin assembly who is also a Methodist minister.

Other groups that made major contributions to hunger awareness were those that deal with the distribution of emergency food, particularly Second Harvest. Such groups are familiar with creating awareness about hunger

---

*This case study was adapted and expanded from "Developing a Hunger Bill in Wisconsin" by Dr. Jane Voichick, Professor of Nutritional Sciences at the University of Wisconsin-Madison, which appeared in *Food Security in the United States: A Guidebook for Public Issues Education,* Leidenfrost NB and Wilkins JL, Eds. Published and distributed by the Cooperative Extension System, November 1994.

issues and fund raising, so their expertise is invaluable. This is an area in which diverse perspectives abound. Many community nutrition professionals feel that provision of emergency food is not an ideal long-term solution to the hunger problem, favoring instead those programs that will lead to sustained change. In contrast, those unsupportive of government programs to feed the hungry usually favor such emergency food provision efforts because they are independent of government "control."

There were no data gathered in Wisconsin specifically to document the prevalence and severity of the hunger problem. The sense of need arose from a combination of people's personal experiences and findings from other states. The FRAC, an advocacy group based in Washington, D.C., conducted a series of studies throughout the United States starting in 1989. The findings from the first set of studies in the Community Childhood Hunger Identification Project (CCHIP)[2] were quite helpful to those in Wisconsin who used these data in building their case.

Individuals and groups working on the hunger issue in Wisconsin felt that the problem could be best addressed and rectified by taking a "policy" course of action. They believed that passing a law would lead to more sustainable change and would bring resources along with a policy commitment.

Agenda Setting

Because of his familiarity with the Wisconsin assembly, the Rev. Harvey Stower (the Methodist minister mentioned earlier) became a spokesperson for legitimizing the hunger issue and addressing it through policy means. In addition to a number of prominent citizens who called for a study of the hunger problem in Wisconsin, sixteen legislators supported the effort. One of these was Spencer Black, a representative from Madison, who had a long history of being responsive to such issues; he had previously introduced legislation on this issue, but his effort had been defeated. No organized group opposed the addition of "hunger" to the policy agenda at this time.

Policy Formulation

One of the key policy "gatekeepers" in the Wisconsin legislature is a specific committee called the "Legislative Council." It consists of twenty-one members, including the presiding officer of each house, speaker pro tempore of the assembly, senate and assembly majority and minority leaders, the two cochairpersons, and the ranking minority members from each house on the Joint Committee on Finance. In addition, five senators and five representatives are appointed as members of the Council.

It is this "Legislative Council" that is charged with the responsibility for considering various problems of state and local government in Wisconsin and presenting its recommendations in the form of bills to the entire legislature for subsequent action. Study topics are selected from requests presented to the Council by law, joint resolution, or requests from individual legislators. After research and public hearings, the Council study committee drafts proposals and submits them to the council. The Council must approve those drafts it wants introduced in the legislature as council bills. In general, council bills are more likely to be passed by the full legislature than bills brought up by individual legislators.[5]

Just getting a topic selected to be studied by the council requires promotion by individuals interested in specific issues. While there were no outright protests about moving the issue of hunger onto the policy agenda, the problem was one of competition for attention by the council. Support letters from seventeen legislators coupled with a very effective letter-writing drive from concerned citizens throughout Wisconsin requested that his particular topic be addressed. In 1992, over a hundred topics were suggested, and twenty—including the one on hunger prevention—were chosen by the Council for further study. Modest media attention was directed at the hunger issue at the start of the study by the Council.

The Legislative Council appointed a bipartisan study "Committee on Issues related to Hunger Prevention." This special committee was composed of one Senator, four Representatives, and thirteen public members. The committee was chaired by a representative and staffed by lawyers who were employed by the Council. The study committee also included representatives from hunger advocacy groups, the food industry, the state university, the county government, the faith community, Head Start, the County Commission on Aging, the Wisconsin Farmers Foundation, and school food service directors. The charge to the committee was to (1) review the extent and cause of hunger in Wisconsin, (2) examine current programs directed at alleviating hunger, and (3) develop initiatives to reduce the incidence of hunger and lack of adequate nutrition in Wisconsin's population.[4]

During the 1992 to 1993 year, the committee held five meetings at the state capital in Madison and two public hearings, one in a rural area of the state and one in Milwaukee. The first meetings were arranged to obtain information about state and federally funded food and nutrition programs administered by the state department of education (Wisconsin Department of Instruction) and the state Department of Health and Social Services (DHSS). In the two public hearings, the committee solicited specific testimony on the extent of hunger and malnutrition and how existing federal and state programs could be improved to better meet the needs of citizens. Thirty people provided testimony at the committee. Those who advocated the policy change and were organizing the hearings recognized that the most salient—and convincing—testimony usually comes from those experiencing the problems firsthand. Therefore, presentations at the hearings were from members of advocacy organizations as well as from citizens who had experienced food insecurity as well as from volunteers who worked at local emergency food providers such as food banks and shelters for the homeless. In the final meetings, the committee reviewed preliminary motions and subsequent drafts related to a variety of topics. The variety of perspectives provided by members of the committee greatly enriched the outcomes of the discussions. The Special Committee developed ten drafts, which were then combined into a single bill, *1993 Assembly Bill 582*. The bill was introduced by the Legislative Council in June 1993 and it was referred to the Assembly Committee on Children and Human Services. This committee held hearings on the bill, adopted two amendments, and recommended passage. Then the bill was referred to the Joint Committee on Finance, which held an executive session on the bill in March 1994; this committee also recommended passage of the bill with substitute amendments. Also in March 1994, the assembly passed the bill with amendments. Subsequently, the Senate Committee on Health, Human Services and Aging and the full Senate concurred on the bill. The bill was signed into law by the governor on March 28, 1994 and took effect April 12, 1994, just about two years after the first requests for the study committee to be constituted had been made. Highlights of Act 168 include:

- The establishment of a Board on Hunger with the DHSS
- The creation of a community-based hunger prevention grants program
- The establishment and funding of a food stamp outreach program
- A directive to the DHSS to assist school districts in the direct certification of children's eligibility for free and reduced-price nutrition programs

- The creation of a school breakfast grant program
- A proposal to pay food stamp benefits in Milwaukee through electronic benefit transfer.

Policy Implementation

As a result of the "Hunger Bill" in Wisconsin, a Hunger Board was established to monitor hunger prevention efforts, review proposals, and award grants. Two cycles of grant-making occurred between mid-1994 and mid-1996. Administrative responsibility for the Hunger Board and management of the Community-Based Hunger Prevention Program Grants was assigned to the Division of Economic Support in the DHSS. In the first year after passage, the division had a total of $375,000 available for start-up projects, for which applicants could compete for grants of up to $20,000. Altogether, $250,000 was available for grants during calendar year 1996. Grants were given out for some very diverse projects, all locally originated and managed.

Policy Evaluation

In the interest of "streamlining" government, there is a movement in Wisconsin to greatly reduce the number of advisory committees and boards; at present, the Board on Hunger (along with a number of others) is being considered for elimination. The decision has been put "on hold" but will be reviewed soon. It is incumbent on those who fought so hard to create the legislation to fight equally hard to obtain new appropriations to continue to support the community hunger grant program.

Because of the need for improved public understanding of the hunger issue, many in Wisconsin are working together to increase awareness of the problem and commitment to solving it among local groups. A program has been developed to accomplish this goal; included among the program's component are a TV documentary on hunger in Wisconsin to be aired on the state public TV network, a satellite videoconference aimed at training and empowering local community groups, a training conference on skill-building, and another conference linking university researchers with community groups who need assistance with monitoring and evaluating program progress. Those associated with the effort for a number of years believe it is all "very exciting!"

Certainly, there are some common goals as well as unique talents spread among the diverse constituencies—advocates, academics, the food industry, the religious and philanthropic communities, public relations, and communications and media specialists—all working in the name of preventing and alleviating hunger. The "trick" for those working in these groups is to respect each others' unique contributions and identify common goals on which all can agree. The key words—consensus, coalitions, and compromise—will serve this cause well in the future. Progress often comes slowly—but, it comes.

REFERENCES

1. *Anatomy of legislatures*. In Bagwell M, Clements S, editors: *A political handbook for health professionals,* Boston, 1985, Little, Brown and Company.
2. Food Research and Action Center (FRAC): *Community childhood hunger identification project,* Washington, DC, 1991, FRAC.
3. *The legislative process,* Wisconsin Blue Book, 1995, Dept of Administration—Wisconsin Legislative Reference Bureau, Madison, Wisconsin.
4. Rose L: *New law relating to hunger prevention (1993 Wisconsin Act 168),* Information memorandum 94-3, Madison, 1994, Wisconsin Legislative Council.
5. Wisconsin Legislative Reference Bureau: State of Wisconsin 1993–1994 Blue Book, Madison, 1993, Department of Administration.

DISCUSSION QUESTIONS

1. What role did the community nutrition professional have in helping to create the legislation? Now that the legislation is being implemented, what role(s) should community nutrition professionals be playing? What roles should they play in the future?
2. Identify the networking partners used by the community nutrition professional. Were these coalitions beneficial? Are there food industries that could be supportive of this issue? How could the media be utilized to continue awareness of hunger?
3. What should be the next steps? Advocate for continuance of the Board on Hunger? Lobby for new appropriations to support implementation of the Act? Actively promote (and publicize) evaluation of the funded projects? (Think: what if they are not working?) Other steps? What roles do each of the following groups have in this endeavor: community nutrition professionals, the food industry, university researchers, community advocates, the religious community?
4. What would you consider to be "indicators of success" for this bill as it is evaluated? What would be indicators that would ensure the continuance of its programs? What measures would suggest that the program be discontinued?

CHAPTER SIX

THE CHANGING AND DYNAMIC FOOD SUPPLY
PRODUCT INNOVATION AND FOOD SAFETY

*It should be a goal of our country to provide a sufficient variety
of foods throughout the year to meet the energy and nutrient
needs of its citizens and promote health. Our food supply should
be safe and properly preserved to maintain high quality, yet be
low enough in cost for all to have access to a nutritionally
adequate diet irrespective of income.*

—INSTITUTE OF MEDICINE, NATIONAL ACADEMY OF SCIENCE, 1994

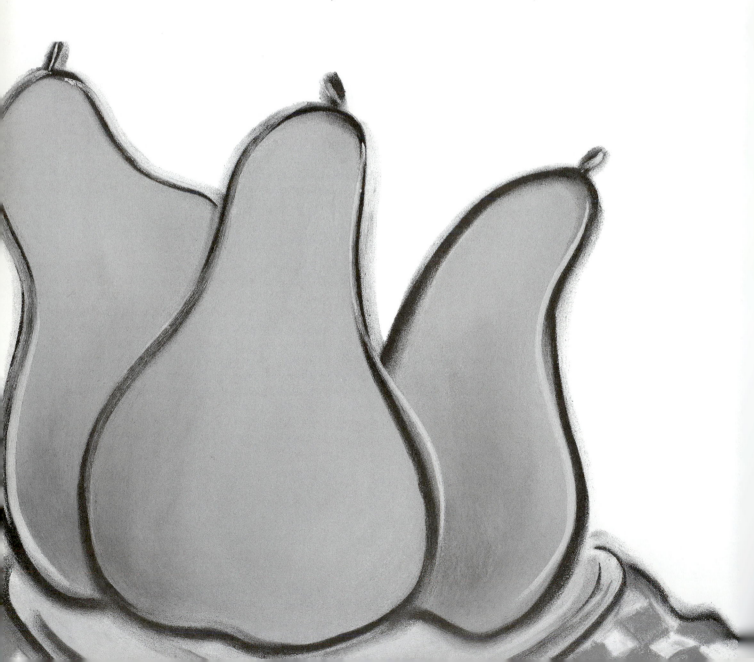

Core Concepts

This chapter addresses the modifications in foods and their ingredients that consumers and the food industry are making to address the relationship between diet and health and the changes in food technologies that will make a greater variety of foods more readily available and safer in the future. In examining the impacts of the diet/health emphasis on the food industry, we also examine the movement toward the use of foods to promote or maintain health and the use of food additives, ingredients, and technologies to modify and improve foods. A summary of the mechanisms that are being used to maintain a safe food supply is included.

Objectives

When you finish chapter six, you should be able to:

~ Describe the major consumer trends affecting food science.

~ Identify the major laws regulating the food supply and their enforcement.

~ Outline the methods by which food additives are approved.

~ Describe the ingredients used to reduce the amount of fat or sugar in foods and their safety.

~ Describe the techniques, advantages, and limitations of food irradiation, modified atmosphere packaging, and biotechnology.

~ Delineate significant types of risks and hazards in the food supply and methods used to reduce them.

~ Define roles for nutrition professionals in serving as advocates for both consumers and the food industry to assure a safe and adequate food supply.

Key Words

Word	Page Mentioned
Organic foods	150
Sustainable agricultural practices	150
Phytochemicals	150
Functional foods	150
Food, Drug and Cosmetic Act	151
Generally recognized as safe (GRAS)	151
Cyclamate	152
Acceptable Daily Intake (ADI)	152
Restoration	152
Fortification	152
Microparticulation	154
Polydextrose	154
Fat substitutes	154
Olestra	154
Structured lipids	155
Engineered fats	155
Nutritive sweeteners	155
Nonnutritive sweeteners	155
Polyols	155
Reduced-calorie sweeteners	155
Aspartame	155
Sucralose	157
Modified atmosphere packaging (MAP)	157
Food irradiation	157
Radura	157
Biotechnology	158
Recombinant DNA (rDNA)	158
Safe	159
Risk	159
Risk assessment	159
Risk management	159
Threshold	160
Infectious dose (ID)	160
Biological hazard	160
Chemical hazard	160
Physical hazard	160
Foodborne infections	160
Foodborne intoxications	160
Hazard Analysis Critical Control Points (HACCP)	164

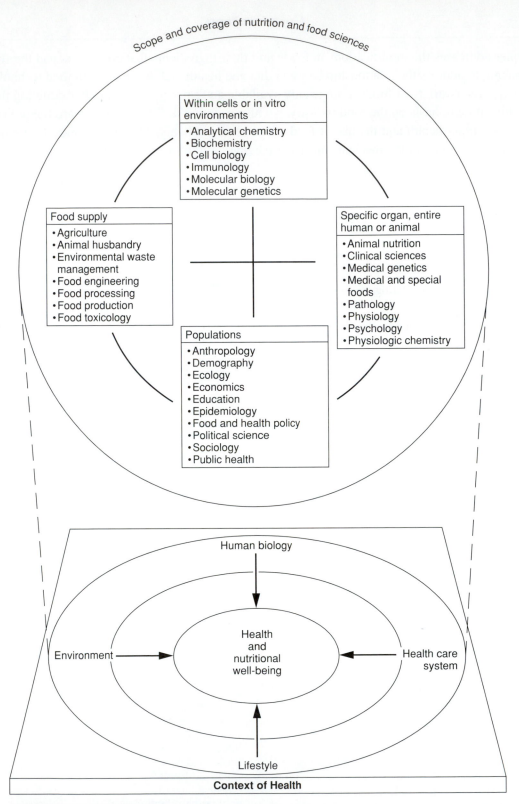

FIGURE 6.1   Context of Health

The scope of nutrition and the food sciences. (*Source:* Top of figure reprinted with permission from *Opportunities in the Nutrition and Food Sciences.* Copyright 1994 by the National Academy of Sciences. Courtesy of the National Academy Press, Washington, DC.)

Nutrition and food science are among the most interdisciplinary of all sciences. They bring together the chemical, physical, biological, medical, agricultural, social, behavioral, and engineering sciences. These sciences are important to determine how food affects health—from the basic molecular and cellular levels to the organ, organism, and even population levels. Another major area of study in these fields is the design of food systems to enhance the physical and economic well-being of individuals and groups as well as the adequacy and safety of their food supply.[23,42]

Community nutrition professionals must have knowledge of nutrition and food science, and their interactions, if they are going to be successful in meeting the nutritional and health needs of individuals and the community. As community nutrition professionals, we must discuss food in relation to nutrition since consumers eat food to obtain the nutrients they need.

Over the years, there has been much discussion about nutrition and food science, however, there is still no single methodology that unites nutrition with food science. Some contend that food science is concerned with food from its production to the point where it is consumed, at which time food becomes the interest of the nutritionist. A more inclusive description of food science and nutrition is that both sciences are a collection of interests centered around food and human well-being and, therefore, are a part of a continuum.

Figure 6.1 describes the scope and coverage of nutrition and food science. Each box represents one focus of the nutrition and food sciences with examples of areas of study.[42] These areas of study are divided into four overlapping areas of concentration within individual cells, specific organs, entire human or animal populations, and the food supply. Each area of concentration and area of study depends on a wide variety of supporting areas. This illustration shows clearly how food science and nutrition are intertwined.

ENHANCING THE FOOD SUPPLY

Food science and the food industry are responding to emerging research findings, changing consumer dietary preferences, and shifting government policies by providing a wide variety of foods that are modified in calorie, fat, cholesterol, and/or salt content. Enhancing the food supply involves producing health-promoting, high-quality, economical, and wholesome foods with reduced adverse effects on the environment and better use of raw materials.

The food industry changes more rapidly each year to meet the demands of the American consumer.[40] In 1998, the Institute of Food Technologists, the professional society of food scientists and technologists, published a list of consumer trends to 2020 and beyond.[38] These trends are listed in table 6.1 and reflect both an increased recognition of the role of food in health and an alteration in lifestyles on the part of the consumer.

Significant shifts in demographics, psychographics and consumer food preferences—taste, price, nutrition, convenience in health and technological innovation—will continue to 2020 and beyond. The fact that consumers have made a strong connection between diet and health is driving many modifications in the food industry, particularly in ingredient use and ingredient technology.[39] Another major impact on the food industry is the necessity to maintain a safe food supply.

TABLE 6.1
Consumer Trends to 2020 and Beyond

1. Eating Occasions Increase
   - Grazing and snacking becoming a way of life.
     Forty percent of consumers eat four or five times a day.
   - Demise of the lunch hour will occur.
     Breakfast eaten in office has doubled since 1990.
   - Number of meals eaten in car will increase.
     Fastest growing segment of food industry is "portable hand-held foods."
   - Packaging will be fundamental.
     Eat in order-controlled easily dispensable and environmentally friendly packaging will be available.

2. Natural Becomes the Norm
   - Desire for fresh, natural and pure products will be stronger than ever.
     Freshness will become the most desired label claim.
   - Artificial will be out.
     Unless the end benefit cannot be achieved any other way.

3. Technologies Will Open Growth Avenues
   - Consumers will embrace new technologies and scientific processes that enhance and protect the food supply.

4. Focusing on Health
   - Concerns over disease prevention, anti-aging, energy, immunity and treatment will get primary attention.
   - Marketing food products for disease prevention and treatment will become commonplace.

Source: From Sloan AE: Food industry forecast: consumer trends to 2020 and beyond, *Food Technology;* 52:37–44, 1998. Used with permission.

USE OF FOODS TO PROMOTE OR MAINTAIN HEALTH

Organic Foods

One of the categories of foods which are considered "healthful" is **organic foods.** Interest in organic foods fits with many of the current trends. Besides being perceived as fresh and healthful, organic foods are selected because they are environment-friendly. There has been a great expansion of organic foods. Organic products represented 6.2 percent of all new product introductions in 1995.[40] In addition to organically grown fresh produce, organic products include milk, pasta, cookies, cereal, baby food, bread, snack chips, spaghetti sauce, chocolate, and coffee. The availability of organic foods has moved from co-ops to mainstream grocery stores and restaurant menus. This trend is due to a combination of factors including growing interest in the environment, an aging population interested in healthful and wholesome food products, and emerging federal and state standards for organic processing and labeling that are opening up the market to more and larger organic food producers and processors.

Organic food production is based on a system of farming that maintains and replenishes the fertility of the soil without the use of synthetic pesticides and fertilizers. A certified organic food is produced using **sustainable agricultural practices** based on ecologic principles, without residual toxic chemicals at any stage of agricultural production, handling, storage, or processing. Certification requires strict documentation by the producer or processor and inspection at least annually by a third-party certification organization. National standards, initiated by the Organic Food Production Act of 1990, and implemented by the USDA through the National Organic Standards Board, guide the regulation and certification of organic growers and processors. These standards, which became effective in 1997, categorize practices and substances as permitted, regulated, and prohibited.[16] For a food product to be labeled organic, it must have at least 95 percent organic ingredients. For a food product to be labeled "Made with organic ingredients," it must have at least 50 percent organic ingredients. Certification and labeling of organic foods will help differentiate them from natural foods, of which there is no regulation and no standard definition.[16]

Fruit and Vegetable Consumption

Another aspect of Americans' diets that is considered "healthful" is eating more fruits and vegetables. Although Americans are not meeting the 5-a-day recommendations for fruits and vegetables, they do report trying to eat more of these foods. Consumption of fresh, frozen, and canned fruits and vegetables has increased. Convenience forms of these foods, such as fresh cut, prepeeled "baby" carrots, snack packs, and frozen vegetable-based meals, have been successful in the marketplace.[39] Questions about vegetarianism are among the top ten questions asked of the National Center for Nutrition and Dietetics Hotline,[1] indicating more of an interest in traditional vegetarianism, at least in some segments of the population. Restaurants and college food service operations report a dramatic increase in interest in vegetarian items—or at least in the use of meat as an accompaniment.[39]

PHYTOCHEMICALS, MEDICAL FOODS, AND ENERGY-ENHANCING FOODS

Another category of foods that are considered "healthful" are those containing **phytochemicals.** Examples of phytochemicals are given in table 6.2 These chemicals, produced by plants, are being investigated for their possible involvement in reducing risk of developing or treating cancers, diabetes, and cardiovascular disease; in boosting the immune system; and in preventing and/or treating neural tube defects, osteoporosis, abnormal bowel function, and arthritis. There are currently no recommendations on appropriate intakes of phytochemicals and much discussion and research centers around optimal intakes, efficacy of supplementation, and designing or engineering foods with selected phytochemical composition.[6]

In addition to the popularity of phytochemicals, other similar categories of "health-promoting foods" have arisen. Examples include designer or **functional foods,** which are foods that have specific nutrients added for a health benefit; and medical foods, which are solutions for enteral feeding that have been used within the medical community for many years as a part of treatment for specific diseases.

In general, to be considered a medical food by the FDA a product must, at minimum, meet the following criteria:

- The product is a food for oral or tube feeding.
- The product is labeled for the dietary management of a medical disorder, disease, or condition.
- The product is labeled to be used under medical supervision.[43]

Use of these categories of foods, and especially oral nutrient supplement beverages, may continue to increase

TABLE 6.2
Examples of Phytochemicals: Possible Health Benefits and Food Sources

Phytochemicals	Possible health benefits	Food source
Carotenoids	Provide antioxidant action	Dark green and yellow fruits and vegetables
Plant sterols	Decrease risk of cancer, decrease cholesterol absorption	Cruciferous vegetables, eggplant, tomatoes, soy products, whole grains
Allyic sulfides	Induce protective enzymes, inhibit cholesterol synthesis, anti-inflammatory activity	Garlic and onions
Genistein	Deters proliferation of cancer cells	Soy products
Coumarin	Delay blood clotting	Parsley, carrots, citrus fruits
Phthalides	Induce detoxification enzymes	Parsley, carrots, celery

as the population ages and becomes increasingly health conscious.

Consumers are also very interested in the energy-enhancing properties of foods and there has been a dramatic growth in this food category, which includes powders, pills, bars, and drinks. These products are being used by the serious and not so serious athlete and, increasingly, by consumers who believe that stressed-out people need extra energy and extra nutrition. Many, but not all, of these products have a high caloric density. Some contain other putative "energy-enhancing" compounds, such as ginseng, guarana, or caffeine.[39]

The primary legislation for approval of food ingredients in the United States is the **Food, Drug and Cosmetic Act** of 1938. This act emphasized administrative procedures, gave authority for plant inspections, established standards of identity for individual food products, and granted authority to obtain federal court injunctions against violators. Although it has been amended several times, the primary objectives of this legislation have not changed from the original ones of ensuring the safety and wholesomeness of the food supply, preventing economic fraud or deception, and informing consumers about the nutritional content of foods.[18] The primary agencies charged with enforcing the provisions of the Food, Drug and Cosmetic Act are delineated in table 6.3.

USE OF FOOD ADDITIVES, INGREDIENTS, AND TECHNOLOGIES TO IMPROVE/MODIFY FOODS

Any discussion of innovation in the food supply would be remiss without the inclusion of a description of the process by which food ingredients are approved for use in the United States. In the early part of the twentieth century, public demand for the approval of food ingredients and regulation of food processes resulted from the demonstration of the prevalence of food adulter-

TABLE 6.3
Federal Agencies Charged with Enforcement of the Food, Drug and Cosmetic Act of 1938 and Its Amendments

Department of Health and Human Services Public Health Service
Food and Drug Administration

Department of Agriculture
Food Safety and Inspection Service
Animal and Plant Health Inspection Service

Environmental Protection Agency

ation by Dr. Harvey M. Wiley of the U.S. Department of Agriculture, the publication of the novel *The Jungle* by Upton Sinclair, and the political advocacy of Theodore Roosevelt.[18]

The Food Additive Amendment of 1958 defined a food additive as

any substance the intended use of which results or may reasonably be expected to result, directly or indirectly, in its becoming a component or otherwise affecting the characteristics of any food (including any substance intended for use in producing, manufacturing, packing, processing, preparing, treating, packaging, transporting or holding food; and including any source of radiation intended for any such use), if such substance is not generally recognized among experts qualified by scientific training and experience to evaluate its safety, as having been adequately shown through scientific procedures (or in the case of a substance used in food prior to January 1, 1958, through either scientific procedures, or experience based on common use in food) to be safe under the conditions of its intended use.[31]

The 1958 amendment also gave us the term **generally recognized as safe (GRAS)** and led to the development of a list of substances that were considered to be GRAS. GRAS ingredients have been shown to be safe based on a long history of common usage in food. Typical GRAS substances are common spices, natural seasonings, and flavoring materials. Just because a food is on the GRAS list does not mean that it is no longer subject to control. For example, **cyclamate,** an artificial sweetener, was considered GRAS but was banned after a research report linking consumption with cancer.[11]

New food ingredients are approved for use only after extensive FDA review. Companies wishing to market a new food ingredient must file a petition with the FDA for use of an additive in a given situation, which includes the results of the following kinds of tests:

1. Acute toxicity testing in at least two different species of mammals is designed to reveal indications of harmful effects that might occur within hours or days of exposure.
2. Subacute toxicity testing in at least two different species of mammals is designed to find the maximum level that does not produce an adverse effect and to determine the possible effects of higher levels. The highest level of the proposed additive that produces no adverse effects (the no observable effect level [NOEL]) is divided by a safety factor of 100 or more to set the maximum daily intake level allowed for humans, which is called an **acceptable daily intake (ADI).**
3. Chronic toxicity testing in at least two different species of mammals throughout their lifetimes is designed to reveal development of chronic disorders and to determine potential carcinogenicity of the proposed additive.
4. Pharmacokinetic studies are used to determine the absorption, distribution among tissues and organs, metabolism, and elimination of the proposed additive.
5. Reproductive tests are used to determine the effects on male or female fertility or on litter size, litter weight, number of viable young, and teratogenicity.
6. Appropriate analytical methods are used for the proposed additive and for any metabolites of the proposed additive.[11]

In granting approval for the use of an additive, the FDA sets limits with respect to the kinds of foods in which the additive may be used and the maximum concentrations that may be used within each of those kinds of food. The amount that may be used within foods is based on typical consumption patterns and are to be less than the ADI. At present, over 3,000 food additives can be used in foods within the limits that have been deemed safe by the FDA.[19]

Another role of the FDA has been to monitor the addition of nutrients to the U.S. food supply through **restoration, fortification,** or enrichment. Restoration is the replacement of nutrients lost during processing to levels comparable to the original levels. Fortification is the addition of nutrients at levels higher than those found in the original or comparable product. Enrichment is the addition of nutrients to achieve concentrations specified by the standards of identity for the food.[19] In the 1940s and 1950s, when nutrient deficiencies were still relatively common in the United States, the FDA established standards of identity for enriched staple foods such as flour, bread, rice, and cornmeal and specified enrichment levels for thiamin, riboflavin, niacin, and iron in these foods. These cereal and grain products were considered to be appropriate vehicles for fortification because they were consumed by most people and provided a significant amount of the daily energy intake. Since then, emphasis in food policy in the United States has shifted from preventing deficiency diseases to minimizing risk of development of chronic diseases and to addressing concerns about overfortification of foods with nutrients such as iron and, recently, folate. This shift has been afforded by the success of the fortification policies in reducing occurrence of deficiency diseases.[13] The current FDA policy is voluntary and states that decisions relative to food fortification should be based on

1. Achieving and maintaining a desirable level of nutritional quality in the food supply
2. Correcting a dietary insufficiency recognized by the scientific community to exist and known to result in a nutritional deficiency
3. Restoring nutrients to levels representative of the food before storage, handling, and processing
4. Balancing the vitamin, mineral, and protein content of a food in proportion to its total caloric content
5. Avoiding nutritional inferiority in a product that replaces a traditional food in the diet
6. Discouraging random fortification that could result in nutrient imbalances
7. Discouraging deceiving or misleading claims
8. Not encouraging indiscriminate addition of nutrients to inappropriate foods such as fresh produce, sugars, snack foods, candies, and carbonated beverages.[3,19]

Nutrient addition is appropriate when the nutrient is stable in the food under customary conditions, is physiologically available from the food, is present at a level that will not result in overconsumption, is suitable for the intended purpose, and is in compliance with applicable regulations.[19] The American Medical Association has endorsed addition of nutrients to foods with the following recommendations:

1. The intake of the nutrient is below the desirable level in the diets of a significant number of people.
2. The food used to supply the nutrient is likely to be consumed in quantities that will make a significant contribution to the diet of the population.
3. The addition of the nutrient is not likely to create an imbalance of essential nutrients.
4. The nutrient added is stable under proper storage conditions.
5. The nutrient is physiologically available from the food.
6. There is a reasonable assurance against excessive intake to a level of toxicity.[19]

CONSUMER DEMANDS FOR FOOD SUBSTITUTES AND REPLACEMENTS

As consumers are becoming increasingly conscious of fat and carbohydrate intakes and their impact on energy intake, weight status, and subsequently, on risk of developing chronic diseases, the demand for substitutes or replacements has increased. These substitutes and replacements are regulated as food additives by the FDA. The sales of low-fat foods were $32 billion in 1991, and are expected to reach $55 billion in 1996.[24]

Reduced Fat/Fat-Free Products

In addition to being an essential nutrient and a carrier for fat-soluble vitamins, fat provides satiety and, as such, may assist with regulation of energy intake. Fat also contributes to the sensory experience of eating by contributing to the odor, flavor, texture, appearance, and mouthfeel in foods. The Dietary Guidelines for Americans and recommendations by the American Heart Association and the American Cancer Society are that Americans consume 30 percent or less of our calories from fat. Decreasing the amount of fat in the American diet from its current 34 percent to not more than 30 percent is desirable in terms of decreasing the risk of developing certain chronic diseases such as cardiovascular disease and some types of cancers.

The simplest method for lowering the fat content of the diet is, of course, to select foods that are naturally low in fat, such as most fruits and vegetables. From a food-processing viewpoint, lowering fat content of multicomponent systems, such as frozen meals or entrées, is easily achieved by simply increasing the proportion of low-fat ingredients within the meal or entrée. The success of this approach is illustrated by the 22 percent increase in sales of frozen meals and/or entrées in the 300 to 400 kcal range between 1989 and 1993.[24] Another highly successful approach to lowering the fat content of diets has been to breed and raise cattle and swine to have lower fat contents. The average cut of beef and pork sold in the United States today has about 20 percent less fat than it did about twenty years ago. This is a result of alterations in management practices by growers, who no longer "fatten" hogs and cattle prior to slaughter, and consumer demand for meat that has been largely trimmed of visible fat prior to purchase.

The simplest way to lower the fat content of a single food is to directly remove some or all of the fat, as is done in the production of low-fat or skim dairy products. Although this approach is successful in production of low-fat or skim milk or yogurt, it fails with whipping cream or sour cream, since the organoleptic and functional properties of these products are dependent on their fat content.[24]

Use of Technologies Not Normally Used in Preparation of a Full-Fat Food　Many fat-free and reduced fat products are made by alterations in the technologies by which foods are processed. Since these products use familiar processing techniques, they do not require FDA approval. For example, the fat content of mozzarella cheese has been lowered from 21 to 10 percent by reducing the cooking temperature of the cheese. This lower cooking temperature results in a cheese with a high moisture content, softer texture, and melting characteristics similar to regular mozzarella.[26] This approach is also illustrated by the introduction of snack chips that have been baked instead of fried, resulting in a familiar product with a much lower fat content.

Use of Functional Ingredients Such as Proteins, Carbohydrates, Emulsifiers, and Stabilizers　Another common method used to manufacture fat-free and reduced fat products is to substitute functional ingredients such as proteins, carbohydrates, emulsifiers, and/or stabilizers for all or part of the fat. Table 6.4 lists many of the approved fat replacements, caloric contributions, and uses. In many instances, these

TABLE 6.4
Fat Replacements, Their Structural Alterations, Caloric Contribution, and Uses

Replacement	Structural alterations	Caloric contribution (kcal/g)	Food uses
Protein based	Microparticulated	1–2	Spreads, salad dressings, frozen and refrigerated desserts, dairy products
Carbohydrate based			
Dextrins	Hydrolyzed	1–2	Spreads, salad dressings, frozen desserts, baked goods, cereals, sour cream, frosting, fillings, processed meats, soups, snacks
Polydextroses	Hydrolyzed	1	Baked goods, chewing gum, salad dressings, frozen desserts, gelatins, puddings, candies, confections, frostings
Microcrystalline cellulose	Acid treatment	0	Baked goods, spreads, salad dressings
Gums		0	Baked goods, spreads, salad dressings
Olestra	Sucrose polyester	0	Chips, savory snacks
Caprenin and salatrim	Short- and long-chain fatty acid triglycerides	5	Soft candy, coatings, spreads

ingredients may be heated, acidified, and/or blended to replicate the textural properties of fat prior to their incorporation into the food. Some commercially available food products for which ingredient substitutions are made include fat-free bakery products, processed cheese products, frozen desserts, yogurts, salad dressings, and spreads.

Protein-based fat replacements are usually made from milk and/or egg white proteins, water, sugar, pectin, and citric acid. Since the replacement is typically used as a solution containing about 25 to 50 percent protein, the replacements contribute 1 to 2 kcal/g. Simplesse®, one of the most common of the protein-based fat replacements, is produced by a process called **microparticulation.** In this process, the protein is heated and blended to result in 0.1-to 3-μm spheres. Food particles in this size range are not detectable as discrete particles by the mouth; instead, the sensation is one of creaminess, a textural property usually attributed to fat. The microparticles are stable to cold temperatures, but coagulate at high temperatures, leading to a loss of the perception of creaminess. Because of this lack of heat stability, microparticulated proteins are not suitable for processes involving the application of heat, such as frying or baking. The FDA has ruled that these protein-based fat replacements are GRAS substances and, therefore, no approval is needed. They may be used to replace fat in mayonnaise, sour cream, salad dressings, frozen and refrigerated desserts, yogurt, and cheese.[4,14,24]

Carbohydrate-based fat replacements include dextrins, modified food starches, **polydextrose,** cellulose, and gums. These ingredients are heat stable, not subject to oxidation, and contribute up to 4 kcal/g. The FDA has ruled that these carbohydrate-based fat replacements are GRAS substances and, therefore, no approval is needed.[4,14,24]

Use of Fat Substitutes   Fat substitutes are synthetic compounds that possess many of the properties of fats. There is only one noncaloric fat substitute that has been approved for use in the United States. **Olestra** (sucrose polyester) is formed by the esterification of sucrose with six to eight long-chain fatty acids. It resembles fats in appearance, taste, texture, and function in foods and, because it is heat stable, can be used in frying, cooking, and baking. Olestra is not absorbed, although it may decrease absorption of fat-soluble vitamins and carotenoids, particularly lycopene. In some people, olestra can lead to flatulence, cramping, and loose stools. The FDA approved the use of olestra in salted snacks and crackers in January 1996. Foods containing olestra must be fortified with vitamins A, D, E, and K and must have the following statement on the label,

This product contains olestra. Olestra may cause abdominal cramping and loose stools. Olestra inhibits the absorption of some vitamins and other nutrients. Vitamins A, D, E, and K have been added.[15]

Other reduced-calorie fat substitutes that are being introduced are termed **structured lipids** or **engineered fats.** Structured lipids are fats in which the triglyceride molecules are rearranged into new lengths, combining short- and long-chain fatty acids to obtain desired functionalities and lower caloric values. Three of these structured lipids that have received FDA approval as GRAS substances and are currently on the market are Caprenin, Salatrim, and medium-chain triglycerides. Caprenin is a triglyceride composed of two medium-chain fatty acids and one very long-chain fatty acid, behenic acid (C-22). Since behenic acid is only partially absorbed and, therefore, contributes very little to the caloric value of the lipid, caprenin has only 5 kcal/g. Salatrim is also a triglyceride composed of one of four basic combinations of short-chain fatty acids and stearic acid. The short-chain fatty acids, acetic, propionic, and butyric, are used in various combinations with the stearic acid to obtain the desired functional properties. As a result of triglycerides containing short-chain fatty acids having fewer calories per gram than triglycerides containing long-chain fatty acids, Salatrim contributes only 5 kcal/g. Both Caprenin and Salatrim have functional properties similar to those of cocoa butter and are potentially used for soft candy, confectionary coatings, spreads, and other intermediate and low-moisture foods.[4,25,27]

In the Future

Other synthetic compounds in various stages of research and development as fat replacers include esterified propoxylated glycerol (EPG), carboxy-carboxylate esters, malonate esters, alkyl glyceryl-ethers, alkyl glyceride fatty acid polyesters, esterified polysaccharides, polyvinyl oleate, ethyl esters, and polysiloxanes.[24]

NUTRITIVE AND NONNUTRITIVE SWEETENERS

Nutritive sweeteners have no nutritional value other than as an energy source. Americans consume an average of 11 percent of their average daily energy intake as nutritive sweeteners,[7] which is within the recommended range of 10 to 15 percent. Those Americans with a high intake of added sugar consume an average of 83 to 126 g added sugar per day. These consumers fall into one of two groups: those who add sugars to a reasonably balanced diet, and those who tend to substitute sugar-rich foods for more nutritious foods. Increased body weight is

not associated with a high consumption of added sugars, since this population tends to have lower fat intakes than the general population.[29] Therefore, individuals who are trying, or have been told, to reduce or control their energy intakes frequently use **nonnutritive sweeteners** to adjust their energy intake without eliminating energy sources that may contribute additional nutrients.

Nutritive Sweeteners

Nutritive sweeteners include sucrose, fructose, lactose, honey, invert sugars, high-fructose corn syrup (HCFS), fruit juice concentrates, and **polyols** (sugar alcohols).

Polyols or sugar alcohols, include sorbitol, mannitol, xylitol, isomalt, hydrogenated starch hydrolysates, lactitol, and maltitol. Although historically, these polyols have been considered to provide 4 kcal/g, the FDA now allows use of lower calorie values for them. The European Economic Community allows use of 2.4 kcal/g of polyol for nutritional labeling. Thus, these products may be considered to be **"reduced-calorie" sweeteners.**[26] Table 6.5 lists the relative sweetness, caloric contribution, and uses of polyols.

Nonnutritive Sweeteners

Nonnutritive sweeteners are also referred to as intense sweeteners, very low calorie sweeteners, or alternative sweeteners. Currently, saccharin, **aspartame,** and acesulfame K three are approved for use in the United States. FDA approval is being sought for sucralose, alitame, and cyclamates. Table 6.5 includes a listing of the relative sweetness, caloric contribution, and uses of intense sweeteners.

Aspartame (NutraSweet®) is the methyl ester of aspartic acid and phenylalanine. It has a clean, sweet taste, but is not heat-stable. It has 4 kcal/g, however, because very small amounts are needed to achieve the desired sweetness, it is considered a noncaloric sweetener. Aspartame is metabolized to aspartic acid, phenylalanine, and methanol, which are then metabolized normally. The FDA approved aspartame as a food additive in 1981 with an ADI of 50 mg/kg body weight. In spite of extensive preapproval testing of the safety of aspartame and its history of safe consumption in many European countries, there were many complaints filed with the FDA detailing adverse effects from aspartame use, especially migraine headaches. In 1984, after reviewing 517 consumer complaints related to the use of aspartame, the

TABLE 6.5
Intense Sweeteners—Their Intensity, Caloric Contribution, and Uses

Sweetener	Sweetening power (sucrose = 100%)	Caloric contribution (kcal/g)	Food uses
Polyols			
Sorbitol	50%	2.6	Candies, chewing gum, jams, jellies
Mannitol	50%	1.6	Bulking and dusting agent
Xylitol	100%	2.4	Candies, chewing gum, pharmaceuticals, oral health products
Hydrogenated starch hydrolysates	25–50%	3.0	Confectionery products
Isomalt	45–65%	2.0	Candies, jams, jellies, desserts, beverages, fillings, frostings
Lactitol	30–40%	2.0	Baked goods, candies, frostings, frozen dairy desserts, jams, jellies
Maltitol	90%	3.0	Confectionery products
Nonnutritive			
Saccharin	30,000%	0	Beverages, table-top sweetener, cosmetics, pharmaceuticals
Aspartame	20,000%	4.0	Beverages, table-top sweetener, frozen desserts and novelties, puddings, fillings, frostings, yogurts, baked goods, candies, gelatins
Acesulfame K	20,000%	0	Beverage mixes, table-top sweetener, gelatins, puddings, dairy product analogs, candies, baked goods and mixes, desserts, sauces, toppings, syrups, alcoholic beverages
Alitame	200,000%	1.2	Petition for approval filed with FDA
Cyclamate	3,000%	0	Petition for approval filed with FDA
Sucralose	60,000%	0	Petition for approval filed with FDA

Centers for Disease Control and Prevention (CDC) found that the complaints "do not provide evidence of the existence of serious widespread, adverse health consequences attendant to the use of aspartame.[7] To consume an amount of aspartame equal to the ADI, a 120-lb adult would need to consume seventeen 12-oz diet soft drinks or seventy-eight packets of table-top sweetener and a 50-lb child would have to consume seven 12-oz diet soft drinks or thirty-two packets of table-top sweetener. In clinical studies in which three to four times the ADI were given in bolus doses, no adverse effects were noted. People with phenylketonuria (PKU) should restrict their intake of aspartame, and all products containing aspartame are required to have a statement on the label that it is not appropriate for these individuals. Labels of all foods containing aspartame must contain the following statement:

Phenylketonurics: Contains phenylalanine

In the Future

There are three low-calorie sweeteners currently under consideration for approval by the FDA. Alitame is a sweetener formed from the amino acids L-aspartic acid and D-alanine and a novel amine. The aspartic acid component is metabolized normally, while the alanine amide is passed through the body largely unchanged. It has a clean, sweet taste; is readily soluble; and is stable at elevated temperatures and over a broad pH range. It has the potential to be used in almost all areas where sweeteners are presently used and in toiletries and pharmaceuticals.

Cyclamate is also being considered for approval by FDA and is approved in over fifty countries. Although most people do not metabolize cyclamate, a small proportion do metabolize some of the cyclamate. It is stable to a range of temperatures and has good shelf life. It is the "least sweet" of the commercially available intense sweeteners. Cyclamates were once widely used in the United States and were on the GRAS list; however, based on research findings that cyclamate consumption led to cancer, it was banned in the United States in 1970. In 1984, the Cancer Assessment Committee of the FDA reviewed the scientific evidence and reached the following conclusion: "The collective weight of the many experiments . . . indicates that cyclamate is not carcinogenic."[7] That conclusion was affirmed in 1985 by the National Academy of Science, which noted, "the totality of the evidence from studies in animals does not indicate that cyclamate or its major metabolite cyclohexylamine is carcinogenic by itself."[7]

Sucralose (SPLENDA®) is a noncaloric sweetener derived from the selective substitution of three chlorine atoms for three hydroxyl atoms on sucrose. It is not metabolized in the body. It has good water solubility, but it will hydrolyze in solution over an extended period of time and under extreme conditions of acidity and temperature. It can be used virtually anywhere sugar can be used.[7,10]

Do Fat and Carbohydrate Replacers Help?

One question regarding the use of fat or sugar replacements is whether people will compensate for their presence by increasing their energy intake. Young children[9] and young adult males[35] who were fed one meal a day containing a fat substitute consumed less fat than subjects who did not consume the fat substitute. However, twenty-four-hour energy intakes remained constant, reflecting an increased consumption of carbohydrate when fed the fat substitute. Results with obese adults were that use of a fat substitute decreased energy as well as fat intake.[20] It has been suggested that, although children and lean adults may be able to compensate for the calories fed as olestra, obese adults may lack this compensation.[20] Similar results have been obtained using the nonnutritive sweeteners. Rolls[34] emphasized that the effect of voluntary substitution of a reduced-calorie product for one higher in calories depends on the individual's motivation. If a person uses the consumption of a reduced-calorie product as an excuse to indulge in a higher calorie product, there will be no net change in energy intake. However, if a person uses the consumption of a reduced-calorie product as part of a weight-control program, reduction in energy intake is likely to occur.

FOOD PRESERVATION

A position paper published by the American Dietetic Association[5] emphasized that nutrition professionals have the responsibility to educate consumers about food and nutrition issues, including such new technologies as food irradiation, and to serve as the advocate for the consumer with the food industry and food regulatory agencies.

In this century, the technology of food preservation has progressed from drying and salting to heat and cold preservation to preservation by "minimal processing" methods, such as irradiation and **modified atmosphere packaging (MAP).** A common characteristic of these latter methods is that the shelf life of the products is extended, but not indefinitely, with the retention of the "fresh" characteristics of the products.

"Fresh" tops the list of the most desirable food claims, even ahead of "fat-free."[39] The demand for fresh foods is forcing manufacturers to use processing technologies and packaging materials to make foods appear to be as fresh as possible and to put freshness dates on all products. **Food irradiation** is a relatively new processing technology that extends the shelf life and improves the safety of "fresh" foods. Modified atmosphere packaging has made possible the wide availability of fresh pasta, sauces, and salsas as well as precut salads, fruits, and vegetables, which are even being sold in vending machines.

Food Irradiation

Irradiation is regulated in the United States as a food additive, that is, by the FDA. In addition, the Food Safety and Inspection Service (FSIS) of the USDA develops standards for the safe use of irradiation on meat and poultry products, and the Animal and Plant Health Inspection Service (APHIS), also within the USDA, monitors programs designed to enhance animal and plant health. In 1963, the FDA approved irradiation-sterilized bacon; this approval was revoked in 1968. In the 1970s, the National Aeronautics and Space Administration (NASA) began using irradiation to preserve some of the foods used by the astronauts, a practice that continues today. In 1983, the FDA approved irradiation as a means of controlling microorganisms on spices, and in 1985, the FDA extended that approval to foods such as strawberries, poultry, ground beef, and pork. There are currently thirty-eight countries worldwide that permit irradiation of food. Irradiated foods are also routinely given to people who have received bone marrow transplants and other immunocompromised patients. All irradiated foods sold in the United States must be labeled with a **radura** (see figure 6.2), the international symbol for irradiation and the words "treated by irradiation" or "treated with radiation." Products that contain irradiated ingredients, such as spices, are not required to be labeled.

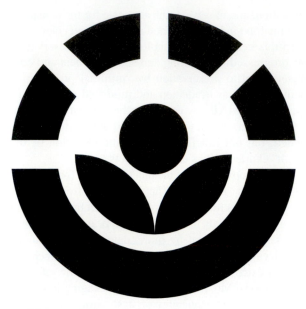

FIGURE 6.2　Radura, the International Symbol for Irradiation

Currently, the term food irradiation is generally understood to mean processing with isotopes that produce either gamma or beta rays. The isotope most frequently used in food irradiation is cobalt 60 (Co-60), a gamma ray emitter, which is derived from nonradioactive cobalt. In theory, other radiation sources for food irradiation could be derived from approved spent fuel elements after their use in a nuclear reactor. Gamma or beta ray emitting isotopes are chosen because they have penetrating power but do not produce radioactivity in treated foods; just as having a magnetic resonance imaging (MRI) or computed tomography (CT) scan does not make a person radioactive, irradiated foods are not radioactive. Irradiation also does not produce significant heat in foods, and so the additional term "cold sterilization" has been applied to this kind of food preservation. The appropriate dose of radiation for foods depends on the intent of the radiation and on the food. The dosage used takes into account safety and organoleptic quality damage, resistance to microorganisms, resistance of food enzymes, and cost.[30,36,41]

Modified Atmosphere Packaging

Modified atmosphere packaging is used for such products as fresh pastas, salads, precut and ready-to-eat vegetables, snacks, and precooked meats. The development of this technology has allowed the market for minimally processed foods to develop, because MAP products have an increased shelf life while retaining their "fresh" characteristics. Successful application of MAP involves controlling the product throughout processing, packaging, distribution, and marketing. In modified atmosphere packaging, a package made of a selected type of packaging material is filled with the food product and the container is flushed with a gas, such as nitrogen. The type of packaging material is carefully selected for its gas and moisture permeabilities as well as for its strength, durability, and suitability to the machinery. For example, fresh produce needs to "breathe" and an appropriate packaging material would maintain reduced oxygen and relatively high carbon dioxide concentrations within the package. The reduced oxygen concentration also slows chemical and microbial spoilage. It is important that the product not dehydrate or overhydrate, therefore, moisture permeability of the packaging material is also carefully controlled. Although MAP coupled with refrigeration slows the growth of pathogenic and spoilage organisms, they do not destroy them. Temperature abuse of MAP products or destruction of the integrity of the packaging material results in an increased likelihood of growth of any pathogenic or spoilage organisms that may be present.[11,32,33] The USDA has the following recommendations to help consumers use MAP appropriately:

1. Read the label. Handling and cooking temperatures may be different for every product, and only proper handling can ensure product safety.
2. Look for a time-temperature indicator. Some of the new products have one. It is usually a strip or dot that changes color if the product is past its expiration date or has been held at an improper, above-refrigeration temperature.
3. Check the "use by" date stamped on the package. You take a chance when you use old products.[11]

Biotechnology

Even though **biotechnology** is not a food processing technology, it is increasingly impacting the food industry. Biotechnology is the application of technology to biological processes. In its most commonly used syntax, it refers to the methods of **recombinant DNA (rDNA)** technology or so-called genetic engineering, in which genes are transferred from one organism to another or in which gene expression is enhanced or inhibited in the same organism.

Currently, relatively few products or processes using biotechnology are being marketed in the food and agricultural sector. The products or processes of biotechnology now in use include embryo transplants; microbial inoculants for soil, silage, and hay; biopesticides; recombinant animal vaccines; monoclonal antibodies for diagnostic uses; yeasts for fermentation processes and products; a genetically engineered enzyme in corn syrup production; growth promotants in the dairy and pork industry; and genetically engineered crops.

Among the first commercially available vegetables produced by genetic engineering is the FlavrSavr® slow-ripening tomato developed by Calgene, Inc., in which the gene for polygalacturonase, the enzyme responsible for softening, is turned off. This tomato can be allowed to ripen on the vine and develop the flavor associated with ripening while retaining a firmness that allows for packing and shipping.

Another commercial application of biotechnology in foods is the use of a recombinant bovine somatotropin (bST) in lactating cows; bST is a protein hormone necessary for milk production. In a system analogous to the production of the human insulin given to individuals with diabetes, the recombinant bST is produced by a bacteria and is then given to cows to increase milk production. The FDA approved the use of recombinant bST in cows based on findings that it is species-specific for cows, is digested in the human digestive tract, does not increase beyond normal limits in milk with supplementation, does not change milk composition, and has not been found to promote growth in a variety of species. The FDA has not altered its decision for approval of bST in spite of intense pressure from groups concerned that the milk supply will be adulterated, that the hormone will be present in the milk in high levels, and that the long-term risks of consumption of bST milk are not known. The eventual extent of availability of milk from bST-supplemented cows in the food supply will reflect the outcome of the political and social debate on this topic, rather than the regulatory and scientific process.

Commercial applications of biotechnology employing microbes have developed faster than those for plants or animals. These genetically engineered microbes are being used to produce a variety of products used in food manufacture. These products include amino acids for synthesis of aspartame, chymosin for cheese manufacture, alpha-amylase for conversion of corn starch into high-fructose corn syrups, and lactase for production of low-lactose milk.

In the future, biotechnology innovations may lead to improvements in shelf life, texture, color, taste, and fat or protein concentrations or composition in foods; increased productivity due to disease-, drought-, and insect-resistant plant species; and decreased need for use of pesticides and herbicides. It is expected that biotechnology will be used to improve detection of foodborne pathogens, toxins, and contaminants; to detect reductions in product quality; to indicate temperature abuse; and to convert waste products into usable products or energy.

In deciding about the regulation of foods produced through genetic engineering techniques, the FDA ruled that these foods required no specific, unique regulation, since traditional breeding techniques involve many of the same concepts. If there is any possibility of introduction of potential allergens or other harmful compounds into a food, however, the company must ask the FDA for a ruling on that product.

Labeling genetically engineered foods is a concern for some consumers. The Food, Drug and Cosmetic Act requires that labels be both true and not misleading. For example, the introduction of a potential allergen into a genetically altered food would require a label alerting consumers to that alteration; failure to do so would be considered misleading labeling. A producer of a cheese made with chymosin produced by genetically engineered bacteria could include on the product label the statement, "Made with microbial enzymes; no animal rennet used." It would be considered misleading, however, to state that a food was or was not produced with genetic engineering technology if there is no difference between the genetically engineered food and its traditional counterpart. To say that "this milk was derived from cows not injected with bST" implies that milk from bST-supplemented cows is less wholesome and is, therefore, misleading. This could be corrected by adding an additional statement that there is no difference between the milks.[2,21,44]

FOOD SAFETY

To understand what food safety means, it is necessary to define the terms safe, hazard, and risk. **Safe** means that nothing harmful results from an action, that is, the absence of effect. A hazard is the capacity of an action to cause harm. **Risk** is the probability of occurrence of harm from a particular action. The process of identifying hazards and estimating their size is termed **risk assessment.** The process of deciding whether or not the risk is acceptable is called **risk management.** Related to these terms is the effective dose (ED) or **threshold,** which is the amount of a chemical that causes an observable effect, and the **infectious dose (ID),** which is the number of organisms required to start an infection. The no observed effect level is the maximum level of consumption at which there is no effect. For populations, the ED-50 is the amount of a chemical agent that causes an observable effect in half of a population; the ID-50 is the number of organisms required to start an infection in half of a population. For example, the ED-50 for vitamin C would be the average requirement for that population.[11]

Hazards Associated with Foods

There are four general categories of hazards associated with foods. These are **biological hazards, chemical hazards, physical hazards,** and nutrition-related diseases. This section focuses on biological hazards, chemical hazards, and physical hazards.

Biological Hazards   Biological hazards include bacterial, fungal, viral, and parasitic organisms and/or their toxins. In 1994, the Council for Agricultural Science and Technology (CAST), a nonprofit organization whose mission is to identify agricultural issues and to interpret scientific research for use in public policy decision making, issued a report concluding that the biggest food safety problem in the United States today is controlling microbiologic hazards to reduce the risks of foodborne illness.[12] Interestingly, consumers surveyed by the Food Marketing Institute also listed contamination by bacteria or germs as their number one concern about safety of the food supply.[17] Conservative estimates are that there are at least 6.5 million cases of foodborne illness each year in the United States, with an estimated economic cost of between $6 and $8.4 billion.[8]

Approximately two-thirds of foodborne illnesses from microbiologic sources are caused by bacteria such as the *Bacillus, Campylobacter, Clostridium, Escherichia, Listeria, Salmonella, Shigella, Staphylococcus, Streptococcus, Vibrio,* and *Yersinia* species and parasites of the genus *Trichinella.* Adding to these microbiologic challenges are several microorganisms that were not previously recognized as important foodborne pathogens. These emerging pathogens include *Campylobacter jejuni* and *Escherichia coli* 0157:H7. Detecting these pathogens in foods is complicated by the absence of widely available tests for their presence. Tests for *E. coli* 0157:H7 are becoming more available with the advent of the new inspection system for meat and poultry mandated by the USDA in 1996.

There are two types of foodborne disease from microbial pathogens: infections and intoxications. Infections result from ingestion of live pathogenic organisms, which survive the digestive process and overcome the host's natural defenses. Intoxications occur when toxins produced by pathogens are consumed and survive the digestive process. **Foodborne infections** usually take eight hours to several weeks to present. It takes this amount of time for microorganisms to penetrate body defenses, reproduce, and cause symptoms involving the immune system, such as fever. By contrast, acute symptoms from **foodborne intoxications** typically occur within one to seven hours of consuming the offending food. Table 6.6 lists the most prevalent microorganisms that cause foodborne illnesses, symptoms of the illnesses, typical foods contributing to outbreaks, and prevention and control measures.

Of the 237,545 outbreaks of foodborne illness reported to the Centers for Disease Control and Prevention between 1973 and 1987, 79 percent involved improper food handling in commercial establishments. The remainder could be traced to food preparation and storage errors in peoples' homes. The most common handling errors were improper storage, inadequate cooking, and poor personal hygiene. The top twelve factors contributing to foodborne illness are listed in table 6.7. For example, improper storage was the factor most often associated with outbreaks caused by *B. cereus, C. perfringens, Salmonella* species, *S. aureus,* and group A *Streptococcus* species. Lack of handwashing and personal cleanliness were most often associated with cases of *shigellosis,* hepatitis A, gastroenteritis caused by Norwalk virus, and *giardiasis.*[23]

Most of the hazards associated with fungi are intoxications resulting from mushrooms and mycotoxins. Over fifty toxins have been identified from mushrooms; commercial varieties are considered safe, but safety of "wild" mushrooms cannot be assured. The toxins are tasteless and odorless and some are heat stable, so it is impossible to determine in advance whether a mushroom is contaminated or to state that cooking increases the safety. The most familiar mycotoxins are the aflatoxins, produced by mold growth on grains and legumes. The aflatoxins are among the most potent carcinogens known.[11]

Chemical Hazards   Chemical hazards associated with foods can be subdivided into naturally occurring, indirectly added, and directly added. Toxic chemicals can

TABLE 6.6
Common Foodborne Diseases Caused by Bacteria

Disease (*causative agent*)	Principal symptoms	Typical foods	Prevention and control measures
Food poisoning, diarrhea (*Bacillus cereus*)	Diarrhea, cramps, occasional vomiting	Meat products, soups, sauces, vegetables	Cook all potential food sources thoroughly, serve at correct temperature, cool rapidly.
Food poisoning, emetic (*B. cereus*)	Nausea, vomiting, sometimes diarrhea and cramps	Cooked rice and pasta	Minimize hot holding times.
Botulism; food poisoning (heat-labile toxin of *Clostridium botulinum*)	Fatigue, weakness, double vision, slurred speed, respiratory failure, sometimes death	Types A&B: vegetables; fruits; meat, fish, and poultry products; condiments; Type E: fish and fish products	Purchase commercially processed foods, serve foods sauteed or infused in oils, promptly discard leftovers.
Botulism; food poisoning infant infection (heat-labile toxin of *C. botulinum*)	Constipation, weakness, respiratory failure, sometimes death	Honey, soil	Do not feed honey to infants.
Campylobacteriosis (*Campylobacter jejuni*)	Diarrhea, abdominal pain, fever, nausea, vomiting	Infected food-source animals	Cook animal foods thoroughly, cool rapidly, avoid cross-contamination, use pasteurized milk.
Food poisoning (*Clostridium perfringens*)	Diarrhea, cramps, rarely nausea and vomiting	Cooked meat and poultry	Cook animal foods thoroughly, cool rapidly, avoid cross-contaminations.
Foodborne infections, enterohemorrhagic (*Escherichia coli*)	Watery, bloody diarrhea	Raw or undercooked beef, raw milk	Cook animal foods thoroughly, cool rapidly, avoid cross-contaminations.
Foodborne infections, entroinvasive (*E. coli*)	Cramps, diarrhea, fever, dysentery	Raw foods	Teach food handlers good hygiene practice, have food handlers wear gloves, minimize holding time.
Foodborne infections, enterotoxigenic (*E. coli*)	Profuse watery diarrhea; sometimes cramps, vomiting	Raw foods	Teach food handlers good hygiene practice, have food handlers wear gloves, minimize holding time.
Listeriosis (*Listeria monocytogenes*)	Meningoencephalitis; stillbirths; septicemia or meningitis in newborns	Raw milk, cheese, and vegetables	Use pasteurized milk, cook foods thoroughly.
Salmonellosis (*Salmonella* species)	Diarrhea, abdominal pain, chills, fever, vomiting, dehydration	Raw, undercooked eggs; raw milk, meat and poultry	Cook animal foods thoroughly, minimize hot holding times, chill foods rapidly, avoid cross-contamination.
Shigellosis (*Shigella* species)	Diarrhea, fever, nausea; sometimes vomiting, cramps	Raw foods	Cook animal foods thoroughly, minimize hot holding times, chill foods rapidly, avoid cross-contamination.
Staphylococcal food poisoning (heat-stable enterotoxin of *Staphylococcus aureus*)	Nausea, vomiting, diarrhea, cramps	Ham, meat, poultry products, cream-filled pastries, whipped butter, cheese	Restrict food handlers with skin lesions or respiratory infections from handling foods.
Streptococcal foodborne infection (*Streptococcus pyogenes*)	Various, including sore throat, erysipelas, scarlet fever	Raw milk, deviled eggs	Use pasteurized milk, teach food handlers good hygiene practices, chill foods rapidly.
Foodborne infection (*Vibrio parahaemolyticus*)	Diarrhea, cramps; sometimes nausea, vomiting, fever, headache	Fish and seafoods	Cook fish and seafood thoroughly, minimize hot holding time.

TABLE 6.7

Top Twelve Factors Contributing to 345 Outbreaks of Foodborne Disease Caused by Mishandling and/or Mistreatment of Foods in Homes in the United States, 1973–1982.

Rank	Contributing factor	Percentage*
1.	Contaminated raw food/ingredient	42.0
2.	Inadequate cooking/canning/heat processing	31.3
3.	Obtained food from unsafe source	28.7
4.	Improper cooling	22.3
5.	Lapse of twelve or more hours between preparing and eating	12.8
6.	Colonized person handling implicated food	9.9
7.	Mistaken for food	7.0
8.	Improper fermentations	4.6
9.	Inadequate reheating	3.5
10.	Toxic containers	3.5
11.	Improper hot holding	3.2
12.	Cross-contamination	3.2

*Precentage exceeds 100 because multiple factors contribute to single outbreaks.
Source: From Food Borne Illness: Role of Home Food Handling Practices, *Food Technology,* Chicago, 1995, Institute of Food Technologists. Used with permission.

occur in foods at levels that cause acute food poisoning symptoms or intoxications or at lower levels, which represent chronic or long-term risks.

Examples of naturally occurring compounds that are considered chemical hazards include scombrotoxin, ciguatoxin, and phytohemagglutinin. Ciguatoxin contaminates more than 400 species of fish; those most important in the United States are grouper, skipjack, and red snapper. The toxin is produced by marine plankton and enters the food chain as fish consume the plankton and other contaminated fish. Scombrotoxin usually contaminates mahi-mahi, tuna, and bluefish. It is a mixture of metabolites resulting from the bacterial action of *Morganella morganii* on the skin of fish to metabolize histidine to histamine, suarine, and other similar compounds. These toxins are not usually detectable in foods and are not destroyed by cooking. However the likelihood of contamination with scombrotoxin may be reduced by appropriate refrigeration.

Directly and indirectly added chemical hazards include heavy metals, agricultural chemicals, prohibited substances, toxic compounds, and food additives. Heavy metals include copper, zinc, cadmium, tin, lead, arsenic, and mercury. Sources of heavy metals in foods include food equipment and tools, environmental contaminants, and agricultural chemicals. Contact of acidic foods with metallic equipment or tools causes the metals to dissolve in the foods. This may be beneficial in the case of iron, but undesirable in the case of heavy metals.

Lead migration into food is a hazard for portions of the population and warrants special attention. Chronic dietary exposure to lead results largely from water and glazed ceramic containers. Lead in drinking water is largely from lead pipes or leachable lead solder. Pottery intended for decorative purposes may have significant amounts of lead and should not be used for food. Even safely glazed ceramic containers may become sources of lead as the glaze chips and erodes during washing. In the past, some lead entered the food supply through use of lead solder in cans, but this has been eliminated in foods processed in the United States. Some people are still exposed to environmental lead from lead-based paints, parts from automobiles that used leaded gasoline, and gasoline-contaminated soils.

Another heavy metal that warrants special mention is mercury, which can contaminate foods in several ways. It is often used in fungicides that protect seed grains during storage. Inorganic mercury may also migrate from contaminated soils, water or air into foods and levels rarely exceed 50 ng/g of food. Fish may contain methyl mercury at levels of 10 to 1,500 ng/g of fish. This organic mercury may enter lakes from the breakdown of chloroalkali plants. As a result of a major outbreak of mercury poisoning in which at least 700 people were affected by contaminated fish and shellfish from Minamata Bay in Japan, the Food and Agriculture Organization (FAO)/World Health Organization (WHO) Expert Committee established a provisional weekly intake of 0.3 mg of mercury. The United States, Canada, Finland, Sweden, and Japan have established marketing limits of 0.4 to 1.0 mg mercury per kilogram of fish. In the United States, the estimated yearly per capita intake of mercury from seafood is 1.8 to 3.6 mg.

Pesticides are considered indirect food additives. That is, they are not intentionally added to food, but they become a part of the food as a result of their use in its production. Manufacturers seeking approval for a pesticide must submit data required for food additive petitions and the pesticide is then subject to the same regulations as an additive. The FDA annually tests more than 15,000 shipments of food for pesticide residues. Of the tested foods, 96 to 99 percent are below tolerances. In addition, the

FDA conducts the Total Diet Studies in which foods that have been purchased in grocery stores are analyzed for more than 150 pesticide residues. The amount of pesticides has consistently been within tolerances and has been steadily declining for the past twenty-five years.[11]

Physical Hazards   Physical hazards in foods include stones, seeds, glass fragments, small bits of metal, and insects and animal parts. These elements can become part of foods from the natural environment in which they are grown or they may be contaminants from processing and packaging.[11,31] Tolerance levels for specific physical hazards in some foods are established by government policy.

Controlling Potential Foodborne Illnesses by Processing

Control points for foodborne illness include vehicle, time, temperature, and pathogen (figure 6.3). If the food product is a potential vehicle for pathogenic bacteria, removing conditions that are favorable to growth of the pathogen or destroying the pathogen are commonly used processing techniques. Conditions favorable to the growth of microorganisms include abundant water, an energy source, appropriate oxygen, and desirable pH.

Most food preservation methods are based on altering the conditions favorable for growth of pathogenic and spoilage microorganisms. Preserving foods by adding salt or sugar and by freezing or drying are based on removal of available water. Preserving foods by canning, vacuum packaging, and modified atmosphere packaging removes available oxygen. Pickling or fermentation decrease pH to levels at which most bacteria do not grow.[31]

Salting and sugaring to preserve foods is one of the oldest food preservation methods. Country bacon and hams are still preserved by salting. Syrups and jellies have high concentrations of sugar, which retards bacterial growth; however, molds and yeasts require less water for growth and may grow on the surface of these products. "Dietetic" jellies, which have reduced sugar levels, may support growth of bacteria that will not grow in traditional jellies and so require different processing methods and different storage conditions. For these reasons, it is important to read all instructions on new products.

Freezing crystallizes water, making it unavailable to support bacterial growth. Drying removes free water. In some regions, a dried food must be kept packaged correctly to avoid rehydration from humidity. The bacteria

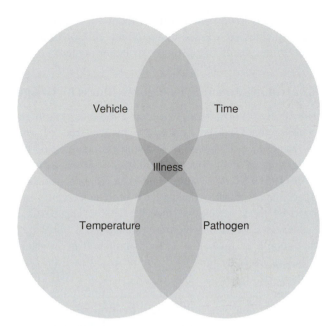

FIGURE 6.3   Control Points for Foodborne Illness

that may be present in frozen or dehydrated foods are not destroyed and will grow at their normal rates once water is again available. For this reason thawing frozen foods at room temperature is not recommended. Some salted, frozen, or dried foods have an additional level of preservation through the use of antimicrobial agents, such as sodium nitrite in cured meats and sulfiting agents.

Preservation methods such as canning are based on the fact that the temperature at which a food is held determines the survival of parasites, viruses, and bacteria. Recommendations for cooking methods and times are based largely on the ability to eliminate or lower the pathogen level. Very limited bacterial growth occurs at temperatures less than 40°F or above 140°F, therefore, temperatures between 40°and 140°F is referred to as the "danger zone," and holding of foods in this temperature range is to be minimized.

Pickling and fermentation are based on lowering the pH of foods to below 4.6, at which point pathogen growth and toxin production is impaired. Therefore, recommendations for processing methods of foods may be based on the pH; fruits with a pH of above 4.6 (low-acid foods) require more extensive heat processing than high-acid fruits (foods with a pH of less than 4.6). Alternatively, the pH may be lowered by fermentation or by the direct addition of an acid. The fermentation of milk to form yogurt lowers the pH from about 7.0 to about 4.5. Many pickles are formed by the direct addition of acetic acid (vinegar), although some may be fermented.

Controlling Potential Foodborne Illness by Design

During the 1960s, NASA needed a reliable system for ensuring that food sent on space flights was free of harmful bacteria, safe, and wholesome and cooperated on the development of the **Hazard Analysis Critical Control Points (HACCP)** system. The HACCP programs for good manufacturing practice have been successfully utilized by food processors since the 1980s. The HACCP system is a series of seven interrelated steps (table 6.8) that should be taken for all foods prepared in an establishment from the time foods are procured until they are consumed. There are two major parts in the HACCP systems—hazard analysis and critical control points.

Hazard analysis is the identification of microbial, chemical, and physical hazards in each ingredient and process that increases the risk of foodborne illness.

Critical control points are factors that can be controlled to reduce risks, such as acquisition, storage, preparation, holding, processing, and distributing. The potential for microbial, chemical, and physical hazards at each control point should be considered. Assessing, monitoring, and controlling potential hazards at purchasing, storage, preparation, and service points reduce the risk of foodborne illness. After identification of the critical control points, acceptable limits for each must be established and a plan for monitoring them developed. When monitoring criteria are not met, corrective action must be taken.

HACCP plans are currently being used in many food industries and the industry is requesting federal guidance and mandates in developing appropriate HACCP plans. Food service establishments, such as food-market deli operations and airline catering, are also beginning to develop HACCP plans.[11,28,31] A sample HACCP plan is included in figure 6.4. The HACCP concept is also useful in institutions as a method of fostering quality improvement, safety and risk management, quality of patient care, and compliance with standards of the Joint Commission on Accreditation of Healthcare Organizations standards. For clinical and community nutrition professionals, HACCP systems can be particularly useful in dealing with clients who are receiving enteral formulas and those whose immune systems are compromised.[37]

T A B L E 6 . 8
The Seven Steps of a HACCP Plan

1. Identify hazards and assess their severity and risks.
2. Determine critical control points (CCP) in food preparation.
3. Determine critical control limits for each CCP identified.
4. Monitor critical control points and record data.
5. Take corrective action whenever monitoring indicates critical limit is exceeded.
6. Establish effective record keeping system to document HACCP system.
7. Establish procedures to verify that HACCP system is working.

The same general hazard assessment activities that apply in commercial food processing industries apply in food service. Some typical hazard assessment activities are delineated in table 6.9. In designing HACCP plans for food service operations, critical control points include procurement and receiving, storage, thawing, cooking, handling, hot holding, cooling, reheating, serving, cleaning and sanitation, and worker hygiene.[37] The relative importance of these critical control points differs based on the type of food service. For example, in an assembly/serve food service, procurement of foods from safe sources is the major critical control point, while in a conventional food service, cooking and hot holding are additional critical control points. Some researchers have suggested that a HACCP approach would also be useful in the home.[22]

Controlling Potential Foodborne Illness by Education

In a July 1996 report, the American Meat Institute (AMI) summarized many research findings that consumers are worried about microbiological hazards in their food, however, they do not understand the risk factors associated with foodborne illness. Consumers tend to view visible signs of spoilage and lack of freshness as risk factors, without realizing that food contaminated with microbial pathogens need not appear spoiled in any way.[8] In a Scientific Status Summary, the Institute of Food Technologists (IFT) reported that even though some people consider the home the least likely place for food safety problems to occur, a significant amount of foodborne illness in the United States results from problems in the home. Most of these illnesses result from contaminated raw foods or ingredients;

Process step	Potential hazard	Description of CCP	Critical limits or criteria	Monitoring	Person responsible	Corrective action	Records	Verification
Receiving raw shrimp	Chemical	Concentration of sulfites	Less or equal to 100 ppm	Testing all incoming shrimp lots for sulfites	Quality control manager	Reject all lots exceeding the critical limits	Receiving records indicating testing results	Review records as often as necessary Collect three samples/supplier/year
	Undeclared food allergen	Labels indicating presence of sulfur dioxide	All labels declaring sulfites	Check all labels for declaration	Labeler	Reject unlabeled containers	Receiving records	Review records as often as necessary

This is a step in the process where a CCP exists, based on an analysis including the use of the CCP decision tree.

These are the identified potential hazards.

This is the description of the hazard itself or a factor related to the control of the hazard.

These are the limits established to control all hazards. Laws and regulations, as well as previous experience, may dictate these limits.

These are instructions on what to do and how often to monitor CCPs. It could be batch or continuous monitoring.

Persons responsible to monitor.

Actual and realistic action to be taken to correct a deviation from critical limits.

Specific records for each potential hazard in a CCP. Records may be legal evidences.

These may be *sporadic* or *distanced* activities to verify that potential hazards are kept under control. Notice that verification is not monitoring.

Note: Standard operating procedures (SOPs) need to be written to indicate how to monitor CCPs, how to take corrective actions, and how to do verifications. SOPs should be written in a very *simple* and *clear* way. Without SOPs it would be difficult to implement HACCP plans.

FIGURE 6.4 Sample HACCP Plan
This one shows a typical critical control point in shrimp processing.

TABLE 6.9
Sample Hazard Analysis Activities and Potential Risks That Could Be Avoided

Activity	Purpose
Review purchasing procedures	Purchase foods from approved vendors to minimize risks of initial contamination.
Review recipe selection	Identify ingredients and steps that have potential hazards
Observe and measure preparation	Measure food temperatures during preparation, avoid use of bare hands, avoid use of unclean equipment, avoid cross-contamination
Observe service	Avoid use of bare hands during service, avoid use of unclean equipment, avoid cross-contamination, avoid incorrect holding temperatures and times
Observe practices during cooling	Avoid cooling foods in large or tightly covered containers, monitor refrigerator temperatures, monitor spacing of foods on shelves

inadequate cooking, canning, or heat processing; food obtained from unsafe sources; improper cooling; lapse of twelve or more hours between cooking and eating; or an infected person handling food.[30] Both the AMI white paper[8] and the IFT status summary[30] also stated that societal changes have led to the failure of many children and young adults to learn basic principles of safe food preparation and suggested that educational efforts be targeted toward the problems outlined above.

Many of the societal changes of concern in terms of minimizing risk of foodborne illness are the same as those discussed earlier in this chapter as driving the food markets today—changes in family lifestyles that lead to less time for food preparation. People are not being taught proper methods of food handling and preparation. For example, of respondents to a survey in 1992, 58 percent knew that *Staphylococcus aureus* infection was associated with infected cuts of food preparers, 65 percent would refrigerate a roasted chicken breast immediately, 29 percent would leave roasted chicken breast out until it reached room temperature, and 18 percent would not be concerned or were not sure about the safety of cooked meat left at room temperature for over four hours. In the same survey only 54 percent would wash a cutting board with soap and water between cutting fresh meat and fresh vegetables.[8]

As interest in decreasing the incidence of foodborne illness grows, there is also more interest in developing and implementing educational methods for food handlers and the consumer. Many government agencies (such as the USDA and the FDA), trade industry groups (such as the American Meat Institute), professional organizations (such as the Institute of Food Technologists, the National Restaurant Association, and the American Dietetic Association) are developing and implementing educational programs. Illustrations similar to the one presented in figure 6.5 have been developed by the FDA and can be used to educate consumers about potential sites of contamination.

In 1989 the USDA[22] applied the HACCP concept in developing a consumer education guide. They identified five "educational critical control points" that should be recognized to prevent foodborne illness but that are not widely understood by consumers. Those critical control points are acquisition, storage, preparation, service, and handling leftovers. The advice based on these control points is:

1. When you shop, buy cold food last and get it home fast.
2. When you store food, keep it safe, refrigerate it.
3. When you prepare food, keep everything clean and thaw in refrigerator.
4. When you serve food, never leave it out over two hours.
5. When you handle leftovers, use small, shallow containers for quick cooling.
6. When in doubt, throw it out.

IMPLICATIONS FOR COMMUNITY NUTRITION PROFESSIONALS

Consumers have received the message about the connection between diet and health and are trying to incorporate this message into their food choices. There is an increased use of foods that are perceived as healthful, such as organic foods, fruits, and vegetables; foods containing phytochemicals; and reduced fat and calorie foods. The widespread availability of foods containing fat substitutes or nonnutritive sweeteners has the potential for altering the typical food patterns either positively or negatively. Nutrition professionals can provide guidance in the appropriate use of these foods within the context of a balanced food plan. To provide this guidance to consumers and to the food industry, nutrition professionals must remain aware of the influences on food choices and the trends in the marketplace.

Spreading foodborne disease

Whether it's in your house or a restaurant, the kitchen is the number one place where foodborne illness is spread. Here's a look at where it comes from and how to prevent the spread of disease:

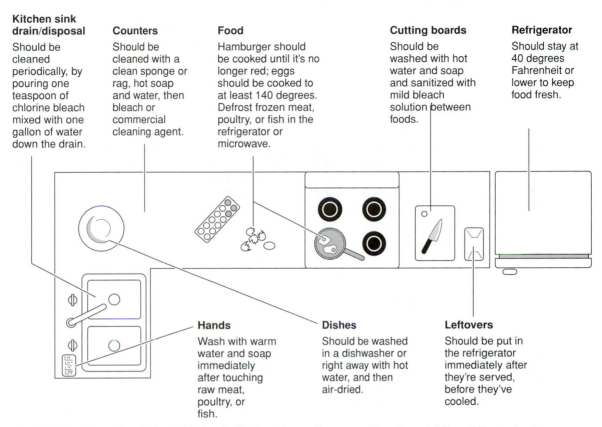

Kitchen sink drain/disposal

Should be cleaned periodically, by pouring one teaspoon of chlorine bleach mixed with one gallon of water down the drain.

Counters

Should be cleaned with a clean sponge or rag, hot soap and water, then bleach or commercial cleaning agent.

Food

Hamburger should be cooked until it's no longer red; eggs should be cooked to at least 140 degrees. Defrost frozen meat, poultry, or fish in the refrigerator or microwave.

Cutting boards

Should be washed with hot water and soap and sanitized with mild bleach solution between foods.

Refrigerator

Should stay at 40 degrees Fahrenheit or lower to keep food fresh.

Hands

Wash with warm water and soap immediately after touching raw meat, poultry, or fish.

Dishes

Should be washed in a dishwasher or right away with hot water, and then air-dried.

Leftovers

Should be put in the refrigerator immediately after they're served, before they've cooled.

FIGURE 6.5 **Illustrations Such as This Can Be Used to Educate Consumers About Potential Sites of Contamination**

Consumers also want food that is fresh or that maintains its freshlike characteristics and is convenient. The food industry is responding to these challenges by the introduction of new food technologies, such as irradiation, modified atmosphere packaging, and genetic engineering. Each of these technologies has advocates and detractors, just as each has advantages and disadvantages. Nutrition professionals need to seek out information on both the science and the consumer perception of these technologies and help consumers make informed choices, just as with other choices related to foods.

Foods may get through the production and distribution systems as safe, fresh, and nutritious products, but may have risks introduced by consumer handling practices. Therefore, appropriate food handling practices for families and for those serving food to others are imperative.

The efforts to control foodborne illness in the United States will require research, legislation, inspection, and education. Nutrition professionals can become involved in each of these efforts, and each nutrition professional is also a food safety educator in the practice setting. It is also important to recognize that certain subgroups within the population—including infants, pregnant women, the elderly, organ transplant recipients, and HIV/AIDS patients—are much more susceptible to foodborne illness.

Consumers trust nutrition professionals to provide accurate food and nutrition information. In that role, nutrition professionals have an obligation to remain aware of the trends in the marketplace from both the consumer and the industry viewpoints. Nutrition professionals are the logical choice for being advocates for both the consumer and the food industry.

COMMUNITY NUTRITION PROFESSIONALS IN ACTION

- A consumer called your office today after reading a newspaper article on phytochemicals and a magazine article on chemical hazards from plant foods. He was confused about the difference between the two. How would you respond?
- Outline basic food safety considerations for an adult day-care center, a child day-care center, a church supper, and a community cookout. Summarize the differences and similarities among the plans.
- Examine the labeling requirements for olestra, saccharin, aspartame, irradiated foods, and genetically engineered foods. What is the consistent theme in the rulings on these labels?
- The local school district has proposed serving wheat cracker prepared with olestra as an option at lunches. This is a topic on the agenda for an opening meeting of the school board and you have been invited to attend to help answer questions. They have been allowing diet soft drinks in the vending machines for many years and have also included fat-free salad dressings on the salad bar. What questions do you anticipate and how will you respond?
- Nutrition professionals have been challenged to play a lead role in communicating consumer issues and concerns to the food industry. Select a topic from this chapter and develop a strategy for explaining potential consumer concerns to the owner of a food company based in your community.
- Nutrition professionals frequently work on teams to address community issues, such as lead poisoning or an outbreak of foodborne illness. For each of these examples, what other professionals would you expect to be involved and what would you expect your role to be?

GOING ONE STEP FURTHER

- Identify a need to improve the American diet and explore actions and controversies related to food product innovation and food safety to address that need, for example, fortification of the food supply with folic acid to prevent neural tube defects, approval of fat substitutes to reduce fat intake, and food safety in day-care centers.
- Stage a mock hearing for approval of a new fat substitute that has no calories and does not interfere with absorption of other nutrients. It is synthe-

sized by genetically engineered bacteria. What needs to be prepared for the company submitting the petition and what questions will be asked by the FDA, consumer groups, the medical community, and consumers.
- Review several issues reported in the *FDA Consumer*. How could you as a community nutrition professional be involved in detection, prevention, and consumer education about these issues?

ADDITIONAL INFORMATION

Professional societies develop statements, scientific status summaries, commentaries, and position papers to clarify issues on which the particular society has expertise and experience. Several of the Institute of Food Technologists Science Communications documents and the American Dietetic Association (ADA) Position Statements are relevant to chapter 6. These are as follows:

IFT Science Communication Documents

1. Assessing, managing and communicating chemical food risks, *Food Technology* 51:85, 1997.
2. Scientific status summary: medical foods, *Food Technology* 46:87, 1992.
3. Scientific status summary: effective management of food packaging; food production to disposal, *Food Technology* 45:225, 1991.
4. Scientific status summary: organically grown foods, *Food Technology* 44:123, 1990.
5. Summary of current information: *Perspectives on food irradiation,* Chicago, IL March 1987, IFT.
6. Backgrounders of IFT (a) genetically engineered foods, October 1996 and (b) bovine spongioform-encephalopathy (BSE), April 1996.

ADA Position Statements

1. Food and water safety, *J Am Diet Assoc* 97:184, 1997.
2. Food irradiation, *J Am Diet Assoc* 96:69, 1996.
3. Biotechnology and the future of food, *J Am Diet Assoc* 95:1429, 1995.
4. Fat replacements, *J Am Diet Assoc* 91:1285, 1991.
5. Use of nutritive and nonnutritive sweeteners, *J Am Diet Assoc* 93:816, 1993.

REFERENCES

1. American Dietetic Association: *ADA 1995 nutrition trends survey,* Chicago, 1995, American Dietetic Association.

2. American Dietetic Association: Position of the American Dietetic Association: biotechnology and the future of food, *J Am Diet Assoc* 95:1429, 1995.

3. American Dietetic Association: Positions of the America Dietetic Association: enrichment and fortification of foods and dietary supplements, *J Am Diet Assoc* 94:661, 1994.

4. American Dietetic Association: Position of the American Dietetic Association: fat replacements, *J Am Diet Assoc* 91:1285, 1991.

5. American Dietetic Association: Position of the American Dietetic Association: food irradiation, *J Am Diet Assoc* 96:69, 1996.

6. American Dietetic Association: Position of the American Dietetic Association: phytochemicals and functional foods, *J Am Diet Assoc* 95:493, 1995.

7. American Dietetic Association: Position of the American Dietetic Association, use of nutritive and nonnutritive sweeteners, *J Am Diet Assoc* 93:816, 1993.

8. American Meat Institute: Putting safe food handling on the table: the pressing need for food safety education, Washington, DC, 1996, American Meat Institute.

9. Birch LL, Johnson SL, Jones MB, Peters JC: Effects of a nonenergy fat substitute on children's energy and macronutrient intake, *Am J Clin Nutr* 58:326, 1993.

10. Calorie Control Council: The secret to good-tasting light foods and beverages, *Calorie Control Commentary* 17(2):1, 1995.

11. Cody MM, Keith M: *Food safety for professionals: a reference and study guide,* Chicago, 1991, American Dietetic Association.

12. Council for Agricultural Science and Technology: Foodborne pathogens: risks and consequences, a report of a task force of the Council for Agricultural Science and Technology, Ames, IA, 1994.

13. Crane NT, Wilson DB, Cook DA, Lewis CJ, Yetley EA, Rader JI: Evaluating food fortification options: general principles revisited with folic acid, *Am J Public Health* 85:660, 1995.

14. Drewnowski A: The new fat replacements: a strategy for reducing fat consumption, *Postgrad Med* 87:111, 1990.

15. *Federal Register:* Food additives permitted for direct addition to food for human consumption: Olestra; final rule, 21 CFR 172, January 30, 1996.

16. *Federal Register:* National Organic Foods Production Act, Proposed Rule. December 16, 1997. 7 CFR, Part 205.

17. Food Marketing Institute: *1995 trends in the US: consumer attitudes and the supermarket 1995,* Washington, DC, 1995, Food Marketing Institute.

18. Gallagher CR and Allred JB: *Taking the fear out of eating: a nutritionists' guide to sensible food choices,* New York, 1992, Cambridge University Press.

19. Giese J: Vitamin and mineral fortification of foods, *Food Technol* 49:110, 1995.

20. Glueck CJ, Hastings MM, Allen C, Hogg E, Baehler L, Gartside PS, Phillips D, Jones M, Hollenbach EJ, Braun B, Anastasis JV: Sucrose polyester and covert caloric dilution, *Am J Clin Nutr* 35:1352, 1982.

21. Hayenga ML: Food and agricultural biotechnology: economic implications, *Am J Clin Nutr* 58(suppl):313S, 1993.

22. Institute of Food Technologists: Foodborne illness: role of home food handling practices—a scientific status summary, *Food Technol* 49(4):119, 1995.

23. Institute of Medicine, National Academy of Sciences, National Research Council: *Opportunities in nutrition and food sciences,* Washington, DC, 1994, National Academy Press.

24. Jones SA: Fat replacers, the broad perspective, *The World of Ingredients* May–June:8, 1995.

25. Kevin K: The next generation of fat replacers, *Food Processing* 56:64, 1995.

26. Kinzel B: Cheese pizza—hold the fat, *Agricultural Res* 42(9):14, 1994.

27. Kosmark R: Salatrim: properties and applications, *Food Technol* 50:98, 1996.

28. LaVella B, Bostic JL: *HACCP for food service: recipe manual and guide,* St. Louis, MO, 1994, LaVella Food Specialists.

29. Lewis CJ, Part YK, Dexter PB, Yetley EA: Nutrient intakes and body weights of persons consuming high and moderate levels of added sugars, *J Am Diet Assoc* 92:708, 1992.

30. Murano AI: Irradiation of fresh meats, *Food Technol* 49:52, 1995.

31. Potter NN, Hotchkiss JH: *Food science,* ed 5, New York, 1995, Chapman and Hall.

32. Rice J: How do you spell opportunity? M-A-P, *Food Processing* 56(7):67, 1995.

33. Rice J: Produce packaging gets fresh, *Food Processing* 56(2):76, 1995.

34. Rolls BJ: Effects of intense sweeteners on hunger, food intake, and body weight: a review, *Am J Clin Nutr* 53:872, 1991.

35. Rolls BJ, Pirraglia PA, Jones MB, Peters JC: Effects of olestra, a noncaloric fat substitute, on daily energy and fat intakes in lean men, *Am J Clin Nutr* 56:84, 1992.

36. Satin M: *Food irradiation: a guidebook,* Lancaster, PA, 1993, Technomic Publishing Co., Inc.

37. Schiller MR, Catakis A: Hazard analysis critical control points: implications for clinical nutrition service delivery, *Top Clin Nutr* 7(4):52, 1992.

38. Sloan AE: Food Industry Forecast: Consumer Trends to 2020 and Beyond: *Food Technol,* 52:37–44, 1998.

39. Sloan AE: America's appetite '96. The top 10 trends to watch and work on, *Food Technol* 50:53, 1996.

40. Smith RE: Food demands of the merging consumer: the role of modern food technology in meeting that challenge, *Am J Clin Nutr* 58(suppl):307S, 1993.

41. Thayer DW, Josephson ES, Brynjolfsson A, Giddings GG: Radiation pasteurization of food. An issue paper on the Council for Agricultural Science and Technology, No. 7, April 1996.

42. Thomas PR, Earl R: Creating the future of the nutrition and food sciences, *J Am Diet Assoc* 94:257, 1994.

43. U.S. Food and Drug Administration: *Compliance program guidance manual*, Ch. 21, Program No. 7321.002, Washington, DC 1989–1991,

44. Zimmernan L, Kendall P, Stone M, Hoban T: Consumer knowledge and concern about biotechnology and food safety, *Food Technol* 48(11):71, 1994.

NUTRITION PROFESSIONALS WORKING WITH THE FOOD INDUSTRY

DESCRIPTION

This case study illustrates challenges of nutrition professionals working with the food industry. Nutrition professionals in this work setting are frequently asked to develop products for specific market segments. These products need to be available for the consumer before the competition gets a similar product to market and, ideally, just as the consumer realizes a need for the product. A vital part of developing any product is marketing it and, of course, making a profit.

METHODOLOGY/TEACHING OBJECTIVES

The main questions raised in this case study have to do with identifying a need for a specific product line, developing those products that can still be incorporated into a balanced food plan, marketing those products, ensuring their safety, and creating satisfied customers. This case study can be used for individual students or for groups of students. It is suitable for use as an out-of-class project followed by in-class presentations.

THE CASE

You have recently been hired by a small supermarket chain as a consultant. This supermarket chain, Eat Well, has twelve locations in rural communities in the Southeast and has built its customer base by providing service and a variety of foods not typically found in these communities. The owner of the company, Mr. Wood, is a dedicated, hard-working man who recently lost his father to heart disease. He has realized that many people in the twelve communities where Eat Well stores are located eat out at least once a week, and that frozen or refrigerated foods are the major items sold in each of his stores.

Mr. Wood has decided to replace part of the deli space in each of his stores with a take-home entrée section that would feature a variety of entrées. He wants consumers to be able either to have the entrées fully prepared in the store or to take them home and finish preparation. He also wants the entrées to fit within the context of a balanced food plan, even though he knows that many of his customers are not extremely adventurous in their food choices. Mr. Wood is fully aware of the potential food safety issues associated with this project. He has hired you to formulate the entrees, recommend types of packaging materials, develop a plan for ensuring safety of the entrees, and devise a marketing plan for the entrees.

SOME QUESTIONS

1. What types of entrées would be popular in these communities?
2. What other types of considerations would enter into your recommendations?
3. What types of existing products would be potential competitors? How would your products differ from them?
4. How would you market the products to the consumer? Could this be an opportunity to provide an additional service (i.e., nutrition education) to the customers? How could you do that?
5. What types of considerations would be needed with regard to packaging?
6. What are the potential food safety issues involved? How could you address them?
7. What other experts could be involved to help you in this project?

CHAPTER SEVEN

NUTRITION BEHAVIOR
IMPLEMENTING CHANGE IN COMMUNITIES

Surely every medicine is an innovation; and he that will not apply new remedies must expect new evils; for time is the greatest innovator; and if time of course alter things to the worse, and wisdom and counsel shall not alter them to the better, what shall be the end? . . . It were good therefore that men in their innovations would follow the example of time itself; which indeed innovateth greatly, but quietly . . .
—SIR FRANCIS BACON

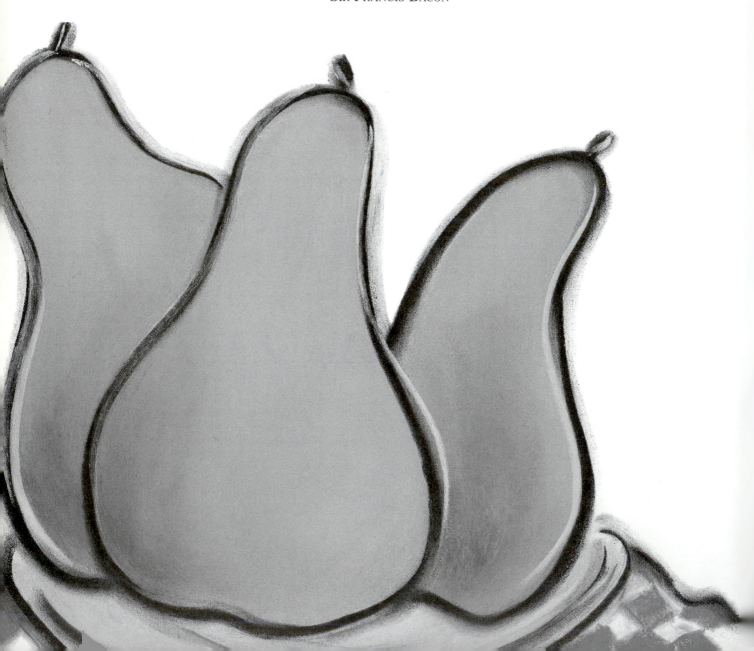

Core Concepts

Successful nutrition intervention in the community involves learning about nutrition behavior and how factors such as personal beliefs and experiences, social ties, and environmental influences can affect eating behaviors. This chapter describes the multilevel, ecological perspective for understanding how people make food choices and change eating behaviors, introduces several models and theoretical frameworks that are relevant to eating behavior change interventions, and presents the principles of social marketing. Applications of these models and theories to nutrition intervention are described throughout the chapter and illustrated in a case study that applies the multilevel approach in a worksite intervention program.

Objectives

When you finish chapter seven, you should be able to:

~ Explain the importance of using behavior change theories and models to design community nutrition intervention programs.

~ Articulate definitions of "theory" and "conceptual model."

~ Identify and describe the five levels of the multilevel ecological model.

~ Describe at least one model aimed at the intrapersonal (individual), interpersonal, and community levels of change.

~ Give examples of how theories and models of behavior change can guide program design and evaluation.

~ Describe at least three social marketing principles that can be applied to the design of eating behavior change interventions.

Key Words

Word	Page Mentioned
Theory	174
Conceptual model	174
Multilevel, ecological perspective	175
Intrapersonal or individual level	178
Interpersonal or social network level	178
Community level	178
Self-efficacy	179
Stages of change	180
Reciprocal determinism	182
Social networks	184
Support systems	184
Lay health advisor	185
Diffusion	186
Community organization	188
Empowerment	188
Social marketing	189
Market segmentation	189

UNDERSTANDING BEHAVIOR AND BEHAVIOR CHANGE

Promoting healthy eating behavior is the central goal of nutrition intervention. For nutrition intervention to be effective, the nutrition professional must understand behavior change theories and transform that knowledge into useful strategies to enhance health. This understanding then needs to be combined with technical knowledge about nutrition and dietary recommendations. It also needs to be put into practice in the community, because healthy dietary patterns can be truly effective only if they are sustained over the long term. This means that attention must be directed not only at influencing people to initiate change but also mobilizing community and environmental supports that will increase the likelihood of maintaining positive changes. These supports can include social support from family and friends, increasing availability of healthy foods in the environment, and policy and institutional changes to support healthy eating.

As is the case for many lifestyle influences on health and disease, diet-related health problems develop gradually and usually do not present immediate or dramatic symptoms. Motivating people to adopt healthier eating patterns requires an understanding of health behavior change. Programs and interventions that are based on an understanding of health behavior theories and that use effective communication strategies (addressed in chapter 17) have a much greater chance of producing positive change. As shown in figure 7.1, this chapter explores theories behind lifestyle behaviors and lays the ground work for designing nutrition interventions to maximize nutritional health and well being.

What Behavior Theories Can Do for Us

Theories are important in any program designed to foster behavior change. A **theory** is a set of interrelated concepts, definitions, and propositions that present a systemic view of events or situations in order to explain and predict future events or situations. Theories are helpful in framing the public health problem, analyzing its antecedents and consequences, informing the needs assessment, and developing the intervention. They can explain the dynamics of the behavior, the processes for changing the behavior, and the effects of external influences on the behavior. They are a behavioral map to better understand and therefore predict behaviors. Theories can help us identify the most suitable targets for intervention programs, the methods for accomplishing change, and the outcomes for evaluation.

Health promotion programs attempt to improve health; reduce disease risks; manage chronic illnesses; and improve the well-being of individuals, families, organizations, and communities. The programs that are most successful are based on a clear understanding of the targeted health behaviors (for example, high-fat diets) and their environmental contexts (for example, a person's family). No one theory provides "all of the answers." Therefore, many different theories have been developed to explain different aspects of people's behaviors. Familiarity with the major health behavior theories can help us be effective nutrition professionals and best serve the populations with whom we are working. They also can tell us why change may not occur despite our efforts, and therefore may help us avoid frustration and "burn-out." Too often, community nutrition professionals focus on operating programs and giving information, forgetting that characteristics of the target audience, such as readiness to change, are determinants of whether the programs will succeed. Theories help us view change as a dynamic interaction, and help us generate new ideas and questions that can improve our effectiveness.

Application of Theories

It is important to note that there are some limitations in using theories because they cannot possibly address all of the complexity of issues related to a public health problem. But as discussed throughout this chapter, theories are useful tools. No single theory can sufficiently explain every health behavior. Often, it is useful to integrate concepts from a number of theories into a **conceptual model** that is relevant to a particular behavior, a specific population, and a defined environmental situation or context. A conceptual model is a framework or diagram of proposed causal linkages among a set of concepts believed to be related to a particular public health problem.[11] A conceptual model for a worksite program to improve diets of workers identified with elevated cholesterol is illustrated in table 7.1.

It is important to remember that theories were developed and modified based on the experiences of researchers' work with individuals, groups, organizations, and communities. Therefore, as a community nutrition professional, it is important to use your common sense and personal experience when selecting theories to use in your programs targeting behavior change. This chapter describes several different theories and models and discusses how they are used in specific situations.

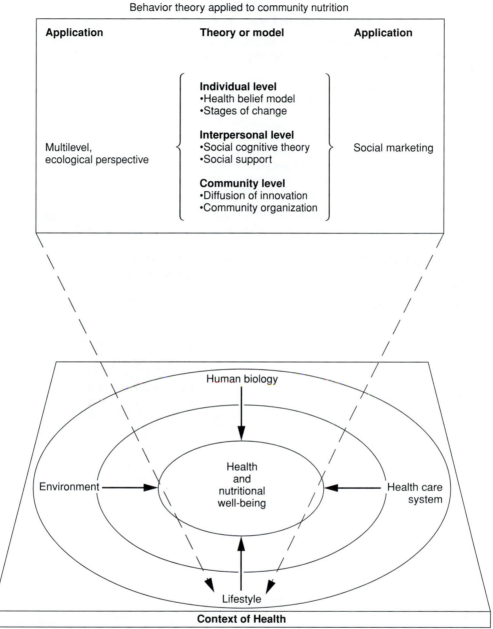

FIGURE 7.1   **Context of Health**
Implementing nutrition behavior change in communities.

MULTILEVEL, ECOLOGICAL PERSPECTIVE TO BEHAVIOR CHANGE

Most health educators believe that a **multilevel, ecological perspective** is needed for understanding and explaining health-related behaviors.[16] This perspective implies that behavior is affected by, and affects, multiple levels of influence. Nutrition intervention in the community includes not only instructional activities directed to individuals and groups, but also organizational efforts, community-level programs, and policy directives. The development, maintenance, and change of eating patterns are determined not only by individual factors but also by many social, cultural, and environmental influences. The idea that individuals are singularly responsible for their

T A B L E   7 . 1
Using Behavior Change Theory to Build a Conceptual Model

Setting: Worksite health promotion center in large manufacturing facility.
Situation: Employees participated in health screening and 19 percent had elevated cholesterol plus one or more risk factors for cardiovascular disease.

Behavior change theory	Health belief model	Diffusion of innovations
Program component	Individual instruction • Highlight perceived susceptibility • Define specific food substitutions to reduce fat intake that are relevant to employee's lifestyle and preferences • Clarify expected effect of behavior changes on weight and serum cholesterol	Self-help materials • Booklet on heart-healthy lifestyle • Pocket guide to low-fat cafeteria selections • Discount coupon for heart-healthy cafeteria item
Outcome expected	Employees recognize risk and begin to understand changes they can make.	Easy ways to substitute low-fat foods are disseminated. Incentives given to induce employees' trial behavior.

Behavior change theory	Social support	Organizational development (social planning) Diffusion of innovations
Program component	Group activities • Worksite walking club • Weight loss competition between work groups	Nutrition professional works with cafeteria managers to have: • Daily heart-healthy menu items featured • Catchy health messages on posters and table tents • Low-fat items in all vending machines
Outcome expected	Coworkers support and challenge each other to continue new behaviors.	Technical assistance empowers cafeteria manager to change eating environment. Low-fat choices are visible and readily available. Posters and menu cue selection of lower fat item.

dietary choices ignores the many influences that affect an individual's diet and often results in victim-blaming. Behavioral choices are influenced by multiple factors that create a web of influence on the individual (see figure 7.2). Health promotion programs that take into account the complexity of influences are most likely to produce lasting behavior change.

Physiological and psychological factors, acquired food preferences, and knowledge about foods are significant individual determinants of food intake. Interpersonal or social factors are also important. For most people, family ties and other close relationships often affect food purchase, preparation, and consumption. Socioeconomic status, economic change, and social support have an important impact on eating patterns that are associated with the prevalence of nutrition-related diseases. Culture, geography, and food availability may increase or limit the range of food choices. Therefore, in developing nutri-

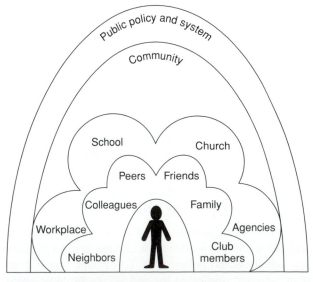

FIGURE 7.2   Multilevel Ecological Perspective

tional interventions, it is important to think about the specific levels of the socioecological model that can be targeted to promote health-inducing behaviors.

A multilevel, ecological perspective is necessary for a broad understanding of dietary behavior. McLeroy and associates[26] have identified five distinct sets of factors that comprise an ecological perspective on health promotion; these factors are summarized in table 7.2.

This chapter focuses on intrapersonal, or individual interpersonal, and community factors that relate to eating behavior. These levels are frequently referred to as individual, group and community or environmental by other writers. For a discussion of institutional and public policy factors, see chapter 5.

The most basic level of health education practice is the individual level focusing on intrapersonal factors. All other levels including groups, organizations, communities, and nations, are comprised of individuals. Therefore, individuals are ultimately a part of every health promotion program at the interpersonal, institutional, community, and policy levels. However, a *multilevel,* interactive perspective has the advantage of empowering people to improve health through a combination of behavioral and environmental strategies (box 7.1). For example, a program aimed at individuals to increase fruit and vegetable intake might be more effective in addressing barriers to change if family and friends are included in the intervention, and if grocers, restaurants, and cafeterias are involved. A multilevel approach increases the likelihood of long-term maintenance of a diet filled with five fruits and

TABLE 7.2
Levels of Change from an Ecological Perspective

Intrapersonal factors	*Individual* characteristics that influence behavior such as knowledge, attitudes, beliefs, and experiences
Interpersonal factors	Interpersonal processes, and primary *groups* including formal and informal *social network* and *social support* systems, including family, work groups, and friends
Institutional factors	Rules, regulations, policies, and informal *organizational* structures that may constrain or promote recommended behaviors within institutions such as workplaces, agencies, or schools
Community factors	Social networks and norms, or standards, that exist as formal or informal "rules" among individuals, groups, institutions, and networks that make up *communities* within defined geographic or other boundaries
Public policy factors	Local, state, and federal laws and policies that regulate or support healthy actions and practices for disease prevention, early detection, control, and management at the broad *system* level

BOX 7.1

ENVIRONMENTAL STRATEGIES

Assessing and then improving the food environment is often an effective way of helping people make dietary changes. Here are a few examples:

PROBLEM

Employees of a small company identify vending machine foods as a problem; food choices are high in fat, sugar, and salt.

Community residents feel that there are no restaurants in the area that serve "healthy" foods.

Church members have many social functions where food is served, but the foods are typically fried or heavily seasoned with fat.

ENVIRONMENTAL STRATEGY

Work with the vendor to offer healthier foods in the machine, such as fruit, juice, and low-fat snacks.

Visit local restaurants and identify healthy menu items. Encourage restaurants to label these items as "healthy" choices and to add more healthy options. Advertise that these restaurants are participating in your program.

Work with the church kitchen committee to plan healthier alternatives and additions to the menu while still serving some "favorite" foods.

vegetables, and has far-reaching effects on other healthy dietary habits. Health promotion is most successful when problems are analyzed and programs are planned on various levels of influence. These levels often overlap and should be considered as working together. Each successively "higher" or "larger" level incorporates concepts from the "lower" or "smaller" level; thus groups are made up of individuals, and communities are composed of individuals and groups. Comprehensive community nutrition intervention efforts draw on understanding strategies from each level.

Individuals are shaped by the communities in which they live, particularly their peer and social networks. These networks provide immense support to individuals, and can greatly influence a person's beliefs, attitudes, and ultimately behaviors. Public health interventions utilize social networks in an effort to normalize targeted behaviors. For example, it is futile to educate individuals about eating low-fat foods if their families and friends are criticizing their efforts to eat these foods. Promoting interventions at the interpersonal level where the social network is involved will build on peer support and foster positive change.

Environmental influences are also strong determinants of dietary choices. For example, foods available in the marketplace impact the entire community. The food supply in the United States has changed dramatically in the past thirty years (see chapter 6 for discussion of this). Using a multilevel ecological perspective, the community nutrition professional could plan an intervention to include healthful foods in grocery stores and restaurants (community); distribution of specially designed informational materials to individuals at work, school, or medical clinic (individual); and activities that foster peer support such as cooking classes, walking clubs (groups).

THEORIES AND MODELS FOR INFLUENCING EATING BEHAVIOR

This section presents several models that are particularly useful for understanding the determinants of dietary behavior and for designing and evaluating dietary intervention programs to improve health. Using a multilevel approach, models are presented that focus on the intrapersonal (individual), interpersonal (group, social network), and institutional-community (organizational or whole community) levels of change.

At the **intrapersonal or individual level,** cognitive-behavioral models help explain the psychosocial factors that may foster or inhibit behavior change. Psychosocial

factors include awareness, knowledge, beliefs, expectations, attitudes, and intentions. Some of these models, such as the *health belief model,* assume that people make rational decisions about health behaviors by weighing the expected benefits versus the costs. These types of models are termed "value-expectancy" models because it is assumed that behavioral decisions stem from an assessment of the value of the behavior and the expected results. Another way of looking at behavior change from a cognitive-behavioral perspective is to examine the process of changing over time. Stages-of-change models visualize behavior change as a series of steps or stages, rather than a decision made at one point in time. At each stage, different cognitive processes and strategies are thought to be important in helping individuals advance toward and then maintain action. The Prochaska and DiClemente transtheoretical model[31] is the most widely used stages-of-change model at present, and it has been applied to a number of health behaviors including eating behavior change. *Social cognitive theory* (SCT) focuses on learning as a cognitive process that includes both intrapersonal and interpersonal factors.[3] SCT views learning new behavior as an interactive process that is influenced by characteristics of the individual, the behavior, and the environment.

At the **interpersonal or social network level,** *social support* theories provide a framework for understanding how social ties influence health behavior and how these ties can be mobilized for health promotion. One application of social support to health is the lay health advisor model, in which natural helpers already present in a community are trained to provide support and encouragement for making healthy behavior changes. Peer breast-feeding support is an example of this.

At the institutional and **community levels** of change, two models—*diffusion of innovations* and *community organization*—help explain how healthier eating habits and related lifestyle behaviors can be initiated, promoted, and sustained in populations. Diffusion of innovations is informative to nutrition professionals, helping them understand how new ideas, products, and practices are adopted in various segments of a population. This understanding can aid in planning more effective programs and responding to societal trends that affect food choices. Community organization models provide tools for community nutrition professionals to work *with and involve* the community in planning programs and determining priorities, rather than imposing program goals from a professional, outsider perspective.

Social marketing is not a theory but rather a set of strategies and techniques that inform the design of effective interventions aimed at individuals and groups. The social marketing approach applies marketing principles to health issues. It emphasizes the role of formative evaluation to determine the priorities and interests of the target audience as a basis for planning programs. It is described in a later section.

For each of the theories and models, a brief description of the central elements of the theory is presented, followed by examples that illustrate how it can be applied to eating behavior change strategies. The case study at the end of the chapter illustrates a community-based nutrition intervention program that attempted to use a multilevel approach.

Health Belief Model

Description What makes people decide to engage in a health behavior change? Knowledge is necessary, but it is not sufficient for helping people to follow guidelines for healthy eating. According to the health belief model, people must believe that they have a risk of developing a particular health problem, that dietary change will decrease their risk, and that the benefits of changing outweigh the costs. Using fear tactics is one way of convincing people to change, however, this may backfire if it results in raising fears to the point where paralysis and fatalism set in. The health belief model examines many of these issues and provides a framework for conveying health information effectively.

The health belief model was one of the first models that specifically adapted concepts from psychology and behavioral science to health problems, and it is still one of the most widely used models for understanding preventive health activities.[33] It was originally developed in the 1950s by a group of psychologists working for the U.S. Public Health Service. The issue of concern was screening for tuberculosis by promoting chest X-rays. The researchers found that a substantial number of people did not obtain chest X-rays despite efforts to convey risk information and to reduce barriers to getting this procedure. They found that one reason people did not obtain the test was the high fear level associated with discovering a serious disease. The researchers identified a set of components of the model that seemed to predict whether individuals would decide to take a preventive health action (see table 7.3). Perceived *susceptibility* to a health problem and perceived *severity* or seriousness of the condition and its consequences combine to form the perception of *threat*. Effective health communications should convincingly present the threat

along with a strategy to reduce threat by taking the recommended action. In addition, individuals weigh the perceived *benefits* of the advised action (what will I gain?) against the perceived *barriers* to change (what makes it hard and/or what will I lose?) before deciding to act. Barriers can be very important inhibitors of behavior change. Examples of barriers to healthy eating include the financial cost of purchasing items such as fresh fruits and vegetables, lack of transportation to supermarkets that sell healthy foods, and unwillingness of other family members to eat healthy foods.

If and how the individual decides to respond to the threat is determined by a number of things. *Cues to action* serve to activate behavior by promoting awareness and reminding individuals to take action. Cues to action include prompts such as a point of sale message on grocery store shelf, reminder card from the health professional, television public service announcement, or flyer advertising a free screening. **Self-efficacy** (confidence) regarding one's ability to perform the behavior is sometimes considered part of the model.[33] The concept of self-efficacy is discussed later in this chapter.

Application There are many ways that the components of the health belief model can be applied to nutrition intervention. The model provides a set of concepts that, if applied, can help make nutrition intervention materials and messages more effective. For example, a program promoting lower fat diets to prevent heart disease might first assess the perceived susceptibility and perceived severity of heart disease in the target group. One might expect that these perceptions would be quite high among a group of cardiac rehabilitation patients, but low among adolescents and young adults. Messages for younger audiences could be designed that presented information to raise threat perceptions along with strategies to cope with the threat through healthy changes. Next, the perceived benefits of changing to a low-fat diet, such as feeling better, controlling weight, or avoiding heart disease, must be compared to the perceived barriers of such a change (such as the cost of low-fat foods, not liking the taste of these foods, or not having time to prepare them). Depending on the relative strength of benefits and barriers, program strategies could target either the benefits of change or overcoming the barriers. Finally, cues to action could be incorporated into the program, such as having a health fair with cholesterol screening or distributing a news article about a celebrity who had a heart attack and then successfully made dietary changes.

TABLE 7.3
Health Belief Model

Concept	Definition	What the client is thinking	Application for professionals
Threat			
Perceived susceptibility	One's opinion of chances of getting a condition	Does it affect me?	Define population(s) at risk, risk levels. Personalize risk based on a person's features or behavior. Heighten perceived susceptibility if too low.
Perceived severity	One's opinion of how serious a condition and what its sequelae are	If I got it, how bad would it be?	Specify consequences of the risk and the condition.
Determining the response			
Perceived benefits	One's opinion of the efficacy of the advised action to reduce risk or seriousness of impact	Would changing now really make any difference?	Define action to take: how, where, when. Clarify the positive effects to be expected.
Perceived barriers	One's opinion of the tangible and psychological costs of the advised action	How hard would it be for me to change?	Identify and reduce barriers through reassurance, incentives, and assistance.
Cues to action	Strategies to activate "readiness"	What do I have to do?	Provide how-to information. Promote awareness, reminders.
Self-efficacy	Confidence in one's ability to take action	Can I do it?	Provide training, and guidance in performing action.

Source: Adapted from Glanz K, Rimer BK: *Theory at a glance: a guide for health promotion practice,* Washington DC, 1995, Dept. of Health and Human Services, Public Health Service, and National Institutes of Health.

Stages of Change

Description Changing dietary habits involves many kinds of decisions. People may or may not be "ready" to try a specific change at a given time. For example, even though someone may be aware that eating high-fat foods can contribute to elevated serum cholesterol levels, he or she may not be ready to switch to lower fat alternatives. This may be true for many reasons. It may be that, because of competing demands and the need to set priorities, the person has decided that other health actions are more important, such as quitting smoking. The person may have tried unsuccessfully in the past to make dietary changes. Or perhaps the individual is ready to change but lacks knowledge or skills to plan and prepare low-fat meals.

A great deal of research in the area of smoking cessation and substance abuse has indicated that people vary in their "readiness" to change. Emerging research on adop-

tion of healthful eating behavior including low-fat, high-fiber, and high-fruit-and-vegetable diets, suggests that this idea also applies to nutrition behavior.[5,7,10,13,15,39] Irrespective of medical needs or medically diagnosed risk, people may be at various stages of receptivity for learning and using nutrition advice. The health education literature indicates that "one size fits all" programs fail to motivate large segments of the population who are at different stages of readiness.[15] By applying this idea to the process of eating behavior change, interventions can be tailored to the needs and concerns of individuals at each stage of the change process. The intervention is different depending on the stage.

The **stages-of-change** transtheoretical method was developed by Prochaska and DiClemente in the context of smoking cessation behavior, and has its roots in earlier stage models of health behavior.[17,30] The model is called "transtheoretical" because it incorporates key elements of a number of social psychological models of health behav-

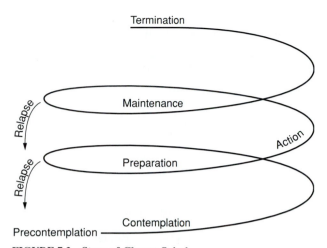

FIGURE 7.3   Stage-of-Change Spiral
(Source: Adapted from Prochaska J: In search of how people change. *American Psychologist,* 47(9):1104, 1109, 1992.)

ior. The model's central assumption is that behavior change is a dynamic process involving several cognitively distinct stages. This is in contrast to a value-expectancy model such as the health belief model, where behavior change is viewed as stemming from a decision based on factors that can be measured at one point in time. According to the stages-of-change approach, people can be categorized according to their readiness to change. The stages constitute a spiral (see figure 7.3) rather than a linear progression, and people can enter or exit the change process at any point. For example, individuals may progress to action but then relapse and go through some of the stages several times before succeeding in maintenance. The stages include: precontemplation (unaware, not interested in change), contemplation (thinking about changing, usually within six months), preparation (ready to change soon, e.g., in the next thirty days), action (currently trying to change), maintenance (maintaining the new habits for at least six months), and relapse (returning to the old behavior) or termination (new behavior is so established that relapse is not an issue).

The stages of change help us to understand *when* shifts in intentions and behaviors are likely to occur. Another important dimension of the model is the *processes* of change, which help us understand *why* these shifts occur.[31] Processes of change are activities that people engage in when they are attempting to change behaviors. Different processes of change are used more often in some stages as compared to others. For example, people who are just starting to consider a behavior change (con-

templation) are most likely to respond to the processes of "consciousness raising" or "self-reevaluation." Table 7.4 illustrates the change process used by the client and the community nutrition professional at each stage of change.

Application   The stages-of-change model has direct application to nutrition intervention. Program strategies will probably be more effective when they are designed to match individual's stage in the change process. Mismatching may result in lack of results or actually discouraging the individual from considering change. For example, if someone with high cholesterol who is consuming a high-fat diet has not even begun to think about changing, there is no point in providing detailed nutrition information and food preparation tips. The person is not ready to make use of this information and may feel overwhelmed or alienated by that approach. It would be more appropriate to focus on increasing that person's awareness and personal health concerns before introducing action-oriented strategies. On the other hand, someone who is engaged in switching to a low-fat eating style may be looking for specific information or resources such as recipes to support that behavior. It would be frustrating for this person to receive educational materials that focus on increasing awareness of risks associated with high serum cholesterol.

The stages-of-change model has important implications not only for planning nutrition intervention strategies but also for evaluating the impact of these activities. By staging individuals at various points in a program, two important evaluation components are gained. From a process evaluation perspective, the stage information can serve to guide program development. For example, a baseline survey at the beginning of a program might show that there is a large percentage of contemplators in the group, but relatively few people who are in action or maintenance. The program planners may then decide to first offer program activities that are designed to move contemplators forward to action. Later, if a midpoint survey shows that there are now more people who have initiated changes, subsequent activities might focus on shifting from action to maintenance while still offering some program pieces for those who have not yet progressed. From an outcome evaluation perspective, assessing stages of change can provide intermediate measures of program effectiveness that may contribute to understanding whether and why the program worked. For example, a final survey can assess overall impact of the program in moving people forward through the stages, as

TABLE 7.4

Change Process Used by Client and Professional in Each Stage of Change

Stage	Helpful behavioral actions of client	Application for professionals
Precontemplation Unaware, not interested in change	Consider risks of current behavior and benefits of change	Increase awareness by clearly identifying problem area, explain why change is important, advocate specific change.
Contemplation Starting to think about change, but ambivalent; could change within six months	Lists positive reasons to move ahead; lists things that make it difficult Think about how these could be handled	Tip the balance in favor of change. Acknowledge positive incentives of old behavior. Emphasize benefits of new behavior. Strengthen client's belief in ability to change. Help overcome barriers.
Preparation Definitely planning to start within a month	Sets realistic and attainable goals; plans rewards; picks start date	Provide specific information about how to change—tailored to client's situation. Give choices. Help client determine best course of action.
Action Doing it	Tells others; enlists support Rewards self for meeting small goals	Provide encouragement; add step-by-step information about incorporating new behavior into life patterns. Initiate contact to check progress and reinforce.
Maintenance Continuing to use what worked in action stage	Sets new goals and rewards; tries variations of new behavior	Reinforce progress made. Teach strategies to prevent relapse.
Relapse Shifted back to old behavior	Is aware of situations that undermine success; recalls reasons to change	Review past-achievement; help client avoid discouragement. Renew above processes.
Termination Behavior is now established habit		

well as looking at typical outcome measures such as dietary intake or weight loss. Sample stages-of-change questions adapted from the 5 a Day for Better Health community research studies are shown in figure 7.4.

Social Cognitive Theory

Description   How do people learn new ways of healthier eating? Is what we eat determined by habits developed from childhood, and must we use rewards and punishments in order to break "bad" habits and form "good" ones? Or do we develop new skills and make choices about what we eat based on interactive learning? According to social cognitive theory, learning results from a complex set of factors within individuals, in interactions with other people, and in the environ-

ment.[2,3] People's personal knowledge and beliefs, their abilities and opportunities to learn and perfect the behavior, and the accessibility of foods all influence what they eat. The social environment includes support from family, friends, and others involved in the process, and is important for initiating and maintaining dietary changes.

SCT postulates dynamic relationships among personal factors, the social and physical environment, and observable behavior. These dynamic relationships are conceptualized in the central construct of **reciprocal determinism,** which means that learning occurs not in isolation but via constant interaction and feedback between the person and the environment. Proponents of operant conditioning and behavior modification techniques would say that learning involves systematized reinforce-

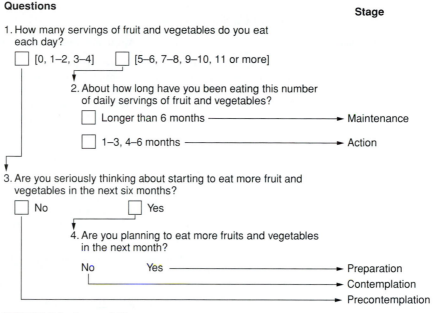

FIGURE 7.4 Stages of Change
Questions regarding fruit and vegetable consumption.

ment of desirable behavior through rewards and positive feedback and extinction of undesirable behavior through negative reinforcement or punishment. Behavior modification techniques can be effective and are often used as parts of nutrition intervention programs. An example is giving positive reinforcement (such as stickers or praise) to reinforce children's participation in activities. Social cognitive theory, however, comes from a long tradition of learning theory that has placed increasing emphasis on cognitive processes as important forces along with behavioral responses to external reinforcements. SCT incorporates the basic concepts of behavior modification in conjunction with cognitive, interpersonal, and environmental influences on behavior.

Social cognitive theory includes many concepts, only a few of which are highlighted here (see table 7.5). They include environment, observational learning, reinforcement, feedback, self-control, and self-efficacy. Environment is defined as all factors physically external to a person that can influence behavior. These factors might include, for example, access to healthy food options or social support for losing weight. Observational learning takes place when someone watches another person's behavior and notices the outcomes of that behavior. It suggests the use of credible role models to demonstrate performing the behavior and to give "testimonials" as to its positive results.

Reinforcement is the response to a person's behavior, which can be positive reinforcement ("reward") or negative reinforcement (no external reward). Reinforcement can be internal to a person, such as a feeling of pride or accomplishment, or it can be external. External feedback can be a strong reinforcer. For example, when a nutrition professional gives praise or shows a person that his or her fat intake is decreasing, the behavior is reinforced. Self-control of behavior involves a person observing his or her own behavior, setting personal goals, initiating action, evaluating achievement of goals, and rewarding himself or herself. Behavioral self-regulation techniques, such as setting specific goals, gradual change, and self-monitoring, are activities based on self-control that are common features of weight management and nutrition counseling programs.

The concept of self-efficacy is one of the most useful parts of SCT in terms of predicting behavior change and informing the kinds of activities that will lead to positive change. According to SCT, behavioral performance is strongly affected by two kinds of beliefs: beliefs about how capable one is of performing a behavior, and beliefs or expectations about what the results or outcomes of the behavior will be. Self-efficacy is defined as an individual's confidence in his or her ability to perform a specific type of behavior. Self-efficacy is not the same thing as self-confidence. Self-efficacy is specific to the behavior of interest. It includes degree of confidence, strength of persistence in the face of obstacles, and commitment

TABLE 7.5
Social Cognitive Theory

Concept	Definition	Application for professionals
Reciprocal determinism	Behavior changes result from interaction between person and environment; change bidirectional	Involve the individual and relevant others; work to change the environment, to reinforce positive action.
Behavioral capacity	Knowledge and skills to influence behavior	Provide information and training about action.
Expectations	Beliefs about likely results of action	Incorporate information about likely results of action in advance.
Self-efficacy	Confidence in ability to take action and persist in action	Point out strengths; use persuasion and encouragement; approach behavior change in small steps.
Observational learning	Beliefs based on observing others like self and/or visible physical results	Point out others' experience, physical changes; identify role models to emulate.
Reinforcement	Responses to a person's behavior that increase or decrease the chances of recurrence	Provide incentives, rewards, praise, encourage self-regard; decrease possibility of negative responses that deter positive changes.

Source: Adapted from Glanz K, Rimer BK: *Theory at a glance: a guide for health promotion practice,* Washington DC, 1995, Dept. of Health and Human Services, Public Health Service and National Institutes of Health.

to continuing the specific behavior in different situations and over time.[25]

Application Social cognitive theory suggests concrete ways to use interactive teaching and learning to alter behavior and it is an important model for designing and implementing nutrition intervention and counseling programs. Behavioral and cognitive strategies to increase self-efficacy include setting small goals at first and gradually increasing the challenge, modeling behavior changes, offering opportunities to practice the behavior, giving constructive feedback, and encouraging positive "self-talk." Perry and colleagues have used interventions based on SCT to improve eating behaviors in children participating in school- and home-based cardiovascular disease prevention and alcohol prevention programs.[29,30] The Go for Health project, a diet and physical activity program for elementary school children in Texas, used SCT to plan and evaluate a program that combined classroom activities with environmental changes in cafeteria offerings.[37] In group programs, activities such as hands-on cooking classes, group problem-solving sessions, and modeling by people who have succeeded in behavior change can also provide opportunities to increase self-efficacy by practicing skills, observing healthy eating patterns, and receiving feedback and social support for new habits. In individual level interventions, self-help and computer interactive strategies can be designed to increase self-efficacy by allowing individuals to select goals, obtain feedback on their progress, and learn concrete skills that are needed to succeed with

the behavioral change. An example is the StampSmart Program, which demonstrated increased self-efficacy as a result of using SCT concepts in a computer-tailored nutrition intervention program to teach low-income women how to lower dietary fat.[6]

Social Support

Description Individuals are shaped by interactions with others in their **social networks,** such as their families, peers, friends, and coworkers. These networks provide immense support to individuals, and can be a great influence on improving individual's beliefs, attitudes, and ultimately behaviors.

Support systems are attachments among individuals or between individuals and groups that serve to improve individuals' ability to deal with short-term crises and life transitions as well as long-term challenges and stresses.[20] There is evidence that lay support systems play an important role in helping individuals decide whether a health concern is serious, gain health information, decide on a course of action, and follow through with health actions. A lay support system is defined as an enduring pattern of continuous or intermittent ties that plays a significant part in maintaining the psychological and physical integrity of the individual over time. Lay helping systems are distinct from professional helping systems in that they are naturally formed roles within communities. Lay helping systems are hidden health care systems that can lead to long-lasting support for positive healthy behaviors among individual community members.

TABLE 7.6
Functional Social Support Categories Applied to Breast-Feeding Support

Instrumental support	Tangible aid, money, resources	WIC vouchers for food for lactating mother, breast pump rental
Informational support	Advice, education, referrals, and information	Printed directions and demonstration how to position baby
Emotional support	Love, care, concern, friendship, listening	Caring, understanding by peer counselor
Appraisal support	Affirmation, feedback for self-reevaluation	Positive feedback for choosing to breast-feed and sticking with it, show evidence that baby is thriving (weight gain, acts satisfied, wet diapers)

Public health interventions can utilize these networks in an effort to improve the adoption of targeted behaviors. For example, it is difficult for an individual to consistently eat low-fat foods if his or her family and friends routinely select high-fat foods. Dietary interventions aimed at change among peers and social groups at the interpersonal level can build on the support provided by existing networks and will usually be more successful for achieving maintenance of eating behavior change than just focusing on the individual.

Social support, provided by social networks, is a way in which individuals are linked to the society at large. Sociological theories provide important concepts and models about how social interactions can influence health.[18] Social support can have positive and negative effects on individual health outcomes, and can actively reduce stress.[8] There are several characteristics of social support. The first is *structural* support, which describes objective characteristics of a support system, such as size and density. This characteristic is concerned with the existence and interconnectedness a person has with their social ties.[35] An example could be the number of different ties to relatives, friends, church, social groups, and work. *Functional support* characteristics are more subjective in nature. They relate to a person's perception of the access and availability of resources provided by a support network. The four types of functional support are defined in table 7.6, and illustrated with an example from breast-feeding support programs. The importance of social support is very evident in breast-feeding. Women who have a circle of relatives and friends who have breast-fed feel more able to deal with problems faced when initiating and continuing to breast-feed. Breast-feeding women without this support often lack confidence and experience higher stress. Awareness of a lactation consultant or peer educator could be a buffer when a problem occurs.

Social support assumes that an individual's health is enhanced by the existence and depth of support in a person's life. It also assumes that social systems are impor-

tant mediating structures for individuals' connection with the society at large. Therefore, it assumes that the resources provided by social ties and the intensity of the relationship with those ties are a positive thing. Several key studies have shown that individuals with more social support do have lower morbidity and mortality rates from chronic diseases compared to those with lower support.[20]

The **lay health advisor** model is an extension of social support theory to health-related interventions that involves tapping into existing lay support systems. Lay health advisor (LHA) programs build on existing support provided by natural helpers already present in social networks. LHAs are a source of help internal to a community.[12] They are trusted individuals to whom people turn to for advice. LHAs naturally provide instrumental, informational, emotional, and appraisal support to individual network members. An LHA intervention seeks to identify the natural helpers in the community and provide them with added information and skills to disseminate health messages through their existing social ties. By talking to community or network members, a program planner can identify the natural helpers, invite them to participate, and provide the appropriate training. A key challenge of LHA programs is to enhance the LHAs' knowledge and credibility without altering their natural role or co-opting them into becoming part of "the system." The LHA model has been used extensively in the development of breast-feeding support programs.

Application   Interventions that utilize LHAs can occur in a workplace, place of worship, community organization, or neighborhood. Depending on a program's objectives, lay health advisors can be used to provide any combination of social support functions (instrumental, informational, emotional, and appraisal support). There are many different lay health advisor roles that can be utilized in nutrition prevention programming. LHAs can serve to support community members' efforts to increase healthy eating by providing information or by giving

TABLE 7.7
Characteristics of Successful Innovations

Concept	Definition	Application for professionals
Complexity	How difficult the innovation is to understand and/or use	Create program/idea/product to be uncomplicated, easy to use and understand.
Compatibility	How consistent the innovation is with values, habits, experience, and needs of potential adopters	Tailor innovation for the intended audience's values, norms, or situation.
Relative advantage	Degree to which an innovation is seen as better than the idea, practice, program, or product it replaces	Point out unique benefits: monetary value, convenience, time saving, prestige, and the like.
Flexibility	Range of settings and situations the innovation can be adapted to fit	Demonstrate how the innovation can be used in a variety of circumstances.
Trialability	Extent to which the innovation can be experimented with before a commitment to adopt is required	Provide opportunities to try on a limited basis, for example, free samples, introductory sessions, money-back guarantees.
Observability	Extent to which the innovation provides tangible or visible results	Assure visibility of results; feedback or publicity

Source: Adapted from Glanz K, Rimer BK: *Theory at a glance: a guide to health promotion practice,* Washington DC, 1995, Dept. of Health and Human Services, Public Health Service, and National Institutes of Health.

positive feedback. LHAs can also help individuals obtain resources such as WIC or food stamps by telling them about these resources or by providing instrumental support, such as transporting someone to the agency or clinic. Also, LHAs can be agents of social change by helping to mobilize community attention and resources around health issues, such as organizing an event to promote healthier food choices for young children.

It is important to note that lay health advisor programs do not replace the role of trained professionals. Rather, LHAs can work collaboratively with professionals, such as nutritionists, toward mutually beneficial goals. LHAs can extend the reach of typical agency-based programs and can help professionals gain access into "hard-to-reach" segments of the population.[36] LHAs can provide valuable insights into why certain programs do not work or are not sustained. For example, a program may be rejected because it is perceived as using "outsiders" to come in and tell people what they are doing wrong. Utilizing the natural roles and functions of LHAs can increase trust and acceptance of program messages, and can increase community members' sense of empowerment and control over their own health.

Diffusion of Innovations

Description   Why do some new ideas and products take off in popularity right away, while others, sometimes better, ideas achieve little or no attention? Diffusion of innovations theory helps to explain the factors that influence the adoption and maintenance of new

products and practices in society. Diffusion has occurred when a new nutrition curriculum is adopted by a school system, when shoppers buy a new product at the grocery store, when a woman goes for her first mammogram, and in countless other health-related examples.

Diffusion is defined as the process through which an innovation is communicated through channels over time among members of a social system.[32] An innovation is an idea, practice, service, or object that is considered new by an individual or social group. According to diffusion theory (table 7.7), certain characteristics of innovations increase the chances that they will be widely adopted. An innovation must be understandable to get the interest of the target audience. Innovations are more likely to succeed if they are perceived as compatible with existing value systems and lifestyles of the target audience. The new approach must offer a relative advantage over existing methods. People and groups are more likely to try a new program if it is flexible, adaptable to different settings and situations, trialable (can be tried out on a pilot basis), and reversible (can go back to the old way if not satisfied with the new idea). Using the innovation must produce tangible results. Successful innovations usually are perceived to have greater benefits than their costs, and the risks of changing are not seen as prohibitively high. The stages that typically occur in the diffusion process, whether applied to an individual, a group, or an organization are awareness, interest, evaluation, trial, and finally adoption. Personal experience and the experience of those in social networks are also important to the continued use of an innovation.

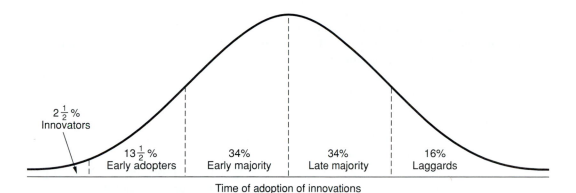

FIGURE 7.5   Adoptor Categorization
Certain types of people and groups tend to adopt innovations faster than others. (*Source:* Adapted from Kotter, P. *Marketing for nonprofit organizations,* Englewood Cliffs, NJ, 1982, Prentice Hall.)

Diffusion does not occur uniformly in society. The pattern of diffusion for an innovation depends on its characteristics and the speed with which it is disseminated either actively or passively. In addition, certain types of people and groups in society tend to adopt innovations faster than others (see figure 7.5). The "early adopters" usually are more highly educated, affluent, and actively use information-seeking processes. They tend to be risk takers and are sometimes viewed as outlandish by others in the social group. Media sources (such as broadcast media, print materials, and the Internet) are effective in promoting awareness and interest in trying new things among the early adopters. Later adopters tend to be less advantaged in society and may have significant barriers, such as education or finances, that impede their trying and using an innovation. Interpersonal sources of communication, especially from respected individuals and peers, tend to be more influential in promoting new health practices and programs among later adopter groups.

Application   Innovations are constantly entering the nutrition field in the form of new food products, supplements, health advice, medical tests, and so on. Consumers are interested in nutrition but are often confused about which innovations are worth trying because of the speed with which media report and debunk nutrition recommendations. Disseminating sound nutrition programs requires an understanding of the diffusion process. In working with organizations such as schools and worksites, it is important to build in the characteristics that predict successful adoption, for example, emphasizing the flexibility and trialability of the new program. Community nutrition professionals often use programs and materials that appeal to people who are information seekers but may fail to reach

TABLE 7.8
Attributes of Communities

Membership	Sense of identity and belonging
Common symbol systems	Similar language, rituals, and ceremonies
Mutual influence	Influenced by each other, share needs and committed to meet them
Shared emotional connection	Common history, experiences, and mutual support

the majority of individuals who are more receptive to interpersonal strategies. Thus, we may often find ourselves "preaching to the choir" because the information seekers are likely to adopt new practices anyway and having our message "fall on deaf ears" because the majority do not yet see the relevance of the innovation. Using an interpersonal model such as the lay health advisor approach to diffuse information might be more effective in fostering innovation among less-advantaged groups in society.

Community Organization

Description   A community can be defined by geographical, political, or organizational boundaries, by heritage or ethnic group, or by shared interests and concerns. Individuals are a part of many communities. Some geographically defined areas, such as a city, might be filled with many ethnic communities that identify more strongly with their ethnic group than with the geographic community. A community is a locale or domain that is characterized by several elements,[19] as shown in table 7.8.

Community-level health promotion initiatives are the heart of public health programming. Interventions at this level do not single out "high-risk" members of the populations based on certain characteristics (such as age, gender, or disease risk), rather, the community as a whole is the target for the intervention. The collective well-being of communities can be fostered by creating structures and policies that support healthy lifestyles and by reducing or eliminating hazards in social and physical environments.

Community organization is the participatory process by which community groups are helped to identify common problems or goals, mobilize resources, and in other ways develop and implement strategies for reaching goals.[27] Central concepts in community organization include empowerment, development of community competence, participation, community-based issue selection, and critical consciousness (see table 7.9).[27] Community organization is not a single theory, rather it is derived from an amalgamation of theories and processes of social change, including social support, political action, and other perspectives.

Community organization uses several social change models, often identified using Rothman's typology: locality development (or community development), social planning, and social action.[34] *Social planning* is task oriented and focuses on problem solving with assistance from outside experts. The experts provide technical assistance to community members around a specific health issue. *Community development* uses a broad cross section of people in the community to identify and solve their own problems. It is process oriented and stresses consensus development, cooperation, capacity building through leadership development, and building a group identity. *Social action* is skill-building and outcome oriented and aims to increase a community's problem-solving ability. Its goal is to achieve concrete changes, often for a group that is considered disadvantaged. Social action for community organizing often involves political action and conflict with the status quo to achieve needed changes. Community organization approaches should empower communities to control and guide their lives.[19] Through the process of **empowerment,** individuals gain problem-solving ability and the power of critical consciousness to examine the causes of other problems existing in the community.

Application   Different models of community organization require various levels of involvement and direction by nutrition professionals. A social-planning strategy might include professionals from different agencies advising community leaders to determine the health priorities and change strategies to be employed. With a community development approach, a nutrition professional may act as a behind-the-scenes organizer, provide training, be a participant, and/or offer technical assistance. In many community development programs, community advisory boards and/or coalitions are formed that consist of key community representatives. Nutrition professionals might help organize or serve on a coalition that had a mission to improve nutrition among vulnerable groups in the community. Social action often requires the health professionals to take a back seat and be available to provide assistance and encouragement only when the community wants it.

SOCIAL MARKETING

Description

The term social marketing was introduced to describe application of commercial marketing principles and technologies to advancement of a social cause, idea, or behavior[20] (such as the 5-A-Day campaign to increase

TABLE 7.9
Community Organizing Concepts

Empowerment	The process of gaining mastery and power over one's self/one's community, to produce change: empowerment can be achieved by giving individuals and community tools and responsibility for making decisions that affect them.
Community competence	Community's ability to engage in effective problem solving: community competence can be achieved by working with a community to identify problems, create consensus, and reach goals.
Participation	Organizing must start where the people are. The individual's or community's "felt needs" and concerns must guide the agenda. When issues are selected by the community itself a real sense of "ownership" can emerge.
Issue selection	A good issue must be winnable, simple, and specific. It should affect many people and unite members in a meaningful way. Surveys, group process, and discussion are ways to increase participation and identify issues.
Critical consciousness	Through problem-posing dialogue, the community develops an understanding of the root causes of the issue being addressed. Health concerns should always be considered in the broader social background in which they occur.

consumption of fruit and vegetables). **Social marketing** is the analysis, planning, implementation, and evaluation of programs that seek to increase the acceptability of a social ideal or cause in a target audience. It is not a theory, but a set of concepts and techniques that form a framework for planning and managing effective health interventions.[28] In public health, social marketing is used to influence the behavior of target audiences in order to improve their physical and mental well-being and/or that of the society of which they are a part. When applied appropriately, social marketing empowers individuals to be involved and responsible for their well being.[23]

Social marketing approaches are consumer oriented and rely on concepts of market segmentation, market research, concept (or message) development and tailoring, communication channels, facilitation, incentives, and voluntary exchange to maximize target group response. Descriptions of key principles follow.

Consumer Orientation Social marketing programs take a consumer-driven, audience-centered approach to determining the needs, concerns, wants, and priorities that will be the focus of the health program.

Voluntary Exchange Similar to purchasing a commercial product, consumers and organizations have a certain amount of resources that they will voluntarily exchange for goods or services that they value. Applied to health, this implies that the "product" or idea being advanced must have high perceived benefit or value to the audience, so that the resources of time, effort, inconvenience, or restriction of pleasure (such as limiting favorite foods) are considered worth the benefit of adopting the new idea or behavior. Most preventive health activities are undertaken voluntarily, rather than by mandatory laws or coercive approaches, therefore this principle is important to keep in mind.

Market Segmentation Social marketing assumes that populations are heterogeneous and differ according to factors such as sociodemographic characteristics, concerns, needs, desires, lifestyles, barriers, and motivations to act. These factors can be identified and analyzed to differentiate more homogeneous subgroups (target audiences) within the population. This is called **market segmentation.** For health campaigns, certain market segments or target audiences may be especially important because they are particularly vulnerable to a health problem or have not responded to more general educational efforts. Figure 7.6 illustrates market segmentation for

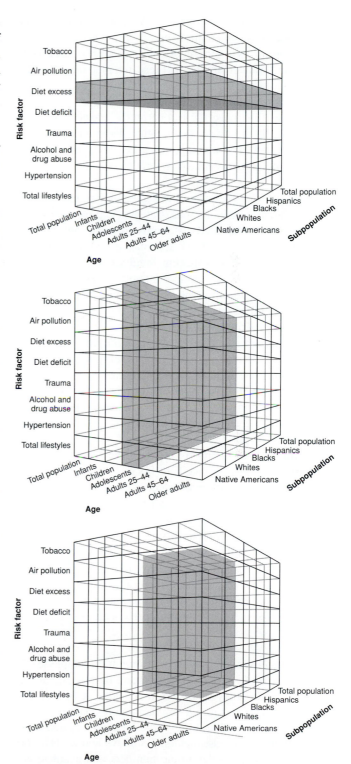

FIGURE 7.6 Market Segmentation by Health Risk Factor, Age Group, and Ethnic Group
(*Source:* From US Department of Health and Human Services, Public Health Service, Office of Disease Prevention and Health: *Integration of Risk Factor Interventions.*)

health promotional programs. Programs are designed specifically to meet the needs of the target audience based on an assessment of the audience's perceived needs and wants using market research methods of audience analysis and formative evaluation.

Message   The message is a carefully selected, concise set of words or images that capture the main idea to be disseminated. The message must be clear, memorable, and personally relevant to the target audience.

Tailoring   Based on market segmentation and formative evaluation, educational strategies and messages are developed and targeted differently for each subgroup to enhance the potential for acceptance and adoption of ideas or behaviors. Tailoring involves fitting the message to a person's or group's interests, lifestyle, behaviors, barriers, and motivators that are most likely to affect behavior change. Information that is pertinent to the needs and interests of a particular audience would be highlighted and other information might be omitted. Typically, nutrition professionals perform individual tailoring of the dietary change program in one-on-one patient counseling sessions with high-risk individuals. Social marketing uses tailoring to match information to the specific needs of the target audience.

Channels   A channel is the medium through which the message will be received. Social marketing is typically associated with mass media campaigns, which use channels such as television, radio, and print materials to reach consumers. Channels can also be places where people frequently go for work, school, recreation, or access to goods and services. Examples include worksites, schools, churches and synagogues, supermarkets, beauty salons, and social service agencies. New technology and computer-based applications offer new channels for the delivery of tailored health messages to various audiences.[38]

Market Research   Market research encompasses a wide range of methods to understand the needs, wants, motives and behavior of the target population and the preferred ways to reach them.[1] Commonly used methods are described in table 7.10. Audience analysis often uses quantitative methods, including surveys and analysis of secondary data, to determine numbers and characteristics of people who have the problem, engage in certain practices, and are aware of options. It provides information about demographics, lifestyle practices, knowledge,

attitudes, and beliefs. Quantitative data helps planners determine the scope and focus of the needed programs.

Formative evaluation is used to guide the selection and development of specific program components including the message, communication channels, materials, and strategies. Qualitative methods are used in formative evaluation to understand what the target audience is thinking, what worries them, who they listen to, the words they use when talking about the problem, and so on. Qualitative methods used in market research include ethnographic studies such as participant observation, and participatory rapid appraisal, in-depth interviews of opinion leaders and representative members of the target population, and focus groups. Focus groups are a commonly used technique for message development.[4,22,40] Chapter 17 describes this process.

Audience analysis and formative evaluation are used to plan the social marketing program. This is followed by pretesting, which is a hallmark of social marketing. Market research methods used during pretesting can include focus groups; theater testing; individual interviews; mail, phone, or intercept surveys; and readability tests. Pretesting results are used to revise and/or refine the program and prepare for expanded implementation. After the program is implemented, qualitative and quantitative methods are used to monitor the number and demographics of persons reached; their responses to the message; and its impact on their knowledge, attitudes, intent to change, and actual behavior.

Social Marketing Process   The process of social marketing involves several steps that are often repeated many times as a program is formulated, refined, implemented, and evaluated. Figure 7.7 shows the six parts of the social marketing process.[14] In the first steps, planners clarify need, differentiate potential target audiences, assess their health-related needs, develop informative and persuasive messages, select health education and promotion strategies, and determine communication channels likely to be used by and to influence the target population and its subgroups. Chapter 3 on epidemiology, chapter 13 on planning, and chapter 17 on communication provide information related to these steps. Latter steps focus on implementing and evaluating the intervention. These management topics are addressed in chapters 14 and 15. The challenge of social marketing is linking an understanding of how people make behavior choices—behavior theories and models—with program planning, implementations, and evaluation to have a positive impact on important public health problems.

TABLE 7.10

Market Research Methods Used in Audience Analysis, Formative Evaluation, and Pretesting

Quantitative methods

Surveys
  Mail
  Telephone
  In person, at home, at program
  Customer intercept
	Structured question format using forced-choice responses; attention given to contacting a representative sample of the population of interest

Analysis of secondary data	Reanalysis of existing data that was gathered for some other purpose or from a larger population (e.g., examine local trends in using census data)

Qualitative methods

Ethnographic studies Observation (participant or nonparticipant)	Spending time in the target setting and population; watching and participating in activities
Case studies	In-depth study and description of one person's, group's, or agency's characteristics and experiences related to the issue or program of interest
Review of documents and materials	Gathering and studying information that sheds light on the issue of interest, such as educational materials already developed or in use, letters, planning documents, evaluations, annual reports, newsletters, meeting minutes, and agendas
Participatory rapid appraisal	Actively involves target population in providing, gathering, and interpreting data about needs and acceptable intervention approaches; uses multiple methods over a shorter period of time than traditional ethnographic studies

In-depth interview
  Key informants
  Community leaders
  Clients
  Potential participants
  Service providers
	One-to-one interviews guided by open-ended questions (i.e., do not have categorical (yes/no) answers); exploratory interviews to find out what issues are important, what people think, in person or by phone

Focus groups	Small discussion groups of similar people, discussion led by trained moderator following a semistructured question guide

Pretesting methods

Readability tests	Use of formulas to predict the approximate educational level a person must have to understand written materials (e.g., SMOG Readability Formula[1])
Theater testing	A large group invited to a central location (school, senior citizen center), to preview and react to materials presented in a simulated situation; participants complete a questionnaire with close-ended questions; data gathered usually includes recall of key messages, reactions, and demographics
Surveys	As above
Interviews	As above
Focus groups	As above

Application

Social marketing principles have been used in a number of nutrition education programs including the 5 a Day for Better Health campaign.[24] Nutrition professionals should apply social marketing principles when developing new programs and updating existing ones. The processes of formative evaluation and feedback via pretesting and evaluation are especially valuable for designing and improving interventions. Keeping an audience-centered approach helps to assure that the program you are planning will not "miss the mark" by focusing on issues or messages that are not important to your audience. Social marketing methods are not meant to replace theories but to be used in combination with selected theories such as the ones discussed in this chapter.

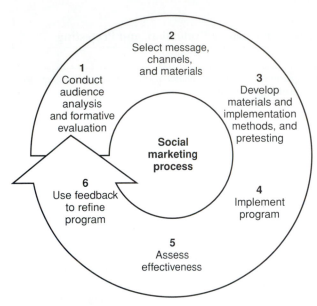

FIGURE 7.7   Social Marketing Process
(*Source:* Adapted from Glanz K, Rimer BK: Theory at a glance: a guide to health promotion practice, Washington, DC, 1995, Department of Health and Human Services, Public Health Service, and National Institutes of Health.)

EFFECTIVENESS OF BEHAVIOR CHANGE THEORY IN NUTRITION INTERVENTION

A comprehensive review of nutrition interventions conducted since 1980 found that effective programs were behaviorally focused and based in appropriate theory.[9] This was true for all audiences studied: preschool, school-aged, adult, pregnant women, older adults, and in-service providers. The special issue of the *Journal of Nutrition Education* that reports these findings is an important reference for examples of well-designed nutrition interventions. Key findings from the review have important implications for community nutrition professionals. Strategies that should be routinely applied to nutrition interventions are shown in box 7.2. Numerous other guidelines for program implementation and challenges for future nutrition program policies and research are given in the report.

Researchers and experienced practitioners agree that effective eating behavior change interventions are multifaceted and ongoing. Improving the dietary behaviors of individuals and communities is not short-term work; it progresses through stages of change. Competition for attention is a challenge. Numerous environmental forces encourage people to eat in nonhealthful ways, thus, motivators and reinforcers of healthful dietary be-

haviors need to be continually updated, re-energized, and made relevant to people's lifestyles.

IMPLICATIONS FOR COMMUNITY NUTRITION PROFESSIONALS

A central goal of nutrition intervention is to promote healthful eating behaviors in individuals, groups, and communities. Successful nutrition intervention in the community involves understanding why people behave the way they do and using this understanding to develop appropriate and effective interventions.

This chapter has presented a multilevel ecological approach for planning behavioral change programs and has demonstrated how this approach can be translated into strategies for facilitating change in eating behaviors. The ecological perspective includes several levels: intrapersonal factors, such as knowledge, beliefs, self-efficacy, and skills; interpersonal factors, including social networks and support systems of families, friends, lay advisors, and coworkers; community factors, including features of social organizations and institutions and their interrelationships.

Of the many theories for understanding behavior, several theories or models have been described that are most useful for understanding factors affecting nutritional behaviors and the processes of improving them. The models at the individual level are the health belief model, and the stages-of-change transtheoretical framework. The health belief model provides information about the factors that influence preventive health actions, including beliefs about susceptibility and severity of health conditions, the benefits of and barriers to engaging in behavior change, and the role of cues to action. The stages-of-change model has as its central premise the idea that behavior change decisions involve a series of steps and that people may be at various levels of readiness to change. The model suggests that interventions will be more effective if information and activities are tailored to the appropriate stage of change, rather than offering a "one size fits all" program for an entire group.

Social cognitive theory incorporates both individual and interpersonal concepts. SCT postulates reciprocal relationships between individuals, their environments, and behavior. It incorporates concepts of behavior modification such as goal setting, self-monitoring, and reinforcement, and emphasizes the role of self-efficacy for successfully achieving behavior change. Social support theories attempt to explain the importance of significant others and social networks in health promotion. Social

BOX 7.2

STRATEGIES FOR EFFECTIVE NUTRITION INTERVENTIONS

STRATEGIES FOR ENHANCING AWARENESS AND MOTIVATION

- Pay attention to motivators and reinforcers that have personal meaning for the particular population group.
- Build in feedback through personalized self-evaluation or self-assessment in relation to recommendations to enhanced motivation.
- Include active participation.
- Use a systematic, audience-centered planning approach such as social marketing to increase awareness of anticipated consequences of diet behaviors.
- Develop highly targeted messages focused on specific food behaviors to produce behavior change.

BEHAVIORAL CHANGE STRATEGIES

- Use the systematic behavioral change process most likely to bring about changes in behaviors. Effective strategies include the following: *for young children,* exposure to food in a positive social context, modeling by peers and adults, and appropriate use of rewards, and *for older children and adults,* self-assessment, learning behaviors for healthful eating, clarifying expectations and values, choosing among alternatives, personal goal setting, learning skills to achieve goals, monitoring progress, incentives, reinforcements, and supportive changes in the food environment.

- Tailor interpersonal counseling and education, whether individual or in small groups, to the built-in social support system because it plays an important role for all population groups.
- Use an empowerment approach to improve self-efficacy and enhanced sense of personal control.

ENVIRONMENTAL INTERVENTION STRATEGIES

- Use point-of-choice interventions in grocery stores and eating establishments to produce short-term change in purchase intentions and behavior.
- Foster changes in the food environment in schools, worksites, and communities for long-term change.
- Assure the availability and accessibility of healthful foods in restaurants and other settings to support the maintenance of change.

COMMUNITY ACTIVATION AND ORGANIZATION STRATEGIES

- Foster active participation of community leaders through community organization and empowerment to improve long-term effectiveness.
- Foster employee participation in the design and implementation of interventions to enhance success.

support includes instrumental support, informational support, emotional support, and appraisal support. Working to strengthen the supportive capacity of existing social networks, such as using a lay health advisor model, can be an effective way to promote behavior change.

Community organization and diffusion of innovations are important foundations for achieving population-wide impact. Community organization concerns ways to activate communities and foster their sense of ownership of health-enhancing efforts. Diffusion of innovations addresses ways to optimize communication and adoption of new ideas and programs in populations.

Social marketing principles can guide intervention development at each level of change. Social marketing applies marketing techniques to health and social issues and emphasizes a consumer orientation, formative evaluation, and constantly feeding back information from consumers to program developers to refine and improve programs.

Community nutrition professionals have the responsibility of designing, implementing, and evaluating nutri-

tion intervention programs that are effective. Using behavior change skills and collaborating with other professionals and community members, community nutrition professionals can help to improve health in population groups and communities. Applying behavior change theories and models to nutrition problems greatly enhances the abilities of community nutrition professionals to design effective programs and demonstrate how and why nutrition interventions can make a difference.

COMMUNITY NUTRITION PROFESSIONALS IN ACTION

- Select a current nutrition issue or recommendation. Survey class members regarding their stage of change in relation to this behavior (see for example, figure 7.4 questions measuring 5 a Day stages of change). In a class setting, break up into small groups according to stages of change for this behavior. Each group can discuss why they feel they are in that stage, what factors would cause them to progress to action or to maintain action, and what factors are keeping them from changing. Summarize results with the entire class.

- Think about your own social networks, including your family, friends, fellow students, colleagues, and the like. Whom would you identify as natural helpers in your networks? Why? How might these individuals be provided with information or skills to help those in your networks deal with a particular health issue (e.g., encouraging and helping a mother to breast-feed successfully or supporting someone's efforts to quit smoking).

- Research the diffusion of a new food product in the marketplace (e.g., frozen low-fat entrees, potato chips made with olestra). What has been the rate of diffusion and who is or is not using the product? What factors seem to be influencing diffusion?

GOING ONE STEP FURTHER

Select a nutrition problem, a target population, and a channel for intervention (e.g., schools, day-care centers, worksites, mass media). Design at least one program component aimed at the intrapersonal, interpersonal/social network, and community levels of change. Base each of your program components on appropriate theories and models from the chapter. Think about how principles of social marketing could be used in the design and dissemination of your program.

REFERENCES

1. Andreasen AR: *Marketing social change,* Jossey-Bass. 1995, San Francisco.
2. Bandura A: Human agency in social cognitive theory, *Am Psychol* 44(9):1175–1184, 1989.
3. Bandura A: *Social foundations of thought and action: a social cognitive theory,* Englewood Cliffs, NJ, 1986, Prentice-Hall.
4. Basch C: Focus group interviews: an underutilized technique for improving theory and practice in health education, *Health Educ Q* 14:411–448, 1987.
5. Campbell M, DeVillis B, Strecher V, Ammerman A, DeVellis R, Sandler R: Improving dietary behavior: the effectiveness of tailored messages in primary care settings, *Am J Public Health* 84:783–787, 1994.
6. Campbell MK, Farrell D, Honess-Morreale L, Gosnell L, Carbone E: Improving dietary behavior among families receiving food stamps: development and evaluation of the StampSmart Program, Paper presented at the annual meeting of the American Public Health Association, San Diego, CA, 1995.
7. Campbell MK, Symons M, Polhamus B, Demark-Wahnefried W, Bernhardt J, McClelland JW, Washington C: Stages of change and psychosocial correlates of fruit and vegetable consumption among rural African American church members, *American Journal of Health Promotion* 12(3):185–191, 1998.
8. Cohen S, Syme L: *Social support and health,* Orlando, FL, 1985, Academic Press.
9. Contendo I: The effectiveness of nutrition education and implementation for nutrition education policy, programs, and research: a review of research, *Journal of Nutrition Education* 27(6):277–418, 1995.
10. Curry S, Kristal A, Bowen D: An application of the stage model of behavior change to dietary fat reduction, *Health Education Research* 7(1):97–105, 1992.
11. Earp J, Ennett S: Conceptual models for health education research and practice, *Health Education Research* 6(2):163–171, 1991.
12. Eng G, Young Y: Lay health advisors as community change agents, *Family and Community Health* 15(1):24–40, 1992.
13. Glanz K, Patterson R, Kristal A: Stages of change in adopting healthy diets: fat, fiber, and correlates of nutrient intake, *Health Educ Q* 21:499–519, 1994.
14. Glanz K, Rimer B: *Theory at a glance: a guide for health promotion practice,* Washington, D.C., 1995. U.S. Department of Health and Human Services, Public Health Service, and National Institutes of Health.
15. Greene G, Rossi S, Reed G, Willey C, Prochaska J: Stages of change for reducing dietary fat to 30% of energy or less, *J Am Diet Assoc* 94(10):1105–1110, 1994.
16. Green, LW, Kreuter MW: *Health promotion planning: an educational and environmental approach,* ed 2, Mountain View, CA, 1991, Mayfield.
17. Horn D: "A model for the study of personal choice health behavior," *International Journal of Health Education* 19:89–98, 1976.
18. Israel B: Social networks and social support: implications for natural helper and community level interventions, *Health Educ Q* 12(1):65–80, 1995.
19. Israel BA, Checkoway G, Schulz A, Zimmerman M: Health education and community empowerment: conceptualizing and measuring perceptions of individual, organizational, and community control, *Health Educ Q* 21(2):148–170, 1994.
20. Kark J, Shemi Y, Friedlander O, Martin O, Manor O, Blondheim S: Does religious observation promote health? Mortality in secular versus religious kibbutzim in Israel, *Am J Public Health* 86(3):341–347, 1996.
21. Kotler P, Andreasen AR: *Strategic marketing for nonprofit organizations,* ed 5, Englewood Cliffs, NJ, 1995, Prentice-Hall.
22. Kruger R: *Focus groups: a practical guide for applied research,* Newbury Park, CA, 1994, Sage.

23. Lefebvre RC, Lurie D, Goodman LS, Weinberg L, Loughrey K: Social marketing and nutrition education: inappropriate or misunderstood, *J Nutr Educ* 27(3):146–150, 1995.

24. Lefebvre RC, Doner L, Johnston C, Loughrey K, Balch GI, Sutton SM:*Use of database marketing and consumer-based health communication in a message design: an example from the Office of Cancer Communication's 5 a Day for Better Health Program.* In Maibach E, Parrott RL, editors: *Designing health messages: approaches from communication theory and public health practice,* Thousand Oaks, CA, 1995, Sage, pp. 217–246.

25. Maibach E, Murphy D: Self-efficacy in health promotion research and practice: conceptualization and measurement, *Health Education Research* 10:37–50, 1995.

26. McLeroy KR, Bibeau D, Steckler A, Glanz K: An ecological perspective on health promotion programs, *Health Educ Q* 15:351, 1988.

27. Minkler M, Wallerstein N: *Improving health through community organization and community building.* In Glanz K, Lewis FM, Rimer BK, editors: *Health behavior and health education,* ed 2, San Francisco, 1997, Jossey-Bass.

28. Novelli W: *Applying social marketing to health promotion programs.* In Glanz K, Lewis F, Rimer B, editors: *Health behavior and health education,* San Francisco, 1990, Jossey-Bass, pp. 342–370.

29. Perry CL, Luepker RV, Murray DM, Kurth C, Mullis R, Crockett S, Jacobs DR Jr: Parent involvement with children's health promotion: the Minnesota Home Team, *Am J Public Health* 78:1156–1160, 1988.

30. Perry CL, Williams CL: Project Northland: outcomes of a communitywide alcohol use prevention program during early adolescence, *Am J Public Health* 86(7):956–965, 1996.

31. Prochaska J, DiClemente C, Norcross J: In search of how people change: applications to addictive behaviors, *Am Psychol* 47(9):1102–1114, 1992.

32. Rogers EM: *Diffusion of innovations,* ed 3, New York, 1983, The Free Press.

33. Rosenstock I, Strecher V, Becker M: Social learning theory and the health belief model, *Health Educ Q* 15(2):175–183, 1988.

34. Rothman J: *Three models of community organization practice, their mixing and phasing.* In Rothman J, Erlich JL, Tropman JE, Cox FM, editors: *Strategies of community intervention: macro practice,* ed 5, San Francisco, 1997, Jossey-Bass.

35. Scott J: Trend report: social network analysis, *Sociology* 22:109–127, 1988.

36. Service C, Salber E, editors: *Community health education: the lay health advisor approach,* Durham, NC, 1979, Health Care Systems.

37. Simons-Morton BG, Parcel GS, Baranowski T, Forthofer R, O'Hara NM: Promoting physical activity and a healthful diet among children: results of a school-based intervention study, *Am J Public Health* 81:986–991, 1991.

38. Skinner C, Strecher V, Hospers H: Physicians' recommendations for mammography: do tailored messages make a difference? *Am J Public Health* 84:43–49, 1994.

39. Sporny LA, Contento IR: Stages of change in dietary fat reduction: social psychological correlates, *Journal of Nutrition Education* 27:191–199, 1995.

40. Strauss A, Corbin J. *Basics of qualitative research,* Newbury Park, CA, 1990, Sage Publications.

DESIGNING AND IMPLEMENTING A BEHAVIOR CHANGE INTERVENTION FOR THE WORKSITE

DESCRIPTION

This case study describes a multilevel dietary intervention program that was designed using behavior change theories. It is hypothetical but is based on several real projects being conducted in North Carolina communities. The case illustrates the use of theories at the intrapersonal, interpersonal, and community levels of change. The project sites are in six rural counties with at least 30 percent minority population, primarily African-Americans. The project focuses on implementing a dietary intervention to increase fruits and vegetables and decrease fat intake to reduce morbidity and mortality from cancer and chronic diseases. The case illustrates some of the challenges of planning, implementing, and evaluating a large-scale eating behavior program in community settings.

METHODOLOGY/TEACHING OBJECTIVES

One major concept illustrated in the case study is how elements of several theories can be combined in a single project to address the various levels of change that impact eating behavior. A second major concept is the importance of formative evaluation to determine how to focus the interventions. Sometimes, the formative evaluation findings are unexpected or even contradictory to what nutrition professionals have planned to provide in a program. Listening and responding to this information can lead to more innovative and effective approaches. Failure to consider the formative evaluation may lead to an ineffective program.

This material will best be used in the order it is presented, so that the case unfolds as students read each paragraph, answer the questions, and then think about what the next step will be. Small group class discussions would be an alternative method of using this material. By breaking the class up into several groups, each group could be assigned one part of the case study to discuss, and then the groups could present their decisions to the whole class.

THE CASE

Part 1

"Health for Life" is a three-year federally funded community-based intervention study that aims to improve health and prevent disease among blue-collar workers in manufacturing industries in rural North Carolina. The project focuses on dietary behaviors that relate to preventable causes of morbidity and mortality, specifically high-fat and low fruit and vegetable intake. The project team, from the University and local health departments, chose to use worksites as a channel for health promotion because most adults are employed either full or part time and therefore the worksite is a place where people spend much of their day. In addition, the team believes that the worksite might be a good place to implement interventions that build on social support. Coworkers may be friends or they may form natural work teams that constitute small social networks. Worksites also form an environment for health behavior change to be facilitated. For example, some have vending machines or cafeterias and some have exercise facilities. There are twelve eligible worksites, employing a total of 2,000 workers, in the study. Sites were randomly assigned to either receive the intervention or be a control site for the duration of the study.

In year 1 of the program, focus groups were conducted at all six of the intervention worksites. Separate focus groups were held for men and women. The focus groups were held during work time at 3 to 5 P.M. and interested workers were asked to sign up to attend. A $15 incentive was offered for participation, to compensate workers for their input. Questions were asked about health and nutrition concerns, health beliefs, interest in participating in a nutrition intervention program, and other related issues. The project team hoped to get good representation from all major job categories and shifts in the worksite. The time of 3 P.M. was chosen because the first shift ended at 4 P.M. and the second shift started then; management had said that workers could use work time to attend the focus group at either the beginning or end of their shift.

Unfortunately, the only people who attended the first round of focus groups were managers and supervisors. Among the men, fitness was the biggest health promotion issue of concern. They did not do much food preparation and were not interested in attending cooking classes but were interested in taste tests and tips on eating out. They mentioned exercise as a health promotion need. Among the women, there was interest in controlling weight as a reason for wanting to improve dietary habits. Cooking classes and taste tests were a popular idea. They were concerned about their children's nutrition also. Barriers focused on lack of availability of healthy foods at the worksite and not having enough time or will power to cook healthy foods. Women also thought exercise should be part of a health program. Both men and women liked the idea of getting printed health information. They cited newspapers, magazines, and their doctors as sources of health information.

Questions

1. Why do you think the focus groups attracted only the managers and supervisors?
2. What could you do to gain participation of other workers in the focus groups?
3. Based on the information gained so far, how would you proceed with program planning?

Part 2

The project team was concerned about the lack of representation in the focus groups from workers on the line. They received permission to conduct a second round of focus groups. Before they proceeded, the planners asked a few workers about why they had not attended the groups the first time. The workers said that they did not think they were allowed to miss an hour of work, and that they did not feel comfortable talking in focus groups where managers were present. Based on this input, the focus groups were offered again with time off work formally approved by management, and workers were assured that no managers would be present in the groups. This time attendance was much better. Similar motivations for behavior change were expressed by men and women, however, some of the barriers were different. In these groups, cost emerged as a major barrier to eating healthy foods, as well as lack of access to supermarkets that carry low-fat products

and good fresh produce. Workers were concerned that the vending machines at the worksites offered only "junk food" choices such as sodas and chips. Time was a consistent barrier in all groups. Several health issues emerged from the focus groups with workers alone, including stress, back pain related to standing for long periods on the job, and chronic diseases such as diabetes. Again, exercise was mentioned as a behavior people wanted to improve. Some of the workers were interested in receiving printed materials but most cited television as their major source of health information. They generally did not go to doctors for preventive health information, only for acute and chronic illness.

Questions

1. How does the new information from the second round of focus groups compare to the earlier information?
2. What conclusions would you draw regarding the different sources of health information cited in the focus groups?
3. The line workers mentioned health concerns the team had not planned to address in the program. Would you respond to any or all of these concerns?
4. What mistakes might have been made in program planning if only the first round of focus groups had been held?
5. Based on the information gained so far, how would you proceed with program planning now? What behavior change theories would you use as you plan?

Part 3

The project team selected several theories to guide the program. At the *intrapersonal* level, *social cognitive theory* and *stages of change* were chosen. Program materials were developed based on these theories. A baseline survey was developed that assessed stage-of-change for improving eating habits. The survey also assessed current dietary behavior using a food frequency questionnaire. Self-efficacy, outcome expectations, and social support were also measured. Following completion of the surveys, individual workers received a personal dietary profile and a nutrition intervention manual tailored to their stage of change. The manual for people at the precontemplation stage included information about the link between diet and disease, and the benefits of changing to healthier eating habits. The manual for people thinking about or planning to change (contemplation) included information such as suggestions for low-cost healthy foods, quick recipes, and tips for healthy choices when eating out. People already in the action and maintenance stages received information designed to help maintain behavior change, such as recipes, grocery lists, and education about label reading. A videotape was also provided to each worker that focused on skill building and setting attainable goals to increase self-efficacy for healthy eating.

At the *interpersonal* level, a *lay health advisor* intervention was planned to train several workers at each site as peer helpers. Three lay health advisor training sessions were conducted at each worksite, focused on giving the LHAs nutrition information and skills to provide social support for healthier eating among the workers.

At the *community* level of change, the group chose to follow a *social planning* approach, providing technical assistance to worksites in collaboration with nutritionists and health educators from county health departments. The objective was to promote linkages between the worksites and local health agencies to create more local control of the program and therefore help sustain it after the funding ended. During the second and third years of the project, worksites were encouraged to work with local health department staff to continue promoting "Health for Life." The team of trained LHAs were designated as contacts.

Questions

1. What rationale do you think the project team had for its choice of behavior change theories?
2. What are the strengths and limitations of each of the interventions that were chosen by the project team?
3. What other intervention strategies might have worked better? Why?
4. In what ways did the project team use the focus group's information effectively? What information did they ignore? What impact did you think these decisions would have on program effectiveness?

Part 4

So, what happened? About 70 percent of employees completed the baseline surveys and received the dietary profiles, manuals, and videos. At five of the six worksites, the people who attended the lay health advisor training were mostly female supervisors or "pink-collar" (secretarial/administrative) workers. The project did not succeed in attracting line workers to the LHA trainings. In most cases, the health department personnel did not participate in the technical assistance part of the project due to factors such as lack of time and not having enough personnel to take on additional program functions. Technical assistance ended up being provided by the project staff and focused on improving vending machine choices at the worksites and advertising a list of community resources for healthy eating classes.

After twelve months of program implementation, a follow-up survey was conducted in all worksites. Evaluation data at the end of the project comparing intervention and control worksites showed modest improvements in behavior. Significant changes in snack food consumption were reported at worksites where the vending machine choices had been improved. Workers reported liking the program and said that it was helpful. Over 80 percent reported reading the nutrition manual when they received it; however, a majority said they did not currently know where their manual or video was located. A large percentage of workers were not aware that there had been a lay health advisor program.

Questions

1. What program elements appear to have succeeded? What parts did not seem to have worked?
2. What errors in program implementation may have led to limited program success?
3. Do you think that this program will be continued in the worksites? Why or why not?

PART TWO

FACING THE CHALLENGE
COMMUNITY NUTRITION ACROSS
THE LIFE CYCLE

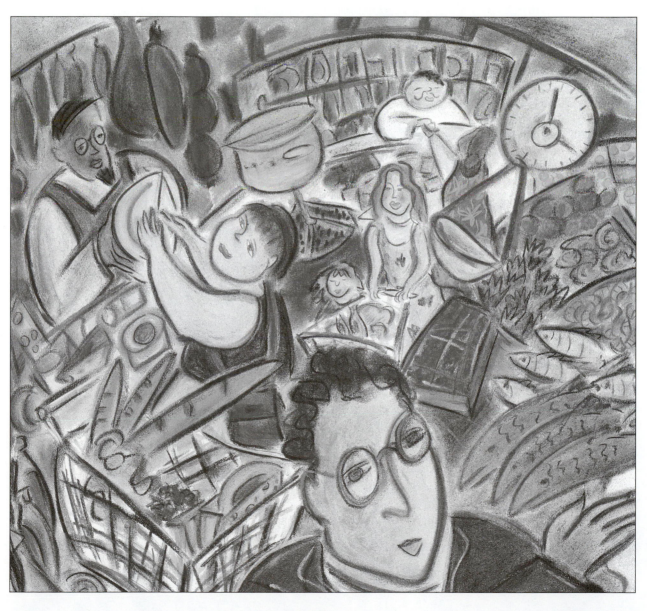

CHAPTER EIGHT

MATERNAL NUTRITION

*Nutrition is probably the single biggest factor in the health and
well-being of a woman at any stage of her life.*
—BERNADINE HEALY, MD

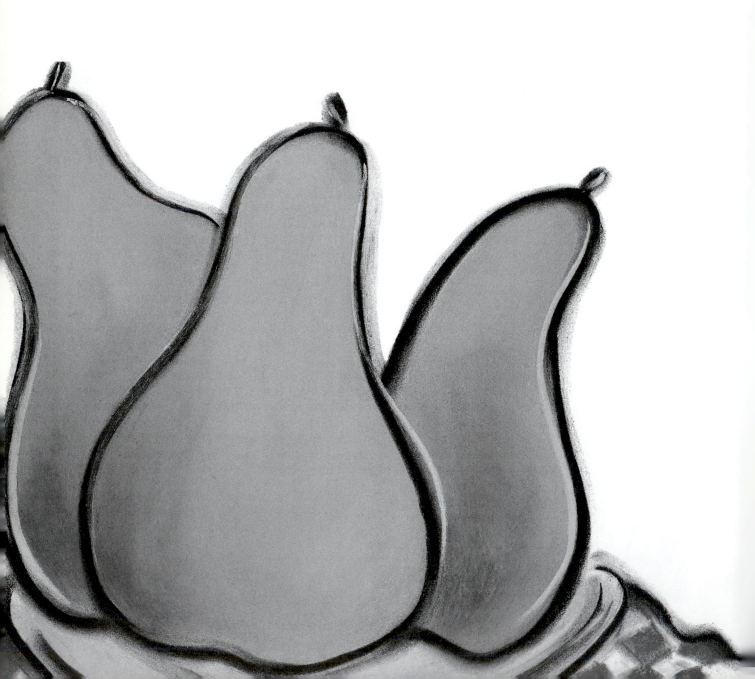

Core Concepts

Adequate nutrition is necessary to support the health and well-being that enables women of all ages to enjoy life and carry out important roles in the family, work, and the community. A special time is reproductive years (fifteen to forty-five) when women conceive, carry an infant, deliver, and care for the infant and family. Maternal nutrition is widely appreciated as a significant factor in a healthy pregnancy and during lactation. The first part of the chapter presents an overview of the status of outcomes of pregnancy in the United States. Relationships between maternal nutritional status, the course and outcome of pregnancy, and nutrition and lactation are then summarized. Nutritional needs of women during and after pregnancy are highlighted. Risk factors for reproductive problems and specific recommendations for patient management are included in this chapter. Health policies and guidelines related to maternal nutrition are summarized, and model programs for service delivery are described.

Objectives

When you finish chapter eight, you should be able to:

~ Cite examples of Healthy People 2000 objectives as they relate to maternal health.

~ Identify the key nutritional factors that influence pregnancy outcome and lactation.

~ Outline nutritional guidelines and recommendations for women during pregnancy and lactation.

~ Identify public policy goals and guidelines that bear directly on the development and delivery of maternal nutrition services.

~ Discuss existing maternal nutrition programs and services and outline ways to improve the effectiveness of nutrition services to pregnant/lactating women in the future.

Key Words

Word	Page Mentioned
Pregnancy outcomes	202
Infant mortality rate	202
Fetal growth retardation	202
Prematurity	202
Low birthweight	202
Prepregnancy weight	202
Prenatal weight gain	202
Body mass index	202
Neural tube defects	202
Folate	202
Anemia	206
Fetal alcohol syndrome	207
Pica	207
Supplements	210
Nutritional risk	211
Lactation	214
Letdown reflex	214
Rooting reflex	214
Nonnutritive substances	216

PREGNANCY OUTCOMES
IN THE UNITED STATES

Improving the nutritional health of women before and during pregnancy is important not only because it has implications for women's health in later years but also because of the link between maternal nutrition and infant health and hence **pregnancy outcomes** (figure 8.1).

The Status of Infant Health in the United States

Infant mortality rates (the number of liveborn infants who die within the first year of life per 1,000 births) are used as an indicator to rank the health status and quality of health care and social systems in countries (table 8.1). Between 1900 and 1950, infant mortality rates in the United States and other industrialized countries dropped substantially, primarily because of improvements in the quality of life—reflected in standards of housing and health care, sanitation, nutritional health, income, and education. Around 1970, declines achieved in the rate of infant mortality in the United States began to reflect advances in neonatal intensive care and the saving of infants who would have had little chance for survival in previous years. The rate of decline in infant mortality in the United States began to slow in 1981.

Birthweight and Health

Birthweight is by far the strongest predictor of infant well-being and is related to death and illness through the early childhood years. The average birthweight of full-term Black infants is 240 g less than that of White infants. Infants born small are at far greater risk of death and disorders than are normal-sized infants. Their smallness is mainly due either to **fetal growth retardation** or to **prematurity** (delivery before 37 weeks of gestation), or a combination of both. In 1995, 7.3 percent of all U.S. infants born had **low birthweight** (LBW) (< 2,500 g or < 5.5 lb) (figure 8.2). The LBW rate among Blacks (13.0 percent) is double that in Whites (6.2 percent), although the rate of LBW among Black infants is decreasing.[5] Some 13 percent of 1994 births in the United States were to mothers less than twenty years of age.[32] One reason for the relatively poor infant mortality rate in the United States is the excess proportion of infants with LBW.

Healthy People 2000 Objectives Related to Maternal Health

Table 8.2 summarizes the Healthy People 2000 objectives as they relate to pregnant and lactating women. These objectives are used by many state and local health departments in developing and refining maternal nutrition programs and services.

NUTRITION-RELATED HEALTH PROBLEMS
OF PREGNANT WOMEN

The nutritional status of women before and during pregnancy exerts important influences on maternal health and fetal growth and development. Of the potential relationships among measures of nutritional status and fetal growth and development, the effects of **prepregnancy weight; prenatal weight gain;** and levels of intake of calories, protein, zinc, iron, and folacin have received the most attention.

Prepregnancy Weight Status and Prenatal Weight Gain

Body weight-for-height or **body mass index** (BMI) prior to pregnancy and rates of weight gain in the second and third trimesters of pregnancy are factors strongly associated with infant birthweight. The best pregnancy outcomes are achieved by women who begin pregnancy at normal weight (BMI between 20 and 25 kg/m^2) and who gain some 14 to 16 kg (30 to 35 lb) during pregnancy. Entering pregnancy underweight (BMI < 19.8 kg/m^2) clearly increases the risk that infants will be born small. Overall, women with low gestational weight gain and low prepregnancy BMI are at highest risk for delivering a LBW infant.[30] Approximately one half of infants born to low-income, underweight women who gain less than 9 kg during pregnancy are at risk of being born with low birthweight.[10]

Women who are obese (BMI > 29 kg/m^2) at the beginning of pregnancy are more likely to have infants with **neural tube defects** (NTD) and this association is independent of **folate** intake.[28,33] Maternal obesity has been shown to be a risk factor for diabetes mellitus, hypertension as well as for urinary tract infection, preeclampsia, and cesarean delivery.[17] Obesity is more prevalent among women of low socioeconomic status, itself a risk factor for less favorable pregnancy outcome. Further risk for high birthweight (> 4,500 g) increases

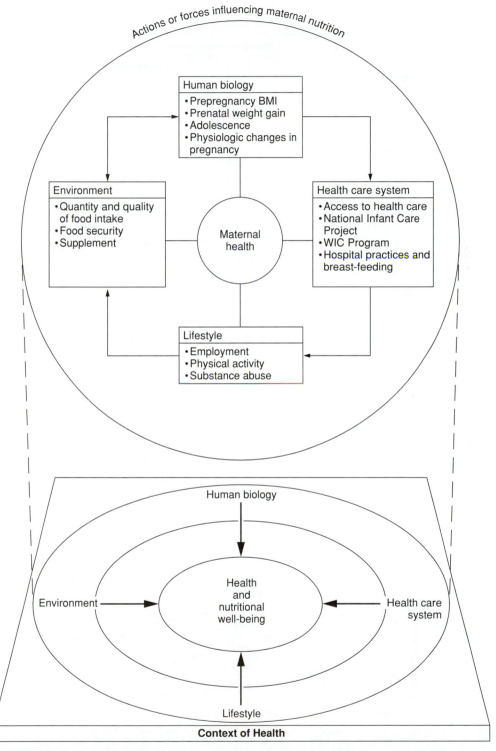

FIGURE 8.1   Context of Health
Influences on maternal nutrition.

TABLE 8.1
Infant Mortality Rates

| Country | Births | Infant mortality rates | | | Percentage of 1994 births to mothers under twenty |
		1930	1994	Percentage decrease	
Japan	1,258,237	124	4.2	96.6	3
Singapore	49,602	—	4.3	—	2
Sweden	112,257	58.5	4.4	92.4	3
Hong Kong	71,646	—	4.5	—	2
Finland	65,922	97.6	4.7	95.2	2
Norway	59,200	54.6	5.0	90.8	4
Switzerland	82,900	54.0	5.1	90.5	2
Netherlands	185,600	50.9	5.6	89.0	3
Germany	765,852	96.4	5.6	94.2	3
Denmark	69,684	82.9	5.7	93.1	2
Australia	258,247	47.2	5.9	87.6	5
Ireland	47,928	67.9	5.9	91.3	6
United Kingdom	750,671	60.0	6.2	89.7	6
Canada	386,350	89.3	6.2	93.0	8
Austria	91,588	117.0	6.3	94.6	6
France	57,747	96.0	6.5	93.3	2
Italy	57,193	124.8	6.6	94.7	4
Spain	39,193	123.0	6.7	94.5	8
New Zealand	3,493	34.5	7.2	79.1	3
Belgium	10,080	92.8	7.6	91.8	6
Israel	5,383	—	7.8	—	4
United States	3,952,767	64.6	8.0	87.6	13

Source: From Wegman ME: Infant mortality: some international comparison, *Pediatrics;* 98:1020–7, 1996.

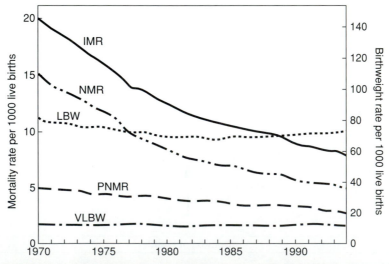

FIGURE 8.2   Infant (IMR), Neonatal (NMR), Postneonatal (PNMR) Mortality and Low (LBW) and Very Low (VLBW) birthweight, United States, 1970–1994
(*Source:* From Guyer B, Strobino DM, Ventura SJ, et al: Annual summary of vital statistics—1995, *Pediatrics;* 98:1007–19, 1996. Reprinted by permission of *Pediatrics.*)

TABLE 8.2
Healthy People 2000 Objectives Related to Maternal Health

Objectives	Base prevalence (year)	Current prevalence (year)
Health status objectives		
Reduce infant mortality rate to no more than 7 per 1,000 live births	10.1 (1987)	8.0 (1994)
Special population targets		
Blacks	18.8 (1987)	11.0 (2000)
Native Americans	13.4 (1984)	8.5 (2000)
Puerto Ricans	12.9 (1984)	8.0 (2000)
Reduce the incidence of fetal alcohol syndrome to no more than 0.12 per 1,000 live births	0.2 (1987)	
Special population targets		
Native Americans	4.0 (1987)	2.0 (2000)
Blacks	0.8 (1987)	0.4 (2000)
Reduce incidence of spina bifida and other neural tube defects to 3 per 10,000 live births	6 (1990)	
Risk reduction objectives		
Reduce LBW to an incidence of no more than 5 percent of live births	6.9 (1987)	
Special population targets		
Black	13.0 (1987)	9.0 (2000)
Puerto Ricans	9.0 (1990)	6.0 (2000)
Increase to at least 75% the proportion of mothers who breast-feed their babies in the neonatal period	54 (1988)	56 (1993)
Special population targets		
Low-income mothers	32 (1988)	
Black mothers	25 (1988)	
Hispanic mothers	51 (1988)	
Native-American mothers	47 (1988)	
Increase to at least 50% the proportion of mothers who continue breast-feeding until their babies are five to six months old	21 (1988)	21 (1993)
Special population targets		
Low-income mothers	9 (1988)	
Black mothers	8 (1988)	
Hispanic mothers	16 (1988)	
Native-American mothers	28 (1988)	
Reduce iron deficiency to less than 3 percent among women of child-bearing age	5 (1980)	
Reduce anemia to 20% among low-income Black women (third trimester of pregnancy)	41 (1988)	
Increase calcium intake so at least 50% of pregnant and lactating women consume three or more servings daily of foods rich in calcium	22 (1986)	
Increase to at least 85% the proportion of mothers who achieve the minimum recommended weight gain during pregnancy	67 (1980)	
Services and protection objectives		
Increase to at least 90% the proportion of all pregnant women who receive prenatal care in the first trimester	76 (1987)	
Special population targets		
Black women	61 (1987)	
Native-American	58 (1987)	
Hispanic Women	61 (1987)	

with increasing weight gain, particularly weight gains of more than 17 kg (~ 37 lb), as shown in figure 8.3.

Nutrient Needs During Pregnancy

The growth and development of the fetus depend largely on the quality and quantity of food consumed by women throughout pregnancy. If a woman fails to consume sufficient calories, protein, vitamins, and minerals to maintain her own health and nutrient stores, the fetus cannot receive adequate amounts of nutrients needed for optimal growth and development. This biological fact stands in contrast to the misperception that the fetus is a parasite that obtains needed nutrients regardless of what the mother consumes in her diet.

Calories   Diets that provide fewer than about 1,800 calories per day are considered "low calorie" during pregnancy. Without enough calories to meet a pregnant woman's need for energy, dietary protein is diverted from use in synthesis of new tissue to meet energy needs. The requirement for energy is the body's first priority; only when the mother's energy needs are met can dietary protein be used for the mother's and the baby's tissue growth and maintenance needs. Low-calorie diets do not supply enough energy to meet the needs for normal fetal growth and lead to fetal growth retardation. Diets that fail to supply enough calories may also provide inadequate amounts of essential micronutrients, further compromising fetal growth and development.

Protein   Most women in the United States consume between 70 and 90 g of protein per day during pregnancy, levels that exceed the 1989 recommended dietary allowance (RDA) and appear to be adequate to meet needs.[23,30]

Folacin   Deficiencies of folacin around the time of conception have been associated with neural tube defects such as spina bifida. Folacin deficiency during pregnancy causes megaloblastic **anemia** in women and reduces fetal growth. As many as 15 percent of low-income women in the United States develop a deficiency of folacin during pregnancy.

Iron   Iron deficiency is the most common nutrient deficiency in pregnant women in the United States. Iron deficiency anemia during pregnancy is defined as a hemoglobin level of less than 110 g/L in the first trimester, less than 105 g/L in the second trimester (reflecting in part

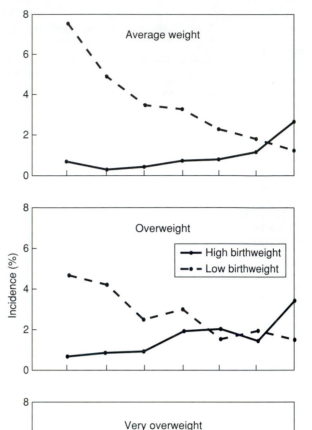

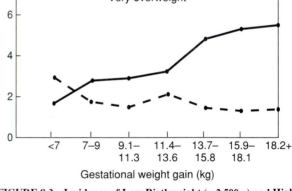

FIGURE 8.3   Incidence of Low Birthweight (< 2,500 g) and High Birthweight (> 4,500 g) by Prepregnancy BMI and Gestational Weight Gain (*Source:* From Cogswell ME, Serdula MK, Hangerford DW, Yip R. Gestational weight gain among average weight and overweight women—what is excessive? *Am J Gynecol;* 172:705–12, 1995. Used with permission.)

the expansion of plasma volume), and less than 110 g/L in the third trimester of pregnancy.[30] In 1990, prevalences of iron deficiency anemia of 10, 14, and 33 percent in the first, second, and third trimesters of pregnancy, respectively, were found for low-income women.[13]

Women who develop iron deficiency anemia in the first trimester are more likely to manifest low gestational weight gain and to deliver infants who are small.[25,30] Infants who are small at birth (premature or LBW) are at greater risk of becoming iron deficient during the first year of life than are full-term infants. This is true whether or not the infant's mother was iron deficient during pregnancy.

Zinc   High-dose iron supplementation (> 100 mg/day) may contribute to the development of zinc deficiency.[30] Zinc deficiency during pregnancy has been associated with abnormally long labor and with the delivery of small infants.

Alcohol and Pregnancy

The detrimental effects of alcohol on babies were not fully acknowledged until the 1970s, when several research reports described a condition called **fetal alcohol syndrome.**[11] Drinking in the first half of pregnancy is closely associated with the birth of malformed, small, mentally impaired infants. When excessive drinking occurs only in the second half of pregnancy, infants are still likely to be small and to manifest abnormal mental development. These conditions are lasting; they cannot be fully corrected with special treatment, and the child does not outgrow them. No amount of alcohol has been found to be absolutely safe during pregnancy.[6,15]

Reactions to Excessive Vitamin and Mineral Intakes

A fetus is generally much more susceptible to the ill effects of vitamin and mineral overdoses than is a pregnant woman, primarily because of the small size and rapid growth and development of the fetus. Overdoses of vitamin and mineral supplements produce the most serious threats to infant health when they occur early in pregnancy, when the fetus's organs are developing.

Vitamins   A deficiency of vitamin C has been observed in infants whose mothers have taken excessive amounts of vitamin C during pregnancy. The excretion mechanisms that rid the fetus of the high levels of vitamin C appear to continue after birth, even though large amounts of vitamin C are no longer being received. Consequently, the newborns excrete too much of the vitamin and develop signs of scurvy within a few weeks

after birth. Such infants can be protected from the effects of vitamin C deficiency if they are supplemented with vitamin C and then gradually weaned from it. As little as 25,000 IU of vitamin A taken daily in the early months of pregnancy has been associated with central nervous system and bone abnormalities in newborns.[4] The increasingly popular use of vitamin A–like (e.g., retinoic acid) compounds for the treatment of acne, wrinkles, and other skin conditions has lead to new warnings about their use by women who are or may become pregnant.[14]

Daily doses of supplemental vitamin D at levels five times the RDA (2,000 IU) have been associated with the birth of infants who are mentally retarded and have heart abnormalities. There is also evidence to indicate that megadoses of vitamin E may result in spontaneous abortion.

Minerals   Intake of zinc in supplements exceeding the RDA for several months may lead to copper deficiency and impairment of some immune responses.[23] The consequences of iodine overdose in pregnancy include development of goiter and mental retardation in infants.

Fiber

Constipation is a problem for many women during pregnancy. It can be alleviated to some extent by increasing intake of whole grains, fruits, and vegetables to increase intake of dietary fiber in the diet, for a total of about 20 to 30 g. Fluid intake should increase along with the increased dietary fiber.

Pica

Pica is defined as the regular consumption of nonfood substances. Women at high risk for pica are more likely to be Black, to live in rural areas, and to have a history of childhood pica or a family history of pica. About 20 percent of high-risk women have pica.[8]

The regular ingestion of clay or laundry starch can cause problems. Clay may contain bacteria and other harmful substances, and it may reduce the amount of minerals absorbed from foods. Also, it may cause intestinal obstruction. Laundry starch may contain contaminants because it is not manufactured for consumption as a food. The body ingests and absorbs laundry starch just as it does food starch, hence, laundry starch can become a significant source of empty calories.

Shifts in Food Preferences

An interesting and common effect of pregnancy is changing food preferences. Food preferences have been noted to change in about three fourths of pregnant women. Foods such as fish, beef, fried foods, alcoholic beverages, diet soft drinks, and coffee are often reported to taste or smell unpleasant during pregnancy, whereas ice cream, chocolate, salty snacks, milk, and fruit are reported to taste better. Pregnant women are less sensitive to the taste of salt; they prefer stronger salt solutions than they do after pregnancy.[1]

Results of Dietary Intake Studies in the United States

Results of a number of studies that estimated caloric level and intakes of up to sixteen nutrients of U.S. women during pregnancy were summarized in 1990 by the Institute of Medicine (IOM).[30] Mean caloric levels and mean intakes of vitamins D, E, and B_6 and folacin, iron, zinc, calcium, and magnesium were less than the 1989 RDAs for pregnant women in nearly all studies. Mean intakes of protein; vitamins A, B_{12}, and C; and thiamin, riboflavin, and niacin tended to exceed the RDAs in these studies.

PHYSIOLOGICAL CHANGES IN PREGNANCY

Several physiological changes occur during the course of pregnancy (see box 8.1).

Increase in Blood Volume

Blood volume increases by almost 50 percent so that enough oxygen can be available to support growing maternal and fetal tissues. Thus, there is an increased need for those nutrients most important for generating blood: protein, iron (hemoglobin is an iron-containing protein), folic acid, and vitamin B_6. If a woman has a normal BMI, is not iron deficient at the time of conception, and has sufficient dietary intake of these nutrients during pregnancy, she will make this adjustment with little problem; otherwise, anemia may result.

Changes in the Gastrointestinal Tract

Increased progesterone production leads to decreased tone and motility of the smooth muscle of the gastrointestinal tract. Hence, food moves through the gastrointestinal tract more slowly. This may be associated with

---

BOX 8.1

PHYSIOLOGIC CHANGES DURING PREGNANCY

Increase in blood volume
Increase in cardiac output
Increase in body water
Increase in glomerular filtration rate
Increase in respiratory tidal volume
Decrease in gastrointestinal motility

---

constipation. In early pregnancy, women also experience nausea and vomiting. Excessive vomiting (hyperemesis gravidarum) sometimes occurs during pregnancy. It can become a serious problem because of electrolyte imbalance and dehydration.

Changes in Renal Function

Blood flow through the kidneys and the glomerular filtration rate are increased to facilitate clearance of urea and other waste products from the mother and the fetus. Normally, most of the glucose, amino acids, and water-soluble vitamins that are present in the glomerular filtrate are reabsorbed in the tubules. However, during pregnancy, substantial quantities of these nutrients are excreted in the urine suggesting that the increased glomerular filtration rate is not compensated for by a comparable increase in tubular reabsorption. Hence, the need to ensure adequate intakes of calories, protein, and water-soluble vitamins.

Increase in Breast Tissue and Fat Stores

The mammary glands in the breast begin to enlarge during pregnancy to allow the milk ducts to prepare for lactation. Fat stores increase in preparation for breast-feeding.

Changes in Weight

The woman gains weight as both her tissues and the tissues of the fetus increase and develop. Additional nutrients are required to build this new tissue and to maintain them. Some of the more striking increases in nutrient needs are those for protein, folate, vitamins C and B_6, and iron. Satisfactory progress with regard to weight gain is essential to the well-being of the developing fetus. It also serves as a major indicator to the health care provider that the pregnancy is proceeding normally.

NUTRITIONAL NEEDS OF PREGNANT WOMEN

Pregnancy represents a period of high nutrient needs. With careful choices, a pregnant woman can meet her nutrient needs with common foods. Regardless of the pregnant woman's age and whether or not she is a vegetarian, her diet should contain:

- Sufficient calories for adequate weight gain
- A variety of foods from each food group
- Regular meals and snacks
- Sufficient dietary fiber (20 to 30 g/day)
- Eight or more cups of fluid each day
- Salt to taste
- No alcoholic beverages

Planning the diet around the basic food groups is the most straightforward approach to meeting nutrient needs for pregnancy (table 8.3). Compared to nonpregnant adult women, pregnant women should consume an additional serving of milk or milk products and an additional serving of meat or meat alternatives. Consuming only the minimum number of servings from each food group does not provide the needed calories.

Nutrient Needs

According to the 1989 RDAs shown in table 8.4, healthy pregnant women need approximately 300 more calories per day (than before pregnancy) during the second and

TABLE 8.3
Recommended Servings of Food Groups During Pregnancy

Food group	Minimum number of servings per day
Breads and cereals	6
Vegetables and fruits	
Vitamin A rich	1
Vitamin C rich	1
Other	2
Milk and milk products	3
Meats and meat alternatives	3
Miscellaneous	Based on calorie needs

Source: Modified from National Research Council: *Diet and health: implications for reducing chronic disease risk,* Washington DC, 1989, National Academy Press.

TABLE 8.4
Recommended Levels for Individual Intake of Nutrients

Energy and nutrients	Women <19	Women 19–50	Pregnant <19	Pregnant 19–50	Lactating <19	Lactating 19–50
Energy (kcal)	2,200	2,200	2,500*	2,500	2,700	2,700
Protein (g)	46	50	60	60	65	65
Vitamin A (µg RE)	800	800	800	800	1,300	1,300
Vitamin D (µg)	5	5	5	5	5	5
Vitamin E (mg α-TE)	8	8	10	10	12	12
Vitamin K (µg)	60	65	65	65	65	65
Vitamin C (mg)	60	60	70	70	95	95
Thiamin (mg)	1.0	1.1	1.4	1.4	1.5	1.5
Riboflavin (mg)	1.0	1.1	1.4	1.4	1.6	1.6
Niacin (mg NE)	14	14	18	18	17	17
Vitamin B_6 (mg)	1.3	1.3	1.9	1.9	2.0	2.0
Folate (µg)	400	400	600	600	500	500
Vitamin B_{12} (µg)	2.4	2.4	2.6	2.6	2.8	2.8
Calcium (mg)	1,300	1,000	1,300	1,000	1,300	1,000
Phosphorus(mg)	1,250	700	1,250	700	1,250	700
Magnesium (mg)	360	320	400	360	360	320
Iron (mg)	15	15	30	30	15	15
Zinc (mg)	12	12	15	15	19	19
Iodine (µg)	150	150	175	175	200	200
Selenium(µg)	55	55	65	65	75	75

*Energy need during pregnancy varies based on activity and on prepregnancy BMI.
NE, niacin equivalents; RE, retinol equivalents; TE, tocopherol equivalents.
Sources: Data from National Research Council: *Recommended dietary allowances,* ed. 10, Washington, DC, 1989, National Academy Press, and for selected nutrients, data from Institute of Medicine: *Dietary reference intakes for calcium, phosphorus, magnesium, vitamin D, and fluoride,* Washington, DC, 1997, National Academy Press; and, data from Food and Nutrition Board, National Academy of Sciences—Institute of Medicine: *Recommended levels for individual intake of B vitamins and choline,* Washington, DC, 1998, National Academy Press (see chapter 2 and inside back cover).
Note: There are differences between the 1989 RDAs and the 1997/1998 recommended levels for individual intake of nutrients with respect to methods of derivation and age-groupings. However, space does not allow separate tables for the 1997/1998 recommended levels for individual intake of nutrients. Accordingly, the authors devised this table to summarize currently available data. It is not an official document developed or approved by the Food and Nutrition Board, Institute of Medicine, National Research Council, National Academy of Sciences.

third trimesters of pregnancy. This figure is an average. Women entering pregnancy underweight need more calories, and those entering overweight need fewer. In addition, physically active pregnant women require higher caloric intakes than these averages. It is generally easier and more accurate to monitor the adequacy of caloric intake by tracking weight gain than by counting calories.

The protein content of a woman's body increases by about 450 g during pregnancy in the expansion of the mother's uterus, breasts, and blood volume; a comparable amount is deposited in fetal tissues.

With the exception of vitamins A and D, calcium, and phosphorus, nutrient allowances for healthy pregnant women are 10 to 100 percent higher than for nonpregnant women (see table 8.4). The relatively high requirements for many nutrients mean that pregnant women should increase their intake of nutrient-dense foods more than they increase their consumption of calorie-rich foods.

Water

Water requirements increase substantially during pregnancy. It is generally advised that women stay well hydrated during pregnancy and that women living in hot climates pay special attention to fluid intake. For most women, a daily intake of 8 to 10 cups of fluids is sufficient.

Vitamins and Mineral Supplements

Current recommendations for prenatal **supplements** call for the routine use of iron during pregnancy. Specifically, the IOM recommends that pregnant women receive 30 mg ferrous iron daily beginning at about week 12 of gestation.[30] Other supplements are necessary when dietary counseling fails to lead to the needed improvements in diet (see box 8.2).

If a vitamin/mineral supplement is indicated, one similar to that shown in table 8.5 is suggested.

BOX 8.2

SUMMARY OF RECOMMENDATIONS FOR MATERNAL NUTRITION

- Routine assessment of dietary practices is recommended for all pregnant women in the United States to allow evaluation of the need for improved diet or vitamin or mineral supplements.
- Where possible, poor dietary practices should be improved by nutrition education, counseling, and referral to food assistance programs. If, in the judgment of the clinician, such interventions are likely to be or have been unsuccessful, then recommendation of a multivitamin/mineral supplement may be the only practical strategy to improve nutrient intake.
- To prevent iron deficiency, the subcommittee recommends the routine use of 30 mg of ferrous iron per day beginning at about week 12 of gestation, in conjunction with a well-balanced diet that contains enhancers of iron absorption (ascorbic acid, meat).
- Zinc supplementation is recommended when 30 mg of supplemental iron is administered per day.
- If a zinc supplement is administered, however, the subcommittee recommends that a 2-mg copper supplement also be given.
- Younger women (less than 25 years) with low calcium intakes (< 600 mg/day) should either increase their intake of food sources of calcium, such as milk or cheese or, less preferably, add a supplement that provides 600 mg of calcium per day.

- When dietary sources of water-soluble vitamins are inadequate, daily supplementation with 300 mg of folate, 2 mg of vitamin B$_6$, and 50 mg of vitamin C is recommended.
- Pending further research, the subcommittee considers it prudent to supplement the diet with low amounts of folate if there is any question of adequacy of intake of this nutrient.
- For women at high risk for inadequate vitamin B$_6$ intake, for example, substance abusers, pregnant adolescents, and women bearing multiple fetuses, the subcommittee recommends a daily multivitamin supplement containing 2 mg of vitamin B$_6$.
- For women at risk of deficiency (users of street drugs and cigarettes, heavy users of alcohol, long-term users of oral contraceptives, regular users of aspirin and salicylates, and women bearing more than one fetus), an ascorbic acid supplement of 50 mg/day is recommended if increased consumption of fruits and vegetables is unlikely.
- For complete vegetarians, a daily vitamin B$_{12}$ supplement of 2 mg is recommended.

Source: From Subcommittee on Nutritional Status and Weight Gain During Pregnancy, Institute of Medicine: *Nutrition during pregnancy,* Washington, DC, 1990, National Academy Press.

TABLE 8.5
Composition of Multivitamin/Mineral Supplement Recommended for Nutritionally At-Risk Pregnant Women

Nutrient	Amount	Percentage of 1989 RDA for pregnant women
Iron	30 mg	100
Zinc	15 mg	100
Copper	2 mg	(no RDA)
Calcium	250 mg	20
Vitamin B$_6$	2 mg	90
Folate	300 µg	75
Vitamin C	50 mg	75
Vitamin D	5 µg	50

Source: From Subcommittee on Nutritional Status and Weight Gain During Pregnancy, Institute of Medicine: *Nutrition during pregnancy,* Washington, DC, 1990, National Academy Press.

Which Pregnant Women Are at Nutritional Risk?

Predictors for poor pregnancy outcomes are shown in box 8.3 and a set of circumstances that place women at **nutritional risk** is given in box 8.4.

It seems likely that a majority of women in the United States are at "nutritional risk." Approximately one third of women in the United States smoke cigarettes before pregnancy (about one third of smokers quit for a portion of the pregnancy), illicit drugs are used by between 6 and 25 percent of women, and 70 to 75 percent of Black and 5 to 20 percent of White women are "intolerant" of lactose and may voluntarily restrict their intake of milk and dairy products. Of all births in the United States, 12 percent are to adolescents.

Weight Gain Recommendations for Pregnancy

No specific amount of weight gain during pregnancy is right for everyone. How much a woman should gain depends on her weight before pregnancy (see table 8.6). Weight gain should be gradual and continue in an upward direction, even for women who enter pregnancy overweight or obese. All guidelines assume that weight gain is achieved by eating high-quality diets.

Appetite and food intake fluctuate widely during pregnancy, and increases in food intake usually do not produce the smooth rate of maternal weight gain shown in the weight gain graphs. There are spurts in food intake and in weight gain. Appetite, food intake, and weight gain generally are greatest in the second trimester. The calorie and nutrient stores that develop as

BOX 8.3

MATERNAL PREDICTORS OF POOR PREGNANCY OUTCOME

- Poverty
- Limited education
- Substance abuse (cocaine, heroin, alcohol, tobacco)
- Young age (less than sixteen years)
- Obesity, gestational diabetes, low pregnancy weight gain, suboptimal nutrition, anemia
- Underweight
- Poor or no prenatal care
- Clinical complications (placenta previa, abruptio placenta, pregnancy-induced hypertension)
- Chronic and acute diseases and disorders (hypertension, diabetes, infection)

BOX 8.4

WOMEN DEFINED AS NUTRITIONALLY AT RISK DURING PREGNANCY

- Women who do not ordinarily consume an adequate diet
- Women carrying more than one fetus
- Women who use cigarettes, alcohol, or illicit drugs
- Women who are underweight or overweight at conception or who gain inadequate or excessive weight during pregnancy
- Adolescents
- Women with poor knowledge of nutrition or who have insufficient financial resources to purchase adequate food

TABLE 8.6
Guidelines for Weight Gain During Pregnancy

BMI (kg/m^2)	Weight gain (kg)
< 19.8 (underweight)	12.5–18
19.8–26 (normal)	11.5–16
26–29 (overweight)	7–11.5
> 29 (obese)	> 5.9
Twin pregnancy	16–20.5

Source: From Subcommittee on Nutritional Status and Weight Gain During Pregnancy, Institute of Medicine: *Nutrition during pregnancy,* Washington, DC, 1990, National Academy Press.

a result of the increased food intake are used to support the high rate of fetal growth that occurs in the last trimester. Thus peak food intake and rate of weight gain precede the time of the largest gains in fetal weight.

Teen Pregnancy

Each day nearly 1,400 babies are born to U.S. teenagers.[29] The pregnancy rate among teenage women age fifteen to nineteen years increased 23 percent between 1972 and 1990 and is now at its highest level in nearly twenty years (117 pregnancies per 1,000 females age fifteen to nineteen years). The major problems related to teen pregnancy are the high incidence of health problems in the babies (LBW and prematurity) and the impact of the pregnancy and parenthood on the mother's educational and economic future. More than 80 percent of adolescents who give birth are low income.[10] Few teenagers are psychologically and economically prepared to succeed in securing a healthy future for themselves while being the primary source of support for one or more children. Regardless of their age, teenage mothers who have healthy lifestyles— those who generally consume balanced diets, gain the recommended amount of weight during pregnancy (young teens may need to gain weight at the high end of the recommended weight gain ranges to accommodate their own growth needs), and do not smoke or use drugs—tend to be healthier and to remain healthier during pregnancy than other teenage mothers.

The infants of healthy teenage girls also tend to be healthier. Nevertheless, growing adolescents have significantly smaller infants compared with same-age peers who did not themselves grow while pregnant, all other things being equal.[26] Fetal growth retardation in adolescent mothers who are still growing may reflect maternal/fetal competition for limited nutrients or to decreased placental blood flow or both. The effects of maternal growth on maternal tissue stores and birthweights of infants have been examined in pregnant growing adolescents.[27] Body composition differences associated with maternal growth appeared after twenty-eight weeks gestation and included accumulation of subcutaneous fat (triceps and subscapular) and greater postpartum retention of gestational weight gain. Scholl and associates[27] concluded that "despite an apparently sufficient weight gain and the accumulation of nutrient stores during pregnancy, young growing women appeared *not* to mobilize stores after 28 weeks gestation to enhance fetal growth, reserving them instead for their own continued develop-

TABLE 8.7

Recommended Weight Gain in Adolescent Pregnancy

Prepregnant BMI (kg/m^2)	Trimester 1 (kg)	Trimesters 2 and 3 (kg/week)	Total (kg)
Low (< 19.8) (underweight)	2.3	0.5	13–18
Normal (19.8–26.0)	1.4	0.5	11–16
High (26.1–29.0) (overweight)	0.9	0.3	7–11
Very high (> 29) (obese)	0.7	0.2	7 +

Source: From Subcommittee on Nutritional Status and Weight Gain During Pregnancy, Institute of Medicine: *Nutrition during pregnancy,* Washington, DC, 1990, National Academy Press.

ment." Recommended weight gains during adolescent pregnancy are summarized in table 8.7.

Unique recommendations for nutrient intakes do not exist for pregnant adolescents except for calcium (1,300 mg), phosphorus (1,250 mg), and magnesium (360 mg) as summarized in table 8.4. Those who begin pregnancy underweight (BMI < 19.8 kg/m^2) *and* are still growing *and* physically active clearly need additional energy intake. The level of energy intake that will maintain the appropriate weight gain (see table 8.7) is the proper one. If the pregnant adolescent consumes a balanced diet providing adequate energy and 55 to 70 g protein per day, this should be sufficient.[30]

Both adolescent growth and pregnancy impose substantial needs for iron because of the synthesis of new tissue (muscle and red blood cells) and expansion of blood volume. Iron-deficiency anemia in the first trimester is a significant risk factor for prematurity and LBW.[25] In 1990, some 11 percent of pregnant adolescents were anemic in the first trimester.[13] If the pregnant adolescent is found to have iron-deficiency anemia (hemoglobin < 110 g/L or hematocrit < 33 percent), she should be treated with 60 to 100 mg of ferrous iron per day until she is no longer anemic. At the same time, she should receive supplementary zinc (15 mg) and copper (2 mg) daily because high doses of iron may reduce absorption of copper and zinc.[30] If the pregnant adolescent is found to be iron-deficient (serum ferritin < 20 µg/L) but not anemic (hemoglobin > 110 g/L) in the first trimester, an iron intake between 30 and 60 mg per day may be sufficient to prevent development of anemia and to correct the iron deficiency.

Adolescents who do not eat breakfast and who consume limited amounts of fruits and vegetables may not have adequate folate intake. Further, those women who have used oral contraceptives for more than a year just before pregnancy are at risk of folate deficiency. Therefore, consumption of folate-rich foods (providing 400 µg/day) is an important preventive measure.

Available data suggest that calcium intake in the range of 1,200 to 1,500 mg/day during adolescence might result in higher peak adult bone mass.[19] It seems appropriate for the pregnant adolescent who is still growing to achieve a calcium intake of 1,500 mg/day.

Weight Loss After Pregnancy

It does not appear that women whose weight gains are close to the recommended levels are any more likely to retain excess weight one year after delivery than are women who gain less than recommended (table 8.8). On the other hand, women who gain more than recommended (for their prepregnant BMI) substantially increase their chances of retaining 4 kg (9 lb) or more compared with those who follow the recommendations.[12] Some 25 percent of White and 60 percent of Black women who gained more than recommended retained 4 kg or more approximately a year after delivering a full-term infant. This observation is of some importance in view of the recommendation that Black women should strive for prenatal weight gain at the upper end of the recommended range for prepregnancy BMI.[7,30] While striving to improve fetal outcome, we may be promoting obesity among women. Attention needs to be given to the individual pregnant woman in terms of her prepregnant BMI and medical and obstetric history as well as to diet, physical activity, weight gain during pregnancy, and weight management in the months after pregnancy.[3,21] On average, a woman loses approximately 7 kg during delivery and the first postpartum week and an additional 15 to 16 kg by the fourteenth week postpartum. Breast-feeding is generally associated with a slightly more rapid postpartum weight loss.[22]

LACTATION

Before 1900, nearly every mother breast-fed her infant. By 1920, however, evaporated milk and later commercial infant formulas became widely available in the United States, and for a time they were perceived to be better for infants than human milk. Rates of breastfeeding fell sharply from 1920 to 1955 but then rose sharply when post–World War II baby boomers began having families. In 1985, the overall rate of breast-feeding in the newborn period was close to 60 percent.[24]

Advantages of Breast-Feeding

Infants Human milk provides the infant with nutrition plus a number of immunoprotective substances that safeguard the nursing infant against various infectious organisms (bacterial, fungal, protazoal, and viral).[31] Infants continue to receive passive immunity against a number of infectious agents as long as breast-feeding continues. The protection against various infectious diseases is particularly important to infants living in situations where the preparation and handling of formulas may be unsatisfactory (contaminated water supply, inappropriate techniques in preparing formulas from concentrated liquid or from powder, lack of refrigeration, etc.). In these circumstances, infants may be exposed to infectious agents introduced into the formula, and at the same time these infants do not receive the protective substances in human milk.

Mother Breast-feeding offers advantages to mothers as well as to infants. Bonding between mother and infant is facilitated by breast-feeding. Breast-feeding causes the release of oxytocin, a hormone that stimulates the muscles of the uterus to contract. Contraction of the uterus helps stop the bleeding caused by the detachment of the placenta from the wall of the uterus during delivery. There is

TABLE 8.8
Percentage Distribution of Mothers by Retained Weight after Delivery and According to IOM Weight Gain Recommendations

| Weight gain | Lost weight | Retained weight (kg) | | | |
		0–1.7	1.8–4.0	4.1–6.3	6.4+
Less than recommended	31.9	30.8	16.0	12.3	9.1
As recommended	25.6	31.0	21.1	11.1	11.1
Greater than recommended	18.7	23.5	19.2	13.2	25.4

Source: Adapted from Keppel KG, Taffel SM: Pregnancy-related weight gain and retention: implications of the 1990 Institute of Medicine Guidelines, *Am J Public Health;* 83:1100–3, 1993.

some evidence that breast-feeding may be associated with a lower risk of premenopausal breast cancer.[18]

Although the great majority of women are biologically capable of breast-feeding their infant, not all women are psychologically able to do it successfully. Breast-feeding can fail if the mother does not receive social and emotional support for her decision to breast-feed. Women who are exposed to high levels of stress and women who suffer depression or other psychological disorders also may be unable to breast-feed successfully. Breast-feeding is a very natural process, but problems do occur, and generally they can be overcome with supportive guidance. The importance of breast-feeding has led to the policy in many European countries of having mothers stay in the hospital with their babies until breast-feeding is successfully established (see chapter 9, pp. 236–237).

Breast-feeding limits the participation of fathers in feeding their infants and intensifies the mother's responsibilities and commitment. Because most infants eat every two or three hours around the clock during the first month or so, their mothers can become exhausted. These disadvantages can be overcome to an extent if the mother's workload is reduced by other family members so she can devote herself nearly full time to feeding and caring for the new infant. If the mother expresses her milk (by hand or with the aid of a breast pump) and stores it for later use, this practice allows the father or other caregivers to feed the baby occasionally during the early weeks. The anti-infective components of human milk help it stay fresh when stored in the refrigerator for as long as twenty-four to thirty-six hours. Once **lactation** and breast-feeding have been successfully established, periodic feeding of expressed milk or formula by bottle can be done without negatively impacting lactation or milk production.

The Process of Lactation

The mother's body prepares for breast-feeding during pregnancy. Fat is deposited in breast tissue, and networks of blood vessels and nerves infiltrate the breasts. Ducts that will channel milk from the milk-producing cells forward to the nipple—the milk-collection ducts—also mature. Hormonal changes that occur at delivery signal milk production to begin. Because delivery, not length of pregnancy, initiates milk production, milk is available for infants born prematurely. The milk produced during the first 3 days or so after delivery is different from the

milk produced later. Called colostrum, this early milk contains higher levels of protein, minerals, and antibodies than does "mature" milk. These antibodies help newborns remain healthy after making the transition from a germ-free environment to a germ-filled one.

Milk is present in the breasts as "fore milk" and "hind milk." Before a feeding, fore milk is present in the milk-collection ducts that lead from the milk-producing cells to the nipple. It is readily available to the infant. Fore milk contains less fat and protein—and therefore fewer calories—than hind milk. Hind milk is produced and stored in the milk-producing cells and is not initially available to the infant. It is released (let down) by oxytocin, which causes the milk-producing cells to contract and thereby release the hind milk.

The Letdown Reflex

The **letdown reflex** is unique as a physiologic process in that it can be initiated by either physical or psychological stimuli. Normally, the letdown reflex is triggered shortly after the infant starts sucking at the woman's breast. It can also occur when the mother hears her infant cry in hunger or when the thought occurs to her that it is time for a feeding. The physical or psychological stimulus signals the mother's brain to release oxytocin into the bloodstream. When the oxytocin reaches the milk-producing cells, they contract and let down the hind milk. Oxytocin is normally released within a minute after breast-feeding starts.

Certain physical and psychological stimuli can prevent the letdown reflex from occurring. Stress, pain, anxiety, and other distractions can block the release of oxytocin. If the mother is distracted by pain or pressured for time, for example, the letdown reflex may not occur, and the infant will consume less nutrient-dense hind milk, not get enough to eat, and is soon hungry again. If this happens often enough, the infant will be hungry most of the time and the mother may think she does not have enough milk for her baby and may decide to switch to bottle-feeding. Oxytocin inhalers are sometimes used to turn on the letdown reflex.

The Rooting Reflex

Humans, like other mammals, are born with a **rooting reflex.** When an infant's face touches the mother's breast, he or she instinctively "roots around" for the nipple. Once the nipple is felt, the hungry infant places his or her mouth around it and begins to suck vigorously. If the flow of milk is not limited the infant feeds until full and then loses interest in eating.

Infants demonstrate that they are hungry in a number of ways: they move their head toward a breast if they are being held, they act irritable, and they cry. They also demonstrate it by the way they start to feed. Hungry infants start to feed with intensity and with their fists tightly clenched. They gradually loosen their fists as their hunger is satisfied, and their hands are fully relaxed and open when they have had enough to eat.

Milk Production

While consuming one meal, an infant is "ordering" the next one. The infant's sucking and the emptying of the breasts during a feeding causes the hormone prolactin to be released from the mother's brain. Prolactin stimulates the production of milk. It generally takes about two hours for the milk-producing cells to produce sufficient milk for the next feeding.

Infants grow in spurts, not at a constant rate. Growth spurts occur frequently between an infant's third and seventh weeks of life, but less often after that. There is an increase in hunger associated with a growth spurt and for about a day, the infant will want to feed more often than usual because he or she is not completely satisfied. Although the mother may spend much of her day (and night) breast-feeding an infant who is entering a growth spurt, she may feel that she does not have enough milk to satisfy the baby and may give the baby a bottle with formula. However, because milk production is determined by how much and how often an infant nurses at the breast, bottle-feedings, which may lead to a decrease in milk production, are not recommended. It is very rare that a lactating woman cannot produce enough milk. As long as an infant is allowed to nurse at the breast as often as desired, the mother's production will catch up with the baby's need for milk.

MATERNAL NUTRITIONAL NEEDS DURING LACTATION

The RDA for calories is about 25 percent higher for lactating women than for women who are not lactating (see table 8.4). The actual increase in caloric need is higher than the RDA, around 40 percent. Energy supplied from fat stores that normally accumulate during pregnancy contributes to meeting energy needs during lactation, so not all of the calories must come from the mother's diet. The RDA calls for increasing caloric intake by 500 calories per day over that of the nonpregnant woman. An additional 300 calories are needed to support lactation, but this energy is assumed to be provided by maternal fat stores.

The average increases in nutrient allowances for lactation are generally higher than the increases for pregnancy. As during pregnancy, proportionately higher amounts of nutrients than calories are required, which indicates the need for a nutrient-dense diet. As can be seen in table 8.4, the RDA for nutrients for lactating women increase to varying extents.

The current RDA for calcium intake during pregnancy and lactation is 1,000 or 1,300 mg/day depending on age. It has been recommended that lactating adolescents and young adults should ingest up to 1,500 mg calcium per day.[19]

The RDA for iron is not increased during lactation. Only small amounts of iron are secreted into human milk (< 1.5 mg/L), and the lactating woman generally does not resume menstrual periods until the infant begins weaning from the breast. The resulting iron savings reduce the lactating women's need for dietary iron.

Dietary Recommendations for Lactation

The additional calories and nutrients needed by the lactating woman can be obtained from a varied diet that includes foods from each of the basic food groups. The amounts of foods needed to meet the additional energy and nutrient requirements of lactation are shown in table 8.9.

Increases in hunger and food intake that accompany lactation generally take care of meeting caloric needs. If the diet includes at least the recommended minimal number of servings from each food group and sufficient calories, the lactating woman is helping to assure an adequate diet for herself and her infant. Failure to consume enough calories from food can decrease milk production. Weight loss that exceeds 0.5 kg/week—even in woman with a good supply of fat stores—can reduce the amount of milk produced.

Maternal Diet and Breast Milk Composition

Rather than the energy content of milk being diluted in response to a low-calorie diet, the volume of milk is decreased. The amount of carbohydrate, protein, and fat in human milk varies only slightly in response to maternal diet, but the type of fat present can vary substantially. If

TABLE 8.9
Amounts of Food Needed to Meet Additional Nutritional Needs of Lactating Women

Suggested foods	Amounts	Energy (kcal)	Protein (g)	A (IU)	C (mg)	B_1 (mg)	B_2 (mg)	Niacin (mg)	Ca (mg)	Fe (mg)
2% Milk	2 cups	290	18	700	—	0.14	0.82	0.4	576	—
Meat, round steak	2 oz.	150	13	35	—	0.04	0.11	2.8	6	1.7
Vegetables, dark green or yellow	3/4 cup	20	2.5	1990	70	0.07	0.15	0.6	68	0.6
Other vegetables	1/2 cup	45	1	10	44	0.05	0.02	0.2	19	0.5
Citrus fruit	1/2 cup	60	1	275	60	0.11	0.01	0.5	12	0.1
Enriched bread	1 slice	65	3	—	—	0.09	0.03	0.8	24	0.8
Total		630	38.5	3010	174	0.5	1.14	5.3	705	3.7

Source: Adapted from Worthington-Roberts B, Williams SR: *Nutrition in pregnancy and lactation,* ed 5, St. Louis, MO, 1993, Mosby.

a woman consumes more vegetable oils than animal fats, her milk contains a high proportion of unsaturated fats. If she fasts, her milk contains the type of fat present in her fat stores.

The water-soluble vitamin content of human milk corresponds more closely to maternal intake than is the case for the energy-yielding nutrients. The amounts of the B vitamins, folate, and vitamin C in breast milk, for example, vary with the types of food and supplements that the mother ingests. The zinc and iodine content of human milk reflect the mother's diet.

Nonnutrient Substances in Breast Milk

Foods contain many substances in addition to nutrients, and other substances enter the body through drugs, medications, and other ingested nonfood substances. All of these **nonnutritive substances** may end up in human milk.

When a lactating woman drinks coffee, her infant receives a small dose of caffeine. Breast-fed infants of women who are heavy coffee drinkers (10 or more cups per day) may develop "caffeine jitters." Alcohol also is transferred from a woman's body to milk, and therefore alcohol consumption during lactation should be restricted.

Nearly any drug or toxin that enters the mother's blood may be detected in her milk. Many environmental contaminants are fat-soluble, and if they are ingested they may be stored in a woman's fat tissues. When the fat stores are later broken down for use in production of milk, the contaminants stored in the fat may enter her milk. For example, environmental contaminants such as DDT, chlordane, PCB, and PBB have been found in human milk.

Maternal Diet and Infant Distress

Some infants may be sensitive to components of certain foods a mother consumes that are transferred into her milk. Peanut butter, chocolate, egg whites, and nuts contain substances that enter human milk and cause some infants to develop a rash, wheezing, or a runny nose. Onions and foods from the cabbage family such as cabbage, broccoli, and brussels sprouts also are suspected to cause adverse reactions in some breast-fed infants.

Why some infants are sensitive to certain components of the foods in their mothers' diets is not known. The general advice for lactating women is to experiment with small amounts of the potentially offending foods to see if the nursing infant is sensitive. If the infant does not appear to be, these foods do not need to be omitted from the mother's diet.

Nutrition recommendations during lactation are summarized in box 8.5.[2]

INTERVENTION

The goals of nutrition intervention before, during, and after pregnancy are to help women achieve and maintain optimal nutritional status for delivery of a healthy infant, successful lactation, and to foster positive health status during the adult years. Community nutrition professionals work toward these goals through community-wide services as well as direct delivery of individual nutrition care services.

Communitywide Services

• Establishment of a plan to assure access to quality perinatal nutrition services for all women in the community

BOX 8.5

RECOMMENDATIONS FOR NUTRITION DURING LACTATION

- Breast-feeding is recommended for all U.S. infants under ordinary circumstances.
- If breast-feeding is not possible, feeding an appropriate formula is an acceptable alternative.
- Lactating women should be encouraged to obtain their nutrients from a well-balanced, varied diet rather than from vitamin and mineral supplements.

  Need for vitamin and mineral supplements should be individually established.

  Fluids should be consumed to meet thirst.

  Remove foods suspected of causing adverse reactions in infants for a trial period.

- Health care should include nutritional assessment and provide dietary guidance.
- Breast-feeding guidance should be provided prenatally, after delivery in the hospital, and during the early postpartum period.
- Anticipatory guidance on weight loss during lactation should be given.

  The average loss is 1 kg/month from months 1 to 6.

  Approximately 20 percent of women do not lose weight.

  Rapid loss (> 2 kg/month) after first month is not recommended.

- Caloric intake less than 1,500 kcal per day is not recommended.
- Use of illicit drugs should be actively discouraged.
- Limit alcohol to no more than 0.5 g/kg body weight per day (e.g., a 60-kg women should have no more than 2 drinks per day).
- Infant nutrition:

  Give 0.5- to 1-mg injection or 1 to 2-mg oral dose of vitamin K after birth.

  Give 5- to 7.5-μg vitamin D per day if exposure to sunlight is limited.

  Give low-dose iron supplement by six months.

- Development of a referral system and referral procedures for pregnant women in need of food, health, social, and other resources
- Development of standards (protocols or guidelines) for nutrition assessment, education, and counseling, and indicators for monitoring nutrition services during pregnancy and lactation; and development and provision of assessment tools and material to enable health professionals to implement the standards
- Provision of in-service education, technical assistance, and consultation for individuals and groups of professionals and associated health personnel caring for or serving women in their child-bearing years (e.g., physicians, nurses, community workers, food service managers, school nurses, detention facilities, etc.)
- Conduction or promotion of out-reach activities in the community to encourage consumption of an adequate diet before and during pregnancy, including intake of folacin
- Conduction or promotion of breast-feeding support programs in the community
- Participation in the coordination of teen pregnancy and high-risk pregnancy services
- Establishment of a data collection system and a nutrition monitoring system to determine the need for

perinatal nutrition care services in the community and to evaluate the effect of such services.

Individual Nutrition Care Services

- Conduction of nutrition assessments on every pregnant woman by the second prenatal visit and in each trimester according to established protocols
- Based on assessment, development and implementation of a nutrition care plan that includes food access, weight gain, diet during pregnancy, and management of risk factors identified
- Provision of education and counseling in a manner consistent with cultural, linguistic, and literacy needs of the woman
- Referral to necessary food assistance (e.g., WIC, food stamps), education (e.g., food management, child birth education), health or social services when needed
- Provision of breast-feeding education and support during and after pregnancy
- Conduction of periodic evaluations to assess the acceptance and effectiveness of prenatal nutrition services and the outcomes of pregnancy for all women served.

Nutrition assessment and intervention guidelines for pregnant and lactating women are summarized in table 8.10.

TABLE 8.10

Nutrition Assessment and Intervention Guidelines for Pregnant and Lactating Women

Assessment components	Methods	Risks/problems indicated	Intervention guidelines	Referral sources
		Pregnant		
Anthropometric Prepregnancy BMI (kg/m^2)	Weight (kg): beam balance; height (m): vertical bar	Underweight: BMI < 19; overweight: BMI > 27	Adjust weight gain to higher than average for underweight and lower than average for overweight	
Prenatal weight gain	Plot weight gain on appropriate grid	Inadequate or excessive rate of gain (see tables 8.3 and 8.9); excessive gain may indicate fluid retention	Adjust food intake and activity level to correspond with desired rate of gain; salt restriction *not* indicated for treatment of physiologic edema	Maternal and Infant Care Project; WIC Program; Food Stamps Program
Biochemical Hemoglobin (Hgb g/L) Hematocrit (Hct, %)	Standard laboratory techniques	Anemia—first trimester: Hgb < 110, Hct < 33; second trimester: Hgb < 105, Hct < 32; third trimester: Hgb < 110, Hct < 33	Ferrous iron intake 60 to 120 mg per day plus multivitamin/ mineral supplement containing 15 mg Zn and 2 mg Cu	Maternal and Infant Care Project; WIC Program
Ferritin (μ/L)	Standard laboratory technique	Iron deficiency in first trimester without anemia: ferritin < 20, Hgb > 110	Ferrous iron: 30 to 60 mg per day to prevent development of anemia	
Urinalysis	Dip stick for glucose, ketones, protein	Gestational diabetes Preeclampsia		
Blood glucose (mg/dl)	Standard laboratory techniques	Glucose > 140: should have three-hour glucose tolerance test		
Dietary Quantity and quality of food intake	Twenty-four hour recall; food record; food questionnaire frequency	Inadequate or excessive nutrient intake; excessive consumption of caffeine-containing beverages	Adjust dietary intake to meet nutrient needs; caution regarding use of caffeine-containing beverages	Maternal and Infant Care Project; WIC Program
Pica	Diet history	Ingestion of nonfood items	Discontinue practice if possible	
Dietary supplements	Diet history	Imbalance in nutrients or excessive amounts of some nutrients	Supplements indicated in following situations: pregnancy with multiple fetuses; poor nutrition history; poor dietary intake	Maternal and Care Projects; WIC Program; Family physician; Ob/Gyn clinic

TABLE 8.10—CONTINUED

Assessment components	Methods	Risks/problems indicated	Intervention guidelines	Referral sources
		Pregnant (continued)		
Clinical Obstetric history	Interview	History of pregnancy involving fetus/infant with NTD; less than one year between pregnancies; history of inadequate prenatal weight gain (< 1 kg/month) or excessive weight gain (> 3 kg/month) after first trimester; anemia; prior oral contraceptive use	Repletion of nutrient stores with adequate diet and supplements if necessary; adjust diet to include good sources of iron folic acid and vitamins C and B_6 as indicated	Maternal and Infant Care Project; WIC Program; maternal child health clinic; EPSDT Program; health departments
Substance abuse	Interview	Alcohol, smoking, drugs (prescription, OTC, illicit)	Multivitamin supplement with vitamins C, B_6, and folate is indicated	
		Lactating		

Anthropometric
  Maternal weight
  loss
	Standard beam balance	Excessive rate of loss (> 2 kg/month) may compromise lactation; inadequate rate of loss (< 0.5 kg/month) may lead to obesity over time	Monitor weight loss of mother and weight gain of nursing infant; adjust maternal dietary intake and level of physical activity	Maternal and Infant Care Project; WIC Program; Food Stamps Program

Dietary
  Quantity and quality
  of food intake
	Standard; twenty-four hour recall; food record; food frequency questionnaire	Energy intake > 1,500 kcal/day; try to obtain all nutrients from diet	Monitor maternal weight loss and infant weight gain; adjust dietary intake to meet needs and provide vitamin/mineral supplementation if necessary	

Based on the IOM reports on nutrition in pregnancy[30] and nutrition in lactation,[9] the Public Health Nutrition Practice Group of the American Dietetic Association developed quality assurance criteria for maternal nutritional care.[2]

PUBLIC FOOD AND NUTRITION PROGRAMS

The major food and nutrition program for low-income women in the United States is the Special Supplemental Nutrition Program for Women, Infants and Children, better known as WIC. In addition, the Food Stamp Program and the Commodity Distribution Program also support food access needs for low-income women.

The WIC Program

The WIC program was enacted in 1974 to help reduce the incidence of low birthweights and to improve maternal and child health by providing nutrition education and food supplements. The program, administered by state health departments, has proven to be effective and has grown in funding each year.[19]

Pregnant women and children up to the age of five who live in poverty and are assessed as being at risk of poor nutrition are generally eligible for the program. The nutrition risk criteria used in the WIC program serve both as indicators of nutrition and health *risk* and also as indicators of nutrition and health *benefit*[10] (see box 8.6). Once enrolled in WIC, pregnant and lactating women and their infants and toddlers receive an assessment of their nutritional status, nutrition education, and coupons for foods to supplement their existing diets. Specific nutrient-dense foods provided by the WIC program are limited to milk, infant formula, eggs, dried beans, cheese, peanut butter, and 100 percent fruit juices (plus carrots and tuna fish for lactating women).

Women who enroll in WIC during pregnancy are less likely to deliver LBW infants and to experience iron deficiency than are women who are eligible but do not participate. Participation in WIC has also been shown to improve diet quality and to reduce significantly the prevalence of iron deficiency in infants and young children.[20] Breast-feeding of WIC infants has been found to reduce WIC and Medicaid costs.[16]

Almost all programs available in communities to assist pregnant adolescents emphasize early and consistent prenatal care, counseling (individual and group), and continuing maternal education. Community nutrition professionals can obtain special multidisciplinary training in adolescent health through the Maternal and Child Health Bureau (MCHB) of the U.S. Department of Health and Human Services. The MCHB assists in coordinating efforts of coalitions of agencies (public and private) and professionals groups to improve nutritional care and education.

IMPLICATIONS FOR COMMUNITY NUTRITION PROFESSIONALS

Infant outcomes in the United States are poorer than expected, given the resources of this nation. Improvements in maternal and child health will, in part, depend on our ability to improve the nutritional status of women before and during pregnancy and during lactation and the interconception period. For this challenge to be met, scientifically based and uniform standards for nutrition services as well as supporting activities such as assurance that adequate diets and knowledge about them are available to all pregnant women must become a reality. Whether efforts to improve maternal nutrition and infant outcomes are successful will largely depend on the ability of the community nutrition professional and others within local agencies to deliver effective nutrition services to women during pregnancy and lactation.

COMMUNITY NUTRITION PROFESSIONALS IN ACTION

- Acquire vital health statistics for your state for the most recent three years for which reports are available. Examine data for infant mortality rate, low-birthweight rate, prematurity, fertility rate, teenage pregnancy rate for the state and several urban and rural counties. Plot data and note trends over time. Also note demographic data and socioeconomic indicators for the counties. Compare data to the Healthy People 2000 objectives. Which counties have the highest rate of poor pregnancy outcome? How do

BOX 8.6

WIC NUTRITION RISK CRITERIA FOR PREGNANT WOMEN

Determined by	*Risk factor*
Laboratory	Anemia; HIV infection
Anthropometry	Underweight; overweight (obesity) abnormal patterns of weight gain
Nutrition-related medical conditions	Clinical signs of nutrition disorders; metabolic disorders; preeclampsia, ecclampsia
High-risk pregnancy	Adolecence; substance abuse (drugs, alcohol, tobacco); history of neonatal loss, prematurity, LBW, congenital malformations
Dietary deficiencies/inadequate nutrition	Gastrointestinal disorders; chronic or recurrent infections; renal disease; cardiorespiratory disorders; severe trauma

rates differ among racial or ethnic groups? What conclusions can you draw regarding who is having babies and the rates of poor pregnancy outcomes in different counties of the state? What implications do these data have for prenatal intervention priorities and strategies?

- What advice would you give a pregnant woman who has gained 3 kg (6 lb) by the twentieth week of pregnancy and tells you she has restricted her food intake because she is concerned that she will not be able to return to her prepregnancy weight and figure after pregnancy?

- What advice would you give to a low-income woman who would like to breast-feed her baby but plans to go back to work in one month? Her mother and friends are telling her to just bottle-feed like they did.

- A local business that employs a large number of young women has discovered that high-risk pregnancies and LBW infants are the most costly conditions being paid by the company's health insurance. The management is interested in initiating worksite interventions to encourage women to have a healthy pregnancy. Design a worksite nutrition intervention program to propose to the management. Include a rationale for each component you include in the program.

- Review available prenatal education and breast-feeding support resources and select those that would be most suited for pregnant teens.

- Research cultural beliefs and special food practices used during pregnancy by different cultural groups who live in your region. Consider how community nutrition professionals can incorporate these beliefs and practices into nutrition education and counseling.

- Visit a WIC site and observe nutrition assessment of pregnant women. What procedures and tools are used to conduct nutrition assessment? How is nutritional risk for WIC eligibility determined? Why are risk codes for WIC eligibility different from usual definitions of nutritional risk?

- Outline the content for a nutrition session to be included in a program for women and/or couples planning to become pregnant.

GOING ONE STEP FURTHER

- Assess the current status of perinatal nutrition services at a local clinic (e.g., family practice or obstetrics clinic or WIC program site) by conducting a chart audit of prenatal patients or clients. Use indica-

tors defined in *Quality Assurance/Quality Improvement Criteria for Nutritional Care of Pregnant and Postpartum Women and Adolescents*[2] to determine the adequacy of nutrition assessments and education and counseling services, and whether women achieve appropriate weight gain based on their prepregnancy weight status or BMI.

- Consider the stages-of-change model described in chapter 7. In what stage are most women with regard to "eating right" during pregnancy? Develop specific nutrition messages for women early in pregnancy who are ready to make changes. Develop another set of messages for women who have made changes to prevent relapse to unhealthy eating practices after delivery of the baby. Describe how, when, and why these different messages should be used in a prenatal program.

- The local high school is updating its services for pregnant teens. They have come to you for technical assistance regarding nutrition issues and nutrition service policies and procedures. How will you assist them?

- Identify the training requirements to become a certified lactation educator (CLE) or a certified lactation consultant (CLC). Interview a CLE or CLC. What are the most common problems women have in the first few days of breast-feeding? What approaches are successful in enabling women to continue breast-feeding for several months?

- Secure data from the Pregnancy Nutrition Surveillance System for your state or a neighboring state by contacting the state health department. Find out what data are contributed to the surveillance system for the state and how the summary information is used in program planning and evaluation. Discuss the strengths and limitations of the Pregnancy Nutrition Surveillance System from the point of view of the state public health nutrition director and from the point of view of a local community nutrition professional at a clinic site who submits data to the system.

- What services exist in your community to support a healthy pregnancy for high-risk women? Do an inventory of available programs and services. Summarize your findings in the form of a Referral Directory.

- Research dietary assessment methods used in pregnancy. What are the strengths and weaknesses of each method? Based on your review, in what situation would you recommend a food frequency questionnaire, a twenty-four hour recall, a food record or diary?

- Investigate how local hospitals are promoting and supporting breast-feeding. Talk with the lactation consultant and other staff. Have efforts increased the percentage of breast-feeding initiation? What else could hospitals do to facilitate successful breast-feeding?

ADDITIONAL INFORMATION

Professional societies develop statements, scientific status summaries, commentaries, and position papers to clarify an issue in which the particular society has expertise.

The American Dietetic Association (ADA) Position Statements relevant to chapter 8 are listed below:

1. Promotion of Breast-Feeding, *J Am Diet Assoc* 97:622, 1997.
2. ADA Supports National Association of WIC directors position on breast-feeding in the WIC Program, *J Am Diet Assoc* 90:8,1990.
3. Nutrition care for pregnant adolescents, *J Am Diet Assoc* 94:449, 1994.

REFERENCES

1. Brown JE, Tomas RB: Taste changes during pregnancy, *Am J Clin Nutr* 43:414–416, 1986.
2. Caldwell M: *Quality assurance/quality improvement criteria for nutritional care of pregnant and postpartum women and adolescents,* Chicago, 1993, American Dietetic Association.
3. Cogswell ME, Serdula MK, Hungerford DW, Yip R: Gestational weight gain among average weight and overweight women—what is excessive? *Am J Obset Gynecol* 172:705–712, 1995.
4. Costass K, Davis R, Kim N, et al: Use of supplements containing high-dose vitamin A—New York State, 1983–1984, *JAMA* 257:1292–1297, 1987.
5. Guyer B, Strobino DM, Ventura SJ, et al: Annual summary of vital statistics—1995, *Pediatrics* 98:1007–1019, 1996.
6. Hanson JW, Streissguth AP, Smith DW: The effects of moderate alcohol consumption during pregnancy on fetal growth and morphogenesis, *J Pediatr* 92:457–460, 1978.
7. Hicky CA, Cliver SP, Goldenberg RL, et al: Prenatal weight gain, term birth weight, and fetal growth retardation among high-risk multiparous black and white women, *Obstet Gynecol* 81:529–535, 1993.
8. Horner RD, Lackey RB, Kolassa K, et al: Pica practices of pregnant women, *J Am Diet Assoc* 91:34–38, 1991.
9. Institute of Medicine: *Nutrition during lactation,* Washington, DC, 1991, National Academy Press.
10. Institute of Medicine: *WIC nutrition risk criteria: a scientific assessment,* Washington, DC, 1996, National Academy Press.
11. Jones KL, Smith DW: Patterns of malformation in offspring of chronic alcoholic mothers, *Lancet* 1:1267–1268, 1973.
12. Keppel KG, Taffel SM: Pregnancy-related weight gain and retention: implications of the 1990 Institute of Medicine guidelines, *Am J Public Health* 83:1100–1103, 1993.
13. Kim I, Hungerford DW, Yip R, et al: Pregnancy nutrition surveillance system—United States, 1979–1990, *MMWR CDC Surveill Summ* 41(SS-7):26–42, 1992.
14. Lammer EJ, Chen DT, Hoar RM, et al: Retinoic acid embryopathy, *N Engl J Med* 313:837–841, 1985.
15. Little RE: Moderate alcohol use during pregnancy and decreased birth weight, *Am J Public Health* 67:1154–1156, 1977.
16. Montgomery DL, Splett PL: Economic benefit of breast-feeding infants enrolled in WIC, *J Am Diet Assoc* 97:379–385, 1997.
17. Naeye RL: Maternal body weight and pregnancy outcome, *Am J Clin Nutr* 52:273–279, 1990.
18. Newcomb PA, Storer BE, Longnecker MP, et al. Lactation and a reduced risk of premenopausal breast cancer, *N Engl J Med* 330:81–87, 1994.
19. Optimal calcium intake, *NIH Consensus Statement* 12:1–31, 1994.
20. Owen AL, Owen GM: Twenty years of WIC: a review of some effects of the program, *J Am Diet Assoc* 97:777–782, 1997.
21. Parker JD, Abrams B: Differences in postpartum weight retention between black and white mothers, *Obstet Gynecol* 81:768–774, 1993.
22. Potter S, Hannum S, McFarlin B, et al: Does infant feeding method influence postpartum weight loss? *J Am Diet Assoc* 91:441–446, 1991.
23. *Recommended dietary allowances,* ed 10, Washington, DC, 1989, National Academy Press.
24. Ryan AS: The resurgence of breast-feeding in the United States, *Pediatrics* 89:4/e 12, 1997.
25. Scholl TO, Hediger ML: Anemia and iron-deficiency and compilation of data on pregnancy outcome, *Am J Clin Nutr* 59(suppl):492S–501S, 1994.
26. Scholl TO, Hediger ML: A review of the epidemiology of nutrition and adolescent pregnancy: maternal growth during pregnancy and its effects on the fetus, *J Am Coll Nutr* 12:101–107, 1993.
27. Scholl TO, Hediger ML, Scholl JI, et al: Maternal growth during pregnancy and the competition for nutrients, *Am J Clin Nutr* 60:183–188, 1994.
28. Shaw GM, Velie EM, Schaffer D: Risk of neural tube defect–affected pregnancies among obese women, *JAMA* 275:1093–1096, 1996.

29. Story M, Alton I: Nutrition issues and adolescent pregnancy, *Nutr Today* 30:142–151, 1995.

30. Subcommittee on Nutritional Status and Weight Gain During Pregnancy, Institute of Medicine: *Nutrition during pregnancy,* Washington, DC, 1990, National Academy Press.

31. Wagner CL, Anderson DM, Pittard WB: Special properties of human milk, *Clin Pediatr* 35:283–293, 1996.

32. Wegman ME: Infant mortality: some international comparisons, *Pediatrics* 98:1020–1027, 1996.

33. Werler MM, Louik C, Shapiro S, Mitchell AE: Prepregnant weight in relation to risk of neural tube defects, *JAMA* 275:1089–1092, 1996.

CASE STUDY

NUTRITION ASSESSMENT AND INTERVENTION OF PREGNANT ADOLESCENTS

TED FAIRCHILD, MPH, RD

PRESIDENT, T. FAIRCHILD ASSOCIATES

This case study illustrates the range of concerns that need to be addressed when working with women who are pregnant—particularly the needs of pregnant teens. Pregnant teenagers face the challenge of continuing their own physical growth, while at the same time supporting appropriate development of the fetus. In addition, teens are developing their own identities, working on emotional maturation, and dealing with the emotional and social issues related to the pregnancy. The combination of these factors presents a particular challenge to community nutrition professionals.

The main questions raised in this case study have to do with the kinds of interventions that would be most successful in assisting pregnant teens to make appropriate choices for their own and their infant's health and well-being. Questions regarding adequate weight gain for the ideal growth of the fetus and the social considerations of teenagers are presented. Students should review the information available in the case study. They will need to review the biochemical and sociological information presented and make decisions regarding additional information needs and plan interventions that would be appropriate for the teens. Students can analyze the information and discuss possible alternatives in small groups.

THE CASE

A fairly small city in northern Utah has a combination city and county health department. The health director is recognized by the community as a leader in providing appropriate health services for the citizens. Recently, a contract was negotiated with the state to designate the department as a preferred managed care provider in the community. The mission of the department is to be progressive in the provision of preventive services to the community.

One of the primary problems in the community is a high incidence of adolescent pregnancy. The cultural value system of the majority of citizens is very conservative. The schools are not allowed to teach or discuss sex education. The only options for discussion of family planning are abstinence until marriage. The conservative nature of the community has made it difficult to have the adolescent pregnant women receive early pregnancy diagnosis and entrance to adequate prenatal care.

The Adolescent Health Program (AHP) is part of a newly organized unit of the health department. The department has recently implemented multiskilling as a part of its restructuring. You are the community nutrition professional in the department but are assigned as the program manager responsible for the AHP, and consequently, the health needs of adolescents in the community. The health department has primary responsibility for the health of all school-age children and has nurses assigned to each school.

The number of pregnant teenagers in the high school is of primary concern for the AHP. One of the first tasks you are assigned is to assess the situation and implement the necessary programs for pregnant teenagers who attend the alternative high school in the city.

Your responsibility includes not only the special nutrition concerns but also the monitoring of adequate prenatal care. Teens have a higher rate of premature births, growth-retarded infants, preeclampsia, and other obstetrical problems. Lack of prenatal care for teens has been linked to both denial of pregnancy and lack of knowledge of the physiological changes that occur during pregnancy. Early and aggressive prenatal care, including nutrition assessment and intervention are important in prevention of low birthweights and other problems associated with teen pregnancy. Adequate weight gain during pregnancy is of primary concern for teens. Teens frequently are conscious about their weight and do not eat adequately. Weight gain during pregnancy, which will sustain the growth of the fetus and also provide adequate nutrient intake for the mother, should be monitored. Attention should also be paid to iron deficiency anemia. Hematocrits of less than 33 suggest iron deficiency. Adequate intake of calcium is also important. Intakes of at least 1,500 mg of calcium a day should be attained. This is important not only for adult peak bone mass, but recent associations between adequate calcium intake and the prevention of preeclampsia is an important consideration. Folate is also an important nutrient to consider.

There are twenty girls in grades 9 to 12 who attend the special program at the alternative high school. The girls range in age from thirteen to eighteen years. Some of the girls are married, others live with their parents or friends. Three girls are of Hispanic origin; the remainder are Anglo. This distribution reflects the population of the county in general, which has little ethnic diversity.

There are several relevant pieces of information available. The school curriculum for the girls is geared to assist them with life skills necessary for their futures. In addition to the regular required courses, the girls also have one period a day in which health is the main focus. The girls learn about their own growth and development as well as the growth and development of the fetus and later the infant. There is an opportunity for the class to be expanded.

A special evening class is offered to the girls and their partners or parents during the third trimester of pregnancy to prepare them for childbirth. One of the additional services includes a social worker assigned from the local church community who assists single girls in deciding whether they should keep their baby or place the baby for adoption.

The following table presents some information about the teens currently enrolled in the program.

QUESTIONS

1. Which girls were underweight or overweight for height before pregnancy?
2. Which girls have inappropriate weight gain at this point in their pregnancy and what recommendations do you have for them?
3. Consider the girls with low hematocrits. What other determinations could you make to help determine if this is iron deficiency anemia? What nutrients other than iron need to be considered in determining cause of anemia in pregnancy?
4. What are the appropriate recommendations for treatment of iron deficiency during pregnancy?
5. What other pieces of information do you need to make a complete nutrition assessment?
6. What are some methods you should use to gather the information?
7. Who are the key people you could work with in gathering additional information needed for assessment?
8. Design a nutrition intervention program for the pregnant teens. What approaches are likely to be most effective? What behavior change strategies will you use?
9. Many programs designed for adolescent focus on active involvement and participation. Peer counseling also is particularly effective. What kinds of activities would be appropriate for pregnant teens?
10. Will the intervention program be different for teens with special problems such as anemia or inadequate weight gain?

Girl	Age (years)	Weight Prepregnancy (lb)	Current (lb)	Height (in.)	Hematocrit (%)	Gestation (weeks)	Grade
1	14	120	135	65	35	26	9
2	17	90	95	58	30	16	12
3	15	110	140	61	38	20	10
4	16	98	127	62	35	38	10
5	16	85	115	59	36	30	11
6	15	150	162	66	32	30	9
7	17	100	108	63	36	21	12
8	13	96	106	57	29	18	9
9	16	190	185	63	31	28	11
10	17	85	102	57	33	27	12
11	15	100	123	58	34	36	10
12	16	95	101	60	39	14	11
13	15	130	150	61	28	30	9
14	18	105	135	64	36	37	12
15	15	110	127	59	38	25	9
16	16	92	122	56	26	32	10
17	15	130	132	65	36	18	9
18	16	120	130	63	33	20	10
19	17	92	100	56	37	23	12
20	15	125	115	63	34	25	10

CHAPTER NINE

INFANTS, CHILDREN, AND ADOLESCENTS

Well begun is half done.
—HORACE

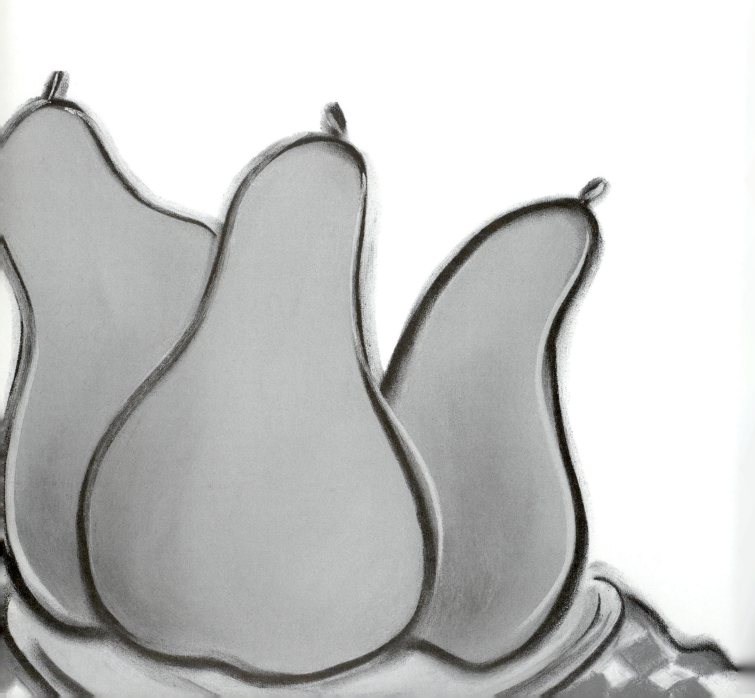

Nutrition is an important component of health care for infants, children, and adolescents. Infants grow rapidly and have requirements for energy, protein, and other essential nutrients that are higher per unit of body weight than at any other time during life. Increase in body size is among the most dramatic developmental changes during the first year of life. Growth rate slows considerably after the first year of life and remains relatively slow during the preschool years. Adolescence is a time of biological, physical, emotional, social, and educational transitions. Adolescents' health and nutritional needs should be viewed in the context of individuals seeking to establish their identity in a changing adult world. Infants, children, and, to a lesser extent, adolescents are dependent on parents and other adults for provision of food and nutrition and health care guidance. During this period of life, attitudes about food, preferences, and behaviors are shaped.

Objectives

When you finish chapter nine, you should be able to:

~ Describe and explain changing and variable nutritional needs of infants, children, and adolescents.

~ Identify and define nutrition risks for infants, children, and adolescents.

~ Outline and implement basic guidelines for nutritional management, including assessment, intervention, and referral.

~ Describe nutrition programs and services available for infants, children, and adolescents.

Key Words

Word	Page Mentioned
Iron deficiency anemia	228
CDC/PedNSS	228
WIC	228
NCHS	228
NHANES	231
Human milk	232
Beikost	232
Fatty acids	233
Immunological benefits	234
AAP	234
HIV infection	234
Nipple confusion	236
Recumbent length	237
Skinfold thickness	241
Bioavailability	243
Fluoride	245
Atherosclerosis	247
Juvenile-onset obesity	247
NCEP	248
Anorexia nervosa	254
NIDDM	255
BMI	255
CATCH	255

NUTRITION-RELATED HEALTH PROBLEMS OF CHILDREN

Nutrition plays a vital role in the growth and development of infants, children, and adolescents, and it is a major factor in promoting health and preventing disease (see figure 9.1). Since the early 1900s, our society has recognized the importance of adequate nutrition during infancy, childhood, and adolescence and has publicly funded a variety of nutrition services and programs for children.

In the national goal to prevent unnecessary disease and disability and to achieve a better quality of life for all Americans, specific actions are needed for children. Specific nutrition objectives to be accomplished by 2000 relating to infants and children are summarized in table 9.1.

IDENTIFYING PROBLEMS IN THE COMMUNITY: THE PEDIATRIC NUTRITION SURVEILLANCE SYSTEM

Table 9.2 outlines the health problems and related nutrition risk factors of children.

Conditions Related to Deficiencies

Iron Deficiency In the first national study of preschool children carried out in the late 1960s, it was found that 28 percent of all toddlers (one to two years old) were iron-deficient (transferrin saturation < 15 percent), while 10 percent were anemic (hemoglobin < 110 g/L). Among those in the lowest socioeconomic group, 45 percent were iron deficient and 19 percent were anemic.[34]

The Centers for Disease Control and Prevention (CDC) Pediatric Nutrition Surveillance System (PedNSS) confirmed that **iron deficiency anemia** was prevalent among low-income preschool children. In an analysis of hemoglobin and hematocrit data for low-income children in the 1970s, it was found that 25 percent of preschool children were anemic (hemoglobin < 110 g/L or hematocrit < 33 %).[31] In 1974 and 1975, the **CDC/PedNSS** started collecting data in six states (Arizona, Kentucky, Louisiana, Montana, Oregon, and Tennessee). Anthropometric and hematologic data were of primary interest because of the prevalence of anemia and evidence of growth retardation among low-income children. The CDC/PedNSS has expanded during the past twenty years so that by 1995, data were being collected from all states. Data were collected from low-income children enrolled in various public health programs (The Special Supplemental Nutrition Program for Women, Infants and Chil-

dren [**WIC**]; the Early Periodic Screening, Diagnosis and Treatment [EPSDT] program; Head Start; and Maternal and Child Health [MCH] clinics).

The risk for anemia decreases for children older than three or four years. This reflects the fact that the rate of growth is much slower than in infancy and the need for dietary iron is less and that the diet has expanded and consumption of iron-containing foods, including meats, has increased. Data from PedNSS for the 1980s shows that the prevalence of anemia in young children participating in public health programs declined substantially.[47] This reflected an emphasis on breast-feeding and on use of iron-fortified infant formula during the first year of life. There is still a significant prevalence of anemia among low-income toddlers (13.5 percent) and three- to five-year-old preschoolers (8 percent), who are eligible but are not participating in WIC or other public health programs.[48]

Growth Stunting The national prevalence of short stature (length or height less than the fifth percentile of the National Center of Health Statistics [**NCHS**] reference), an indicator of chronic undernutrition, was 9.4 percent among low-income children in 1990. Infants less than age one year and, in particular, Black infants had the highest prevalence of short stature for age. This may reflect the greater prevalence of low birthweight among Black infants. In contrast to results for infants, Black children in the PedNSS have the lowest prevalence of short stature by ages two to five years, reflecting a more rapid rate of growth in early childhood (figure 9.2).

In the period from 1980 to 1990, trends from PedNSS suggested that the prevalence of growth stunting among children remained relatively stable except among Asians, who continued to decrease their rate.[49] More recent data indicate that the prevalence of growth stunting among lower income Asian preschool children has nearly doubled the preceding five years and in 1995 was close to 10 percent.[36] Stunting among other low-income ethnic groups has remained around 5 percent.

Conditions Related to Excesses or Imbalances

In the PedNSS 1990 findings, overweight among children increased to its highest rate, 9.5 percent, since 1980. Hispanic and Native-American children had higher overall prevalence of overweight than other ethnic groups, especially at age 1 year. The association between diet, obesity and type II diabetes mellitus is well known and this association is of particular concern among Native Americans. Preliminary data from

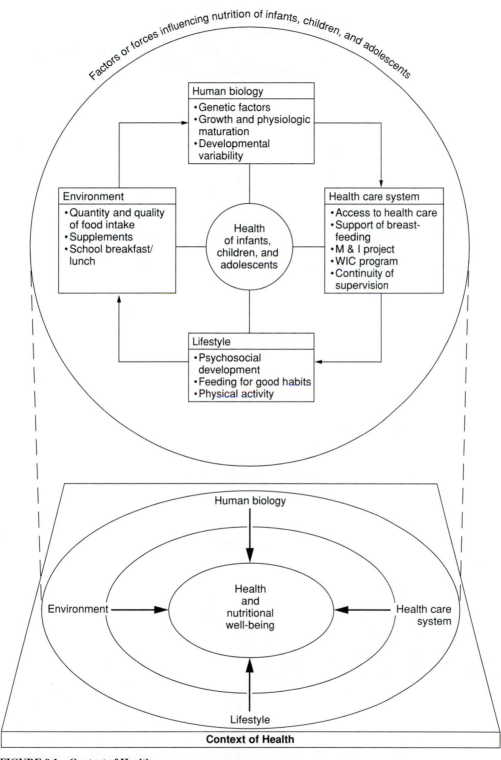

FIGURE 9.1   Context of Health
Influences on the nutrition of infants, children, and adolescents.

TABLE 9.1
Healthy People 2000 Objectives

Objectives	Baseline prevalence (year)	Current prevalence (year)
Health status		
Reduce infant mortality rate to no more than 7 per 1,000 live births	10.1% (1987)	7.5% (1995)*
Special population targets		
Blacks	18.8% (1987)	14.9% (1995)*
Alaskan and American natives	13.4% (1984)	NA**
Puerto Ricans	12.9% (1984)	NA
Reduce prevalence of iron deficiency to less than 3% among children one to four years of age		
All children age one to two	9% (1980)	
All children age three to four	4% (1980)	
Special population targets		
Low-income children age one to two	21% (1980)	4% (1985)
Low-income children age three to four	10% (1980)	3.5% (1985)
Reduce prevalence of anemia among Native Alaskan children to less than 10%	25% (1985)	15.6% (1995)
Reduce prevalence of growth retardation among low-income children under age five years to less than 10%	11% (1988)	6.2% (1995)
Special population targets		
Low-income Black infants	15% (1988)	13.3% (1995)
Low-income Hispanic infants	13% (1988)	7.6% (1995)
Low-income Asian/Pacific islander infants	14% (1988)	9.8% (1995)
Increase to at least 75% the proportion of mothers who breast-feed their babies in the early postpartum period and to at least 50% the proportion who continue breast-feeding until their babies are five to six months old (see table 8.2)		
Increase to at least 75% the proportion of parents or caregivers who use feeding practices that reduce or prevent deciduous tooth decay	55% (1991)	NA
Special population targets		
Parents/caregivers with less than high school education	36% (1991)	NA
Alaskan and American native parents or caregivers	47% (1991)	NA
Blacks	48% (1991)	NA
Hispanics	39% (1991)	NA
Services and protection		
Reduce the incidence of spina bifida and other neural tube defects to 3 in 10,000 live births	6 in 10,000 (1990)	NA
Increase to at least 95% the proportion of newborns screened by state-sponsored programs for genetic disorders and other disabling conditions and to 90% the proportion of newborns testing positive for disease who receive appropriate treatment	70% screened for galactosemia in thirty-eight states reporting	NA
Increase to at least 90% the proportion of children eighteen months of age and younger who receive recommended primary care services at appropriate intervals	NA	NA

Preliminary.
**Data not available.*

TABLE 9.2
Health Problems and Related Risk Factors

Health Problems	Related nutrition risk factors
Infants and children	
Growth retardation	Dietary inadequacies, especially total calories
Iron deficiency anemia	Inadequate intake of iron and too early introduction of cow milk during infancy
Elevated serum cholesterol	Excess fat, saturated fat, and cholesterol in diet
Obesity	Food consumption (caloric intake) exceeds energy needs for growth and physical activity
Dental caries	Nursing caries (prolonged and frequent bottle- or breast-feeding with continuing exposure of teeth to carbohydrate)*
	Insufficient fluoride after age three years
Adolescents	
Obesity	Food consumption (caloric intake) exceeds energy needs for growth and physical activity
Elevated serum cholesterol	Excess dietary fat, saturated fat, and cholesterol intake
Underweight	Food consumption (caloric intake) inadequate to meet energy needs for growth and physical activity
Dental caries	Continuing exposure of teeth to cariogenic carbohydrates
Iron deficiency	Inadequate iron intake

*Dental caries is an infectious disease caused by fermentable carbohydrates, especially sucrose, that are available to bacteria in the mouth. These bacteria, especially *Streptococcus mutans,* produce organic acids that lower pH at the tooth surface and lead to demineralization of enamel, that is, caries.

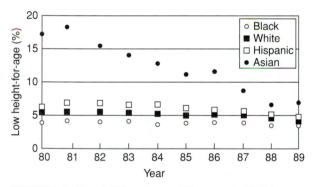

FIGURE 9.2 Trend of Prevalence of Shortness for Children Two to Five Years of Age Among Four Ethnic Groups from 1980 to 1989, PedNSS
(*Source:* From Yip R, Scanlon K, Trowbridge FL: Trends and patterns in height and weight status of low-income US children, *Crit Rev Food Science Nutr,* 33:409–421, 1993.)

the National Health and Nutrition Examination Surveys (**NHANES III**) suggest that one fifth of six- to seventeen-year-old children are overweight. Childhood obesity does not always, but may persist into adult years. At age six years, an obese child has a 25 percent chance of being overweight as an adult; the twelve-year-old obese child's chances are closer to 75 percent. Early identification and intervention are important in management of overweight and obesity in childhood.

The importance of physical activity to increase energy output and achieve energy balance has always been known but seems to be forgotten periodically.

INFANTS

Physical Growth

Increase in body size is among the most obvious developmental changes occurring during the first year of life. Average weight gain in the first year is 7 kg, about half of which occurs in the first four months of life. Infants triple or quadruple their birth weight in the first year. Healthy infants usually increase in length by 50 percent by twelve months of age, double their birth length by four years of age, and triple it by thirteen years of age.

Approximately one third of calories consumed are used for growth during the first four months. This rapid growth in healthy term infants during the first four months of life requires more energy, protein, and other essential nutrients per unit body weight than at any other time in infancy or childhood. Energy and nutrient needs during this phase of rapid growth can be met completely with **human milk** or infant formula.

Between four and six months of age, infants enter a transitional period characterized by a decreased rate of growth and an increased level of caloric expenditure for physical activity. Although total nutrient requirements continue to increase as a result of growth, decreasing requirements for energy and protein intake relative to body weight reflect a progressive decrease in growth rate. By age eight or nine months, foods other than milk (**beikost**) provide significant sources of energy and other nutrients to supplement the basic intake from human milk or formula.

Physiology of Infant Nutrition

The enormously complex, yet efficient, gastrointestinal mechanisms required for digestion of milk (human milk and infant formula) and absorption, utilization, and metabolism of nutrients in milk are well developed at birth. The ability of infants to ingest and process foods other than milk depends on the level of physiological development. Capacities for salivary, gastric, pancreatic, and intestinal digestion increase with age (table 9.3), indicating what may be a natural pattern for introduction of various forms of beikost. Neuromuscular and psychosocial development of infants (up to twelve months) has important implications for feeding.[32] The parent (or care provider)-infant relation during the early weeks and months may have long-term implications for the child's physical and emotional growth.

Nutrient Requirements

In table 9.4, recommended dietary allowances (RDAs) for selected nutrients for infants are summarized. Estimated nutrient requirements for infants younger than six months of age usually are based on the nutrients

TABLE 9.3
Digestion in Infancy

Location	Function	Effect on feeding
Birth to three months		
Salivary	Amylase present in small amounts	Some digestion of starch to maltose and α-dextrins
	Lipase (lingual)	Assists in digestion of triglycerides in stomach
Gastric	HCL and pepsin precipitate casein into curds and acidify whey protein	Beginning of protein digestion
	Secretion of HCL and pepsin quite low during this period	Relatively low levels of HCL and pepsin do not appear to limit protein digestion
	Gastric lipase	Assists in digestion of triglycerides
Pancreas	Little amylase produced in early months of life	Human milk contains amylase, which along with small amount of salivary amylase, allows digestion of some starch to maltose and α-dextrins
	Lipase	Hydrolyzes long chain triglycerides to a 2-monoglyceride and two fatty acids
Intestinal	Pancreatic endopeptidases and exopeptidases and intestinal brush border enzymes break down protein	Digest protein to small peptides (two to three amino acids) and free amino acids, which are absorbed from intestine
	Brush border lactase	Digests virtually all lactose to monosaccharides glucose and galactose for absorption
	Brush border maltase and α-dextrinase	Digest maltose, maltotriose, and α-destrins to glucose for absorption
	Bile salts activate lipase present in human milk	Hydrolyses triglycerides into glycerol and three fatty acids; by age 1 month, infant digests and absorbs 90–95% of human milk fat
Four to six months		
Salivary	Ptyalin and amylase increase	Aid in digestion of starch present in beikost added to diet
Gastric	HCL and pepsin increase	Aid in digestion of protein in beikost
Pancreatic	Amylase secretion increases	Aid in digestion of starch-containing beikost, particularly cereals

Source: Adapted from Fomon SJ: *Nutrition of normal infants,* St. Louis, 1993, Mosby.

consumed by healthy, thriving infants who are breast-fed by healthy, well-nourished mothers.

The RDAs for infants up to six months old are based primarily on amounts provided by human milk (750 ml), but in some cases, allowances may exceed those levels to provide for infants receiving formula.[16] RDAs for infants six months to one year of age are based on consumption of formula (600 ml) and increasing amounts of beikost. RDAs for must nutrients represent values well above the average estimated requirement and encompass the range of variability in individual requirement estimates. In contrast to allowances for spe-cific nutrients, the allowance for energy is based on the average needs of the age group under consideration and no adjustment is made for individual variability.

For infants up to six months of age, average energy needs are met at an intake of 108 kcal/kg per day, and for the six- to twelve-month-old infant, 98 kcal/kg per day. The protein allowance for infants up to six months of age is 2.2 g/kg per day, and for six- to twelve-month-old-infants, 1.6 g/kg per day. Two **fatty acids**—linoleic (18:2 *n*-6) and α-linolenic (18:3 *n*-3)—are essential nutrients for the infant. Human milk contains both in adequate quantities to meet estimated requirements: linoleic (from 1 to 2 percent of total calories) and α-linolenic (0.1 to 0.5 percent of total calories).[16]

TABLE 9.4
Recommended Levels for Individual Intake of Nutrients

Nutrient	0–5 mos	6–11 mos
Protein (g/100 kcal)	1.9	1.5
Protein (g/kg)	2.2	1.6
Vitamins		
A (RE)	375	375
D (μg cholecalciferol)	5	5
E (mg α-TE)	3	4
K (μg)	5	10
C (mg)	30	35
B_1 (mg)	0.2	0.3
B_2 (mg)	0.3	0.4
Niacin (mg NE)	2	3
B_6 (mg)	0.1	0.3
Folate (μg)	65	80
Minerals		
Sodium (mEq)	12	9
Calcium (mg)	210	270
Phosphorus (mg)	100	275
Magnesium (mg)	30	75
Iron (mg)	6	10

RE, retinol equivalents; TE, tocopherol equivalents; NE, niacin equivalents.
Sources: Data from National Research Council, *Recommended dietary allowances,* ed. 10, Washington, DC, 1989, National Academy Press, and for selected nutrients: From Institute of Medicine: *Dietary reference intakes for calcium, phosphorus, magnesium, vitamin D, and fluoride,* Washington, DC, 1997, National Academy Press; and, from Food and Nutrition Board, National Academy of Sciences—Institute of Medicine: *Recommended levels for individual intake of B vitamins and choline,* Washington, DC, 1998, National Academy Press. (see chapter 2 and inside back cover)

Note: There are differences between the 1989 RDAs and the 1997/1998 recommended levels for individual intake of nutrients with respect to methods of derivation and age-groupings. However, space does not allow separate tables for the 1997/1998 recommended levels for individual intake of nutrients. Accordingly, the authors devised this table to summarize currently available data. It is not an official document developed or approved by the Food and Nutrition Board, Institute of Medicine, National Research Council, National Academy of Sciences.

Human Milk Human milk from a healthy mother is considered the ideal food for the infant. Levels of some nutrients secreted in human milk vary with maternal diet, stages of lactation, duration of lactation, and individual biochemical variability among women. Caloric density and relative proportions of protein, fat, and carbohydrate in colostrum, transitional milk, and mature human milk vary considerably. There is a 30 percent decrease in protein content of human milk between the first and sixth months of lactation.[24] During the same interval, lactose content does not change, while concentrations of calcium, phosphorus, zinc, iron, sodium, potassium, and chloride all decrease 10 to 20 percent.[15] Studies of mineral content of milk from women one to thirty-one months postpartum showed levels of some trace metals, particularly zinc, declined substantially over time. Levels of iron and copper decreased only moderately after the first six months.

In healthy, well-nourished women, fatty acid composition of milk fat is determined primarily by maternal diet. Levels of linoleic acid vary between 7 and 25 percent and those of linolenic between 0.3 and 1.9 percent of total fatty acids. Linoleic acid (LA) is a precursor of arachidonic acid (20:4 *n*-6) or AA and linolenic acid (LNA) is a precursor of docosahexanoic acid (22: *n*-3) or DHA. These long-chain polyunsaturated fatty acids are present in human milk in small quantities and are important in the development of the central nervous system. Formulas for healthy term infants do not need to contain AA or DHA so long as they contain adequate amounts of LA and LNA.[1]

Vitamin D is deficient in human milk. Iron content of human milk appears to be low, although it is readily bioavailable. In the United States, vitamin and mineral supplements are commonly used during pregnancy and during the early weeks of the postpartum period, especially during lactation. However, maternal intake of vitamin D (a fat-soluble vitamin) appears to have little effect on the level of this vitamin in human milk. Supplementation of the breast-fed infant with vitamin D is recommended starting sometime during the first month of life unless the infant has adequate exposure to sunlight to ensure endogenous production of this vitamin. Variations in maternal intake of other fat-soluble vitamins (A, E, and K) appear to have little effect on levels of these vitamins in human milk. Variations in maternal intake of water-soluble vitamins (B vitamins and ascorbic acid) are reflected in levels of these vitamins in human milk. Vitamin B_{12} deficiency has been reported in a six-month-old infant breast-fed by his vegan mother. Iron content of human milk is not influenced by maternal intake of iron.

Immunological Benefits of Breast-Feeding   In the past fifteen years, there has been considerable research on the nonnutritional aspects of human milk, especially its **immunological benefits** and other protective constituents which interact with epithelial surfaces or with specific nutrients or potential pathogens in the gastrointestinal tract.[45] Secretory immunoglobulin A (SIgA) in mammary glands and human milk is largely derived from maternal gut-associated lymphoid tissue. SIgA resists the proteolytic action of the infant's gastroenteric secretions and reduces antigen contact with the intestinal mucosa until the infant's own antibody responses develop. Lysozymes, lactoperoxidases, and lactoferrin are protein macromolecules in human milk that may be important host resistance factors for the infant (see table 9.5). The importance of these immunological, cellular, and enzymatic components of human milk to the infant are indisputable. The advantages of breast-feeding, compared with formula-feeding, are discussed later in this chapter.

Other Nonnutrient Components of Human Milk   Drugs taken by lactating women may reach infants through the milk produced. Amounts of drugs secreted into human milk depend on their lipid solubility, mechanisms of transport, degree of ionization, and changes in plasma pH. In general, the higher the lipid solubility, the greater the concentration in human milk.

Human Immunodeficiency Virus Infection   Although an infant's risk of human immunodeficiency virus type 1 (HIV-1) infection by breast-feeding is low in women who were prenatally infected with HIV-1, the American

TABLE 9.5

Immunoprotective Components of Human Milk

Component	Attributes
Secretory IgA	Maternal-specific immunoglobulin to environmental agents
Lactoferrin	Bacteriostatic, iron-binding protein; antiviral
Lysozyme	Bacteriocidal; in synergism with peroxide and ascorbate will kill *Escherichia coli* and some *Salmonella* strains
Bifidus factor	Promotes growth of *Lactobacillus bifidus* and inhibits growth of *E. coli*, *Salmonella* and *Shigella* strains
Lipids	Antiviral, antibacterial, and antiprotazoal properties
Oligosaccharides	Block antigen attachment to gut epithelium
Leukocytes	Phagocytosis of bacteria, viruses, and fungi

Source: From Wagner CL, Anderson DM, Pittard WD: Special properties of human milk, *Clin Pediat* 35:283–293, 1996.

Academy of Pediatrics **(AAP)** recommends that "women who are known to be HIV infected should be counseled not to breast-feed or provide their milk for the nutrition of their own or other infants."[10] Women who are seronegative should be encouraged to breast-feed. However if they or their sexual partner(s) are injection drug users or if their sexual partner(s) is/are known to be HIV-positive, it may be prudent to recommend formula feeding. This is because women who develop primary **HIV infection** while lactating may pose an especially high risk for transmitting the infection via their milk.[35, 51]

Prepared Formula   In the United States, virtually all infants who are not breast-fed are started on commercial infant formulas. Commercial formulas are composed of cow milk protein, lactose, and vegetable oils plus vitamins and minerals. Some infants receive formulas based on isolated soy protein, vegetable oils, and glucose polymers prepared by partial hydrolysis of corn starch. All these products are designed to meet infants' nutritional needs during the first six months of life. Nutrient composition of two widely used infant formulas is given in table 9.6 along with that of mature human milk for comparison. Special formulas designed to meet nutritional needs of infants and children with metabolic and other disorders are discussed in chapter 12 (table 12.1).

TABLE 9.6

Nutrient Composition of Human Milk and Proprietary Infant Formulas and Recommended Levels for Full-Term Infants (per 100 Calories)

Nutrient	Minimum level*	Human milk	Enfamil (Mead Johnson)	Similac (Ross)
Protein (g)	1.8[†]	1.3–1.6	2.1	2.2
Fat (g)	3.3	5	5.3	5.4
Carbohydrate (g)	—	10.3	10.9	10.7
Vitamins				
A (IU)	250	250	300	300
D (IU)	40	3	60	60
E (IU)	0.5	0.3	2	3
K (μg)	4	2	8	8
C (mg)	8	7.8	12	9
B_1 (μg)	40	25	80	100
B_2 (μg)	60	60	140	150
Niacin (μg)	250	250	1,000	1,050
B_6 (μg)	35[‡]	15	60	60
Folacin (μg)	4	4	16	15
Pantothenic acid (μg)	300	300	500	450
B_{12} (μg)	0.15	0.15	0.3	0.3
Biotin (μg)	1.5	1.0	3	4.4
Inositol (mg)	4	20	17	4.7
Choline (mg)	7	13	12	16
Minerals				
Calcium (mg)	60	50	78	75
Phosphorus (mg)	30[§]	25	53	58
Magnesium (mg)	6	6	8	6
Iron (mg)	0.15	0.1	1.9[‖]	1.8[‖]
Iodine (μg)	5	4–9	10	15
Copper (μg)	60	60	75	90
Zinc (mg)	0.5	0.5	1	0.75
Manganese (μg)	5	1.5	15	5
Sodium (mg)	20	24	27	28
Chloride (mg)	55	55	63	66
Potassium (mg)	80	81	108	108
Potential renal solute load (mOsm)	—	11.3[#]	20	15

*Food and Drug Administration: Rules and Regulations. Nutrient requirements for infant formulas (21 CFR Part 107), *Fed Reg* 50:45106–84510, 1985.
[†]Protein quality not less than 70% of casein. Lesser quality requires proportionately greater minimum amount of protein.
[‡]At least 15 μg of vitamin B_6 per gram of protein.
[§]Calcium/phosphorus ratio not less than 1:1 and not more than 2:1.
[‖]Iron-fortified formula.
[#]Calculated by method of Ziegler and Fomon.

Foods Other Than Milk (Beikost)   To meet the nutritional needs of infants, the AAP recommends breast milk or iron-fortified formula up to age one year, with a gradual addition of beikost starting at five or six months. By age six months, healthy infants will have developed fine, gross, and oral motor skills; be able to sit with some support and control the head; and show some hand-eye coordination to consume semisolid foods. During the next six months, as more beikost is introduced, human milk (or formula) provides a progressively smaller share of total calories, so that by age nine to twelve months, between one third and one half of total calories will be supplied by beikost. By the end of the first year, beikost supplies nearly half the total calcium (550 mg), two thirds of the total protein (20 g), and essentially all the iron (10 mg) in the diet of the breast-fed infant.[15] If the infant receives an iron-fortified formula rather than human milk, beikost supplies nearly half the total protein and half the iron in the diet.

Recent Trends in Infant Feeding Practices

During the past twenty-five years, important changes occurred in patterns of infant feeding. From 1971 to 1984, the incidence of breast-feeding in the newborn period increased from 25 percent to nearly 60 percent nationally, with considerable variation among socioeconomic groups. Breast-feeding rates in the United States have always tended to be highest among women who are older, better educated, more affluent, or living in western states and lowest among those who are younger, less educated, have lower income, or are living in the southeastern states.

The vast majority of infants in the United States are born in hospitals and some hospital practices (such as separation of mother and infant, early supplementation, delay in getting the infant to the breast, and short stay in hospital after birth) as well as inadequate training of physicians and other health care professionals may contribute to the lower rates of breast-feeding.[17,46] Successful initiation of breast-feeding is dependent on a number of factors. The most important are (1) maternal desire to breast-feed, (2) appropriate breast-feeding guidance by physicians and nurses, and (3) appropriate hospital practices with respect to breast-feeding on demand (rooming-in) and (4) duration of stay in hospital.[37] In Ontario, it was shown that as infants' length of stay at birth hospital decreased from a mean of 4.5 days in 1987 to a mean of 2.7 days in 1993, their readmission rate during the first postnatal week doubled.[23] Primiparous mothers of five infants admitted to an Ohio hospital with failure-to-thrive and hypernatremia (elevated serum sodium) reported extensive preparation for breast-feeding.[11] These five infants were discharged from the hospital between twenty-seven and forty-eight hours after birth and were readmitted at five to fourteen days of age. None of the families supplemented the infants with water or formula more than once between discharge and readmission. It was suggested that avoiding supplementation in attempts to establish breast-feeding might have exacerbated the problem. Finally, although some of the families had contact with lactation consultants (1/5) or home health nurses (3/5) and telephone conversations with a pediatrician (3/5), none of the infants were weighed or examined by a pediatrician between discharge and readmission. The AAP has stated that all infants should be *seen* by their practitioner within seven days of discharge from birth hospital. Health care providers must be supportive of breast-feeding and, at the same time, be prepared to carefully evaluate any infant with a problem.

There is considerable controversy regarding the use of infant formula to supplement the breast-fed infant during the early days of life. It has been argued that such practice interferes with lactation and leads to "**nipple confusion**" insofar as the infant is concerned but it has been questioned whether "nipple confusion" is a real entity.[14] They argue that the use of the term "nipple confusion" suggests that an artificial nipple on a bottle is somehow equivalent to the nipple on the breast. In fact, babies do not feed from nipples on breasts; they feed from a teat formed (by the baby) from the nipple and the breast with the nipple extending as far back as the junction of the hard and soft palate. If the baby cannot be attached to the breast adequately or successfully by the mother, the priorities are that the mother produces milk (by expressing) and that her baby receives the milk (by bottle). This gives the mother time, with help, to offer the baby the breast until he or she can be attached properly. "In no instance, in these circumstances, has a baby ever refused the breast, even when breast-feeding has been separated by several days of exclusive bottle feeding."[14] Certainly, bottle feeding may be safely introduced two-to-three weeks after lactation has been established.[21]

Schwartz and coworkers[43] noted that participation in WIC during pregnancy was not associated with a decrease in breast-feeding. As shown in table 9.7, it was estimated that 34 percent of newborns participating in WIC throughout the United States were initially breast-fed in 1989 but only 8 percent were still breast-fed at age six months.[41] In contrast, in 1994 and 1995, it was estimated that approximately 47 percent of WIC infants throughout the United States were breast-fed in the neonatal period.[42] Just as there is geographic variation in breast-feeding rates among non-WIC populations in the United States, there are substantial variations in rates of breast-feeding among different WIC programs. For example, the 1994 to 1995 neonatal rate in Arizona, Montana, and Utah was

TABLE 9.7

Recent Breast-Feeding Trends in the United States

Percentage of Infants Breast-Feeding

	1989		1995	
	Newborn	Six months	Newborn	Six months
WIC infants	34	8	47	13
Non-WIC infants	63	24	71	29

Source: Adapted from Ryan AS: The resurgence of breast-feeding in the United States, *Pediatrics;* 99(4), 1997.

approximately 65 percent, whereas in Illinois, Ohio, and Pennsylvania, it was approximately 35 percent.[7]

Based on a recent study of 876 infants (406 breast-feeding and 470 formula-feeding) in Colorado, WIC food costs were calculated taking into account the administrative costs (20 percent is the U.S. average) and formula-manufacturer's rebates.[27] It was found that the monthly WIC food cost for breast-feeding was $6.85 less than for formula feeding. Monthly savings in Medicaid expenditures ($16.98) plus the savings in WIC costs ($6.85) gives a net benefit of $23.83 associated with breast-feeding.

Consequences of Infants at Nutritional Risk

Iron Deficiency   Iron deficiency is one of the most common nutritional deficiencies in North America. Although signs of anemia may appear after twelve months of age, they have their genesis in inadequate iron nutrition during the first year of life. Prolonged iron deficiency eventually results in iron deficiency anemia. In healthy full-term infants, iron deficiency anemia is uncommon before age nine to twelve months because of iron stores present at birth, effective utilization of iron from human milk, and use of iron-fortified formulas.[50]

Obesity   With few exceptions, infantile obesity is secondary to excessive intake of food. Poor infant feeding practices and misuse of beikost, such as introducing beikost too early, mixing cereal with milk in a bottle, and use of sweetened juices as a pacifier, can readily contribute to energy intake greater than energy needs.

Guidelines for Nutrition Care in Infancy

Nutrition care includes assessment, care planning and implementation (including counseling, education, medical nutrition therapy, and referral), monitoring, and follow-up. The expected outcomes of nutrition care for a normal infant include the following:

- Infants maintain acceptable weight- and length-for-age, and weight-for-length between the fifth and ninety-fifth percentiles when plotted on the NCHS growth charts.
- Infants do not deviate more than twenty-five percentile points from their established pattern of growth.

---

*Updated NCHS growth charts will be released sometime in 1998.

- Infants' hemoglobin levels are equal to or greater than 110 g/L or their hematocrit levels are equal to or greater than 33%.
- Infants are breast-fed up to one year of age. If this is not feasible, iron-fortified formula should be used as a replacement for human milk during the first year.
- Infants consume beikost in accordance with stages of neuromuscular readiness and growth.
- Infants' food intake is nutritionally adequate for age or stage of development.

Nutrition Assessment

Nutrition assessment and intervention guidelines for infants, children, and adolescents are outlined in table 9.8.

Anthropometric Assessment   Anthropometric measurements recommended for infants include weight, **recumbent length** (crown-heel), and head circumference. Appraisal of body size and pattern of growth are fundamental parts of pediatric care. Evaluation of growth helps in detection and diagnosis of a host of disorders of infancy and childhood. Discussion of an infant's growth is often the starting point for effective dialogue with that infant's parent or caregiver.

In 1975, the NCHS prepared a series of percentile curves of weight-for-age, length-for-age, weight-for-length, and head circumference-for-age reflecting growth of infants and children in the United States.[19] Figures 9.3 to 9.5 are examples of growth charts for girls from birth to age thirty-six months. The same type of percentile curves are available for boys, birth to thirty-six months, and weight-for-age, height (stature)-for-age, and weight-for-height (stature) for both boys and girls two to eighteen years of age are also available.

The NCHS growth charts have been widely accepted as reference growth charts, although it has been demonstrated that breast-fed infants today tend to grow more rapidly during the first two or three months and more slowly the balance of the first year than as depicted by the NCHS curves.[13]*

Weight   The infant's body weight should be measured to the nearest 10 g (½ oz) using a beam-balance scale. The infant's clothes should be removed before he or she is weighed. The infant should be placed in the center of the weighing surface. Zero should be checked before every session and when the scale is moved. The

TABLE 9.8

Nutrition Assessment and Intervention Guidelines for Infants, Children, and Adolescents in Community Nutrition

Assessment components	Methods	Risks/problems indicated	Intervention guidelines	Referral sources
Infants and children				
Anthropometric				
Birth weight for gestational age	Digital scale; reference standard	Intrauterine growth retardation (IUGR); large for gestational age; prematurity	Adjust feeding to meet nutritional needs based on gestational age and catch-up growth potential in IUGR and in prematurity; rule out hypoglycemia in small and in large newborns.	Private physicians and primary care; regional center for high-risk newborns; WIC program; services for children with special health care needs.
Weight for age Height for age Weight for height Head circumference (FOC) to age two years	Beam-balance scale Measuring board Nonstretch tape NCHS growth charts	Undernutrition, malnutrition Stunting; failure to thrive (height for age < fifth percentile); severe malnutrition (height for age < fifth percentile and FOC < fifth percentile); overweight or obesity (weight for height > ninety-fifth percentile)	Adjust dietary intake to increase weight or stabilize intake until overweight is compensated by increases in height; adjust activity level; refer children and families to food assistance programs; report/refer cases of child abuse.	Children and Youth Program; Title XIX; Head Start; child abuse and neglect centers; Food Stamps; Commodity Supplemental Food Program
Biochemical				
Hemoglobin (Hgb) Hematocrit (Hct)	Standard laboratory techniques	Anemia	Improve dietary iron intake and/or supplement with iron.	

Age (yr)	Hgb (g/L)	Hct (%)
1–< 2	< 110	< 32.9
2–< 5	< 111	< 33.0
5–< 8	< 115	< 34.5
8+	< 119	< 35.4

Assessment components	Methods	Risks/problems indicated	Intervention guidelines	Referral sources
Serum cholesterol*		> 170 mg/dl	Reduce total fat and cholesterol intake.	
Blood lead+		> 10 µg/dl	Environmental intervention for lead.	
Dietary				
Quantity and quality of food intake Motor and feeding development	Twenty-four-hour recall, food record, or food frequency questionnaire	Inadequate or excess intake; abnormal development of motor skills and feeding ability	Adjust dietary intake to meet nutrient needs; progress toward normal feeding developmental milestones.	
Clinical				
Blood pressure	Monitored in children > 3 years	"High normal" pressure	Institute weight management; reduce sodium intake if excessive.	

*Children two years of age and older with a family history of premature cardiovascular disease or at least one parent with high serum cholesterol. Adapted from US Department of Health and Human Services, Public Health Services, National Institute of Health: *Report of the expert panel on blood cholesterol in children and adolescents,* Pub (NIH) 91-2732, Washington DC, 1991, US Government Printing Office; US Department of Health and Human Services, Public Health Services, Centers for Disease Control: *Preventing lead poisoning in young children and adolescents,* Atlanta, 1991, US Government Printing Office.

TABLE 9.8—CONTINUED

Assessment components	Methods	Risks/problems indicated	Intervention guidelines	Referral sources
		Adolescents		
Anthropometric Weight Height	Beam-balance scale Vertical bar and or assess stature using weight and height for age- and weight-for-height growth charts (NCHS) as reference	Overweight, underweight Short stature Anorexia	Adjust dietary intake and level of physical activity.	If pregnant, prenatal care; WIC program; Maternal and Infant Care Programs; Commodity Supplemental Food Program; physical fitness and recreational facilities; physician, psychologist, or guidance center
Biochemical Hemoglobin Hematocrit	Standard laboratory techniques	Anemia	Adjust diet; supplement with iron as indicated.	
Serum cholesterol		> 170 mg/dl	Reduce total fat, saturated fat, and cholesterol intake.	
Dietary Quantity and quality of food intake (nontraditional)	Twenty-four-hour recall; three-day record; food frequency questionnaire	Inadequate or excess intake	Adjust dietary intake to meet nutrient needs.	Adolescent clinic; alternative health center
Clinical Blood pressure	Standard technique	"High normal" pressure	Institute weight management; reduce sodium intake if excessive.	
Dental		Dental caries	Institute oral hygiene; reduce intake of sticky sweets.	Dentist/dental hygienist
Eating disorders	Medical history; close observation	Anorexia nervosa; bulimia	Provide eating disorder referral.	Physician, psychologist, or psychiatrist

Biochemical anemia reference values:

Age (hr)	Hgb (g/L)	Hct (%)
Male		
12–< 15	< 125	< 37.3
15–< 18	< 133	< 39.7
18+	< 135	< 39.9
Female		
12–< 15	< 118	< 35.7
15–< 18	< 120	< 35.9
18+	< 120	< 35.7

scales should be calibrated at least every six months against reference weights.

Length Recumbent length is measured for infants. The measurement should be made on an examining table with a length-measuring device with a headboard and a movable footboard that are perpendicular to the table surface. Length is recorded as the distance between the headboard and footboard when the infant has been positioned properly, as illustrated in figure 9.6. Two people are required to measure accurately an infant's length. Length should be recorded to the nearest 0.1 cm (1/8 in.).

Head Circumference A flexible but nonstretchable tape measure is used to measure the circumference of the head. The tape is applied firmly above the supraorbital (above the eyes) ridge around to the occiput to obtain the maximum circumference. Values are plotted on the growth chart (figure 9.5) for comparison to reference data.

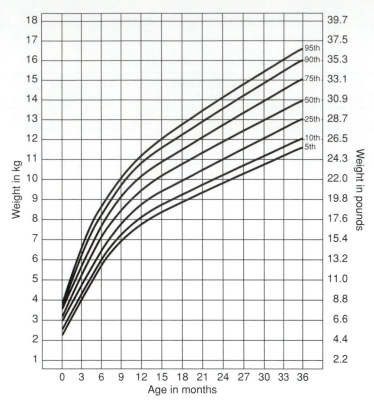

FIGURE 9.3   Weight-for-Age Percentiles for Girls—Birth to Thirty-Six Months

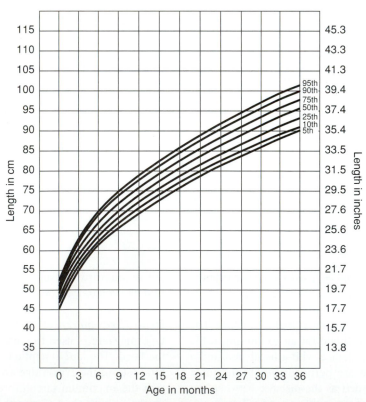

FIGURE 9.4   Length-for-Age Percentiles for Girls—Birth to Thirty-Six Months

240

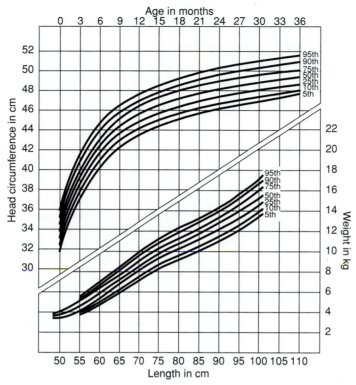

FIGURE 9.5   Head Circumference-for-Age for Girls—Birth to Thirty-Six Months (Top) and Weight-for-Length Percentiles for Girls— Birth to Thirty-Six Months (Bottom)

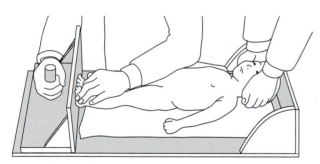

FIGURE 9.6   Two Persons Measuring Infant Length with Measuring Board

Skinfold Thickness   **Skinfold thickness** has been proposed as a useful index of relative fatness of the body because subcutaneous adipose tissue is a major component of body fat.[33] Skinfold thickness is not recommended as a routine screening measurement in well-child care, however, it is useful in follow-up and monitoring of individual infants or children who are identified using weight-for-length charts as having a potential or real problem of overweight or obesity.

Biochemical Assessment   Biochemical and laboratory indicators of current dietary intake and of the nutritional status of young children are presented in tables 9.8 and 9.9. Note that some laboratory tests reflect recent or current intake of nutrients, while others are indicators of longer term nutritional status or chronic intake and/or biochemical adequacy.

Dietary Assessment   It is important to determine if the baby is breast-fed or receives formula or milk. If the baby is breast-fed, how frequently, for how long, and is supplemental formula given. If the baby is formula-fed, what type of formula and how much is and what is the technique of formula preparation. Determine the type (cereal, eggs, dried beans or peas, meat, rice, potatoes, fruits, vegetables, and mixed dishes), frequency, and amount of beikost consumption. Does the infant's caretaker have access to a clean and safe water supply and basic kitchen

TABLE 9.9

Laboratory Indicators of Dietary Intake and Nutritional Status of the Young Child

Nutrient	Current dietary intake	Nutritional status	Comments
Protein	Serum or urine urea nitrogen (UN) Serum retinol-binding protein (RBP)	Serum albumin	Urea nitrogen in serum or urine correlates reasonably well with intake of protein if renal function is normal. UN values in serum < 6 mg/dl or in urine < 8 mg/g creatinine or serum RBP < 15 µg/ml suggest low recent intake of protein. Serum albumin is a rather insensitive and non-specific indicator of protein status but values < 3.2 g/dl suggest poor protein nutritional status.
Iron	Transferrin saturation	Ferritin Hemoglobin (Hgb) Hematocrit (Hct)	Levels of transferrin saturation (iron/total iron binding capacity × 100) < 16% suggest iron deficiency even when the concentration of Hgb is > 110 g/L. Ferritin < 15 ng/ml indicates iron deficiency. Hgb < 110 g/L (Hct < 33%) suggested as lower limit of normal for infants and young children.
Vitamin A	Serum carotene	Serum vitamin A	Approximately one half of total vitamin A intake from foods is supplied by fruits, vegetables, and cereal grains in the form of carotene. A level of serum carotene < 40 µg/dl suggests low net intake of carotene. A level of serum vitamin A < 20 µg/dl suggests low stores of vitamin A or may indicate failure of transport or retinol out of liver into blood.
Ascorbic acid	Serum ascorbate or whole blood ascorbate	Leukocyte ascorbate	At usual levels of intake of ascorbic acid from foods, there is a good correlation between intake and serum ascorbate; levels in serum < 0.3 mg/dl suggest that recent intake has been low. Whole blood ascorbate levels < 0.3 mg/dl indicate low intake and a reduction in body pool of ascorbic acid. Leukocyte ascorbate levels < 15 mg/100 g suggests poor nutritional status.
Riboflavin	Urinary riboflavin	Erythrocyte glutathione reductase	There is reasonably good correlation between intake and urinary excretion of riboflavin. Excretion of < 250 µg/g creatinine suggests low recent intake of riboflavin. Glutathione reductase-FAD (flavin-adenine dinucleotide) effect expressed as a ration > 1.2 suggests poor nutritional status.
Thiamin	Urinary thiamin	Erythrocyte transketolase	Excretion of < 125 µg/g creatinine suggests low intake of thiamin. Transketolase-TPP (thiamin pyrophosphate) effect expressed as a ratio > 15 suggests poor nutritional status.
Folacin	Serum folacin	Erythrocyte folacin Formiminoglutamic acid (FIGLU)	Level of serum folacin > 6 µg/dl suggests low intake. Levels of erythrocyte folacin > 20 µg/dl or increased excretion of FIGLU in urine following a histidine load suggests poor nutritional status.
Iodine	Urinary iodine	Serum protein-bound iodine (PBI)	Urinary excretion of < 50 µg/g creatinine suggests low recent intake of iodine. PBI < 3 µg/dl suggests poor nutritional status.

necessities? Is the infant receiving vitamin drops or iron drops as a supplement? If the infant is on any special diet, what is it and who recommended the diet? Does the infant eat dirt, paint chips, or other nonfood items? What concerns does the respondent have about infant feeding?

The questions are designed to select from among a large group of infants those few (perhaps 5 or 10 percent) receiving a diet potentially deficient or excessive in one or more nutrients and who are in need of more in-depth dietary evaluation and counseling. Information from the dietary assessment is used by the community nutrition professional to provide anticipatory guidance and education of the mother or caretaker. The twenty-four-hour recall method can be used to guide the mother or caretaker through the feeding pattern of a typical day to evaluate this information. The type and quantity of milk and beikost is then compared against recommendations, taking into account cultural food ways.

Clinical Assessment   The physical examination can reveal signs that indicate deficiencies of essential nutrients or malnutrition or other nonnutritional disorders that merit further evaluation and treatment.

Nutrition Intervention and Counseling

Guidelines for Feeding the Normal Infant   Based on current knowledge there is an optimum feeding schedule to match the special nutritional needs and unique physiological characteristics of the infant during the first year of life. The consensus of current research from most sources indicates the need for providing guidelines regarding feeding practices. Two basic principles should be used in guiding the feeding process: (1) necessary nutrients are required, not any specific food, and (2) food is the basis for early learning, both personal development and cultural needs.

The First Six Months   Ideally, human milk should be used as the sole source of food for the first six months. The breast-fed infant should receive supplemental vitamin D, 400 IU daily if sunlight exposure is less than two hours per week, and 7 mg of iron daily from ferrous sulfate or other preparations of high bioavailability after four to six months of age. Infants fed commercially prepared iron-fortified formula do not require supplements. Beikost should not be introduced before five to six months of age.

After Six Months   Human milk should be used up to one year. If breast-feeding is not possible, an iron-fortified commercial formula should be used throughout the first year. At five or six months of age, beikost should be introduced. Iron-fortified dry cereal commercially prepared for infants, beginning with rice cereal, should be introduced first and fed daily until eighteen months of age. Other foods such as fruit and vegetables prepared commercially or at home should then be introduced singly, with no more than two new foods introduced in the same week. When breast-feeding is continued beyond age six months, some foods that are relatively rich in protein (e.g., meat, legumes, and eggs) should be added to the infant's diet. By ten months, bite-size pieces of soft foods can be given, and by twelve months, soft foods from the family table can be given. Table 9.10 outlines typical recommendations for the addition of beikost. Regular or reduced-fat cow's milk is not recommended during infancy. Some suggestions for mothers and caretakers regarding feeding infants are given in box 9.1.

Supplements   Full-term infants born to well-nourished mothers generally have sufficient iron stores (in hemoglobin and liver) that they maintain satisfactory hemoglobin levels during the first three to four months of life. After age four to six months, iron must be provided by the diet to the term infant to ensure adequate hemoglobin production. The usual level of hemoglobin at birth is high, 160 to 180 g/L, and falls normally to a level of 100 to 120 g/L at age three to four months. Low birthweight (1,000 to 2,500 g) infants require iron supplementation of 2 mg/kg per day starting by two months of age, because the hemoglobin level at birth is lower than in the full-term infant and it drops more rapidly during the first two months.

The AAP states that, in the normal infant, the addition of iron-fortified cereal at six months of age will supply adequate amounts of iron to prevent iron deficiency anemia. Three tablespoons of iron-fortified infant cereal mixed with formula, breast milk, or water provides 7 mg of iron, the suggested level of supplementation per day. However, the extent to which the iron in infant cereal is absorbed and utilized by the infant is somewhat controversial.[15] Several factors determine the **bioavailability** of iron in infant cereal products: type of flour (level of phytic acid), type of iron salt, and levels of ascorbic acid).[12] Phytic acid inhibits iron absorption. Phytic acid can be degraded by

TABLE 9.10

Feeding Chart for Baby Six Months to Twelve Months

	Sixth month; daily servings; begin with small servings and gradually increase	Seventh and eighth months; add texture daily; begin to emphasize use of cup	Ninth to twelfth month; continue use of cup; increase texture; add variety
Formula or breast milk	26 to 40 oz (three to five 8 oz bottles)	24 to 32 oz (Avoid giving too much formula or breast milk.)	
Grains: infant cereal, rice, noodles, bread	4 to 8 tablespoons (Begin with thin cereal and thicken gradually.)	Add texture by giving teething biscuits, soft cooked noodles, toasted bread, rice, and the like.	
Fruit juice	4 oz daily	Avoid giving more than 4 oz per day. Use a cup for juice rather than bottle.	
Fruit: peaches, pears, bananas, applesauce, apricots, fruit cocktail	2 to 5 tablespoons; smooth, pureed, or strained	4 to 8 tablespoons (¼ to ½ cup); Gradually add texture. Mash or cut into small pieces.	
Vegetables: potatoes, sweet potatoes, green beans, wax beans, carrots, squash, beets	2 to 5 tablespoons; smooth, pureed, or strained	4 to 8 tablespoons (¼ to ½ cup); Gradually add texture, use soft cooked vegetables chopped not mashed	
Meat and protein: chicken, beef, pork, turkey, baked beans, lentils		2 to 4 tablespoons pureed; Add potatoes if your child doesn't like meat. Gradually decrease the potatoes and increase the meat.	4 to 6 tablespoons; Increase texture. Give tender small pieces of soft cooked meat in sauces, like stews or casseroles.

BOX 9.1

FEEDING FOR GOOD HABITS

- Smile and talk to your baby while you feed him or her. Let the baby know that mealtime is pleasant and that foods are good.
- Eat at the same time as your baby. Let him or her eat with the family. Babies learn a lot from watching others at mealtime.
- Be a good model. Serve and eat a variety of foods. If you never eat vegetables, your baby may not either.
- Serve small amounts and offer seconds. It is good to let your baby decide how much he or she will eat. Do not force your baby to "clean his or her plate."
- Avoid using food as rewards or punishments.
- Establish regular mealtimes each day. Regular eating times give children a sense of safeness and order.

- Plan for nutritious snacks at regular times each day. Most children this age need to eat four to six times a day for best growth.
- Offer foods with good nutrition. Children this age need healthy foods, not sugary or salty snacks.
- Throughout your baby's first year, practice using a cup. Soon after your baby's first birthday, it will be time to wean him or her from the bottle.
- Make changes slowly using small steps. Babies have not experienced much yet. Sudden changes can be hard to handle. Ease changes by mixing the old with the new. Small simple changes will help your baby be happy and healthy.

Source: From The Nutrition Unit, Minneapolis Health Department.

addition of phytase but the inhibitory effect of phytic acid is overcome by ascorbic acid, an enhancer of nonheme iron absorption. Iron from ferrous sulfate, ferrous ascorbate, and ferrous gluconate is more bioavailable than iron in more complex compounds such as ferrous fumarate, ferrous succinate, ferric pyrophosphate, and ferric orthophosphate. An iron supplement also can be in the form of iron drops prescribed by a physician. Except for breast-fed infants, as noted above, the diet should contribute all the nutrients needed by the infant.

Current recommendations of the AAP[9] on **fluoride** supplementation are shown in table 9.11. When prepared with fluoride-free water, concentrated liquid and powder infant formula products will contain less than 0.3 parts per million (ppm) of fluoride (< 0.3 mg/L). Ready-to-use (RTU) liquid products also provide less than 0.3 ppm. The fluoride content of reconstituted products (powder or concentrated liquid) will reflect the fluoride content of the water used. If it isn't possible to use RTU formula, it is recommended that water with low fluoride content be used for preparing formulas, at least during the first six months.[9]

Referral

The food assistance programs available to infants include the WIC Program and the Commodity Supplemental Food Program (CSFP), also called the Mothers and Children (MAC) program in some states. Table 9.12 outlines federally sponsored food programs available to infants and children. The WIC program is discussed in some detail in chapter 5. Other areas for referral include the physician; the EPSDT program, and child abuse and neglect centers.

TABLE 9.11
Recommended Fluoride Supplementation

Age (years)	Concentration of fluoride in drinking water (mg/L)		
	< 0.3	0.3–0.6	> 0.6
0–0.5	0	0	0
0.5–3	0.25	0	0
3–6	0.5	0.25	0
6–16	1.0	0.5	0

Source: From Committee on Nutrition, American Academy of Pediatrics: Fluoride supplementation for children: interim policy recommendations, *Pediatrics;* 95:777, 1995.

TABLE 9.12
Federally Sponsored Food Assistance Programs for Infants, Children, and Adolescents

Program offered	Purpose of program	Administering agencies
Special Supplemental Nutrition Program for Women, Infants and Children (WIC)	Assist pregnant, lactating, and postpartum women and children up to five years of age in obtaining specified nutritious foods and nutrition education	USDA Food and Nutrition Services (FNS) and state and tribal health agencies
Commodity Supplemental Food Program (CSFP)	Provides pregnant, lactating, and postpartum women and children up to six years of age with supplemental foods and nutrition education	FNS and state and tribal agencies
School Lunch Program	Provides nutritious lunch to all children (some free or at reduced prices) attending participating schools; educates children about nutritious food habits	FNS and state educational agencies
School Breakfast Program	Provides nutritious breakfast to all children (some free or at reduced prices) attending participating schools	FNS and state educational agencies
Child and Adult Care Food Program	Provides cash reimbursements and/or commodities for nonresidential child-care institutions including family day care and day-care centers	FNS and state educational agencies and public or private not-for-profit day-care center
Summer Food Service Program	Provides nutritious meals for preschool and school children participating in schools, recreation centers, or camps during the summertime	FNS and state educational agencies; governmental agencies; and public and private not-for-profit residential summer camps
Food Stamp Program	Assist family in providing nutritious meals	FNS and state welfare agencies

CHILDREN

A young child's growth rate slows considerably from the first year of age. Toddlers (one and two years old) gain only from 2 to 4 kg (5 to 10 lb) each year. Preschoolers (three through five years old) have still a slower rate of growth, averaging from 1 to 2 kg (3 to 5 lb) each year. As a result of this significant slowing down in growth, the toddler and the preschooler often require less food and their appetites decrease. Between ages one and two, children learn to feed themselves independently. They progress from eating with their hands to using utensils. Messiness and spilling are the rule during the first half of the second year, but by age two hand-to-mouth coordination has noticeably improved. Children should be allowed to try new skills over and over again. Hallmark characteristics of toddlers are curiosity and independence. Exploration of the environment is enabled by the child's increasing mobility, manipulation, and attempts at various activities. During the preschool years (ages three to five) there is a greater increase in height relative to weight; the "chubby" appearing toddler becomes a leaner preschooler. Each child will grow at his or her own rate as determined by heredity, state of health, and nutritional adequacy of the diet.

Compared to the preschool and adolescent periods, the mid-childhood years (from age six to onset of puberty) are relatively stable with regard to growth rate and behavior. Height and weight vary greatly among children because of genetic and environmental influences, but for an individual child growth is usually slow and steady. In spite of a relatively slow growth rate, nutrition still plays an important role by (1) providing building materials for growth, (2) furnishing the energy needed for the vigorous physical activities of the age group, (3) helping to maintain resistance to infection, and (4) providing adequate nutrient stores to assist in adolescent growth.

Nutritional Requirements

Energy   Energy requirements for a child must allow for basal metabolism, the specific dynamic action of food, losses in excreta, muscular activity, and growth. The average energy requirement for basal metabolism during the first twelve to eighteen months is 55 kcal/kg body weight. Thereafter, the requirement on a weight-specific basis gradually declines to an adult level of 25 to 30 kcal/kg. As children grow older, caloric intake increases because of the larger body size, but the need for energy per unit weight decreases. Recommended energy intakes of children are 102 kcal/kg (1,300 kcal) for ages one to three years, 90 kcal/kg (1,800 kcal) for ages four to six years, and 70 kcal/kg (2,000 kcal) for ages seven to ten years (table 9.13).

Protein   Protein needs for growth decrease as the rate of growth declines. On a weight-specific basis, protein requirements decrease from the first month of life through childhood and adolescence. Safe levels of protein intake, assuming an adequate intake of energy, are approximately 1.2 g/kg per day at ages one to three years, 1.1 g/kg per

T A B L E   9.13
Recommended Levels for Individual Intake of Nutrients

	1–3 years	4–8 years
Weight (kg)	13	20
Energy (kcal)	1,300	1,800
Protein (g)	16	24
Vitamin A (μg RE)	400	500
Vitamin D (μg)	5	5
Vitamin E (mg TE)	6	7
Vitamin C (mg)	40	45
Folate (μg)	150	200
Niacin (mg NE)	6	8
Riboflavin (mg)	0.5	0.6
Thiamin (mg)	0.5	0.6
Vitamin B_6 (mg)	0.5	0.6
Vitamin B_{12} (μg)	0.9	1.2
Calcium (mg)	500	800
Phosphorus (mg)	460	500
Iodine (μg)	70	90
Iron (mg)	10	10
Magnesium (mg)	80	130
Zinc (mg)	10	10

RE, retinol equivalents; TE, tocopherol equivalents; NE, niacin equivalents.
Sources: Data from National Research Council, *Recommended Dietary Allowances,* ed. 10, Washington, DC, 1989, National Academy Press, and for selected nutrients: From Institute of Medicine: *Dietary reference intakes for calcium, phosphorus, magnesium, vitamin D, and fluoride,* Washington, DC, 1997, National Academy Press; and, Food and Nutrition Board, National Academy of Sciences—Institute of Medicine: *Recommended levels for individual intake of B vitamins and choline,* Washington, DC, 1998, National Academy Press. (see chapter 2 and inside back cover)

Note: There are differences between the 1989 RDAs and the 1997/1998 recommended levels for individual intake of nutrients with respect to methods of derivation and age-groupings. However, space does not allow separate tables for the 1997/1998 recommended levels for individual intakes of nutrients. Accordingly, the authors devised this table to summarize currently available data. It is not an official document developed or approved by the Food and Nutrition Board, Institute of Medicine, National Research Council, National Academy of Sciences.

day at ages four to six years, and 1.0 g/kg per day at ages seven to ten years.

Lipids   Linoleic acid is an essential nutrient for children and adults, the estimated requirement being between 1 and 2 percent of total calories in the diet. In children without a family history of hyperlipidemia, it is not clear whether diets low in saturated fats reduce the likelihood of adult **atherosclerosis.** In general, it is recommended that total fat consumption should be an average of no more than 30 percent of total calories and saturated fatty acids should be no more than 10 percent of total calories.

Minerals   During childhood, there is a progressive increase in mineral content of the body. The three major groups of minerals include (1) sodium, potassium, calcium, and magnesium; (2) chlorine, phosphorus, and sulfur; and (3) iron, iodine, and trace elements. Sodium and potassium requirements for growing children are met easily because most foods contain an abundant supply. Calcium required during growth is estimated to be 50 to 70 mg/kg per day. The recommended dietary allowance for calcium in children one to ten years of age is 800 mg/day. Exact magnesium requirements are not known for young children. Almost 16 percent of ingested magnesium is retained with 50 percent deposited in bone. The usual diet is assumed to contain an adequate amount of magnesium. A requirement has been set at 6 mg/kg per day.

The importance of iron in the diets of children has long been recognized. The dietary allowance of 10 mg/day is recommended for children one to ten years of age. Inadequate dietary intake of iron and reduced body stores of iron are reflected first in lower levels of serum ferritin, then in lower levels of serum iron and transferrin saturation, and ultimately in lower levels of hemoglobin. The hemoglobin level should be 110 g/L or higher until age five years and then 115 g/L or higher until age twelve years.

Nutrition-Related Problems

The most common manifestations of nutrition problems during childhood include anemia, obesity, and dental caries. Hyperlipidemia must also be considered.

Anemia   The child who suffers from anemia is usually pale and lethargic, tires easily, has a short attention span and decreased ability to concentrate, and is susceptible to infection. Iron deficiency, the most common cause of anemia among children, is most prevalent between ages one and three years. Iron-deficient children perform poorly on vocabulary, reading, mathematics, problem-solving, and psychological tests. It is important that iron deficiency anemia be prevented in infancy and early childhood so that these problems can be avoided.

Treatment of anemia of childhood usually involves the use of iron salts at levels providing from 3 to 4 mg of elemental iron/kg per day, often in conjunction with supplemental vitamin C, until hemoglobin levels have been restored to normal. This treatment regimen includes a diet high in iron-rich foods such as meat, iron-enriched cereal grain products, and fruits and vegetables.

Obesity   Childhood or **juvenile-onset obesity** is one of the most prevalent nutrition problems among children. There is no single definition of obesity; therefore, prevalence estimates range from 20 to 30 percent. Obesity is often defined as a "weight-for-height" greater than the ninety-fifth percentile according to the NCHS growth charts. An alternative definition is a body weight greater than 120 percent of the median weight-for-height. Using reference charts such as the NCHS growth charts can be a problem because children vary greatly in the timing of weight and height growth spurts. Childhood obesity is best avoided because it is difficult to treat and tends to persist into adult life.

Parents who may unwittingly establish a pattern of overfeeding infants and young children represent part of the problem. Physical inactivity on the part of the children represents another part of the problem. Working with children and parents and caretakers on appropriate food choices and eating habits and increasing physical activity are essential components of management. Encouraging a child to adopt a pattern of eating that allows growth into his or her weight has met with more success than attempting to bring about an actual weight loss. Sound programs for treatment or prevention should be individualized, nutritionally sound, psychologically acceptable, supportive of social needs, diversified, and based on the premise that there is a wide range of acceptable body sizes and shapes.

Dental Caries   Diet and nutrition have an important role in the development of dental caries. Cariogenicity of a child's diet is related more to frequency of intake of sugar-containing foods that remain in the mouth and/or cling to the teeth than to the total amount of sugar in the diet. Preventive actions include restricting sugar-containing foods to mealtime and brushing teeth immediately after eating sugar-containing foods. The practice of putting the infant to bed with a bottle containing milk, formula, or fruit juice (particularly sweet-ened fruit juice) or giving the older infant or young toddler the bottle containing fruit juice as a "pacifier" should simply be avoided.

Atherosclerosis   Available evidence suggest that atherosclerosis may begin in early childhood and that serum cholesterol levels in children are predictors of levels in adult life. Whether there should be universal screening for children's cholesterol levels has been debated. The National Cholesterol Education Program (**NCEP**) Expert Panel on Cholesterol in Children and Adolescents[28] and the AAP[2] recommend two strategies to reduce elevated cholesterol levels: a population approach and an individualized approach. The individualized approach is directed toward identifying and managing individual children and adolescents with elevated serum cholesterol levels and who have a family history of hyperlipidemia and/or premature heart disease. The population approach for dietary intervention for children age two years and older has the following recommendations: nutritional adequacy of the diet should be achieved by using a variety of foods; energy (calories) should be sufficient to support growth and development and to reach or maintain a desirable body weight; daily fat intake should be an average of no more than 30 percent of total calories; intake of saturated fat should be no more than 10 percent of total calories; and consumption of dietary cholesterol should be less than 300 mg/day.

These population recommendations are the same as those for adults and affirm a healthful diet shared by the whole family. Because of the on-going development of the central nervous system, dietary fat should not be limited for toddlers between ages one and two years.

Feeding Patterns

In reviewing the food habits of any child, it is important to keep in mind nutritional requirements, culture, socioeconomic status, and family dynamics as they influence the individual. By age eighteen months to two years, many toddlers are reasonably adept at feeding themselves. Individual dietary preferences appear, and the child should be allowed to choose food he or she likes. Toddlers often prefer small, frequent feedings of finger foods and often reject or simply pick at a prepared meal. This behavior should not alarm the parent or caretaker or be perceived as a challenge to adult authority. Parents who are distraught over the eating

patterns of toddlers often can be reassured that atypical (by adult standards) eating behaviors are normal during this period of exploration and experimentation.

By age five years, children can effectively use knives and forks. There are increased opportunities for socializing through preschool and school experiences with exposures to new foods and new practices. Asking children to assist in preparing or serving a new food often will permit them to overcome reluctance to experiment with new foods. Table 9.14 outlines food intake according to food groups and number of servings at different stages of the life cycle.

Guidelines for Nutrition Care in Childhood

Guidelines for nutritional assessment and intervention in children are described in table 9.8. Nutrition assessment of young children occurs routinely in WIC programs, Head Start programs, and in physicians offices during routine child health visits. Weight and height are commonly monitored in schools for school-age children and in periodic clinic visits.

The expected health outcomes for a normal child include the following:

- Maintains height for age between the fifth and ninety-fifth percentiles on the NCHS growth chart.
- Maintains weight-for-height between the fifth and ninety-fifth percentiles on the NCHS growth chart.
- Does not deviate more than twenty-five percentile points from his or her established growth pattern (height or weight) on the NCHS growth chart.
- Hemoglobin and/or hematocrit determinations are within acceptable levels.
- Consumes types and amounts of foods in frequencies appropriate for age, body size, and physical activity.

Nutrition Assessment

Anthropometric Assessment   Weight and stature (standing height) measurements should be completed for preschool children. Head circumference should be measured until three years of age. From school age through adolescence, anthropometric measurements should include weight and stature. Triceps skinfold thickness is also frequently used in sports physicals and weight management programs.

Weight   Children who can stand without assistance are weighed standing on the scale and wearing only light-

TABLE 9.14
Food Guide for Healthy Children and Adolescents to Meet Nutrient Needs
Recommended Number of Daily Servings

Age Group	Fruits/vegetables	Cereal grain	Dairy*	Animal or vegetable protein+ (oz)	Fats/oils (tsp)
Toddler					
1–2	5–9	7–11	2	3–4	2
2–3	5–9	7–11	2	3–4	6
Children					
4–6	5–9	7–11	2	3–4	8
7–10	5–9	7–11	2	5–7	8
Adolescents					
Female					
11–18	5–9	7–11	3	5–7	8
19–24	5–9	7–11	3	5–7	6
Male					
11–14	7–9	7–11	3	7	8
15–18	7–9	9–11	3	7	10
19–24	7–9	9–11	3	7	8

*Serving size of fluid milk = 8 oz. Use low-fat or nonfat products after age three years.
+Use low-fat or lean protein foods (animal and vegetable).
Note: Physically active children and adolescents going through growth spurts may require larger amounts of foods.
Source: Adapted from Kizer KW: *The California daily food guide: dietary guidance for Californians,* Sacramento, 1990, California Department of Health Services.

weight undergarments. The scale should be located in an area that ensures privacy. The child stands over the center of the platform with heels together. The reading is made when the child is standing still. Weight should be recorded to the nearest 100 g (or ¼ lb). Consistency of equipment, technique, and weight units (i.e., kilograms or pounds) is important to avoid unnecessary sources of error in determining, documenting, and interpreting weight measurements.

Stature   Children between two and three years of age can be measured in the recumbent (see figure 9.6) or standing position, depending on their ability to cooperate during the procedure. It is essential to note whether length (recumbent) or stature (standing height) was measured because length is greater than stature by as much as 2 cm (nearly 1 in.). Thus, interpretation of measurements will be difficult if it is not known (recorded) whether length or stature was measured or if length was measured on one occasion and stature on another.

Children aged three years and older must be measured standing. Measurements of stature require a measuring stick or nonstretchable tape attached to a verti-

cal, flat surface, such as a wall. A guide for a right-angle headboard also is needed. Measuring rods on platform scales should not be used to measure stature. The child should wear only underclothes, so that the stance can be seen clearly. The child should stand with arms at sides and shoulders relaxed, knees should be straight with bare heels together on the floor, and with back of the head, shoulder blades, buttocks, and heels touching the wall (figure 9.7).

The child should be asked to "stand tall," take a deep breath, and look straight ahead so the line of vision is perpendicular to the wall. Then the head board is lowered against the guide onto the crown of the head. The measurer's eyes should be level with the headboard to avoid errors caused by parallax. With the headboard in place, the measurement is made and recorded to the nearest 0.1 cm (⅛ in.). NCHS growth charts (appropriate for age and gender) should be used to monitor the child's growth.*

Triceps Skinfold Thickness   This is a measurement of a double thickness of skin and subcutaneous fat on the back of the upper arm.[33] It is not recommended as a routine screening measurement in well-child care, however, it may be useful in follow-up and monitoring of children who are identified as overweight or obese.

*Updated NCHS growth charts will be released sometime in 1998.

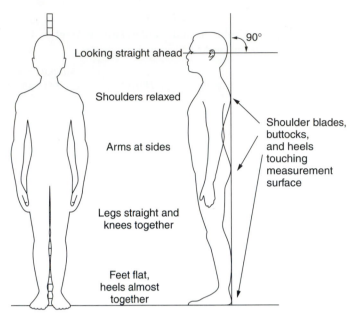

Looking straight ahead

Shoulders relaxed

Arms at sides

Legs straight and knees together

Feet flat, heels almost together

90°

Shoulder blades, buttocks, and heels touching measurement surface

FIGURE 9.7   Positioning Children for Height Measurement

Biochemical Assessment   Because anemia is a problem in one- to three-year-olds, the initial screening should include hemoglobin and hematocrit determinations. Acceptable levels are shown in table 9.8.

When serum lipid levels are determined, 170 mg/dl is used as the cutoff point for total cholesterol and 110 mg/dl for LDL (low-density lipoprotein) cholesterol in children two through seventeen years with familial risk factors.

When blood lead levels are determined on preschool children, a cutoff point of 10 µg/dl is used. Two groups of children are at risk for an elevated blood lead level: (1) those who live near lead mining and smeltering operations and (2) those living in older housing, particularly in older urban communities. Among low-income preschool children living in an urban community, significant positive associations were found between blood lead and fat intake.[25] There is some evidence that stimulation of bile flow during fat digestion may contribute to increased absorption of lead.

Dietary Assessment   Dietary assessment is used to obtain presumptive evidence of dietary deficiencies or excesses in individuals. The most commonly used instruments for assessment of the diet are the twenty-four-hour recall of food intake or some type of food frequency questionnaire. Both techniques have limitations with respect to estimating adequacy of nutrient intakes over time. Variations in food intake over time, including day-to-day variation and periodic variation (day-of-the-week effects and effects related to timing of household income), is the major problem related to use of the twenty-four-hour recall to infer usual intake.

Although most food frequency questionnaires provide some measure of the nutritional quality of the diet and information about food patterns useful in epidemiologic studies, they were not designed to provide estimates of nutrient intakes of individuals. It has been suggested that twenty-four-hour recall and food frequency questionnaires not be used to identify *nutrient inadequacy,* although with modification they may be useful for identifying *inappropriate diet.*[22] Techniques of dietary assessment are discussed in detail in chapter 3.

Clinical Assessment   Screening children for hypertension has become routine in many clinics. Blood pressure during childhood and adolescence varies according to age, sex, and height.[29] Elevated blood pressures are those that are greater than the ninety-fifth percentile for age, sex, and height. More detailed information on assessment of blood pressure is available in the original report.[29]

Nutrition Intervention, Counseling, and Education

Head Start is a model day-care program that was initiated as an eight-week summer program by the Office of Economic Opportunity in 1965. It is now a full-year program administered by the Administration of Children, Youth and Families, Department of Health and Human Services. The goal is to provide low-income preschool children with a comprehensive program based on their special educational, psychological, health, and nutrition needs. Nutrition education is provided to the children and their parents, and the meal service is used as an educational tool.

Major vehicles for nutrition education in elementary and secondary schools are the School Breakfast and School Lunch Programs administered by the USDA and state departments of education (discussed in chapter 5). In 1977, Congress passed Public Law 95-166 as part of the National School Lunch Act and Child Nutrition Amendments, which authorized the Nutrition Education Training (NET) Program to fund projects to teach children about the relation between food and health, train food service personnel, instruct teachers to teach nutrition in their classrooms, and develop and use innovative classroom materials and curricula. The current status of this program is questionable. Use of the Dietary Guidelines for Americans and the Food Guide Pyramid have been emphasized in both classroom and meal service settings during the past several years.

The American Dietetic Association (ADA) has supported the Dietary Guidelines for Americans in child nutrition programs, including school meal programs, but has recommended consideration be given to development of specific dietary guidelines for healthy children that would take into account children's needs for growth and development and support health promotion and disease prevention.[44] A joint position statement is shown in box 9.2.

BOX 9.2

JOINT POSITION STATEMENT

It is the position of The American Dietetic Association, the Society of Nutrition Education and the American School Food Service Association that Comprehensive school-based nutrition programs and services be provided to all of the nation's elementary and secondary students. The programs and services include: effective education in food and nutrition; a school environment that provides opportunity and reinforcement for healthful eating and physical activity; involvement of parents and community; and, screening, counseling and referral for nutrition problems as part of school health services.[39]

Referral

Federal food assistance programs available to children include WIC (preschoolers), School Breakfast, School Lunch, Summer Feeding, Special Milk, and Child Care Food programs. In addition, food stamps and commodity foods are available to families (see pages 130 to 133 in chapter 5).

ADOLESCENTS

Adolescence, the transition from childhood to adulthood, is accompanied by a series of physical, physiological, biochemical, hormonal, and psychological changes. A time of wide variability in norms of growth, adolescence lasts nearly a decade with no specific beginning or end. Progress in the individual is characterized by orderly sequence, but there is marked variation between sexes and between individuals in timing, intensity of change, and deviation in the process. This period is usually described in two phases: pubescence and adolescence. Pubescence, which includes the adolescent growth spurt (average age is nine to thirteen for females and twelve to sixteen for males), begins with the first increase in hormonal secretion and appearance of secondary sex characteristics (increase in breast size in females and external genitalia in males and appearance of pubic hair) and ends when sexual reproduction becomes possible. Adolescence (average age is ten to seventeen years for females and twelve to twenty-one years for males) is the period beginning with the appearance of sexual maturity and terminating with the cessation of growth in stature.

The dramatic increase in physical size and development during the transition from childhood to adulthood creates substantial nutritional demands. In normal healthy girls, on the average, the growth spurt begins at 9.5 years, peak height velocity occurs at age 11.8 years, stage 2 breast development occurs at 11.2 years, and menarche at 12.4 years. Normal variations around the average are noted, as for any biological phenomenon, but menarche before nine years or after age sixteen years is considered outside the normal range. In addition to bone and muscle, a significant component of weight gain in the girl during this growth spurt in girls is adipose tissue. Males begin their pubescent growth spurt approximately two years later than females. Onset of male adolescence, in the nine- to twelve-year range, is accompanied by production of gonadotropin, which stimulates enlargement of the testes. Skeletal growth continues at an accelerated rate, reaching an annual peak of approximately 10.3 cm (4 in.) at age 14.1 years. Associated changes in muscle mass, voice, and physical skills are noted. Linear growth almost ceases at around age eighteen years, although some boys continue to grow taller well into their twenties. Weight gain in males during this period is predominantly an increase in bone and muscle mass.

Hormonal Influences

Although the sex hormones exert a major controlling influence, many other hormones participate in adolescent development. Growth hormone, somatotropin, a polypeptide produced by the pituitary, stimulates protein anabolism at the cellular level. Thyroid hormones influence overall body growth and skeletal maturation. The metabolic effects of the thyroid hormones include increases in oxygen consumption, heat production, nitrogen retention, protein synthesis, glucose absorption, and gluconeogenesis. Insulin has an indirect effect on growth by increasing the uptake and metabolism of glucose and synthesis of fatty acids. It also stimulates transport of amino acids into cells and catalyzes incorporation of amino acids into protein. Estrogen influences development and maintenance of secondary sex characteristics and reproductive functions. Estrogen results in significant morphological, physiological, and behavior changes by regulating the secretion of follicle-stimulating hormone and luteinizing hormone by the pituitary, thereby increasing uterine size and inducing vaginal cornification. Progesterone, secreted by the ovaries, causes changes in the uterine endometrium (lining of the uterus) and is responsible for the cyclic changes in the vagina and also is involved in maturation of breast function.

Nutrient Requirements

Nutrient requirements peak during the years of maximum growth. For practicality, the RDAs during the adolescent period are divided into chronological, rather than maturational or biological, age groups. The RDAs for males and females nine to thirteen and fourteen to eighteen years are shown in table 9.15.

There are a few direct experimental data on which to base nutrient requirements, particularly vitamins and minerals, of adolescents. Except for energy, RDAs for adolescents are extrapolated from adult studies. Nutrient needs are greatest during the adolescent growth spurt and gradually decrease as the individual achieves physical and sexual maturity. The adolescent growth spurt contributes about 50 percent to young adult body weight and 15 percent to final adult height. The peak

TABLE 9.15
Recommended Levels for Individual Intake of Nutrients

	Males		Females	
	9–13	14–18	9–13	14–18
Weight (kg)	45	66	46	55
Energy (kcal)	2,500	3,000	2,200	2,200
Protein (g)	45	59	46	44
Vitamin A (μg RE)	1,000	1,000	800	800
Vitamin D (μg)	5	5	5	5
Vitamin E (mg TE)	10	10	8	8
Vitamin C (mg)	50	60	50	60
Folate (μg)	300	400	300	400
Niacin (mg NE)	12	16	12	14
Riboflavin (mg)	0.9	1.3	0.9	1.0
Thiamin (mg)	0.9	1.2	0.9	1.0
Vitamin B_6 (mg)	1.0	1.0	1.0	1.2
Vitamin B_{12} (μg)	1.8	2.4	1.8	2.4
Calcium (mg)	1,300	1,300	1,300	1,300
Phosphorus (mg)	1,250	1,250	1,250	1,250
Iodine (μg)	150	150	150	150
Iron (mg)	12	12	15	15
Magnesium (mg)	240	410	240	360
Zinc (mg)	15	15	12	12

RE, retinol equivalents; TE, tocopherol equivalents; NE, niacin equivalents.
Sources: Data from National Research Council, *Recommended dietary allowances,* ed. 10, Washington, DC, 1989, National Academy Press, and for selected nutrients: data from Institute of Medicine: *Dietary reference intakes for calcium, phosphorus, magnesium, vitamin D, and fluoride,* Washington, DC, 1997, National Academy Press; and, Food and Nutrition Board, National Academy of Sciences—Institute of Medicine: *Recommended levels for individual intake of B vitamins and choline,* Washington, DC, 1998, National Academy Press. (see chapter 2 and inside back cover)

Note: There are differences between the 1989 RDAs and the 1997/1998 recommended levels for individual intake of nutrients with respect to methods of derivation and age-groupings. However, space does not allow separate tables for the 1997/1998 recommended levels for individual intake of nutrients. Accordingly, the authors devised this table to summarize currently available data. It is not an official document developed or approved by the Food and Nutrition Board, Institute of Medicine, National Research Council, National Academy of Sciences.

energy value for females is at eleven to sixteen years (2,200 kcal), but for males it is of greater magnitude (3,000 kcal) and occurs later, at fifteen to eighteen years. Thus, the male has a higher allowance for energy within which to meet requirements for other essential nutrients. The female, with lower energy needs, must select foods of high nutrient density to meet all of her nutrient needs without consuming more calories than needed.

Energy The requirements for energy vary widely from one individual to another, not only because of different timing and magnitude of somatic growth, but also because of variations in physical activity. Age or weight alone is not a useful predictor of energy needs. The single measurement that best predicts energy needs in adolescence is height, because it usually correlates well with physiological development.

Protein, Carbohydrates, and Lipids Protein allowances, like those for energy and the micronutrients, follow the growth pattern. During adolescence, the highest protein allowance (59 g) for males begins at fifteen years and persists through adulthood; for females, the protein allowance (46 g) peaks at eleven to fourteen years. Most adolescents consume protein in excess of these amounts. Limitation of either protein or energy intakes during the accelerated phase of growth has been repeatedly demonstrated to inhibit growth. Adolescents who restrict intake to control weight, "make weight" for athletic competition (e.g., wrestling), or because of eating disorders are at risk of stunting. No allowances have been established for carbohydrates or lipids. Carbohydrates are of particular importance to the adolescent who participates in athletic competition.

Vitamins and Minerals There is a paucity of information concerning vitamin and mineral requirements of adolescents. Few data are based on measurements of adolescents and recommended levels are extrapolations from adult and child studies with built-in safety factors. With the increase in energy demands, rates of tissue synthesis, and skeletal growth associated with adolescence, it can be expected that vitamin needs are elevated. To meet the increased energy demands, higher-than-normal-adult levels of thiamin (B_1), riboflavin (B_2), and niacin are necessary. Folate and vitamin B_{12}, both required for tissue growth, have increased requirements. In addition, skeletal growth necessitates adequate vitamin D intake. Vitamins A, C, and E are all essential to maintain biologic function of this new tissue.

Calcium Calcium needs are greater during adolescence than in either childhood or adulthood. During the adolescent growth spurt, about 45 percent of the adult skeletal mass is formed. Consequently, the RDA for calcium increases from 800 mg for children four to eight years of age to 1,300 mg for both males and females from nine to eighteen years of age. The need to consume good sources of calcium such as dairy foods is important for bone health during adolescence and beyond.

Iron The need for dietary iron increases during the adolescent growth spurt, particularly for males, because of the expansion of blood volume and muscle mass. Females require less iron for growth but must replace menstrual iron losses. Iron needs are related closely to lean body mass, with males requiring 42 mg/kg of weight gain and females needing 31 mg/kg of weight gain. When growth is rapid in males, they may require more iron than menstruating females, but once growth slows down, the female's iron needs surpass those of males.

The recommended iron intake of 12 mg/day for males nine to eighteen years, an additional 2 mg/day more than in children, is to cover the adolescent growth spurt that occurs between ten and seventeen years. In females, the recommended intake of 15 mg/day, starting at age nine years, an additional 5 mg/day more than children, is to cover the adolescent growth spurt and menstruation and continues through child-bearing years.

Although iron is most easily absorbed from meat (heme iron), absorption from plant (nonheme iron) sources, such as legumes and green vegetables, can be significantly enhanced by eating these foods along with meat and foods high in vitamin C. The major sources of nonheme iron are fortified cereals and bread products. To meet the RDA of 12 to 15 mg, adolescents must consciously select iron-containing foods of high iron bioavailability.

Zinc Zinc is necessary for growth and sexual maturation. The recommended allowance for males is 15 mg/day and for females is 12 mg/day. It has been shown that many adolescents consume less zinc than they need, especially girls, who often consume less than half the RDA.

Psychological and Environmental Influences and Health Consequences

The nutritional health of American youths is better than in past decades. Except for iron deficiency, overt nutrient-deficiency diseases are not a public health problem. Problems of dietary imbalances and excesses are more common than nutrient deficiencies.[8,49] Certain dietary habits among adolescents may continue into adulthood, and along with other factors, increase the risk for chronic diseases (e.g., osteoporosis, heart disease, and some types of cancer). Inadequate nutrition during adolescence may retard or stunt linear growth, lower resistance to infections, impair learning ability and performance, adversely affect the ability to function at peak physical capacity, and diminish quality of life and life span for those with chronic illness. Many factors impinge on and modify the adolescent's diet. Most teenagers are preoccupied with physical appearance, body shape and size, and peer acceptance. A strong desire to be lean and to have a particular body image can result in inappropriate weight reduction, dietary aberrations, and selective widely distributed nutrient deficiencies. Chronic dieters are at high risk for inadequate nutrient intake, depleted nutrient stores, and malnutrition. In adolescent females, such behavior may lead to the serious eating disorders **anorexia nervosa** and bulimia nervosa.

Obesity   Overweight in adolescents is significantly associated with elevated levels of blood pressure, blood lipids, and plasma insulin and other factors known to be risk factors for obesity-related disease in adults.[4,5,8] Obesity appears to cluster in families so that intervention plans need to center around the family to include teaching appropriate dietary habits and physical activity and attention to body image rather than a restrictive dietary program.

Atherosclerosis   Major modifiable risk factors associated with atherosclerosis (hyperlipidemia, cigarette smoking, inactivity, hypertension, and diabetes) have their origins and behavioral development during adolescence. Altering smoking behavior, controlling blood pressure in hypertensive individuals, preventing obesity through physical activity and weight control, and modifying dietary fat intake to reduce serum cholesterol require more emphasis with adolescents.

Anorexia Nervosa   Anorexia nervosa is an eating disorder with serious underlying developmental and psychological disturbances. It is a syndrome of self-induced starvation characterized by voluntary refusal to eat because of a fear of becoming obese, as well as by extreme weight loss, amenorrhea, and body image disturbances. Surveys establish the prevalence at about one case per 100 adolescent girls. Management of adolescent females with anorexia nervosa depends on the stage and severity of the problem. Interventions include nutritional, medical, and psychological support. There is strong resistance to treatment, with a high incidence of relapse or only partial recovery.

Bulimia Nervosa   This disorder is distinct from anorexia nervosa. This syndrome is characterized by recurrent episodes of binge eating or engorging followed by self-induced vomiting, abuse of laxatives and diuretics, and vigorous exercise, but also maintenance of normal body weight and body shape. Today, many teenagers use vomiting as a method of weight control. The behavior may be reinforced among girls on athletic squads or when groups of young people, such as college students, live together.

Substance Abuse   Substance abuse among adolescents is a public health problem of major significance. Tobacco, alcohol, and illicit drugs are the substances most used by adolescents. In a 1993 national survey of high school seniors, 64 percent reported alcohol use in the previous 30 days and 4 percent reported daily consumption, 3 percent reported daily marijuana use, and 0.2 percent reported daily cocaine use.[30] More recent figures (1996) indicate the problems persist.[3] Chronic users are more vulnerable to nutrition problems because of either inadequate intake or in the case of alcohol, maldigestion and malabsorption. Alcohol use is as high among females as among males. Of particular concern is the pregnant adolescent who consumes alcohol and may have a marginal diet. She has the risk of producing a child with fetal alcohol syndrome plus nutrient deficiencies. Young people differ from adults in that they tend to drink less regularly but consume larger amounts at a time—binge drinking.

Tobacco   Cigarette smoking continues to be prevalent among teens despite the evidence of negative health effects. Along with perceived social benefits, smoking is recognized by teens for its effect on appetite and controlling body weight. Besides cigarettes, there is increased use of smokeless tobacco by children and adolescents. Complications of regular use of chewing tobacco and snuff include periodontal disease, oral cancer, hypertension, and dependence.

Sports and Athletics   Optimal nutrition is a basic requisite for training and maintaining good physical performance. Diets of athletes must supply optimal amounts of energy, protein, water, fat, carbohydrates, vitamins, and minerals. Energy is needed for growth as well as the extra energy expended in physical activity. Adequate hydration is a principal concern for adolescent athletes to combat fluid loss before, during, and after exercise or competition. A problem associated with excessive activity and inappropriate weight loss in females is amenorrhea, thought to be associated with a change in lean body mass/body fat radio. At particular risk are gymnasts, runners, and swimmers, who train intensely, with loss of body fat and concomitant gain in lean body mass.

Adolescents who exercise infrequently have a greater risk of becoming obese. Lack of exercise, coupled with the boredom that results in increased food intake, puts adolescents in double jeopardy for excessive accumulation of body fat. The increasing prevalence of adolescent obesity in the United States appears to be associated with an increasing evidence of non-insulin-dependent diabetes mellitus (**NIDDM**).[38] In 1994, NIDDM accounted for one third of the diagnoses of diabetes mellitus among adolescents in greater Cincinnati. Mean age of these patients was 13.8 years and mean body mass index (**BMI**) was 37.7 kg/m². As noted by Chua and Leibel,[6] "even transient obesity in adolescence may have a permanent impact on adult susceptibility to diabetes." The importance of physical activity during childhood and adolescence cannot be overemphasized.

The Child and Adolescent Trial for Cardiovascular Health (**CATCH**) was carried out between 1991 and 1994 in some 5,100 third-graders (initially) in ninety-six public schools in California, Louisiana, Minnesota, and Texas.[26] Interventions included school food service modification, enhanced physical education, and classroom health curricula in twenty-eight schools. The same interventions plus family education were carried out in another twenty-eight schools. Forty schools served as controls. In intervention schools, the percentage of energy intake from fat decreased significantly more (from 38.7 to 31.9 percent) than in control school lunches (from 38.9 to 36.2 percent). Intensity of physical activity in physical education classes increased significantly in the intervention schools as did the duration of vigorous physical activity. Although serum total cholesterol decreased slightly in the intervention school children from 170 to 168 mg/dl and in the control school children from 171 to 170 mg/dl, there were no significant differences between intervention and control groups with respect to serum cholesterol, blood pressure, or anthropometric measurements (weight, height, skinfold thickness) at the beginning or at the conclusion of the trial.

The investigators in this major study suggest that the effects of diet and exercise changes on serum total cholesterol and other physiological risk factors may have been obscured by developmental changes. Many of the children entered puberty during the study and "it may be more important for this age group to demonstrate the ability of the

program to modify nutrition and physical activity behaviors in ways leading to lifetime health habits rather than to reduce immediate physiological risk levels."[26]

Fast foods, fad diets, skipped meals, and high-carbohydrate foods are facts of life in our society. Condemnation of such dietary practices does little to win adolescents' confidence. Many fast foods are good sources of energy and selected nutrients. However, continued intake of a single class of foods eliminates variety and balance; further, skipping meals habitually can result in a low intake of selected nutrients or uncontrolled eating binges. Both practices are unhealthy. When nutritional guidance is needed, it should be provided without preconceived or culturally induced biases about the importance or quality of a particular food. A rational approach is to determine the nutritional contribution of the particular food to the adolescent's overall daily needs. Figure 9.8 describes the interrelations of factors influencing adolescent food consumption patterns. A prudent diet in moderation with appropriate snacks provides a diet that meets the nutrient requirements of adolescents.

Guidelines for Nutritional Management

The outcomes expected in working with adolescents include the following:

- Weight and height do not differ by more than twenty-five percentile points from his or her established growth pattern, as plotted on the NCHS growth chart.
- Consume appropriate types and amounts of food to meet energy and growth needs.
- Hemoglobin and hematocrit meet acceptable standards, as shown in table 9.8.

Nutrition Screening and Assessment   Physical examination, including evaluation of stage of sexual maturation, is the first step in medical evaluation. Anthropometric measurements, including weight, height, and skinfold thickness should also be done. Serum lipids should also be determined

Anthropometric   Height, weight, and skinfold thickness measurement should be made at least annually (see p. 249). It has been recommended that BMI should be used routinely to screen for overweight adolescents.[20] Individuals with BMIs greater than the ninety-fifth percentile for age and sex, or > 30 kg/m² should be considered overweight (see figure 9.9).* An approach to assess possible nutritional risk in adolescents in relation

---

*Updated NCHS growth charts will include BMI percentiles (rather than weight-to-height percentiles) for adolescents.

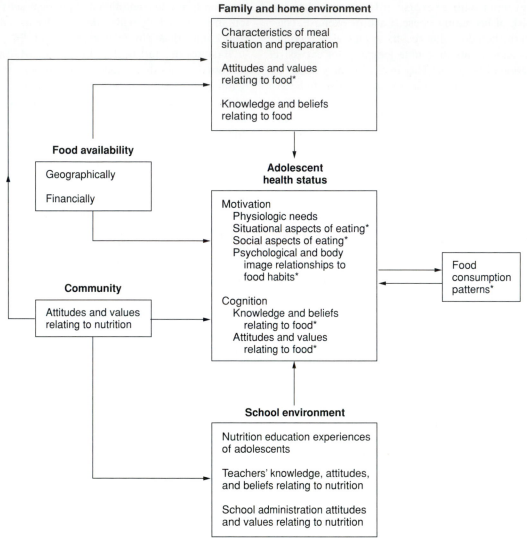

FIGURE 9.8   Interrelations of Factors Influencing Adolescent Food Consumption
*Factors investigated in the survey described and conducted in Edmonton.
Source: Adapted from Lund LA, Burk MC: *A multidisciplinary analysis of children's food consumption behavior,*
University of Minnesota's Agriculture Experimental Station Technical Bulletin 265, 1965, University of Minnesota Press.

to BMI level is shown in figure 9.10. Skinfold thickness (triceps and subscapular) measurements can be compared with reference percentiles.[33]

Biochemical Assessment   Because iron deficiency is still prevalent among adolescents, hemoglobin and/or hematocrit determinations should be made periodically as indicated.

As mentioned previously, the NCEP Children and Adolescents Panel[28] and the AAP Committee on Nutrition[2] have provided guidelines for selective screening

for hypercholesterolemia in children and adolescents: only children older than two years with family histories of hypercholesterolemia (total cholesterol > 240 mg/dl) or early atherosclerotic heart disease should be screened for hypercholesterolemia. The effectiveness of these recommendations was examined in urban African-American adolescents and it was found that more than half of those with increased LDL cholesterol levels could have been missed with the recommended selective screening.[41] In part, this reflects the fact that many of the adolescents in the study came to the clinic alone

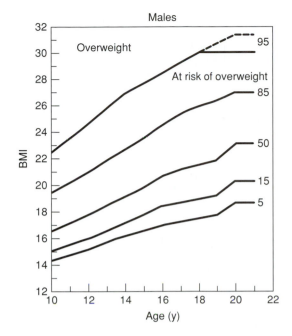

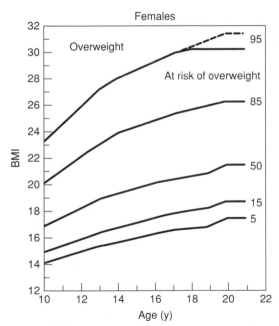

FIGURE 9.9 Recommended Percentiles of BMI (kg/m²) in Adolescents

Source: From Himes JH, Dietz WH: Guidelines for overweight in adolescent preventive services: recommendations from an expert committee, *Am J Clin Nutr;* 59:307–16, 1994. © *Am J Clin Nutr.* American Society for Clinical Nutrition. Reprinted with permission.

(unaccompanied by a parent) and apparently were not aware of the family history of hypercholesterolemia and premature coronary heart disease. Accordingly, these investigators recommended that total cholesterol and high-density lipoprotein (HDL) cholesterol be universally screened in nonfasting adolescents sixteen years of age and older. It will be of interest to determine if similar observations are made in other adolescent population groups.

IMPLICATIONS FOR COMMUNITY NUTRITION PROFESSIONALS

The period from infancy through adolescence is characterized by dramatic changes in body size, physiological functions, psychological development, and a move from complete dependence (infant) to independence (young adult).

The nutrition professional must be able to communicate effectively with parents or caretakers, in the case of infants and young children, and with older children and adolescents to have an early positive influence with respect to development of healthy lifestyles during childhood. Community nutrition professionals must exert more effort to develop and implement nutrition and physical activity interventions not only in preschool and school settings but must also develop and utilize other creative channels of communication in the public and the private sectors. Working with adolescents is particularly challenging. The community nutrition professional must provide pertinent information in engaging ways and be viewed by adolescent clients as helpful and an appropriate role model.

Quality Assurance Criteria set for Pediatric Nutrition Conditions, developed and periodically updated by the Pediatric Nutrition Practice Group of the American Dietetic Association, outline useful guidelines for nutrition services and their outcomes.[40] This criteria set is an important tool for community nutrition professionals in all settings where nutrition needs of infants, children and adolescents are identified and/or managed. Recently, the ADA's emphasis has been focused on medical nutrition therapy (MNT) of various disorders. It is expected that the 2nd edition of "MNT Across the Continuum of Care" will be released by ADA in the summer of 1998.

In the interest of overall child health, the reader may wish to refer to *Bright Futures: Guidelines for Health Supervision of Infants, Children and Adolescents.*[18]

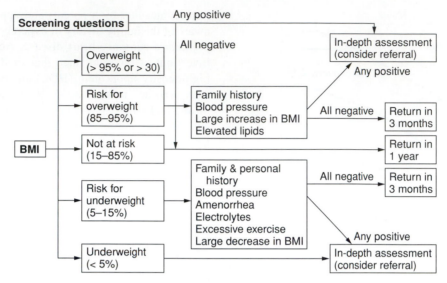

FIGURE 9.10 Algorithm to Guide Assessment for Possible Nutritional Risk in Adolescents
Source: From Skiba A, Loghamani E, Orr DP: Nutritional screening and guidance for adolescents, *AAP Adolescent Health Update;* 9(2), 1997. (Adapted from Himes JH, Dietz WH: Guidelines for overweight in adolescent preventive services: Recommendations from an expert committee, *Am J Clin Nutr* 59:307–316, 1994.

COMMUNITY NUTRITION PROFESSIONALS IN ACTION

- Identify strategies in your community that contribute to accomplishment of the Healthy People 2000 objectives for infants, children and adolescents.

- Which nutritional risks should community nutrition professionals be alert to throughout the stages of infancy, early childhood, school-age, and adolescence? Discuss reasons why nutritional risks change during these ages.

- Pick a controversy in child nutrition from one of the following, conduct a literature review, and discuss the pros and cons. Based on this information, what would you recommend?
  - The use of whole cow's milk until age two years is being challenged. Some research indicates children under two years who drink 2 percent milk grow just fine. Should whole cow's milk or low-fat milk be given to one- and two-year-old children? Why?
  - Iron supplementation in breast-fed infants is a very controversial topic. What is your position on supplementing or not supplementing? Why?
  - Some say juvenile-onset obesity should be aggressively treated to prevent lifelong obesity and its associated psychosocial and medical risks; others

take a conservative approach to see if the child will grow out of the overweight. What stand would you take?

- You have been providing nutrition intervention to a six-year-old boy who weighs 36 kg and is 112 cm tall. You are concerned because, even though his mother says she is following your recommendations, the boy has continued to gain weight during the past month. Determine his ideal weight and his nutritional requirements. Set up a meal plan for him incorporating foods from his school breakfast and school lunch. Should a school nurse become involved in his weight management plan? Is there anyone else at school to get involved? How can the boy's compliance with the meal plan be more closely monitored?

- Investigate the extent to which local hospitals promote and support breast-feeding. Have their past efforts increased the rate of breast-feeding? In view of current hospital management, do you think there is anything more that can be done in hospitals to increase the breast-feeding rate?

- Visit a school lunch program. Observe food preparation techniques and meal service. Interview cooks, servers, and the director, as well as children. What nutrition guidelines and regulations must schools follow? How have these changed over the past ten to fifteen years? How do menu plans match guidelines and students' taste preferences? Analyze the menus for a week. Do they meet guidelines? Based on your observations, what conclusions can you make and what recommendations would you give the school?

- Create a user-friendly directory of food and nutrition programs, projects, and clinical services that could be used as a referral guide when nutrition-related needs and problems of infants, children, and adolescents are identified. Include program eligibility requirements, enrollment processes, service or benefits, and contact persons.

- You have been invited to give a thirty-minute talk on child nutrition to a group of low-income parents. Prepare and outline what you plan to discuss. The organizer has asked you to include recommendations of some good reference books and materials for parents. What would you recommend?

- Ask an adolescent family member, neighbor, or acquaintance to keep a three-day food record. Analyze the nutritional adequacy of the food intake using a computer nutrient analysis program and the Food Guide Pyramid. What can you conclude about this person's dietary intake using these two methods of analysis?

- Interview at least six or eight adolescents aged thirteen to eighteen about their eating habits and food and nutrition concerns. What issues are mentioned most often? Are concerns different among younger and older adolescents? Based on this, what practical advice would you give people planning nutrition programs for adolescents?

- Watch two hours of children's programming on Saturday morning television. What food messages are directed to children in programs and in commercials? Write a letter to the network voicing your concerns or your compliments.

GOING ONE STEP FURTHER

- Identify existing data sources that give clues to nutrition related problems occurring among infants, children, or adolescents in your community. Summarize known information and outline additional data needs to accurately describe nutrition problems and their determinants.

- Review the findings from the evaluation of one of the federal child nutrition programs such as School Breakfast, School Lunch, Child and Adult Care Food Program, or WIC. Based on the evaluation results,

should the program be changed in any way to produce better results? Describe.

- Select a problem that is prevalent among infants, children, or adolescents (e.g., obesity, dental caries, etc.). Outline strategies to combat this problem. Differentiate strategies designed for primary intervention from strategies for treatment (secondary prevention).

- Review the Quality Assurance Indicators for Pediatric Conditions and the Nutrition Guidelines from *Bright Futures*. Which of these indicators and guidelines are relevant for application in community-based programs such as Head Start and WIC?

- Review the evidence for the effectiveness of nutrition education programs directed to children reported in the *Journal of Nutrition Education* in the November-December 1995 issue. Using the findings and recommendations, design a nutrition education program for children.

ADDITIONAL INFORMATION

Professional societies develop statements, scientific status summaries, commentaries, and position papers to clarify an issue in which the particular society has expertise.

The American Dietetic Association (ADA) Position Statements relevant to chapter 9 are listed below:

1. Child food and nutrition programs, *J Am Diet Assoc* 96:913, 1996.
2. ADA Supports National Association of WIC Directors position on breastfeeding promotion in the WIC program, *J Am Diet Assoc* 90:8, 1990.
3. Nutrition services for children with special health needs, *J Am Diet Assoc* 95:809, 1995.
4. Nutrition standards for child care programs, *J Am Diet Assoc* 94:323, 1994.
5. Promotion of breast-feeding, *J Am Diet Assoc* 97:662, 1997.
6. School-based nutrition programs and services, *J Am Diet Assoc* 95:369, 1995. ADA, Society for Nutrition Education and American School Food Service Association Joint Position.

Timely Statements

1. Nutrition guidance for child athletes in organized sports, *J Am Diet Assoc* 96:610, 1996.
2. Nutrition guidance for adolescent athletes in organized sports, *J Am Diet Assoc* 96:611, 1996.

REFERENCES

1. Auestad N, Montalto MB, Hall RT, et al: Visual acuity, erythrocyte fatty acid composition, and growth in term infants fed formulas with long chain polyunsaturated fatty acids for one year, *Pediatr Res* 41:1–10, 1997.

2. American Academy of Pediatrics, Committee on Nutrition: Statement on cholesterol, *Pediatrics* 90:469–473, 1992.

3. American Academy of Pediatrics, Committee on Substance Abuse: Testing for drugs of abuse in children and adolescents, *Pediatrics* 98:305–307, 1996.

4. Baumgartner RN, Siervogel RM, Chumlea WC, Roche AF: Association between plasma lipoprotein cholesterols, adiposity and adipose distribution during adolescence, *Int J Obesity* 13:31–41, 1989.

5. Burke GL, Webber LS, Srimivason SR, et al: Fasting plasma glucose and insulin levels and their relationship to cardiovascular risk factors in children: Bogalusa Heart Study, *Metabolism* 35:441–446, 1986.

6. Chua SC, Leibel RL: An ounce of prevention, *J Pediatr* 128:591–592, 1996.

7. D. Clark (CDC), B. Dobson (Iowa), D. Krauter (Massachusetts), A. Shoemaker (Arizona), personal communication. 1997.

8. Clarke WR, Woolson RF, Lauer RM: Changes in ponderosity and blood pressure in childhood: the Muscatine Study, *Am J Epidemiol* 124:195–206, 1986.

9. Committee on Nutrition, American Academy of Pediatrics: Fluoride supplementation for children: interim policy recommendations, *Pediatrics* 95:777, 1995.

10. Committee on Pediatric AIDS, American Academy of Pediatrics: Human milk, breastfeeding, and transmission of human immunodeficiency virus in the United States, *Pediatrics* 96:977–979, 1995.

11. Cooper WO, Atherton HD, Kahana M, Kotagal UR: Increased incidence of severe breast-feeding malnutrition and hypernatremia in a metropolitan area, *Pediatrics* 96:957–960, 1995.

12. Davidsson L, Galan P, Cherouvrier F, et al: Bioavailability in infants of iron from infant cereals: effects of dephytinization, *Am J Clin Nutr* 65:916–920, 1997.

13. Dewey KG, Peerson JM, Brown KH, et al: Growth of breast-fed infants deviates from current reference data: a pooled analysis of US, Canadian and European data sets, *Pediatrics* 96:495–503, 1995.

14. Fisher C, Inch S: Nipple confusion—who is confused? *J Pediatr* 129:174–175, 1996.

15. Fomon SJ: *Nutrition of normal infants,* St. Louis, 1993, Mosby Year–Book.

16. Food and Nutrition Board, National Academy of Sciences: *Recommended dietary allowances,* ed 10, Washington, DC, 1989, National Academy Press.

17. Freed GL, Clark SJ, Lohr JA, Sorenson JR: Pediatrician involvement in breast-feeding promotion: a national study of residents and practitioners, *Pediatrics* 96:490–494, 1995.

18. Green M, editor: *Bright futures: guidelines for health supervision of infants, children and adolescents,* Arlington, VA, 1994, National Center for Education in Maternal and Child Health.

19. Hamill PVV: *NCHS growth curves for children, birth to 18 years,* U.S. Department of Health, Education and Welfare, Pub. no. PHS 78-1650, Hyattsville, MD, 1977, National Center for Health Statistics.

20. Himes JH, Dietz WH: Guidelines for overweight in adolescent preventive services: recommendations from an expert committee, *Am J Clin Nutr* 59:307–316, 1994.

21. Hopkinson J, James K, Zimmer JP. Management of breast-feeding. In Tsong RC, Zeotkin SH, Nichols BL, Hansen JM (editors) *Nutrition During Infancy: Principles and Practices,* 2nd edition, Digital Educational Publishing, Inc., Cincinnati 1997.

22. Institute of Medicine: *WIC nutrition risk criteria: a scientific assessment,* Washington, DC, 1996, National Academy Press.

23. Lee K-S, Perlman M, Ballantyne M, et al: Association between duration of neonatal hospital stay and readmission rate, *Pediatr* 127:758–766, 1995.

24. Lonnerdal B, Forsum E, Hambraes L: A longitudinal study of protein, nitrogen and lactose contents of human milk from Swedish well-nourished mothers, *Am J Clin Nutr* 29:1127–1133, 1976.

25. Lucas SR, Sexton M, Langenberg P: Relationship between blood lead and nutritional factors in preschool children: a cross-sectional study, *Pediatrics* 97:74–87, 1996.

26. Luepker RV, Perry CL, McKinlay SM, et al: Outcomes of a field trial to improve children's dietary patterns and physical activity: the Child and Adolescent Trial for Cardiovascular Health (CATCH), *JAMA* 275:768–776, 1996.

27. Montgomery DL, Splett PL: Economic benefit of breast-feeding infants enrolled in WIC, *J Am Diet Assoc* 97:379–385, 1997.

28. NCEP Expert Panel on Blood Cholesterol Levels in Children and Adolescents, National Cholesterol Education Program (NCEP): Highlights of the report of the Expert Panel on Blood Cholesterol Levels in Children and Adolescents, *Pediatrics* 89:495–501, 1992.

29. NHBPEP Coordinating Committee: Update on the 1987 Task Force report on high blood pressure in children and adolescents: a working group report from the National High Blood Pressure Education Program, *Pediatrics* 98:649–658, 1996.

30. O'Malley PM, Johnston LD, Bachman JG: Adolescent substance abuse and addictions: epidemiology, current trends, and public policy, *Adolesc Med State Art Rev* 4:227–248, 1993.

31. Owen AL, Owen GM: Twenty years of WIC: A review of some effects of the program, *J Am Diet Assoc,* 97:777–782, 1997.

32. Owen AL, Pipes P, Lee SL: *Infant feeding guide,* Bloomfield, NJ, 1979, Health Learning Systems.

33. Owen GM: Measurements, recording and assessment of skinfold thickness in childhood and adolescence: report of a small meeting, *Am J Clin Nutr* 35:629–631, 1982.

34. Owen GM, Kram KM, Garry PJ, et al: A study of nutritional status of preschool children in the United States, 1968–1970, *Pediatrics* 53(4, Part II):597–646, 1974.

35. Palasanthiran P, Ziegler JB, Stewart GJ, et al: Breast-feeding during primary maternal human immunodeficiency virus infection and risk of transmission from mother to infant, *J Infect Dis* 167:441–444, 1993.

36. Pediatric Nutrition Surveillance: 1995 annual summaries. (Personal communication, S. Lee, Arizona Department of Health Services).

37. Perez-Escamilla R, Pollitt E, Lonnerdal B, Dewey KG: Infant feeding policies in maternity wards and their effect on breast-feeding success: an analytical overview, *Am J Health* 84:89–97, 1995.

38. Pinhas-Hamiel O, Dolan LM, Daniels SR, et al: Increased incidence of non-insulin-dependent diabetes mellitus among adolescents, *J Pediatr* 128:608–615, 1996.

39. Position of ADA, SNE and ASFSA: school-based nutrition programs and services, *J Am Diet Assoc* 95:367–369, 1995.

40. Quality Assurance Criteria Sets for Pediatric Nutrition Conditions. Pediatric Nutrition Practice Group, The American Dietetic Association, Chicago, IL, 1993.

41. Rifai N, Neufeld E, Ahlston, P, et al: Failure of current guidelines for cholesterol screening in urban African-American adolescents, *Pediatrics* 98:383–388, 1996.

42. Ryan AS: The resurgence of breast-feeding in the United States, *Pediatrics* 99:4/e12, 1997.

43. Schwartz JB, Popkin BM, Tagnetti J. Zohoori N: Does WIC participation improve breast-feeding practices? *Am J Public Health* 85:729–731, 1995.

44. Timely Statement of the American Dietetic Association dietary guidance for healthy children, *J Am Diet Assoc* 95:370, 1995.

45. Wagner CL, Anderson DM, Pittard WB: Special properties of human milk, *Clin Pediatr* 35:283–293, 1996.

46. Wright A, Rice S, Wells S: Changing hospital practices to increase the duration of breast-feeding, *Pediatrics* 97:669–675, 1996.

47. Yip R, Binkin, NJ, Fleshood L. Trowbridge FL: Declining prevalence of anemia among low-income children in the United States, *JAMA* 258:1619–1623, 1987.

48. Yip R, Parvanta I, Scanlon K, Borland EW, Russell CM, Trowbridge FL: Pediatric Nutrition Surveillance System—United States, 1980–1991, *MMWR Morbi Mortal Wkly Rep* 41(SS-7):1–24, 1992.

49. Yip R, Scanlon K, Trowbridge FL: Trends and patterns in height and weight status of low-income US children, *Crit Rev Food Science Nutr* 33:409–421, 1993.

50. Yip R, Walsh KM, Goldfarb MG, Binkin NJ: Declining prevalence of anemia in childhood in middle-class setting: a pediatric success story? *Pediatrics* 80:330–334, 1987.

51. Zimmer P, Garza C. Maternal considerations in formulating HIV-related breast-feeding recommendations. *Am J Public Health* 87:904–906, 1997.

CASE STUDY

THE NATIONAL SCHOOL BREAKFAST VIDEO INITIATIVE

KATHY COBB, MS, RD, CD/N
SENIOR NUTRITION CONSULTANT
STATE OF CONNECTICUT DEPT OF PUBLIC HEALTH
HARTFORD, CT

DESCRIPTION

This case study describes the successful building of a national coalition to reduce childhood hunger. Twelve state and national nutrition and antihunger organizations came together through an innovative model video project that promotes school breakfast programs, the School Breakfast Video Initiative (SBVI). This initiative targets parents in an effort to increase the number of School Breakfast Programs (SBPs) and student participation. Because of today's complicated lifestyles and economic challenges, more children are responsible for their own meals and come to school hungry without the benefit of breakfast. To further complicate the problem, SBPs are available to only about half of our nation's schoolchildren and are underutilized by thousands of others. A creative marketing approach to increase school breakfast participation was needed. Implementation of the SBVI has resulted in a national school breakfast promotion that involved over 2,000 professionals in fifty states.

METHODOLOGY

Hungry children cannot learn. Hunger among schoolchildren is a growing national crisis. One out of four children under the age of twelve experiences hunger or is at risk of hunger. Although we rarely see life-threatening starvation in the United States, even mild levels of malnutrition must be taken seriously, especially in young children. One subtle form of malnutrition with serious long-term effect is skipping breakfast. Children who do not eat breakfast suffer twice as many health problems; are absent from school more often; have lower test scores; and exhibit restlessness, lack of attention, sleepiness, and disruptive behavior. *Question to be raised:* If we know that eating breakfast can positively impact children's nutrition, health, growth, behavior, and learning ability, why don't all schools offer School Breakfast Programs?

The limited access to School Breakfast Programs is troubling, but even more so is the underutilization of existing SBPs. To better understand why eligible students in Connecticut were not participating in SBPs, the Hartford Mayor's Task Force on Hunger, School Breakfast Subcommittee conducted a bilingual survey of parents and elementary students. The parent survey showed that 30 percent of parents did not know about the SBP. A colorful bilingual SBP brochure was developed and distributed with student report cards. This parent outreach effort resulted in an immediate doubling of student participation in SBPs. Considering this initial success, the subcommittee sought to further enhance student participation by bringing the message to life through a video program. When the idea of a video was tested with a Hartford focus group of parents, it was seen as an effective way to stimulate parent interest in SBPs as well as to encourage student participation. *Question to be raised:* Why does the video target parents?

THE CASE

Concerned by the compelling reports of hunger in Hartford, the Connecticut Dietetic Association (CDA) began an initiative to reduce childhood hunger within Connecticut. This initiative now reaches children in all fifty states. The initiative grew from a voluntary effort in Connecticut to a national campaign for SBPs. Building and maintaining partnerships with the twelve national professional organizations was key to success. To decide who the initial partners should be, we asked the question, Who in Connecticut would benefit from a school breakfast project? Beside the obvious groups of children, parents, and school and health communities, it was determined that the food industry would also benefit from the sales of breakfast foods. Lender's Bagel Bakery was the first company approached because of their healthy breakfast products and recognized commitment to alleviate hunger. They eagerly became a partner, providing point staff, financial resources, and entree to their national company, Post Cereals. CDA initiated contacts with national nutrition and antihunger organizations to become partners. As the project developed, partnerships were expanded. The partner list is included at the end of the case study.

The core partners were drawn together by mutually shared goals and the recognition of the need to share limited resources. The goals of the initiative were to increase parent and student awareness about School Breakfast Programs, to increase the number of School Breakfast Programs throughout the United States, and to boost student participation in existing programs.

The national partners developed strategies for the video and its production, distribution, and implementation in each state. The state-level partners would determine how to reach parents and communities with the video program. The project coordinator from the CDA led the national coalition and wrote the grants to obtain funding for production of the video and material development and distribution. Lender's Bagel Bakery and Post Cereals, Divisions of Kraft General Foods, Inc.; the National Dairy Council; and the National Dairy Promotion and Research Board funded the various components of the project. The video was produced by Bossert & Company in New York. The Leader's Guide was developed through the national coalition and other supportive materials were identified and acquired, such as the three Public Service Announcements (PSAs). The final program kit was distributed to 1,500 professionals nationwide in March, 1993 and contained the video, "You Can't Learn When You're Hungry"; the Leader's Guide; two reproducible masters of parent "take home" materials; the resource booklet; background information on Hunger and Under-Nutrition in America; a colorful wall poster; and three attention-grabbing Public Service Announcements.

This dynamic video program is shown in school and community settings to generate interest, advocacy, and support for SBPs. The video shows parents and stimulates discussion about how important it is for children to eat breakfast; identifies obstacles to get children to eat breakfast (not enough time, home alone, not enough food); and shows that a solution to these problems can be found in SBPs. The video's theme revolves around three early morning vignettes. Teenaged actors portray the three students' real life morning situations. Each child in his or her own way discovers that breakfast works and that the SBP is a good place to get it. This age group was selected to serve as role models for

younger children to broaden acceptability and appeal of the video. The actors also reflect cultural sensitivity and ethnic diversity. The video program is presented by dietitians and school food service directors because of their expertise in child nutrition and/or SBPs.

At the state level, the CDA joined with the state representatives of the national partners to form a task force to network and develop a state implementation plan. This task force identified thirteen pilot school sites and recruited CDA members to serve as speakers and advocates. A speaker's bureau was established to deliver the school breakfast video program to the parent-school community. Training sessions were held for speakers and included background information about the video, school breakfast facts, parent advocacy tips, and opportunities to role play. Connecticut's task force set the goal to present five parent programs by June 1993 and to reach all of the thirteen pilot communities by January 1994. The first goal was achieved. The second was not, primarily due to difficulties in marketing SBPs to administrators who were cutting academic programs in a period of economic downturn.

Evaluation of the video was conducted at the national level. The distribution of and responses to the video program kits were monitored. To meet the ongoing demand for materials, the American School Food Service Association, through the Emporium, agreed to distribute the SBVI program kit. Since the initial distribution, an additional 515 kits have been sold without advertisement, thus demonstrating the continuing value of the SBVI. Through this initiative, over 2,000 nutrition and school breakfast leaders have been reached in every state. The number of SBPs and participation rates by schools increased from 53.5 percent in 1992 to 58.4 percent in 1993. Utah, one of the states showing the greatest improvement, reported successful use of the SBVI to generate legislative support for SBPs. Both Montana and Utah report that as a result of the SBVI, they have more School Breakfast Programs and fewer hungry children. A more formal evaluation is needed to clearly demonstrate the impact of the SBVI. The increase in numbers of School Breakfast Programs at state and national levels is encouraging, but additional efforts directed to parents and communities are needed to continue this upward trend. Even with this positive momentum, many school children still are not eating breakfast. A recent report found that whether or not SBPs were in place, 12 percent of the students did not eat breakfast. This finding underscores the need for wider use of innovative programs like SBVI for parents and students. Through SBVI's national and state-level points of access, the SBVI is a readily available tool that could and should be used with students. We have not yet targeted teacher or student markets, nor have we determined strategies to reach these populations.

There are lessons to be learned. The SBVI began as a volunteer endeavor with the CDA. As it grew, it moved from a voluntary assignment into a full-time job for the project coordinator, a CDA member working for the State of Connecticut Department of Health. As project coordinator, the author's responsibilities varied from obtaining partner commitment and funding to writing video scripts and materials and gaining partner sign off in key decisions regarding video production and the design, development, and distribution of the kit. The importance of communicating among partners at each step of the way needs to be emphasized. Although extremely time consuming, this proved essential in building trust among the coalition members, which greatly contributed to the overall success of the initiative. One memorable example is that the coordinator left work for the filming of the video before a fax reached her changing a number in the script. To maintain the commitment to the coalition, an entire segment of the video was refilmed.

Although it has been impossible to maintain the original intensity of national partnerships, state and local partners are making headway. In 1995, in response to the threat of federal cuts to SBPs, a Connecticut senator was invited to eat breakfast at school and an attention-grabbing flyer was sent to every CDA member urging their support of SBPs. We know that parents are being reached through SBVI programs conducted in every state. Increases in the number of SBPs as a result have been reported. During the last three years, the SBVI has been able to reach the parent target as well as professionals and students throughout the nation. On going research and additional resources will show the long-term benefit.

STUDENT PROJECT IDEAS OR QUESTIONS:

1. What would be necessary to implement this project at the local level?
2. Who would you choose as your partners?
3. What would it take to maintain the partnerships at the national, state, and local levels?
4. What type of infrastructure might facilitate this and at which level?
5. How will you secure the necessary resources to make this happen?

The twelve partners are the American Dietetic Association; the School Nutrition Services Practice Group; the Association of State and Territorial Public Health Nutrition Directors; the Connecticut Association of Human Services; the Connecticut Dietetic Association; the Connecticut School Food Service Association; the Food Research and Action Council (FRAC); the National Dairy Council; the School Food Service Foundation of the American School Food Service Association; the State of Connecticut, Department of Education, Child Nutrition Programs; the State of Connecticut, Department of Health Services, Child and Adolescent Health Division; the Texas Nutrition Education and Training Program; and the United States Department of Agriculture (USDA) Food and Nutrition Service, Western Regional Office.

CHAPTER TEN

NUTRITION IN THE ADULT YEARS

Americans—the only population that thinks death is optional.
—Anonymous

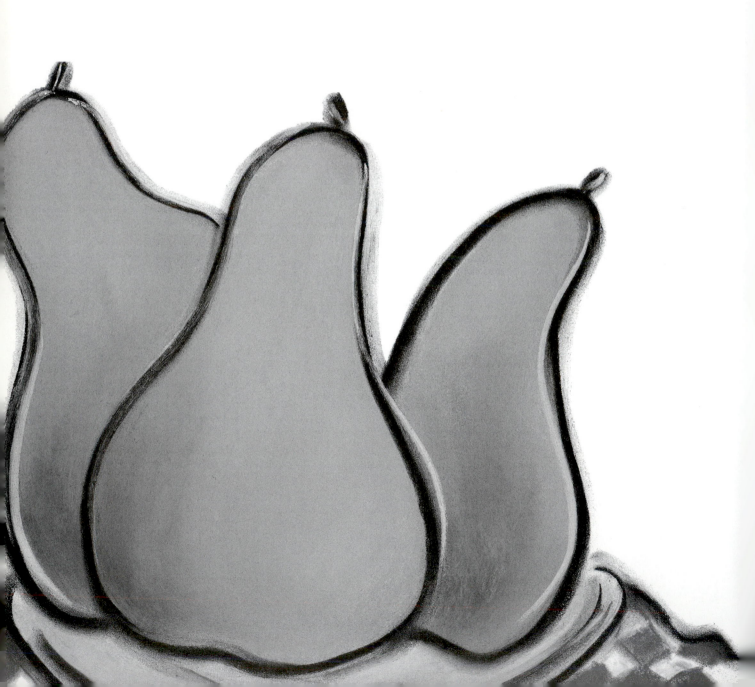

Core Concept

Adulthood, the longest period of the life cycle, interfaces adolescence and the senior years and spans ages twenty-one to sixty. Maintaining health, preventing nutrient deficiency and excess diseases, and reducing the risk of chronic disease are primary nutrition goals for adults. The consequences of many nutrition-related diseases can be avoided, or at least delayed, and the severity lessened, if healthful lifestyle practices are adopted early and followed for a lifetime. This, in large part, is the rationale for the many nutrition interventions targeted to the adult population.

Objectives

When you finish chapter ten, you should be able to:

~ Cite examples of Healthy People 2000 objectives for the United States as they relate to the adult population.

~ Recognize an individual's changing nutritional needs and concerns during the forty years spanning adulthood.

~ Identify the energy and nutrient needs of health adults.

~ List the risk factors for major nutrition-related chronic diseases of adults.

~ Determine the risk factors for women in nutrition-related chronic diseases.

~ Select interventions for chronic disease risk reduction in the adult population.

~ Integrate knowledge of adult nutritional needs with psychosocial concerns.

~ Develop an innovative strategy for nutrition intervention programs in the community.

~ Identify the components of successful nutrition education interventions in the adult population.

Key Words

Word	Page Mentioned
Chronic diseases	268
Adult years	268
Cancer	268
NIDDM	268
Osteoporosis	268
Life expectancy	272
Obesity	273
Yo-yo dieting	276
"Healthier weight"	276
Depression	278
Trans-fatty acids	281
Drug-nutrient interactions	288
Assessment	291
Nutrition education interventions	291
Nutritional status	291
Nutrition education programs	297
Intervention process	298
Intervention context	298
Federal food assistance program	299

HEALTHY PEOPLE 2000 OBJECTIVES FOR ADULTS

Early adulthood is associated with vigor and vitality; however, as people age there is a decrease in physiological functioning. Genetics plays an important role in the development of a number of **chronic diseases** (e.g., obesity, hyperlipidemias, diabetes, hypertension). The incidence and severity of these diseases are influenced by lifestyle choices, including food choices, which play a prominent role. These and other factors affecting nutrition in the **adult years** are described in figure 10.1. A systems review of the interrelations between food supply, consumption, and health is depicted in figure 10.2. Table 10.1 gives a complete listing of Healthy People 2000 objectives for nutrition-related issues specific to adults for both health status and risk reduction, along with baseline prevalences and the most recent figures available as of 1997.

As of 1997, one of the adult nutrition-related objectives—the availability of reduced-fat processed products—far exceeded the original target goal. As table 10.1 shows, progress has also been made in other areas. These include reduction in coronary heart disease and **cancer** deaths; reduction in fat intake; increased use of food label and informative nutrition labeling; increased availability of low-fat, low-calorie restaurant choices and of worksite nutrition and weight management programs. Unfortunately, progress has not been satisfactory for two objectives—decreasing the prevalence of overweight and increasing the use of healthful weight loss practices. In fact, recent data indicate that more Americans are overweight than ever before and are not using sound weight loss programs. For several objectives, there are no new data.

BACKGROUND OF PRESSING PROBLEMS IN THE ADULT YEARS

Today's adults encompass several generations and face a wide range of problems. These include:

- Positioning themselves in the workforce
- Establishing and raising families
- Caring for their aging parents
- Becoming involved with social and community issues

Adults' food choices may be less related to health and nutrition concerns than to their role in their families and in society (figure 10.2). The younger adult who is trying to get through a busy day's schedule balancing work and family needs may base food choices on convenience and cost as well as taste. For older adults, however, the nutritional issues associated with morbidity, mortality, and quality of life that accompany chronic diseases become more pressing and healthfulness plays a greater role in food selections. Socioeconomic and psychosocial concerns may override all other concerns, including health. Health status is strongly associated with family income.[9] In 1993, the percentage of persons with low family incomes (< $14,000) who reported fair or poor health was 5.5 times that for persons with high incomes (> $50,000). Despite their poorer health status, persons with low incomes are more likely to have gone without a recent physician contact than persons with high incomes.

All of these factors affect the delivery of nutrition interventions as well as the specifics of the educational messages themselves. The community nutrition professional must recognize these factors when designing, implementing and evaluating nutrition interventions.

SELECTED NUTRITION-RELATED HEALTH PROBLEMS

Diet is associated with five of the ten leading causes of death in the United States; coronary heart disease, some types of cancer, stroke, non-insulin-dependent diabetes mellitus (**NIDDM**), atherosclerosis, and other disease of the arteries, arterioles, and capillaries.[34] In addition, other chronic diseases such as **osteoporosis** have an associated nutrition component. As expected, death rates increase as the population ages (table 10.2). In addition, there are major differences in death rates between males and females and between Blacks and Whites in the four major age categories on the mid-adult years. While the all-causes death rate is 882.4 per 100,000 estimated population, the highest death rates are from major cardiovascular diseases and cancers.

Advances in medical technology throughout the twentieth century have increased survival rates of adults stricken with chronic diseases in their young and middle adult years while deaths from infectious diseases have decreased. Through personal choices, adults have many opportunities to change established practices and adopt lifestyles that can significantly shape their long-term health prospects. Community nutrition professionals must have a working knowledge of the etiology, prevalence, and treatment of the major nutrition-related chronic diseases to determine the level of intervention needed in their community.

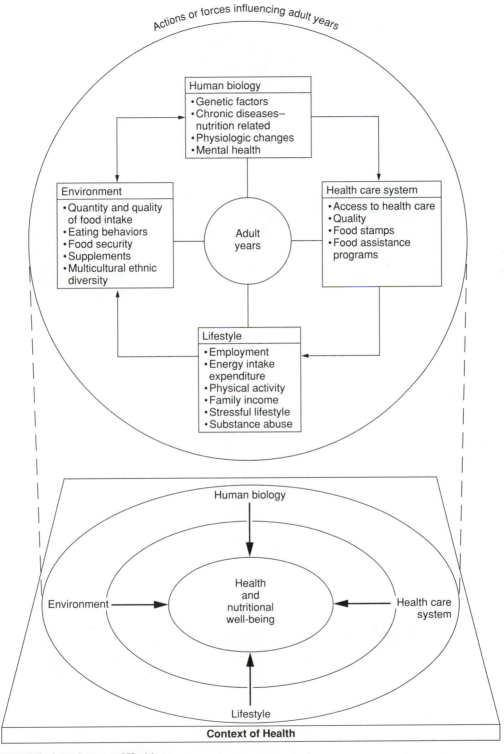

FIGURE 10.1 Context of Health

Influences on nutrition and health in the adult years.

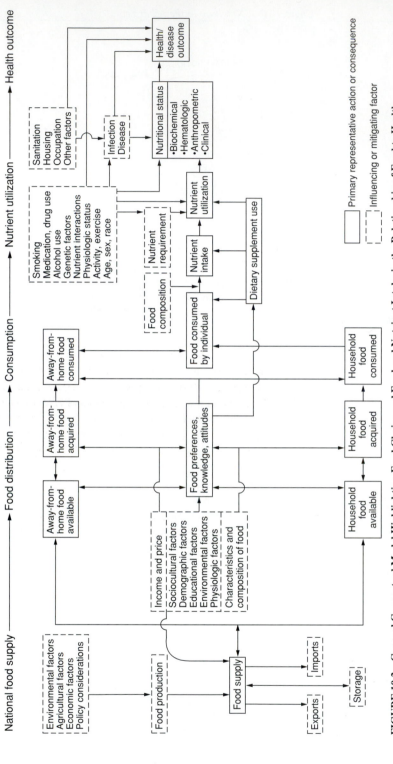

FIGURE 10.2 General Conceptual Model Highlighting Food Choice and Food and Nutrient Intake in the Relationship of Food to Health

(*Source*: From Federation of American Societies for Experimental Biology, Life Sciences Research Office: *Third report on nutrition monitoring in the United States: volume 1.* Prepared for the Interagency Board for Nutrition Monitoring and Related Research, Washington, DC, 1995, US Government Printing Office.)

TABLE 10.1
Healthy People 2000 Objectives for Adults

Objectives	Baseline prevalence (year)	Current prevalence (year)
Health status		
Reduce coronary heart disease deaths to no more than 100 per 100,000 people.	Age-adjusted: 135/100,000 (1987)	114/100,000 (1992)
Reverse the rise in cancer deaths to achieve a rate of no more than 115 per 100,000.	Age-adjusted: 168/100,000 (1987)	151/100,000 (1992)
Reduce overweight to a prevalence of ≤ 20% among people twenty years and older.	25% for people twenty to seventy-four (1976–80); for men, 24%; for women, 27%	For men, 34% (1992); for women, 35% (1992)
Risk reduction		
Reduce dietary fat intake to an average ≤ 30% energy and average saturated fat intake to < 10% of energy among people two years of age and older.	For people twenty to seventy-four (1976–80): 36% from total fat; 13% from saturated fat; 36% and 13% for women, nineteen to fifty (1985)	34% (1989–91) from total fat; 12% from saturated fat
Increase complex carbohydrate and fiber-containing foods to five or more servings daily for vegetables (including legumes) and fruits, and to six servings for grain products.	2½ serving of vegetables and fruits; 3 servings grains for women nineteen to fifty (1985)	Not available from this source
Increase to at least 50% the proportion of overweight people twelve years and older who have adopted sound dietary practices combined with regular physical activity to attain appropriate body weight.	30% overweight women; 25% overweight men aged twenty and older (1985)	19% for women; 17% for men (1993)
Increase to at least 30% the proportion of people eighteen years and older who engage regularly, preferably daily, in light to moderate physical activity for at least thirty minutes per day.	22%, five or more times weekly; 12%, seven or more times weekly (1985)	24% five or more times weekly; 17% seven or more times weekly (1992)
Increase calcium intake so at least 50% of people twenty-five years and older consume two servings daily of food rich in calcium.	23% males; 15% females (1986)	23% males; 16% females (1989–90)
Reduce alcohol consumption by people aged fourteen and older to an annual average of no more than 2 gal of ethanol per person.	2.54 gal per capita (1987)	2.31 (provisional, 1992)
Decrease sodium intake so at least 65% of home meal preparers prepare foods without adding salt, at least 80% of people avoid using salt at the table, and at least 40% of adults regularly purchase foods modified or lower in sodium.	43% of women aged nineteen to fifty who served as main food preparer did not use salt in preparation (1989–90); 60% also did not use salt at the table; 20% of all people eighteen years of age regularly purchased food with reduced salt and sodium (1988)	Not available
Increase to at least 85% the proportion of people eighteen years of age who use food labels to make nutritious food selections.	74% (1988)	76% (1990)
Increase to at least 50% the proportion of worksites with more than fifty employees that offer employees nutrition education/weight management programs.	17% offered nutrition education and 15% offered weight management activities (1985)	31% offered nutrition education; 24% offered weight management; 37% offered nutrition education and/or weight management (1992)

Source: Data adapted from Department of Health and Human Services: *Healthy people 2000: national health promotion and disease prevention objectives, midcourse review,* Washington, DC, 1995, US Government Printing Office.

TABLE 10.2

Provisional Rates of Major Causes of Death in Caucasian and Black Adults in the United States, 1994*

Age (year)	Both sexes			Males			Females		
	All races	Whites	Blacks	All races	Whites	Blacks	All races	Whites	Blacks
25–34	142	123	282	208	128	276	77	64	162
35–44	242	207	531	341	181	417	145	121	322
45–54	456	409	910	588	292	771	330	295	643
55–64	1,149	1,084	1,853	1,479	527	1,233	849	798	1,359

*Annual basis per 100,000 estimated population.
Source: Data adapted from *Monthly Vital Statistics Report;* 42(12):17, 1995.

Women's Health

It has long been recognized that women suffer more illnesses than men do, particularly chronic diseases, even though women live longer.[42] For many years, women's health has been an invisible issue among the general public as well as among health researchers and policy makers. In the late 1980s, the Congressional Caucus for Women's Issues claimed that for years the medical research community had ignored women's important health needs.[45] Women were regularly excluded from clinical and preventive research for several reasons, including the effect of variable menstrual cycles and the potential risk to an unborn fetus.[11]

Resolutions concerning the women's health research gap served as the impetus for a 1990 General Accounting Office (GAO) investigation that showed that despite years of discussions to the contrary, the National Institutes of Health (NIH) had done little to implement policies supportive of women.[29]

The GAO report was the impetus for the laws passed in 1993 mandating an Office of Women's Health within the NIH with a $16.7 billion budget. These laws specify that studies must include women when appropriate and that they must be conducted so that gender differences can be analyzed.[5]

Women's Health Initiative   One of the most significant developments resulting from the NIH's renewed commitment to women's health is the Women's Health Initiative (WHI), a fourteen-year, $625 million clinical study, the largest and most complex epidemiologic study of the century. The research is directed by the NIH and involves forty clinical research centers across the United States. Approximately 163,000 postmenopausal women aged fifty to seventy-nine will participate in one or more components of the WHI.[24] Launched in 1993, this study will address three of the

most common causes of death, disability, and impaired quality of life among postmenopausal women—heart disease, cancer, and osteoporosis.[29] A randomized, controlled clinical trial will explore approaches to prevention that include the effect of a low-fat diet on heart disease and colon cancer; the effect of estrogen replacement therapy on heart disease, osteoporosis, and increased risk of breast cancer; and the effect of calcium and vitamin D supplementation on osteoporosis and colon cancer.

Women in Ethnic Minority Populations   Black American, Hispanic American, American Indian and Alaskan Native-American, and Asian and Pacific Islander American women have higher rates of some chronic diseases in comparison with White, non-Hispanic American women.[28] Cultural and genetic factors may have a role in these less favorable health profiles of minority women. Socioeconomic factors play an important part as a disproportionately large number of women in these ethnic groups face poor access to health care and other poverty-related factors that may contribute to health problems in numerous ways. Minority women have a shorter **life expectancy,** experience higher maternal and infant mortality, and have a high incidence of chronic diseases such as diabetes mellitus and hypertension.[42]

In 1995, the American Dietetic Association (ADA) and the Canadian Dietetic Association (CDA) stated their joint position on the issues of women's health and nutrition (see box 10.1). Central to this position is the concept of total health. Although women's individual risk profiles vary widely, available evidence indicates that the role of nutrition is remarkably similar from disease to disease. Therefore, it is important for women's overall health that community nutrition professionals promote consistent healthful messages as outlined in the U.S. Food Guide Pyramid and the Canadian Food Guide

JOINT POSITION STATEMENT OF THE ADA AND THE CDA

It is the position of the American Dietetic Association (ADA) and the Canadian Dietetic Association (CDA) that because of biological, social and political factors, women are at unique risk for major nutrition-related diseases and conditions including cardiovascular disease, certain cancers, osteoporosis, diabetes and weight-related problems. ADA and CDA strongly encourage health promotion activities, health services, research and advisory efforts that will enable women to adopt desirable nutrition practices for optimal health.[42]

to Healthy Eating.[42] The community nutrition professional must work to increase the public's knowledge about women's health by developing and providing quality health promotion and disease prevention programs.

Obesity and Weight Management

Obesity is associated with the development of cardiovascular diseases, hypertension, NIDDM, osteoarthritis, gallbladder disease, and some cancers.[33] Obesity is related to the risk of these diseases in three ways. First, the expression of genetic predisposition for some diseases and health risks are manifested as weight increases. Second, medical risks of coexisting diseases are heightened when obesity is present. Finally, massive obesity can be considered as an independent risk factor because it is intimately related to many health problems. Distribution of body fat also plays an important role in relation to increased risk of death, stroke, heart disease, and NIDDM. Visceral fat (fat centrally located around the abdomen—the android/apple shape) appears to be more of a health risk than fat peripherally located around the hips (the gynecoid/pear shape).

Environmental factors and genetics are important determinants of the onset and severity of obesity. A genetic predisposition is not absolutely predictive of becoming obese. Thus, prevention is important during the entire lifespan, and in particular during adulthood when healthful lifestyle habits are critical to avoiding weight gain in the middle adult years. Energy intake and energy expenditure are the two major modifiable components that affect body weight. Over the past twenty-five years, most efforts have focused on modifying energy intake. More recently, attention has been given to the health benefits of lifestyle behavior modifications as well as increased physical activity (see chapter 7).

Unfortunately, there is a lack of consensus over definitions of both obesity and healthy weight. A variety of standards have been used to quantify these terms, including weight-for-height tables based on minimal mortality assessed by life insurance companies, body mass index (BMI = weight [kg]/height [m^2]), percentage of body fat (a measurement highly correlated with BMI but more difficult to obtain), waist-to-hip ratio, and weight for body frame size based on a representative sample. Anthropometric measurements, although the easiest to obtain, are gross measures that do not capture functional and psychosocial variables necessary to describe quality of life and define healthy weight.

The fourth edition (1995) of the *Dietary Guidelines for Americans*[37] suggests a range of body weights for height (figure 10.3) with higher weights in the healthy weight range applying to adults with more muscle and bone (predominantly males). At the same time, the Expert Panel on Healthy Weight convened by the American Health Foundation suggested a body mass index (kg/m^2) or BMI of < 25 for adults as a goal.[33] Great attention has been given to the association of excess weight with many health problems by the scientific and health communities as well as by the media. In addition, an estimated $30 to $50 billion is spent annually on weight loss products and services. Despite these efforts, American adults have gotten heavier and moved farther away from the Healthy People 2000 goal. Based on 1990 population estimates, approximately 26 million men and 32 million women are overweight (using a BMI > 27.7 for men and > 27.2 for women as the standards).[25]

Patterns of prevalence vary by gender and race and ethnic group (table 10.3). The prevalence of overweight adult men in minority populations is shown in figure 10.4 and that of overweight adult women in minority populations is shown in figure 10.5.[27] Given that overweight is associated with increased risk of many chronic diseases, the United States could have saved approximately $45.8 billion or 6.8 percent of health care expenditures in 1990 alone if obesity were prevented. When looking at economic and social indices, a healthy body weight appears to be a BMI < 25 and within the range shown in figure 10.3. It should be noted that excessive thinness has also been associated with increased risk of morbidity and mortality. Current recommendations are to maintain a BMI of

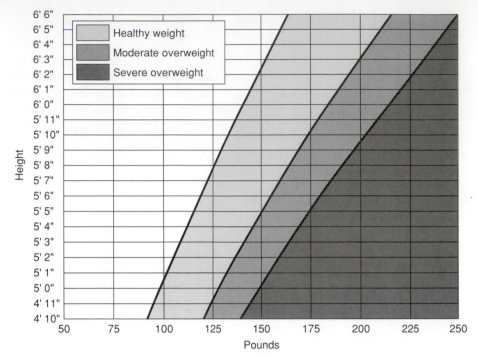

FIGURE 10.3   Body Weight Ranges for Heights in Adults
(*Source: From Nutrition and your health: dietary guidelines for Americans,* ed 4, Washington, DC, 1995, USDA and DHHS, Home and Garden Bulletin no. 232.)

TABLE 10.3

Comparison of Prevalence of Overweight American Adults, 1960–1991*

Population group	NHES I (1960–1962)[†]	NHANES I (1971–1974)	NHANES II (1976–1980)	NHANES III Phase I (1988–1991)
Age 20–74 years	24.3%	25.0%	25.4%	33.3%
Race/sex				
White				
Men	23.0	23.8	24.2	32.0
Women	23.6	24.0	24.4	33.5
Black				
Men	22.1	23.9	26.2	31.8
Women	41.6	43.1	44.5	49.2
Sex/age (years)				
Men				
20–74	22.8	23.7	24.1	31.7
20–29	18.4	15.7	15.1	20.2
30–39	21.8	28.4	24.4	27.4
40–49	25.5	30.2	32.4	37.0
50–59	28.8	27.1	28.2	42.1
60–74	23.0	21.6	26.8	40.9
Women				
20–74	25.7	26.0	26.5	34.9
20–29	10.1	12.5	14.7	20.2
30–39	21.9	22.9	23.8	34.3
40–49	26.8	29.7	29.0	37.6
50–59	35.0	35.5	36.5	52.0
60–74	45.6	39.0	37.3	41.3

*Age-adjusted and age-specific percentages. Pregnant women excluded. NHES indicates National Health Examination Survey; NHANES, National Health and Nutrition Examination Survey.
[†]A total of 0.9 kg was subtracted from measured weight to adjust for weight of clothing.
Source: Data from *JAMA,* July 20, 1994. Vol. 272(3):208.

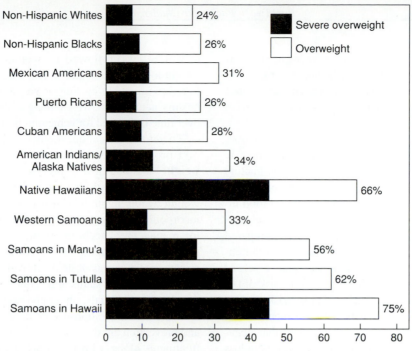

FIGURE 10.4   Prevalence of Overweight Adult Men in U.S. Minority Populations
(*Source:* From Kumanyika S: Special issues regarding obesity in minority populations, *Ann Intern Med;* 199:650–654, 1993. Reprinted with permission from Annals of Internal Medicine.)

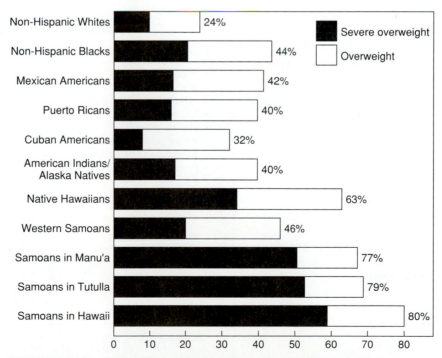

FIGURE 10.5   Prevalence of Overweight Adult Women in U.S. Minority Populations
(*Source:* From Kumanyika S: Special issues regarding obesity in minority populations, *Ann Intern Med;* 119:650–654, 1993. Reprinted with permission from Annals of Internal Medicine.)

at least 19. Thus, weight loss is not recommended if weight-for-height is already within the healthiest range in figure 10.3, if less than 4.5 k (10 lb) has been gained since reaching adult height, and if the person is otherwise healthy.

Given the multifactorial and complex nature of obesity, it may well be impossible to determine specific causes for the observed increase in prevalence. Factors affecting the recent increase in rates of overweight may include inadequate knowledge and awareness of food intake, inadequate knowledge and awareness of food consumption, and increased consumption of foods prepared outside the home. But intake is only one side of the energy balance equation. Irregular and inadequate levels of physical activity also play a critical role in the risk of becoming overweight as well as increasing the risk of mortality associated with obesity, especially for men.

Weight loss will occur with any regimen that negatively shifts energy balance but there are some weight loss programs that are sensible and others that are questionable (see box 10.2). Unfortunately, the vast majority of people who have lost weight relapse and subsequently regain at least the amount lost, and sometimes more. Many go through several rounds of dietary restrictions leading to weight loss, followed by weight gain, then further weight loss, and gain, and so on. Whether this pattern, referred to as weight cycling or **yo-yo dieting,** is itself unhealthy is uncertain. Maintaining a stable healthy weight over time is the goal for achieving best health results.

Therefore, critical questions facing community nutrition professionals are how to facilitate a "**healthier weight**" loss and how to prevent weight gain or regain. Concern over the overwhelming failure to maintain lost weight by relying on food restriction alone prompted the incorporation of increased physical activity and behavior management techniques into weight management programs (see chapter 7). Not surprisingly, these techniques are the cornerstone of lifestyle changes necessary to improve health status and reduce risk of chronic disease in all individuals, obese and nonobese alike.

More recent additions to the field of obesity treatment and prevention are the concept of matching individuals to treatments along with the concept of body size acceptance (table 10.4). Rather than the standard practice of putting every overweight individual on a diet or into a weight loss program, individuals are matched to the most

---

BOX 10.2

WEIGHT LOSS PROGRAMS

CHARACTERISTICS OF SENSIBLE PROGRAMS
- Weight loss of 0.25 to 0.5 kg (½ to 1 lb) per week
- *New* habits stressed
    Increase physical activity
    Low-fat, affordable, practical food choices with energy adjusted to meet individual needs
    Change in food and eating habits
- Positive mental attitude
- Lifetime commitment and monitoring

CHARACTERISTICS OF QUESTIONABLE PROGRAMS
- Author not a nutrition authority
- Forbidden food lists
- Use of supplemental food or pill
- Use of secret scientific formula
- Anecdotal reports
- Fewer than 1,000 calories
- No medical supervision if use drugs or very low calories
- No maintenance plan

T A B L E   10.4

Considerations in Matching Obesity Treatments to Individuals

Client factors	Program factors
• Weight	• Group versus individual setting
• Body composition	• Dietary counseling
• "Healthier weight" goal*	• Behavioral component
• Dieting history	• Structured exercise
• Health status	• Supervised exercise
• Eating patterns (binges)	• Professional versus lay leader
• Readiness to participate	• Meeting frequency
• Psychosocial factors	• Prepackaged foods
	• Dietary supplements
	• Cost and convenience
	• Program length
	• Degree of dietary restriction
	• Drug intervention
	• Surgical procedures
	• Psychotherapy component

*Refers to the body weight achieved by a weight loss of 4.5 to 7 kg (~ 10 to 16 lb) or the equivalent of approximately two BMI units for individuals who are above a BMI of 25.
Source: Data adapted from Brownell KD, Fairburn CG: *Eating disorders and obesity—a comprehensive handbook,* New York, 1995, Guilford Press; Meisler JG, St. Jeor ST: American Health Foundation roundtable on healthy weight, *Amer J Clin Nutr;* 63(3S), 1996.

appropriate intervention depending on health status and readiness to participate. The body size acceptance concept indicates that human beings come in a variety of sizes and shapes; there is no ideal body size or shape or weight that every individual should strive to achieve and that good health is not defined by body size alone. It is also a state of physical, mental, and social well-being.[20]

In 1995, the Institute of Medicine released *Weighing the Options: Criteria for Evaluating Weight Management Programs.*[20] Figure 10.6 presents a framework for the conduct of programs and behavior of individuals that should help consumers choose more wisely from among available weight management programs. Figure 10.6 illustrates the model in such a way that each of its major components is associated with a criterion and each criterion is discussed as it pertains to both weight management programs and to consumers seeking such programs.

In 1994, C. Everett Koop, former Surgeon General, launched a major campaign called Shape Up America to place healthy weight and physical activity high on the national agenda. Involving a broad coalition of industry, media, health, nutrition, physical fitness, and re-lated organizations, the campaign has galvanized support of public policy efforts, community programs, and education needed to effect change.

Obesity: Concerns for Women   Obesity's multiple etiologies pose special concerns for women because of differences in physiology, psychology, and genetics as well as environmental influences. Hormonal factors impart the greatest influence for obesity risk in women. Hormonal changes during critical periods of puberty, pregnancy, and menopause have implications for development of obesity and for treatment. Nearly one half of non-Hispanic Black women (48.6 percent) and Mexican-American women (46.7 percent) are overweight compared with 32.9 percent of non-Hispanic White women. Obesity has been increasing at a greater rate among Black girls and adolescents (six to seventeen years) than among non-Hispanic White girls.[49]

Physical Activity

Regular physical activity is defined in *Healthy People 2000* as "exercise which involves large muscle groups

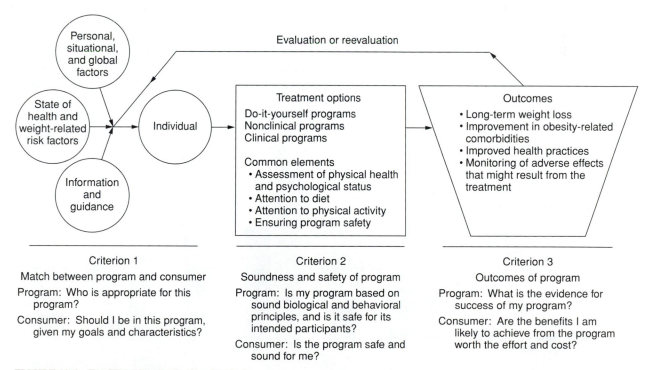

FIGURE 10.6   The Weighing the Options Method
(*Source:* Reprinted with permission from *Weighing the Options: Criteria for Evaluating Weight-Management Programs.* Copyright 1995 by the National Academy of Sciences. Courtesy of the National Academy of Sciences. Washington, DC.)

in dynamic movements for periods of twenty minutes or longer, three or more days a week, and which is performed at an intensity of 60 percent or greater of an individual's cardiorespiratory capacity."[54] Even light to moderate activity (requiring sustained, rhythmic muscular movements) below levels recommended for cardiovascular fitness have significant health benefits. To increase energy expenditure, attain fitness, and potentially increase lifespan, individuals should *accumulate* thirty minutes or more of moderate physical activity on most (preferably all) days of the week.[40] Although they express interest in increasing physical activity, relatively few American adults engage in moderate exercise five or more times a week (24 percent in 1992) and only 14 percent reported exercising vigorously. Most Americans have a very light to light level of activity. Regular physical activity can help reduce the risk of, and manage, coronary heart disease, hypertension, colon cancer, stroke, NIDDM, osteoporosis, obesity, and mental health problems such as **depression** and anxiety. Physically active people, on the average, tend to outlive more sedentary people. There is evidence that moderate and high levels of physical fitness (assessed by a maximal exercise treadmill test) are associated with lower risk of mortality in overweight and normal weight men when compared with their less fit peers. Increased physical activity may favorably affect blood pressure, platelet aggregation, and glucose tolerance. Aerobic exercise enhances cardiovascular function. Exercises to in-

crease muscle strength and flexibility may protect against disabilities and injuries.

Although physical activity and exercise training alone result in limited weight loss, those who engage in routine physical activities can better maintain their body weight. In addition, those who remain overweight benefit from an active lifestyle. As with weight management, no one specific physical activity plan will suit all individuals. Matching personal preferences with appropriate activities is critical to maintaining a regular program of physical activity. Individuals can select from a variety of activities to develop a personalized physical activity plan suited to their own preferences and adapted to meet their own health needs. In addition, they can choose to exercise alone, participate in a structured and/or supervised exercise program, purchase home equipment, or join a club or center. Overcoming the sedentary lifestyle of many American adults and increasing physical activity are challenges that confront community nutrition professionals. Nonetheless, this is a very important health message that has to be communicated to all Americans.

Cardiovascular Disease

Although death rates from heart attacks declined 29.7 percent between 1983 and 1993 (figure 10.7), coronary heart disease (CHD) is still the leading cause of death in the United States. There are approximately 1 million deaths annually from heart and blood vessel diseases and more

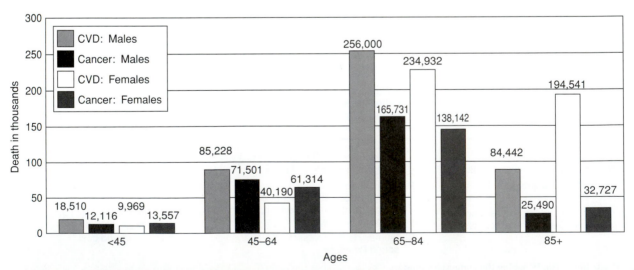

FIGURE 10.7 Deaths from Cardiovascular Diseases and Cancer by Age and Sex
(*Source:* Reproduced with permission. *Heart and Stroke Facts: 1996 Statistical Supplement,* 1995. Copyright © American Heart Association.)

than one in four Americans has some form of CHD. In addition, major disparities and gaps exist among population groups and geographic regions of the United States, with a disproportionate burden of death and disability in minority, low-income, and less-educated populations. As pointed out in chapter 2, whereas the incidence of CHD has decreased in the population as a whole, there has been less of a decrease in disadvantaged groups.

The major modifiable risk factors for CHD are hypercholesterolemia (elevated total and low-density lipoprotein [LDL] cholesterol levels), hypertension, and ciga-rette smoking (table 10.5). Excessive body weight and long-term physical inactivity are other controllable risk factors. A low level (< 35 mg/dl) of high-density lipoprotein [HDL] cholesterol is also a risk factor that can be modified. NIDDM is also a risk factor. The major nonmodifiable risk factors are family history of premature CHD and increasing age for both genders. Recent studies conclude that elevated blood levels of homocysteine, a metabolite that can accumulate when dietary folate, vitamin B_6, and/or vitamin B_{12} are inadequate, is an additional independent risk factor for CHD.[17]

TABLE 10.5
Classification, Assessment, and Action of Coronary Heart Disease

Based on total cholesterol and HDL cholesterol (nonfasting)

Total cholesterol	HDL cholesterol	Assessment	Action
< 200 mg/dl	> 35 mg/dl	Desirable level	Repeat tests in five years; provide education on physical activity and risk factor* reduction.
	< 35 mg/dl		Confer with physician and request a fasting lipoprotein analysis if one is not available.
200–239 mg/dl	> 35 mg/dl *and* fewer than two risk factors*	Borderline high	Provide information on dietary modification, physical activity, and risk factor* reduction. Reevaluate in one to two years.
	< 35 mg/dl *or* two or more risk factors*		Assess fasting lipoprotein analysis.
> 240 mg/dl		High	Assess fasting lipoprotein analysis.

Classification based on LDL cholesterol (nine to twelve hours fasting)

LDL cholesterol	Classification	Action
< 130 mg/dl	Desirable	Repeat total cholesterol and LDL cholesterol measurement within five years. Provide education on dietary modification, physical activity, and risk factor* reduction.
130–159 mg/dl with less than two risk factors*	Borderline high	Provide education on Step I Diet and physical activity and risk factor reduction. Reevaluate lipoprotein analysis annually and reinforce nutrition and physical activity education.
with two or more risk factors*		Clinically evaluate patient (history, physical examination, and laboratory tests). Evaluate for secondary causes and familial disorders. Consider influences of age, sex, and other CHD risk factors. Initiate diet therapy.
> 160 mg/dl	High	Clinically evaluate patient (history, physical examination, and laboratory tests). Evaluate for secondary causes and familial disorders. Consider influences of age, sex, and other CHD risk factors. Initiate diet therapy.

*Risk factors include:
- Age: male older than forty-five years; female older than fifty-five years or premature menopause without estrogen replacement therapy
- Family history of premature CHD: heart attack or sudden death before age fifty-five in father or other male first-degree relative, or before age sixty-five in mother or other female first-degree relative
- Current cigarette smoking
- Hypertension: > 140/90 mm Hg, or on antihypertensive medication
- Diabetes
- Physical inactivity
- High plasma triglycerides (> 400 mg/dl)
- Obesity

Note: A high HDL cholesterol level (> 60 mg/dl) is protective against CHD; when calculating the number of CHD risk factors, count each listed and subtract one if HDL cholesterol level is > 60 mg/dl.

Source: Data adapted from *Heart and stroke facts: 1996 statistical supplement,* Dallas, TX, 1995, American Heart Association.

The National Cholesterol Education Program (NCEP)[35] defines a desirable serum cholesterol level as less than 200 mg/dl, a borderline cholesterol level as 200 to 239 mg/dl, and high cholesterol as more than 240 mg/dl. LDL cholesterol is the unfavorable lipoprotein fraction in the blood (i.e., the fraction associated with increased atherosclerosis) and is classified as follows: a desirable LDL cholesterol is < 130 mg/dl, a borderline LDL cholesterol as 130 to 159 mg/dl, and a high LDL cholesterol level is greater than 160 mg/dl. The average serum cholesterol level for the U.S. adult population is 210 to 215 mg/dl. More than half of adult Americans have a cholesterol level of more than 200 mg/dl, and of this group, approximately one third of them have cholesterol levels of 240 mg/dl or above (figure 10.8).[17] These high cholesterol levels likely have their beginnings early in life as it is estimated that more than one third of American youth age nineteen and under have cholesterol levels of 170 mg/dl or higher. Teens with total cholesterol levels greater than 170 mg/dl are likely to become adults with total cholesterol levels greater than 200 mg/dl. The goal of the NCEP is to reduce the average cholesterol level to less than 200 mg/dl by the year 2000.

Diet, as well as increased physical activity, are the primary treatment regimens for elevated LDL cholesterol levels. The NCEP has recommended that essentially all Americans over two years of age achieve and maintain an ideal body weight by reducing consumption of total fat, saturated fat, and cholesterol and increasing physical activity. The Step I Diet has been recommended for all Americans:

- Less than 10 percent of total calories should come from saturated fat.
- An average of 30 percent or less of calories should come from all fat.
- Dietary energy levels should achieve or maintain a desirable body weight.
- Consumption of cholesterol should be less than 300 mg per day.[35]

Overall, based on 1990 population data, 29 percent of the U.S. population twenty years of age and older are candidates for dietary therapy based on blood cholesterol levels.[47] More men than women are candidates for dietary therapy (32 percent versus 27 percent) when all age groups are considered together. This trend continues until women reach age fifty-five, when almost equal numbers of men and women are candidates for dietary therapy (56 percent for men and 52 percent for women). Adoption of the Step I Diet can result in a 5 to 10 percent reduction in cholesterol levels, which in turn is expected to lead to a 10 to 20 percent or greater reduction in CHD. A Step 2 Diet (less than 30 percent of calories from all fat, less than 7 percent of calories from saturated fat, and less than 200 mg cholesterol per day) is recommended for individuals who need to be treated more aggressively to lower their plasma total and LDL cholesterol levels. Individuals with an elevated plasma

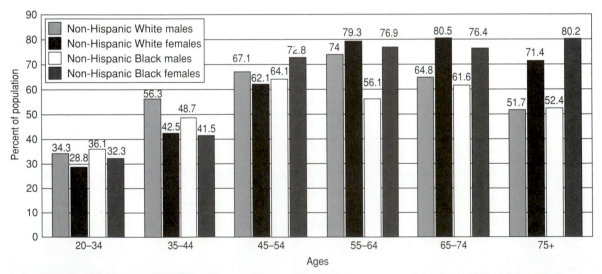

FIGURE 10.8   Estimated Percentage of Americans Age Twenty and Over with Serum Cholesterol of 200 mg/dl or More by Age, Sex, and Race

(*Source:* Reproduced with permission. *Heart and Stroke Facts: 1996 Statistical Supplement,* 1995. Copyright © American Heart Association.)

total and LDL cholesterol should follow a Step I Diet (followed by a Step 2 Diet, if indicated) for at least six months before drug therapy is initiated.

Although the relationship between the development of CHD and both saturated fatty acids and total dietary fat is well established, recent concerns have been raised regarding **trans-fatty acids.** Trans-fatty acids are found in partially hydrogenated vegetable oils, in meat, and in dairy products.[43] Their effect on blood cholesterol levels was examined decades ago but there has been renewed interest in understanding how trans-fatty acids affect blood lipids and lipoproteins. Trans-fatty acids are consumed in small quantities (2 to 4 percent of energy) and have been shown to be modestly hypercholesterolemic in studies that have substituted hydrogenated vegetable oils for nonhydrogenated oils. In contrast, when partially hydrogenated vegetable oils containing trans-fatty acids are substituted for cholesterol-raising saturated fats, blood cholesterol levels are reduced. Since partially hydrogenated vegetable oils are used in place of saturated fat in many food products, these foods can help consumers lower their saturated fat intake to achieve dietary recommendations. Intake of trans-fatty acids does not pose as much of a health concern for Americans as does intake of cholesterol-raising saturated fatty acids. Efforts to decrease trans-fatty acids in the diet certainly can be encouraged, but within the context of a diet that emphasizes reducing total and saturated fats.[43]

A goal of *Healthy People 2000* is for 75 percent of adults to have their blood cholesterol checked during the preceding five years. As of 1995, 71 percent of adults achieved this goal. An additional goal has been incorporated into the established guidelines of the American Heart Association (AHA) and the NCEP to have 30 percent of patients with CHD lower their LDL cholesterol to < 100 mg/dl. The goal of LDL cholesterol < 100 mg/dl is the best estimate of a blood level below which the rate of progression of CHD is likely to be slowed.[54]

Cardiovascular Disease and Women's Health CHD and myocardial infarction (MI) is the most common cause of death in both women and men. Women account for approximately 52 percent of all deaths from major cardiovascular diseases.[24] Numerous studies have shown that in general cardiovascular diseases occur about ten to twelve years later in life in women than in men. The manifestations of CHD differ in men and women—men are more likely to have acute CHD and

women more likely to have chronic CHD that may span periods of time, for example, twenty-five years. Thus, for many women, CHD is a debilitating disease that can adversely affect the quality of their lives for a number of years.[22,23]

The major risk factors for CHD in women are similar to those for men and include hypercholesterolemia, hypertension, and cigarette smoking (table 10.6). Other important risk factors such as age or premature menopause and family history of premature CHD have also been identified.[42] Many of these risk factors increase as women age. The lipid profile most predictive of cardiovascular disease (CVD) risk in women are low HDL cholesterol (< 50 mg/dl) coupled with a high triglyceride (TGC) level (> 400 mg/dl). In addition, a prospective study demonstrated that a high ratio of total cholesterol/HDL cholesterol, left ventricular hypertrophy (indicative of hypertension), or diabetes tended to eliminate the female advantage for CVD over men.[21]

TABLE 10.6
Major Risk Factors for CHD in Women

Risk factor	Cut-point associated with increased risk
Modifiable	
Total cholesterol	> 240 mg/dl
LDL cholesterol	> 160 mg/dl
HDL cholesterol	< 50 mg/dl
Triglyceride	> 400 mg/dl
Hypertension	
Systolic blood pressure	> 140 mm Hg or on antihypertensive medications
Diastolic blood pressure	> 90 mm Hg
Cigarette smoking	Use of cigarettes
Diabetes mellitus	Diagnosis
Overweight	BMI > 27.3 kg/m^2
Sedentary	Lack of at least 30 min of light-to-moderate activity five times per week
Waist-to-hip ratio	> 0.8
Nonmodifiable	
Age	> fifty-five years or premature menopause without estrogen replacement therapy
Family history	Clinical evidence in male or female first-degree relative

Source: Adapted from Krummel DA, Kris-Etherton PM, editors: *Nutrition in women's health,* Gaithersberg, MD, 1996, Aspen Publications.

Women with a BMI > 29 are three times more likely to suffer from both non-fatal and fatal CHD. Women with BMI between 25 and 29 are estimated to have an 80 percent greater risk of CHD than lean women with BMI < 20.[32] Excess body weight predisposes women to other risk factors including hypertension, diabetes mellitus, and increased levels of LDL-cholesterol and TGC. Recent evidence suggests that the distribution of adipose tissue in the abdominal region as measured by waist-to-hip ratio (WHR) > 0.8 is more predictive of CVD risk than is overall obesity.[32]

Menopause presents a unique factor for CVD with implications for both nutritional and pharmacological interventions.[42] Increased risk for CVD after menopause is largely attributable to dropping estrogen levels, which in turn alter a woman's plasma lipid profile. Total cholesterol, LDL cholesterol, and TGC levels increase, whereas protective HDL cholesterol levels remain unchanged or decrease. The ratio of total cholesterol/HDL cholesterol increases, a risk factor positively linked to CVD in women.[26]

Mortality rates and other variables associated with heart disease are considerably less favorable for Black women when compared with White women and other minority women.[28] Of all the risk factors leading to heart disease, hypertension plays a major role and the rates of hypertension are notably higher in Black women. Cholesterol levels are not very different by ethnicity which means they are often as high among ethnic minority women as among women in general. However, obesity in Black women (obesity is twice as prevalent among Black women as among White women) along with the above-average rates of diabetes would seem to contribute substantially to their heart disease risks. Of all the risk factors that place a women at risk for CVD, those that are responsive to nutrition interventions are hypercholesterolemia and excess body weight, which in turn affect the risk of hypertension and diabetes. Thus, nutrition interventions are highly appropriate for women.[23]

Hypertension

Hypertension generally is defined as a systolic blood pressure greater than 140 mm Hg and/or a diastolic blood pressure greater than 90 mm Hg.[2] Approximately 24 percent of adults have hypertension and almost two thirds of these individuals are aware of their condition, but only about one fourth have achieved hypertensive control. The incidence of hypertension is especially high in Blacks, with rates exceeding 50 percent in older individuals. The higher incidence of hypertension in Blacks than in Whites is suggestive of an underlying genetic predisposition.

Several dietary factors are thought to affect blood pressure. Habitual high alcohol intake is related to elevated blood pressure. Some individuals are responsive to a habitual high-salt (high-sodium) diet. A high-potassium diet seems to be protective against development of hypertension. Some evidence suggests an inverse relationship between blood pressure and calcium as well as magnesium intake and the level of physical activity. Caffeine may acutely raise blood pressure in some individuals, but there appear to be no long-term effects. Other dietary factors that have been shown to play some role in the regulation of blood pressure include dietary fat (both quantity and kind), carbohydrate, protein, garlic, and onion.[10]

Blood pressure control is a major objective of the Department of Health and Human Services (DHHS). The goal for the year 2000 is to have blood pressure control in 50 percent of the hypertensive population (up from 24 percent in 1982 to 1984) and to have at least 90 percent of individuals with hypertension taking action to control their elevated blood pressure.

Hypertension and Women's Health   Twenty percent of all women more than twenty years of age have hypertension. The prevalence is higher in older women. This age-related increase in blood pressure is believed to be preventable.[51] A substantial proportion of women with hypertension are overweight.[31] Black women of any age are at the greatest risk for developing hypertension.

Diabetes Mellitus

Diabetes is viewed as two clinically distinct abnormalities in glucose metabolism: NIDDM and IDDM (insulin-dependent diabetes mellitus). Over 90 percent of individuals with diabetes have NIDDM. Approximately 16 million (6 percent of the population) American men, women, and children have diabetes mellitus. However, in 1993, only about 7.8 million people reported knowing they had diagnosed diabetes. NIDDM is associated with unknown genetic factors as well as aging and insulin resistance associated with obesity.[7]

Relative body weight is the only factor that consistently has been related to the prevalence of NIDDM (see box 10.3). A higher calorie and fat intake are posi-

BOX 10.3

RISK FACTORS FOR DEVELOPING DIABETES MELLITUS

- A family history of diabetes (parents or sibling)
- Obesity (body weight more than 20 percent above ideal)
- African-American, Hispanic, or Native-American ancestry
- Age greater than forty years
- Previously identified impaired glucose tolerance
- Hypertension or significant hyperlipidemia (for example, cholesterol > 240 mg/dl or TGC > 250 mg/dl) or the presence of other complications related to diabetes
- In nonpregnant women, a history of gestational diabetes or delivery of a baby weighing more than 4,000 g (9 lb)

Note: Identifying an asymptomatic individual with NIDDM in the general population is very unlikely. However, the chance of developing diabetes increases with any of these factors.
Source: Data from *Diabetes 1996: vital statistics,* Alexandria, VA, American Diabetes Association.

tively related to the incidence of NIDDM, perhaps because of the positive relationship reported between percentage of body fat and percentage of calories from fat. However, the increasingly sedentary lifestyle of Americans may be an important factor as well. The management goal for both NIDDM and IDDM is to achieve normal or near-normal blood glucose levels throughout the day. If the blood glucose levels are not controlled and hyperglycemia is commonly present, then there is a much greater chance for neuropathies, nephropathy, and retinopathy to develop. Therefore, control of blood glucose is critical.

A calorie-restricted diet to lose weight and to maintain weight loss is the primary treatment of NIDDM. Because the leading cause of death among individuals with NIDDM is CHD, diet therapy also entails restricting saturated fatty acids to less than 10 percent of energy and dietary cholesterol to less than 300 mg/day. Energy from total fat and carbohydrate is individualized according to what results in the best clinical outcome for persons. For some, a higher carbohydrate diet is indicated, whereas for others a diet high in total fat is preferable. For persons who need to lose weight, a diet higher in carbohy-

drate (e.g., Step 1 Diet) may be advisable. On the other hand, a diet high in monounsaturated fat, and hence, total fat (e.g., ~ 35 percent of energy) is recommended for the prevention of carbohydrate-induced hypertriglyceridemia as well as further increases in blood glucose and insulin levels. In both instances, these diets typically are implemented using the Exchange Lists for Meal Planning.[8] Recent guidelines recommend using the Exchange Lists along with counting grams of dietary carbohydrate and monitoring blood glucose levels.

The medical nutrition therapy of diabetes involves efforts to restore normal metabolism primarily on blood glucose and plasma lipids. The 1994 American Diabetes Association nutrition recommendations focus on outcomes and no longer advocate an "official diabetic diet."[2]

Diabetes Mellitus and Women's Health Diabetes mellitus is the seventh leading cause of death in the United States. It is a major health problem for women, particularly as they age. It is estimated that women account for more than half of all cases of diabetes. The prevalence rate for diabetes is lower among White women than among women from ethnic minorities in the United States. Black, Native-American, and Hispanic women are 1.5 to 2.5 times more likely to develop diabetes than White non-Hispanic women of comparable age.[55]

In the presence of diabetes mellitus, women face a variety of increased risks, many of which are responsive to nutrition-related interventions. Diabetes mellitus is a powerful and independent risk factor for CVD. The protective effects of premenopausal estrogen are mostly eliminated in the presence of diabetes mellitus.[52] Women with diabetes have twice the risk of heart disease compared with nondiabetic women.

Diabetes mellitus and overweight are interrelated health risks for women. Excess body weight is a known risk for NIDDM.[30] Together, diabetes and overweight are major risk factors for development of CVD. In addition, excess weight negatively affects blood glucose control primarily through its effect on insulin sensitivity. Hypertension, a major risk factor in renal disease and a complication of diabetes mellitus, is more prevalent in women with diabetes than in men with diabetes.[30]

Cancer

The causes of cancer are multifactorial (table 10.7). Although it is not possible to quantify precisely the

TABLE 10.7
Risk Factors for Developing Cancer

Type of cancer	Increase risk	Decrease risk
Lung	Cigarette smoking, exposure to industrial substances, air pollution, radon, second-hand smoke	
Colon and rectal	Family history, physical inactivity, high-fat and/or low-fiber diet	Estrogen replacement therapy, aspirin
Breast	Age, family history, early menarche, late menopause, null parity, first birth at late age	
Prostate	Age, race (African-Americans have higher incidence rates), high-fat diet	
Pancreatic	Age, smoking, high-fat diet	
Cervical	Sexual behavior (first intercourse at an early age, multiple partners), cigarette smoking, low socioeconomic status	
Endometrial	Estrogen, diabetes, gallbladder disease	Pregnancy, oral contraceptive use
Skin	Exposure to ultraviolet (UV) radiation, fair complexion, occupational exposure to certain chemicals, family history	
Ovarian	Age, null parity	Pregnancy, oral contraceptive use
Oral cavity and pharynx	Cigarette, cigar, or pipe smoking; use of smokeless tobacco; excess consumption of alcohol	
Bladder	Cigarette smoking	

Source: Data adapted from *Cancer facts and figures,* Atlanta, GA, 1996, American Cancer Society.

contribution of specific dietary components to individual cancers, it is believed approximately one third of all cancer deaths in the United States may be related to diet. Although the exact mechanisms have yet to be established for either the carcinogenic or anticarcinogenic effects of specific dietary factors, there is strong evidence from both epidemiological and animal studies to suggest that specific food components affect the development of neoplasms.

Cancers of the gastrointestinal tract have been positively associated with alcohol (esophageal and colorectal); salt-cured, smoked, and nitrite-cured foods (esophageal and stomach cancer); and dietary fat (colorectal and prostate cancers). Consumption of fresh fruits and vegetables is inversely associated with stomach cancer. High intakes of vegetables have a strong inverse association with colorectal cancer.

Epidemiological studies from different countries suggest a positive association between prostate cancer and high fat intakes.[6] Whereas, there has been some epidemiological evidence that supports a modest positive relationship between fat intake and breast cancer, a recent meta-analysis of the existing databases concluded that total fat intake is not a risk factor for breast cancer. High alcohol intake is associated with breast cancer.

Consumption of foods contaminated with mycotoxin (e.g., aflatoxin) has been positively associated with the development of liver cancer. Additional food components implicated in the initiation of cancer include heterocyclic amines and *N*-nitroso compounds.[44] Broiling, frying, and barbecuing protein-rich high-fat, low-carbohydrate foods, such as meats, at high temperatures so that the meat burns, can cause formation of heterocyclic amines. *N*-nitroso compounds are formed by the interaction of amines and nitrosating agents such as nitrite or nitrous oxide. This reaction happens in cured meats and salt-dried fish.

Lung and bladder cancer are most clearly associated with exposure to tobacco and certain industrial chemicals. Eating fruits and vegetables high in beta-carotene has been associated with a lowered risk of cancer, however, beta-carotene supplements do not appear to provide the same benefit. Two recent studies suggest that beta-carotene supplementation for smokers can actually be harmful.[1,38] It must be pointed out that these two studies involved long-term smokers who continued to smoke and that their cancers may have already been in the development phase before the study began. It is thought that beta-carotene is only one of several components in fruits and vegetables that reduce the risk of cancer. Many epidemiological and animal studies

TABLE 10.8
Trends in Evidence Associating Diet and Cancers Among Women

Dietary factor	Risk	Cancer sites
Total fat, saturated fat, animal fat	Increase	Colon/rectum, lung, endometrium, ovary
Vegetables: green/yellow, carotenoid-rich	Decrease	Breast, colon/rectum, lung, cervix, ovary
Vitamin C–rich fruits	Decrease	Breast, cervix, lung, colon/rectum
Fiber, grains, cereals, complex carbohydrates	Decrease	Breast, colon/rectum, endometrium, ovary
Vitamin E	Decrease	Breast, cervix
Folate	Decrease	Breast, colon/rectum, cervix

Source: Adapted from Freudenheim JL, Potischman N: Cancer. In Krummel DA, Kris-Etherton PM, editors: *Nutrition in women's health,* Gaithersberg, MD, 1996, Aspen Publications.

strongly suggest that increased carotenoid intakes and blood levels are protective against a variety of chronic diseases, including heart disease, cancers, and cataracts; other specific dietary components identified as possible protective agents include phytochemicals, vitamin C, fiber, and selenium. Phytochemicals are compounds in plants that influence production of certain enzymes involved in detoxifying carcinogens and removing items from the body. When consumed on a regular basis, some phytochemicals may help reduce the risk of cancer and heart disease.

Obesity is associated with an increased risk of the development of cancer of the endometrium and the gallbladder. The underlying biological mechanisms that may account for this are unclear, although elevated estrogen levels, increased energy intake, and increased intake of carcinogens, among others, have been implicated. There is also evidence that supports a positive relationship between obesity and breast cancer.

Epidemiological studies associating specific dietary factors to human carcinogenisis are often inconclusive or conflicting.[16] This inability to determine association may be due to methodological differences associated with measuring nutrient and energy intake, studying people within a country where diet and lifestyles are relatively homogeneous, and being unable to account for lifestyle and cultural differences between populations. Based on the evidence available to date, the National Research Council has issued the following dietary recommendations to lower cancer risk:

- Increase fruit, vegetable, and whole-grain consumption
- Limit total fat intake
- Limit intake of alcohol and salt-preserved and nitrite-cured foods
- Maintain healthy body weight

Cancer and Women's Health   For women in the United States, there are approximately 576,000 new cases and 225,000 deaths from cancer annually.[5] Breast cancer, which is the most frequently diagnosed malignancy in women today, remains a major threat. Known risk factors include age, early menarche, late age of first pregnancy, late menopause, family history, and obesity. The link between nutrition and breast cancer is controversial, particularly the association between dietary fat and development of breast cancer. Findings from animal research and international correlation studies indicate a causal relation between fat intake and breast cancer. Nevertheless, epidemiological studies (case-control and cohort) give conflicting results regarding any causal relation between fat intake and breast cancer. The fact that these studies have failed to consistently show a significant association between fat intake and breast cancer may reflect the difficulty of collecting accurate dietary information and other methodological limitations. Findings are also limited because of the lack of data on the influence of a high-fat diet during childhood.[14]

An area of study that may hold promise in linking diet and breast cancer is the density of breast tissue.[3] Research at the National Cancer Institute (NCI) found that women with very high breast density have a five-fold greater risk of breast cancer. Preliminary research conducted at Canada's Ontario Cancer Institute has demonstrated that breast density as reflected on mammography is decreased with a low-fat diet. A prospective randomized controlled study examining breast density with a diet consisting of only 15 percent fat calories is now underway. This finding, if substantiated, may lead to improvement in diagnosis by mammography and help in lowering the risk of breast cancer.

There is evidence to suggest that there are dietary patterns that are generally associated with a lower risk of cancer (table 10.8). Diets low in fat and high in fruits and vegetables and fiber-rich grains have been shown with some consistency to be associated with lower risk of many of the major cancers affecting women in the United States.[14]

Osteoporosis

Osteoporosis is a multifactorial and complex disorder of the skeletal system characterized by bone loss and increasing skeletal fragility.[15] This disorder is usually not clinically apparent until minimal trauma causes a fracture, most typically in the hip, wrist, or vertebrae. Osteoporosis is a common condition affecting about 24 million Americans, 80 percent of them women. It is the major cause of approximately 1.3 million bone fractures yearly in the United States.

It is estimated that 50 percent of women over forty-five years of age have osteoporosis. The gradual decrease in estrogen secretion following menopause is directly correlated with the reduction in bone mass. Reduced estrogen levels result in reduction of intestinal calcium absorption, as well as in an increase in bone calcium resorption. However, ethnic and genetic differences, decreasing physical activity, cigarette smoking, alcohol intake, adiposity as measured by BMI, reproductive history, and low bone calcium reserves may play selective roles. It is important to note that bone health, and consequently bone mass, is a function of three components: nutrition (primarily calcium), hormones (primarily estrogen), and lifestyle (primarily weight-bearing physical activity). Each component is essential and one component cannot substitute for another (figure 10.9).

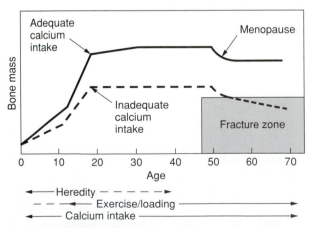

FIGURE 10.9   Bone Mass Lifeline with Some of the Major Controlling Influences
(*Source:* Reprinted with permission from Robert P. Heaney. Copyright 1993.)

Peak bone mass is achieved five to ten years after longitudinal bone growth has ceased. Once peak bone mass is reached, it remains stable until forty to forty-five years of age. Thereafter, bone is lost as a yearly rate of about 0.2 to 0.5 percent, except in women just before and for about ten years after onset of menopause, when the rate increases. Poor nutrition, such as inadequate calcium and vitamin D, high protein/low calcium diet, or inadequate caloric intake can lead to a decrease in bone mass. Absence or marked reduction of estrogen (such as when a woman has an oophorectomy [both ovaries surgically removed] or enters menopause) causes a loss of bone mass due to a reduction in calcium absorption from the intestine. Lack of weight-bearing physical activity also leads to loss of bone mass. Another factor affecting peak bone mass is genetics. There appears to be a strong genetic relationship between mothers and daughters affecting both the level of peak bone mass and the amount of postmenopausal bone loss.

Sufficient dietary calcium must be present to sustain bone density during growth and to maintain skeletal mass later in life. Unfortunately, many Americans consume diets that provide insufficient calcium to attain an ideal peak bone mass and to maintain optimal bone health to prevent age-related bone loss. Adolescent and adult females of most ages and racial and ethnic groups have median calcium intakes from food that are consistently below recommended dietary allowance (RDA) values, and consequently what is considered to be an optimal intake.[39] Therefore, current intake of calcium by these groups may not be adequate to achieve peak bone mass and prevent age-related loss of bone mass.

In the United States, the prevalence of osteoporosis is lower among Blacks than Whites. White women are two to three times more likely to suffer a hip fracture than Black women and men of both races. This difference appears to be related to high bone density, and skeletal calcium content, as well as greater body mass in Blacks, which in all ethnic groups is associated with a lower incidence of osteoporosis.

Although we cannot alter our genetics, which also has an important role in developing bone mass, we can control our nutrition. The following plan provides protection from osteoporosis.[16]

- Diet should provide sufficient nutrients during growth for bone building, both to achieve the full genetic potential for bone mass and to offset daily losses.
- At maturity, the role of nutrition is primarily to preserve the bone mass we have achieved and, secondar-

ily, to help the skeleton recover from the unstable periods of disability, injury, or illness that an adult experiences intermittently throughout life.

- Nutrition plays an important role in susceptibility to fragility in the elderly (particularly hip fracture) and in recovery from fractures.

Thus, primary prevention of osteoporosis lies in achieving peak bone mass during skeletal growth and early adulthood. Secondary prevention lies in the conservation of acquired bone mass during later life stages. Therefore, the strategies to reduce the risk of developing osteoporosis advised in *Healthy People 2000* are: "increase to at least 90 percent the proportion of perimenopausal women who have been counseled about the benefits and risks of estrogen replacement therapy for prevention of osteoporosis . . . [and] . . . increase calcium intake so at least 50 percent of people aged 25 and older consume two or more servings daily of food rich in calcium."[54]

Alcohol Abuse

In the United States, alcohol is the most commonly used psychotropic drug and consequently, alcohol abuse is a major problem.[36] In 1993, half of the U.S. population reported current use of alcohol. Sixteen million (7.5 percent) were daily or almost daily drinkers and 11 million (5.3 percent) reported heavy use of alcohol (drinking five or more drinks per occasion on five or more days in the previous month). Use of alcohol is highest among adults ages eighteen to thirty-four; its use declines among adults over age fifty.[26] The economic costs of alcohol abuse are estimated to be more than $70 billion each year, primarily from decreased productivity. Excessive alcohol consumption increases the risk for heart disease, high blood pressure, neurological diseases, and may other disorders. Alcohol is the major contributor to development of liver cirrhosis, a significant cause of death in the United States, and alcohol is involved in more than half of all motor vehicle accidents and fatal intentional injuries (homicides and suicides). Disproportionately more Blacks and Native Americans suffer from alcohol abuse.

The nutritional consequences of alcohol consumption are related to the amount of alcohol consumed. Light drinkers simply add extra calories, whereas among moderate to heavy drinkers, alcohol may account for half of total energy intake. As consumption of alcohol increases, the percentage of energy from protein, fat, and carbohydrates decreases. Nitrogen excretion increases, resulting in higher protein requirement for alcohol abusers. Dietary nutrient quality declines with significant decreases in intakes of vitamins A and C, thiamin, calcium, iron, and fiber. Alcohol abuse can lead to primary malnutrition, in which alcohol replaces consumption of other food. Alcohol abuse can lead to secondary malnutrition by decreasing digestion, absorption, or utilization, or by increasing nutrient demands.

Some studies suggest beneficial effects of moderate alcohol intake in lowering CHD risk. However, for individuals who do not drink alcohol, it is not appropriate to recommend that they start consuming alcohol primarily because of risk of addiction and other associated problems. If consumed, alcohol intake should be limited to the equivalent of less than 1 oz of pure alcohol per day. This is the amount in two (12 oz) cans of beer, two (5 oz) glasses of wine, or two average mixed drinks (1½ oz of distilled 80 proof alcohol per drink).

Cigarette Smoking

Cigarette smoking is considered to be the single most avoidable cause of death in the United States. In 1995, of the 2.2 million people who died, 512,900 or 24 percent of these deaths could be attributed directly to cigarette smoking.

Cigarette smokers have a higher vitamin C requirement than nonsmokers because smoking increases the metabolism of vitamin C. In addition, smokers absorb 10 percent less vitamin C. The RDA for vitamin C is 100 mg/day for persons who smoke twenty or more cigarettes per day as compared with 60 mg/day for nonsmoking adults.[9]

NUTRITIONAL REQUIREMENTS

Since the 1970s, nutritional concerns have shifted from nutrient deficiencies to nutrient excesses. Chronic disease risk reduction has become a major emphasis of community nutrition professionals.

Nutrient and Energy Allowances

Nutrient allowances for healthy adults are basically the same throughout the adult years with very few exceptions. Older adults (over sixty-five years) need slight increases in fiber, protein, and calcium intakes, while total energy intakes gradually decrease (see chapter 11). Energy needs vary considerably among adults and are functions of gender, body mass, and level of physical activity. Estimates of energy needs for men ages twenty-three to fifty years are 2,700 cal/day and for ages fifty-one to sixty-four years, 2,400 kcal/day. For women ages twenty-three to fifty years, energy needs are estimated at 2,000 kcal/day, and for those fifty-one to sixty-four years, 1,800 kcal/day. A simple method for estimating energy allowance for an individual is to multiply body weight by a predetermined factor for the level of physical activity (table 10.9).

As energy needs decline and nutrient requirements stay essentially the same, it becomes necessary to obtain the required nutrients while consuming a lower energy diet. Therefore, the foods being consumed must be of higher "nutrient density," that is, the ratio of the amount of nutrients to the energy content of the food. An additional way to ensure adequate intake of nutrients while maintaining energy balance is to increase physical activity. This will allow a person to eat a greater variety as well as a larger quantity of foods to obtain needed nutrients.

Drug-Nutrient Interactions

Although some community nutrition professionals consider **drug-nutrient interactions** a problem associated only with the elderly, some younger adults use both prescription and over-the-counter medications for various problems. Thus, community nutrition professionals need to be aware of the potential effects of drug-nutrient interactions in adults of all ages as well as children and adolescents.

Drugs and nutrients can interact in three primary ways: a drug and nutrient can react together to form a new compound, a drug or nutrient can affect the gastrointestinal tract and ultimately the absorption of either, and a drug can impair the metabolism of nutrients (see box 10.4). The occurrence of an interaction is dependent on the drug, the food consumed, and the pattern of food consumption. Risk of interaction can be reduced by adjusting the dosage of drug, the timing of drug intake, and the timing of food intake.[46]

Usually physicians and pharmacists give advice on drug-nutrient interactions. Community nutrition professionals, however, can suggest the following: read labels on and package inserts in prescription and over-the-

TABLE 10.9

Factors for Estimating Daily Energy Allowances at Various Levels of Physical Activity for Men and Women (Ages nineteen to fifty years)

Level of activity	Examples*	Energy expenditure factor[†] (kcal/kg per day)
Very light	Sitting or standing quietly	
Men		31
Women		30
Light	Cleaning house, office work, playing baseball, playing golf	
Men		38
Women		35
Moderate	Walking briskly (3.5 MPH), gardening, cycling (5.5 MPH), dancing, playing basketball	
Men		41
Women		37
Heavy	Jogging (9 min/mile), playing football, swimming	
Men		50
Women		44
Exceptional	Running (7 min/mile), racquetball, skiing	
Men		58
Women		51

*Examples are a rough guide to help categorize individuals; activities should be participated in on a regular basis for an extended period of time. Patterns typical of the U.S. population are in the light or moderate categories.

[†]To calculate estimated daily energy allowance (kcal/day), multiply the individual's body weight in kilograms by the appropriate (for sex and average activity level) energy expenditure factor.

BOX 10.4

DRUG-NUTRIENT INTERACTION

- Long-term use of aspirin can promote chronic gastrointestinal blood loss that can result in iron-deficiency anemia.
- Diuretics can promote loss of body potassium leading to a potential increase in blood pressure.
- Antacids containing aluminum hydroxide can reduce phosphorus absorption and affect calcium balance.
- Dietary calcium can reduce the absorption of the antibiotic tetracycline.
- Carbonated beverages can cause some drugs to dissolve in the stomach rather than in the intestine, where they are more easily absorbed into the blood.
- A combination of alcohol and depressants (tranquilizers, barbiturates, or painkillers) can slow performance skills, judgment, and alertness to dangerously low levels.

counter drugs, question the physician or pharmacist about how a drug may react with food or beverages, and report any unusual symptoms to a physician. Such simple messages can help increase awareness of potential problems and prevent adverse reactions.

Dietary Recommendations

The cornerstone of feeding recommendations for healthy adults are the *Dietary Guidelines for Americans*.[37] The Food Guide Pyramid[53] incorporates the scientific principles linking diet and health and diet and disease. It also integrates the concepts of deficiency disease prevention as established by the RDAs with chronic disease risk reduction as established in the Dietary Guidelines messages. These recommendations are further integrated into the Nutrition Facts panel on food labels. Dietary recommendations are discussed fully in chapter 2.

Dietary recommendations of organizations such as the NCEP, the AHA, and the NCI, to name a few, follow the general concepts embodied in the Food Guide Pyramid. Deviations from these guidelines are made on an individual basis and are structured to accommodate personal differences such as health status, activity levels, and food preferences.

Supplements

Despite statements issued by professional medical and nutrition societies promoting the concept that healthy people can obtain all necessary nutrients by eating a variety of foods, many individuals use dietary supplements. Reasons given for supplement use include uncertainty about nutrient adequacy of foods, a desire to attain perceived improved physical status, and self-treatment for illness. Professionals are concerned about the widespread use of over-the-counter supplements. Overdoses of single nutrients, such as vitamins A and D, can be harmful. Large doses of some nutrients may interact with other nutrients and interfere with their absorption, utilization, metabolism, excretion, and accordingly, their requirements. Additionally, supplementation may mask the diagnosis of some diseases; for example, folate can prevent pernicious anemia caused by vitamin B_{12} deficiency and thereby mask the development of neurological symptoms caused by B_{12} deficiency. Before implementing nutrition education or other intervention activities, community nutrition professionals need to know current dietary patterns and trends (consumer behavior) and the target audience's knowledge and attitudes toward health and nutrition. In addition, they need to be sensitive to any additional environmental factors that might impact on food choices and subsequent health. This information, along with behavior change theories and models that are used to plan interventions are described in chapter 7.

Current Dietary Status

Results from the National Health and Nutrition Examination Survey (NHANES) III survey indicate the median dietary intake of vitamins A, E, and B_6 and the minerals zinc and copper were below recommended values for most age, sex, and racial and ethnic groups.[10] For females age twenty years and older, median dietary calcium intakes were below current recommendations and appreciably lower than the 1,200 to 2,000 mg recommended by the NIH consensus panel. Furthermore, median dietary calcium intakes were below recommended values for non-Hispanic Black males twenty to fifty-nine years of age and for all males sixty years of age and older. Dietary iron intakes were below recommended values for adult females twenty to fifty-nine across all racial and ethnic groups. Dietary intakes of magnesium were below recommended values for all adults. Median dietary folate intakes were below

recommended values for all non-Hispanic Black females older than sixteen years of age and for Mexican-
American females sixty years of age and older.

Intakes of total fat and saturated fatty acids as a percentage of energy have been declining since the 1980s.
Total fat as a percentage of energy decreased from 36 to
37 percent of calories in 1984 to 32 to 34 percent in
1991, whereas saturated fat decreased from 14 percent of
calories to about 12 percent. The intakes for polyunsaturated and monounsaturated fatty acids remained stable at
about 6 to 7 and 13 percent of calories, respectively.

A word of caution is needed regarding the interpretation of dietary trends. Methodological changes have occurred over time in the collection of diet information, in
food composition and analysis, and in sampling the population surveyed. These changes can profoundly alter
the apparent intake of a nutrient over time. For example,
recent advances in cholesterol analysis reveal that previous levels of cholesterol in eggs were overestimated.
Therefore, when community nutrition professionals read
that Americans are consuming less dietary cholesterol,
they must be cautious in concluding that Americans are
consuming lower quantities of cholesterol-containing
foods. The lower levels may simply be an artifact of
changes in measurement.

Other food consumption trends have been noted and
are reflective of generational differences. Breakfast
consumption declined from 86 to 75 percent between
1965 and 1991 for U.S. adults.[13] Breakfast consumption
increases with age, and the nutritional quality of food
consumed at breakfast has improved since 1965. Per
capita consumption of ready-to-eat breakfast cereals
rose from 8.6 lb in 1972 to 11.3 lb in 1992. Snacks contribute approximately 12 percent of daily calories. This
percentage declines as adults get older.

Interesting trends in dietary intake by racial and socioeconomic status (SES) between 1965 and 1991 have
been reported.[41] Although dietary differences have narrowed between SES and race, there has been a reversal
between diet and SES. In 1965, low SES individuals consumed more healthful diets when compared to midrange
persons, whereas high SES individuals consumed diet of
poorer quality (e.g., higher in fat, lower grain consumption). Indeed, diets of lower SES Blacks had the best
overall diet quality in 1965. Although all groups showed
improvements in some areas by 1991, the trends had reversed toward higher SES individuals consuming more
healthful diets. If the trend continues in the same direc-

tion, it is possible that the diet quality of lower SES
groups may not continue to improve as quickly as that
among the higher SES groups. This trend can only serve
to further the morbidity and mortality disparities observed among segments of the U.S. adult population.

Using annual per capita consumption data collected
over a twenty-year time span, it can be seen that American adults are making changes in their food choices. In
addition, many notable differences in food choices exist
within the adult population.

Milk and Milk Products   Between 1972 and 1992, the
annual per capita consumption of whole milk decreased
dramatically (from 200 lb to 81 lb), whereas intakes of
both low-fat and non-fat milk increased (from 39 to 99 lb
and 12 to 25 lb, respectively). Furthermore, consumption
of cheese doubled from 13 to 26 lb. Most striking was
the dramatic increase in yogurt consumption, which rose
from 1.3 lb in 1972 to 4.3 lb in 1992. A greater percentage of Black adults report consuming whole milk,
whereas greater percentages of White adults reported
consuming low-fat and non-fat milks. Black females reported the lowest intake of milk and milk products and
White males reported the highest intake.

Cereal and Grain   Consumption of flour and cereal
products jumped 54 lb per capita between 1972 and
1992, with consumption of rice up 140 percent, corn
products up 126 percent, oat products up 93 percent,
and wheat flour up 26 percent. Much of this growth is
explained by the expansion of the fast-food industry, in-
store bakeries, offerings of grain-based products in the
retail marketplace, and increased interest in ethnic
foods. The percentage of adults reporting intake of
yeast breads and rolls, cereals, and pastas were similar
across race, sex, and income levels.

Meat, Poultry, Eggs, Fish, and Beans   Annual per
capita consumption of red meats decreased slightly
(13 percent) from 1972 to 1992, from 132 to 114 lb.
At the same time, there was a 70 percent increase in
poultry consumption (from 35 to 60 lb) and an 18 percent increase in fish and shellfish consumption (12 to
15 lb). In addition, there was a 23 percent drop in egg
consumption over the twenty years. The 10 percent
decrease in consumption of dry peas and lentils was
offset by an identical increase in consumption of dry
edible beans. Consumption of meat, poultry, and fish

is higher in men than in women. A higher percentage of White than Black adults report consuming beef, whereas a higher percentage of Black adults consumed pork, poultry, seafood, and shellfish. However, adults of any race with higher incomes reported consuming a higher percentage of beef, fish, and shellfish.

Fruits and Vegetables Unfortunately, the change in fruit and vegetable annual per capita consumption was not very dramatic—with 222 lb of fruit and 332 lb of vegetables consumed annually in 1972 and 263 lb of fruit and 379 lb of vegetables consumed in 1992. This represents an 18 percent increase in fruit consumption and a 14 percent increase for vegetables. About 30 percent of adult males and 24 percent of adult females did not eat any fruits and about 6 percent of individuals did not eat any vegetables. A higher percentage of older than younger adults reported consuming dark-green and deep-yellow vegetables, lettuce, and other vegetables.

Fats, Oils, and Sweets Although per capita use of fats and oils climbed 23 percent between 1972 and 1992, the source of the fat changed from highly saturated animal fats to more unsaturated vegetable sources.

Alcohol In 1992, the average per capita consumption of all alcoholic beverages was 2.31 gallons: 56 percent as beer, 31 percent as wine, and 13 percent as distilled spirits. Between 1972 and 1992, per capita consumption of beer and wine among young adults increased 4 percent, while consumption of distilled spirits fell 36 percent. Per capita consumption of beer and spirits reached their peaks in 1981 and have steadily declined since. Wine consumption peaked in 1985 and has also declined steadily since then.

Attitudes and Beliefs About Food and Nutrition

Motivation, attitudes, and beliefs each play a role as significant as knowledge in determining individuals' eating behaviors. Several surveys have been conducted to assess current attitudes and beliefs of American adults regarding food, nutrition, and health. Overwhelmingly, despite adequate knowledge and positive attitudes and beliefs about the relationship of diet and health, taste is the driving force in food choice.

Most often, food selection studies segment respondents based on demographic characteristics such as age, ethnicity, marital status, or income. A unique segmentation approach describing 3,000 Americans according to both their demographic characteristics and their health behaviors, including dietary practices and influences on food choices, was recently reported (table 10.10).[41] In general, many of these Americans were aware of the relationship between diet and health. Some were even motivated to following eating habits consistent with dietary recommendations. However, their food choices demonstrate that awareness and motivation do not automatically translate into action. Community nutrition professionals must determine how these factors influence the communities in which they work, the types of interventions they wish to pursue, and their own attitudes about these issues.

NUTRITION EDUCATION INTERVENTIONS

As awareness of the demographics and key nutrition-related problems in a community as well as within different population groups is important in determining what nutrition **assessment** information is needed in the planning stages of developing **nutrition education interventions.** As described below, there are many different options from which to select to assess the **nutritional status** of a population group. It is also important that community nutrition professionals have current information about standards of care and practice guidelines for health promotion. This information is helpful in guiding decisions about what nutrition assessment measurements to pursue. Collectively, all of the information that is obtained is integrated into the development of the most appropriate nutrition education intervention programs.

Nutrition Assessment

Nutritional assessment is an important part of providing preventive nutrition services. Dietary intake data, anthropometric measurements, biochemical analyses, clinical evaluation, and psychosocial-economic assessment are commonly used to provide an in-depth appraisal of an individual's nutritional status. Comparison of individual assessments with standardized measurements can then be made. Guidelines for assessing nutritional status along with intervention strategies for the adult appear in table 10.11. Involvement and awareness of the adult with whom the community nutrition professional is working at each step of the assessment process are essential.

TABLE 10.10

Segmentation of Americans According to Health Beliefs

Lifestyle descriptor	Proportion	Demographics	General description of health behaviors	Exercise behavior	Dietary intake	Weight control
Physical fantastics	25%	60% female; 76% between eighteen and fifty-four years old; 76% White, 13% Hispanic, 11% Black; > $50,000 yearly	Most compliant with health recommendations	Exercise regularly	Eat healthful foods	Make efforts to control weight
Active attractives	13%	59% men; 80% < fifty-five years old; 77% White, 13% Hispanic, 10% Black; Less likely to have children	Moderately health-oriented; Among the heavier groups	Interested in getting regular exercise but often don't do so	Limit fat intake	Interested in controlling weight but often don't do so
Tense but trying	10%	63% women; 78% between eighteen and fifty-four years old; 75% White, 13% Hispanic, 12% Black	Health-oriented, but smoke; Want to do better	Average level	Average concern about fat	Average concern about weight control efforts
Passively healthy	15%	65% male; 79% between eighteen and fifty-four years old; Average incomes; 74% White, 15% Hispanic, 11% Black	In excellent health primarily because they are young; Indifferent or ambivalent to healthy behaviors	Regular exercise	Don't pay much attention to fat; Don't eat fruits and vegetables	Not interested although they are the thinnest group
Decent dolittles	25%	63% women; 73% between eighteen and fifty-four years old; Above average incomes; 74% married; 80% White, 12% Hispanic, 9% Black	Less health-oriented, although well aware of what they "should" be doing; Most overweight	Unlikely	Unlikely	Unlikely
Hard-living hedonists	6%	82% < fifty-five years old; 73% males; 61% married; 78% White, 14% Black, 8% Hispanic; Lowest incomes	Not at all interested; Least satisfied with their lives; Drink and smoke heavily	Physically active because they are laborers and machine operators	Enjoy eating high-fat foods; No plans to change	No intention
Noninterested nihilists	7%	53% male; 81% < fifty-five years old; Most likely to have children; Incomes < $15,000; 80% White, 12% Black, 8% Hispanic	Least health-oriented; Reject notion people should enhance their health; Smoke heavily	Dislike intensely	Consume high-fat foods; Shun fruits and vegetables	Little effort made

Source: Data adapted from Porter/Novelli. Healthstyles® 1996.

Once the assessment is complete, the community nutrition professional must decide how to proceed.

If no disease is present, nutrition intervention should be directed at removing or limiting risk factors (primary prevention). If disease is symptomatic, early detection, referral, and nutrition intervention to prevent further progression is appropriate (secondary prevention). Finally, if clinical signs of disease are present, nutrition interventions should be aimed at managing the disease and reducing complications (tertiary prevention).

Dietary Assessment Commonly used dietary assessment methods include the twenty-four-hour recall, food records, or diet histories. Food frequency questionnaires also can be used for a less-detailed assessment of an individual's diet. A number of simple tools have been developed that target a specific nutrient (principally fat). After the dietary information has been collected, it must be analyzed and then compared with a standard. Dietary recalls, food records, and diet histories can be analyzed by computer and energy and nutrient intake information are obtained. (see chapter 3 for a detailed discussion of dietary assessment methods.)

Anthropometric Variables Weight, height, and body site measurements are easily obtained and are useful if edema is not present. BMI and waist-hip ratio calculations provide the community nutrition professionals with additional tools for determining counseling strategies. Moreover, collecting information about weight history is helpful in designing appropriate nutrition intervention programs for weight management.

Clinical Assessment Medical history, complete physical examination, blood pressure measurements, chronic disease risk questionnaire, family history, stress factors, physical fitness, smoking history, alcohol consumption information, and dental evaluation are reviewed with the client. Skin, hair, teeth, gums, lips, tongue, and eyes are examined. Because of rapid cell turnover of epithelial and mucosal tissue, the hair, skin, and mouth are susceptible to nutritional deficiencies. However, it is important to note that if nutritional deficiencies are apparent clinically, they are at an advanced stage. Alternatively, a biochemical assessment detects the early stages of a nutrient deficiency.

Biochemical Assessment Examination of a metabolite in blood or urine represents a sensitive measurement of nutritional status. Sometimes tissues such as

hair, fingernails, or even bone and liver are examined. Typically, a complete blood count is used to assess iron status as well as that of other micronutrients, protein status, and liver enzymes. Immunological measurements are useful in assessing malnutrition. Plasma total cholesterol and HDL cholesterol measurements are recommended for virtually all adults, followed by a complete lipoprotein analysis (including HDL cholesterol and LDL cholesterol measurements) when plasma total cholesterol is greater than 240 mg/dl.

Psychosocial-Economic Assessment Information about lifestyle, attitudes about food, nutrition and health, home life, support network, food procurement and preparation facilities, economic situation, literacy level, and ethnicity should be collected. This information is important in establishing an effective counseling relationship with the client.

In addition, tools to determine "stages of change" could be employed to facilitate intervention strategies.[48] The stages-of-change model (described in chapter 7) can be useful to community nutrition professionals as a theoretical framework for designing effective marketing strategies and interventions; to evaluate effectiveness of programming, to alleviate personal frustrations that arise when change is not occurring and that often impair the professional's ability to continue to work effectively; and to facilitate realistic expectations among program participants themselves.

The community nutrition professional needs to remain aware of the many factors affecting each adult to plan intervention programs that help individuals meet their unique nutrition-related needs.

Practice Guidelines

Consensus statements and specific guidelines for prevention management of chronic disease in adults have emerged that incorporate expected health outcomes in a health promotion–disease prevention model. Underlying all nutrition education interventions in the adult years are the Dietary Guidelines.[37] Both the Food Guide Pyramid and the Nutrition Facts Label utilize these recommendations as their base. Healthy People 2000 objectives also are aimed at meeting these guidelines. Community nutrition professionals must be cognizant of the continual updates of the Dietary Guidelines themselves as well as of the yearly monitoring of the health status of the population to maintain and assure program quality. Further, community nutrition professionals

TABLE 10.11

Nutrition Assessment and Intervention Guidelines in Community Nutrition for Adults

Assessment	Methods	Risk or problem indicated	Intervention guidelines	Referral sources
Dietary evaluation: three to four-day food record; twenty-four-hour recall, including one weekend day; food frequency questionnaire	Determine quantity and quality of diet with special consideration given to alcohol, sodium, total fat, saturated fat, cholesterol, and fiber intakes.	Alcoholism; Drug abuse; Marginal intakes of essential nutrients, that could lead to nutritional deficiencies; Excessive intakes of food and/or nutrients that could lead to future nutritional problems	Investigate causal factors in substance abuse and suggest coping mechanism. Adjust diet modifications in relation to other indicators that contribute to dietary amelioration.	Alcoholics Anonymous; Public, private, or voluntary behavioral health agencies/programs; Qualified nutrition professionals
Anthropometric: height, weight, skinfold thickness, arm circumference	Use standardized measurement equipment: balanced scales, steel or nonstretch measuring tapes, calipers; Use standardized height and weight tables to determine weight status (e.g. 1995 *Dietary Guidelines*). Use BMI to determine weight status. Use waist-hip ratio to determine site of fat deposition.	Moderate to underweight: BMI < 16 for men; BMI < 15 for women; Moderate overweight: BMI 25–30 for men; BMI for women: 24–29; Severe overweight: BMI for men: > 30, BMI > 29 for women; Waist-hip ratios: for men: > 1.0 for women: > 0.8	If weight is below healthy range and/or BMI indicated underweight, weight gain may be appropriate. Maintain weight if weight is in healthy range, if less than 10 lb were gained once adult height was reached, and if healthy. If weight is above healthy range and/or BMI > 25, weight loss is necessary. Recommend a weight to achieve a weight approx 2 BMI units lower.	Reputable weight management program; Qualified nutrition professional; Reputable physical fitness program and recreational facilities; Worksite health promotion program
Clinical: medical history; blood pressure; chronic disease risk factor questionnaire (family history, diabetes, and stress); physical fitness; smoking; dental; socioeconomic status	Use clinical assessment and physical examination data to determine if one or more signs indicate nutrition-related diseases. Use questionnaire to determine risk factors for cardiovascular disease. Use a sphygmomanometer and blood pressure procedures established by the Joint National Committee on Detection, Evaluation and Treatment of High Blood Pressure. Use treadmill test for physical fitness. Use lung function test for smoking and other respiratory problems. Examine oral cavity, condition of teeth and gums, and oral hygiene.	Hypertension (blood pressure > 140/90 mm Hg); Risk of heart attack, stroke, and certain cancers (lung, bladder, esophagus) increases with number and severity of risk factors such as overweight, high fat intake, hypertension, elevated cholesterol, smoking, inactivity, and stress.	Encourage adherence to drug and diet modifications. Develop personalized intervention plan on desirable lifestyle modifications that include diet and exercise.	Stop-smoking clinics; Food Stamp Program; Cooperative extension services; Emergency food assistance programs; Qualified nutrition professionals

294

Biochemical: hemoglobin; hematocrit; total serum cholesterol and lipoproteins; blood glucose	Use standardized laboratory equipment and laboratory quality control procedures. Compare values to: • Centers for Disease Control and Prevention standards for hemoglobin and hematocrit adjusted for age, sex, and altitude • National Cholesterol Education Program Guidelines • National Diabetes Data Group, National Institutes of Health	Anemia Elevated cholesterol (>200 mg/dl) Elevated LDL cholesterol (>130 mg/dl) Low HDL cholesterol (<35 mg/dl)	Modify diet to increase number of foods that are high in iron sources. Modify diet to decrease total fat (<30% of energy), saturated fat (<10% of energy), and cholesterol (<300 mg/day). Adjust energy intake as appropriate to achieve and maintain healthy body weight. Adjust personal diet modifications using diabetes exchange lists and carbohydrate counting.	Public, private, and voluntary agencies State and/or local health departments State and/or local heart associations State and/or local diabetes associations Community hospitals Qualified nutrition professionals
Psychosocial: lifestyle; cooking, shopping, eating; family structure; income; ethnicity; literacy level; readiness to change	Determine environmental factors affecting food procurement, choices, and preparation. Determine barriers to change. Determine readiness to change using stages-of-change questionnaires.	Lack of facilities for food purchase and preparation Lack of financial and other resources Lack of awareness of consequences to personal health Lack of motivation to change	Facilitative interventions using behavior change theories to overcome limitations. Use appropriate teaching methods for adult learners.	Public, private, or voluntary agencies

should encourage all American adults to get routine preventive health care services (table 10.12).

The following guidelines serve as recommendations for adults that should be included when planning, implementing, evaluating, and assuring quality adult nutrition interventions:

- Maintain acceptable weight for height based on Dietary Guideline standards.

- Maintain acceptable BMI.
- Maintain acceptable waist-hip ratio.
- Maintain blood pressure < 140/90 mm Hg.
- Maintain plasma total cholesterol < 200 mg/dl.
- Do not smoke.
- Consume no more than one alcoholic drink daily (female) or two drinks daily (male). (One drink equals 12 oz regular beer, 5 oz wine, or 1 1/2 oz distilled spirits.)

TABLE 10.12
Preventive Medicine Tests for Life

Age (years)	Test	People not at high risk	People at high risk*
18–29	Eye	Every two years if there are vision problems	At least once per year
	Dental	Every six months until twenty-one, then once a year	As recommended by dentist
	Cervical (Pap) smear	Annually for women over eighteen and all sexually active women	Once per year
	Blood pressure	Begin at twenty; after twenty, at three- to five-year intervals	Once per year
	Cholesterol	At time of first physical	If abnormal, follow doctor's advice
	Breast	Monthly self-exam	Monthly self-exam
	Rectum/colon	Usually not necessary	Once per year after age twenty
30–49	Eye	Every two years if vision is good, start eye examinations at forty	Once each year
	Dental	At least once per year	As recommended by dentist
	Cervical (Pap) smear	Every one to three years	Once per year
	Blood pressure	Every three to five years	Once per year
	Cholesterol	Depends on results of last test; if normal repeat in five years	If abnormal, follow doctor's advice
	Breast	Monthly self-exam, baseline mammogram at forty, then every one to two years after fifty	Monthly self-exam, mammogram as recommended by doctor
	Rectum/colon	Once a year after forty	Annual digital rectal and fecal blood test, flexible sigmoidoscopy every three to five years
Over 50	Eye	Every two years	At least once per year
	Dental	At least once per year	As recommended by dentist
	Cervical (Pap) smear	Every three to five years	Once per year
	Blood pressure	Once per year	As recommended by doctor
	Cholesterol	Depends on results of last test; if normal repeat in three to five years	If abnormal, follow doctor's advice
	Breast	Monthly self-exam, once per year	Monthly self-exam, mammogram once per year
	Rectum/colon	Annual digital rectal and fecal blood test, flexible sigmoidoscopy every three to five years	Annual digital rectal and fecal blood test, flexible sigmoidoscopy every three to five years

*At high risk: for eye problems, people with diabetes or high blood pressure or who have a family history of glaucoma; for dental or oral difficulties, smokers and tobacco chewers; for cervical cancer (Pap smear), women with herpes or genital warts; for elevated blood pressure, people with a family history of high blood pressure, heart or kidney disease, or stroke and people who are diabetic, overweight, or on contraceptives; for elevated cholesterol, people who have a family history of early-onset heart disease or stroke; for breast cancer, women with a first-degree relative who has had breast cancer; for rectal and colon cancer, people with polyps of the colon or long-standing extensive ulcerative colitis or people with a first-degree relative who has colon or rectal cancer.
Source: Data adapted from The American Medical Association: *Family Medical Guide,* ed 3, 1994, Random House.

- Consume adequate amount of nutrients, fiber, and water with caloric intake to maintain acceptable body weight.
- Maintain hemoglobin level between 120 and 150 g/L.
- Consume appropriate types and amounts of food as defined by the Food Guide Pyramid.
- Consume appropriate amounts of calcium (800 to 1200 mg/day).
- Accumulate thirty minutes or more of moderate physical activity on most (preferably all) days of the week.

TAKING ACTION

As a community nutrition professional, it is a challenge to know how and where to focus professional efforts and activities. Nutrition intervention can consist of provision of food and/or provision of nutrition education. Typically, both are implemented in a community setting. Whereas food assistance programs are for low-income households, programs that feature strictly nutrition education target broader audiences, including those that are not economically deprived. Food assistance programs have specific eligibility criteria and although target populations are defined, priorities usually still must be ap-

plied. Community nutrition professionals must play a major role in making decisions about what **nutrition education programs** should be developed and implemented for both participants of food assistance programs and target populations in the community. In addition, decisions about what populations to target in the community must be made.

With respect to the development and implementation of nutrition education programs, there are many decisions that must be made about the type(s) of program(s) that will be implemented in the community. Based on an assessment of the needs of the community, it is apparent that there are many potential nutrition issues that can be targeted for intervention. Without a doubt, choosing the nutrition education program(s) that will be implemented, identifying target audiences, and selecting the method of delivery are momentous decisions. The provision of nutrition education to adults encompasses a wide variety of approaches for working with individuals, groups, organizations, and communities (table 10.13), and each approach has inherent strengths and weaknesses (table 10.14). The community nutrition professional must use several approaches to be effective. The choice of intervention will be guided by many

TABLE 10.13
Nutrition Intervention Approaches

Approaches for the individual	Approaches for groups/social networks	Approaches for organizations	Approaches for communities
Personalized counseling	Group classes (weight management, blood cholesterol lowering, exercise, cooking, etc.)	Chronic disease risk assessment (via questionnaires, taking measurements such as blood cholesterol and blood pressure)	Mass media approaches: messages on television and radio and in the newspaper
Chronic disease risk assessment			
Personalized nutrition program	Print materials, refrigerator guides, shopping guides	Classes during breaks, lunch hour, and after work	Supermarket and meat market programs that educate consumers about healthful food choices
Personalized fitness program	Blood cholesterol screening with follow-up intervention planned	Video programs shown in the cafeteria	
Supermarket tour		Nutrition information provided for cafeteria, snack bar, and vending food items; provision of healthier alternatives in cafeteria, snack bar, and vending machines	Incentives and coupons
Food preparation instruction (cooking instruction, recipe modification)	Contests (weight loss, recipe, fitness, etc.)		Brochures
Restaurant tour	Family activities		Videos
	Activities in health care provider offices (videos, print materials)		Point-of-purchase nutrition information
	Healthful nutrition potluck dinners	Health celebrations (serve healthful foods at social occasions)	Cooperative extension activities
	Low-fat gourmet clubs	Contests	
	Supermarket and restaurant tours	Column in in-house publications	
		Posters and fliers	

factors such as organizational and personal philosophy, the target population, time, and other available resources. Priorities are set often on the basis of a needs assessment of the community. As described previously, there are many important nutrition issues that are common to the adult population. Furthermore, various target groups of adults have very different needs. This will impact on where the programs are delivered and how they will be delivered. Using obesity as an example of a chosen target area, it will be important to decide on the specific audience (e.g., gender, income, literacy levels, race), the setting (e.g., home, work, grocery store, mall, etc.), and the method of delivery (e.g., classes, mailings, popular press articles, television clips, etc.). Nutrition education program development and implementation approaches are described in further detail in chapter 7. The remainder of this chapter discusses the types of attributes of successful nutrition education programs for adults in a community setting.

Nutrition Education Intervention

Prior to initiating any approach, community nutrition professionals need to recognize the two core components of nutrition education interventions—process and context.[13] The **intervention process** involves getting people's attention, motivating them, and helping them to choose healthy behaviors. Where and how the intervention occurs (the **intervention context**) for example, in the home or a grocery store, in a clinical setting, or even a restaurant, is of great importance in how and whether the education will make a difference, and whether the difference will be observable. Furthermore, it is imperative to recognize the characteristics of the learner in any nutrition education intervention for adults (see box 10.5).

These characteristics suggest that community nutrition professionals must enter the intervention in a manner that acknowledges the learner's experience, stimulates exchange of ideas, as well as disseminates nutrition infor-

TABLE 10.14

Advantages and Disadvantages of Various Nutrition Intervention Approaches

Intervention approach	Advantages	Limitations
Individual	• Highly individual and personalized • Can be intensive with extensive follow-up • Educational materials cost can be very low • Chances for successful behavior modification are good	• Reaches a limited number of people • Small impact on community health • Cost per person is high • Important health or nutrition issues may not be addressed
Group	• Group interactions may facilitate desired behavior change • Important nutrition message(s) can be targeted to individuals within the group who have similar needs or characteristics • Can reach a relatively large number of individuals	• Different learning styles and goals of group members may limit program effectiveness
Organization	• Organization support can facilitate behavior change • Major nutrition problems and issues can be addressed • Can have an impact on the health of an organization's members or employees • Cost per individual can be relatively low	• Intervention is not individualized • Organization support may be too strong and certain related policies (e.g., negative incentives for certain behaviors) may hurt employee or member morale • Organization support may be too weak to facilitate change
Community	• Group interaction and support can facilitate behavior change • Community can be more aware of health and nutrition problems • Target populations can be reached with specific information • Can reach a relatively large number of individuals	• May create awareness but not behavioral change in individuals • May cause change for limited time (while program is ongoing) • Resources may be too limited to cover those in need

mation, and is facilitative and helpful rather than authoritarian in nature. The following sections provide examples of and insights into the role of the community nutrition professional in nutrition interventions for the adult.

Federal Food Assistance and Education Programs for Adults

The Food Stamp Program   The largest and most commonly used **federal food assistance program** for nonpregnant American adults is the Food Stamp Program. Food stamps help low-income households purchase a nutritionally adequate diet. Monthly benefits are based on household size, assets and income, and the cost of the thrifty food plan (table 10.15). This plan represents the least costly of four representative food plans developed by the USDA's Food and Consumer Service. The plan assumes that food for all meals and snacks is purchased at the store and prepared at home. Estimates of amounts of food for each plan are computed from food consumption survey data. Average monthly participation in the Food Stamp Program was approximately 26 million people in 1995, with more than 50 percent of recipients being children. The average length of participation in the Food Stamp Program is less than two years.

Until recently, there were few nutrition education services provided to food stamp recipients directly through the Food Stamp Program. This situation is currently changing. Over the past few years, some states (Wisconsin, Minnesota, Ohio, Virginia, and Washington to name a few) have initiated the Food Stamp Family Nutrition Education Program. Community nutrition professionals coordinate their activities through their state Food Stamp Program office.

Food Assistance Programs   Since 1989, Temporary Emergency Food Assistance Program (TEFAP) funds have been distributed to states for purchase of additional commodities as well as for administrative needs. Money is allocated to the state for distribution to regional food banks as well as to local soup kitchens and other emergency food assistance programs. Local governments often provide supplemental funding for these operations.

In addition to federally funded food assistance programs, many local emergency food programs are privately supported by churches, other nonprofit groups, and

---

BOX 10.5

CHARACTERISTICS OF ADULT LEARNERS

- They are more self-directed than dependent.
- They have an accumulating wealth of personal experiences.
- They orient learning from subject-centered to performance-centered learning (i.e., from knowing to doing).
- They orient their readiness to learn to the tasks of their social roles (e.g., working parent).
- They are motivated by the desire to use (apply) knowledge and skills (practical rather than academic or theoretical).

Source: Adapted from Quigley BA: *Adult learning theory: implications for adult teaching and learning,* Monroeville, PA, 1995.

TABLE 10.15

Cost of Food at Home per Week for Food Plans, June 1995, U.S. Average*

Age group	Thrifty plan	Low-cost plan	Moderate-cost plan	Liberal plan
Family of two				
20–50 years	$53.50	$ 67.50	$ 83.60	$104.30
more than 51 years	$50.30	$ 65.00	$ 80.50	$ 96.60
Family of four				
Couple, 20–50 years				
and children				
1–2 and 3–4 years	$77.70	$ 97.10	$119.00	$146.70
6–8 and 9–11 years	$89.20	$114.20	$143.00	$172.50

*Assumes that food for all meals and snacks is purchased at the store and prepared at home.
Source: Data adapted from *Fam Econ and Nutr Rev;* 8(3):61, 1995.

private industry. Although their primary efforts are to provide food, some agencies provide additional services. These include shelter; referral services to other community agencies; clothing and furniture; and instructional activities including parenting, job training, and nutrition education. Community nutrition professionals frequently volunteer their time and service to these activities.

Government Funded Nutrition Education Services for Adults   A variety of governmental agencies (federal, state, and local), as well as nonprofit groups and private industry, offer nutrition education services to the U.S. adult population. State and local health departments may provide community and individual nutrition intervention programming, including clinical services, participation at local health fairs, and sponsorship of lectures and workshops.

The USDA's Cooperative Extension Service provides education through a variety of programs. Common areas of inquiry for county extension educators include general nutrition topics as well as food safety and food preservation issues. Programs delivered by extension educators include application of dietary guidelines, weight management strategies, child and infant nutrition, and food safety. Many local counties also offer the Expanded Food and Nutrition Education Program (EFNEP) EFNEP, established in 1968, serves low-income households with children under the age of eighteen in both rural and urban areas. Using paraprofessional staffing from within the community, the program provides participant families with the basic information on food purchasing and preparation, nutrition, and food safety. The program assists families in learning how to incorporate this information into menu planning and improving diets. Those states offering the Food Stamp Family Nutrition Education Program coordinate efforts with EFNEP.

Examples of Nutrition Intervention Programs that Work

Three examples of highly successful primary prevention intervention programs targeted to reducing cardiovascular disease risk factors and improving nutrition practices are the National High Blood Pressure Education Program (NHBPEP), initiated in 1973; the National Cholesterol Education Program (NCEP), initiated in 1985; and the National 5 a Day for Better Health Program, initiated in 1992. These programs used mass media intervention campaigns that were based on social marketing principles and were directed to society at large.

The NHBPEP and NCEP are sponsored by the National Heart, Lung and Blood Institute (NHLBI) of the NIH. The purpose of the NHBPEP was to increase awareness in American adults of the consequences of untreated high blood pressure, that high blood pressure is a serious disorder, and that family and social support are essential in the treatment of hypertension. In addition, a major goal of this program was to have Americans know and monitor their own blood pressure and be treated for hypertension, if warranted. Similarly, the initial NCEP intended to get the general public to know their cholesterol number (serum cholesterol concentration). NCEP messages were that high blood cholesterol has no symptoms, that it could affect anyone, and that action can be taken to lower elevated levels.

Both programs have been very successful. There has been an increased awareness of the link between high blood pressure and CVD and between an elevated blood cholesterol level and CHD. Now, almost all Americans (92 percent) are aware of the link between high blood pressure and heart disease. Likewise, most now know that lowering high blood cholesterol levels will lower the risk of CHD. Furthermore, most Americans know their blood pressure and blood cholesterol numbers.

There has been a highly significant decrease in the incidence of CVD since the 1970s and these programs have likely contributed to this trend. The prevalence of high blood pressure among people twenty years and older decreased from 39 percent in 1980 to 23 percent in 1991. With respect to blood cholesterol levels, we are well on the way of achieving an average cholesterol level < 200 mg/dl for the population by the year 2000; in the late 1970s, the average total blood cholesterol level of the population was 212 mg/dl.

The National 5 a Day for Better Health program is jointly sponsored by NCI and Produce for Better Health Foundation. Along with a mass media campaign, this program includes point-of-purchase activities in supermarkets and community interventions. This campaign has been successful in increasing public awareness about the benefits of daily consumption of five or more servings of fruits and vegetables. Within two years, the number of Americans who knew that five or more servings daily of fruits and vegetables were recommended for good health rose from 8 to 29 percent. Moreover, the percentage who believed that eating fruits and vegetables might help prevent cancer rose from 45 to 64 percent.[18]

Examples of two major secondary intervention programs include the Multiple Risk Factor Intervention Trial (MRFIT), a large multicenter study that targeted middle-aged men ($n = 36,000$) at high risk for CVD, and the Women's Health Trial Vanguard Study (WHTVS), which targeted women ($n = 303$) at high risk of developing breast cancer.[19,50] Both of these intervention programs employed individualized counseling and educational approaches, most often in a group setting. In MRFIT, the male study participants and their spouses attended ten weekly sessions on food and behavioral self-management skills, with active participation and frequent follow-ups. The participants of this program made and sustained dietary changes (i.e., decrease in saturated fat and cholesterol, weight loss of 1.5 kg or 3.5 lb). In addition, the intervention resulted in a reduction of plasma cholesterol. In the WHTVS, the nutrition professional served first as a teacher and then as a facilitator and resource person. Sessions were held weekly for the first eight weeks, twice a month during the next six months, and then monthly for the remainder of the program. Each participant also had an individual session with the nutritionist at two and twelve weeks. These women, who were at high risk for breast cancer, quickly attained and then maintained total fat intakes of 22 percent of calories (down from 39 percent) at the end of the two-year study.

With respect to tertiary prevention intervention programs for persons with established disease, there is an impressive database in the area of CVD that has established their dramatic benefits. Because of this, a major emphasis of the second Adult Treatment Panel Report of the NCEP is on rigorous intervention of individuals with established CHD. Typically, these intervention programs entail individual counseling, major dietary modifications (e.g., marked reduction in intakes of saturated fat and cholesterol), and other lifestyle changes along with close monitoring and follow-up. These interventions have proven to be highly effective in markedly reducing subsequent morbidity and mortality form CHD. Based on these most impressive results, this patient-based model will serve as an important paradigm for reducing the morbidity and mortality of other chronic diseases.

Elements of Nutrition Education Programs that Work

Implicit in nutrition education programs is the need for change. Starting with the basic scientific consensus that diet is related to disease, the goals of nutrition interventions are to promote healthful eating patterns and/or to improve health outcomes through direct attempts to influence nutritional knowledge, attitudes, skills, and behavior. The ultimate criteria of success is a change in dietary behaviors and a reduction in disease risk, although many nutrition education interventions, whether directed at the individual, group, or community level, concentrate on delivering knowledge and skills. Although these are critical intervention components, it is unrealistic to assume they will automatically result in behavior change. For example, as a result of the NCEP, most Americans have had their cholesterol level checked; not all who have high levels, however, have successfully altered their lifestyles to accommodate reductions in these levels.

Behavior change, as described in chapter 7, is a complicated continuous process, not a single event. This is particularly true with dietary behaviors. Individuals must change awareness, motivation, and attitudes about the role of nutrition in both health and disease; change the kinds, types, and amounts of foods eaten; change food preparation methods; change sensory perceptions; and even change economic and time commitments. Community nutrition professionals must recognize, facilitate, and accommodate these changes.

IMPLICATIONS FOR COMMUNITY NUTRITION PROFESSIONALS

Adulthood, the longest period in the life cycle, spans the time between adolescence and the senior years. Nutrition becomes a major component of general well-being throughout the adult years. The occurrence and extent of chronic diseases, such as obesity, CHD, diabetes, cancer, and osteoporosis, are determined, in part, by lifestyle choices made during this time. Early adulthood is often accompanied by vigor and vitality; however, the processes of aging and disease are already in progress, although their impact is not often realized until later in life. Physical and psychological changes affect nutritional status; conversely, nutritional status affects physical and psychological well-being. Nutrition intervention during the adult years is designed to reduce the risk and onset of chronic disease. To be effective, nutrition education intervention provided to adults must be perceived as relevant, be easy to use, be disseminated through highly visible and strategically positioned communication channels, and be scientifically and technologically correct.

In the future, community nutrition professionals will be challenged to provide programs and services to diverse audiences in a variety of settings. Workplace intervention programs provide community nutrition professionals with an unprecedented opportunity to positively impact a large number of people. More effort is needed to reach disadvantaged groups, particularly those that are less educated and have lower incomes and thus are disproportionately burdened with disease. These audiences are less likely to be part of the secular trend toward more healthful diets. Nutrition education interventions that have been effective with high-risk groups should be supported and extended to high-risk subpopulations, such as Blacks, Hispanics, and Native Americans as well as women.

Most weight management programs do not result in long-lasting weight maintenance. Success needs to be measured by other health-related standards rather than only by body weight. Community nutritional professionals are indeed challenged in developing strategies to prevent weight gain through the adult years. As audiences become more fragmented, the media have become less "mass" oriented and more targeted in their messages. In addition, interventions that use entertainment (television, radio, print) are another unexploited opportunity for nutrition education.

Finally, some of the most successful interventions involve commercial partners. These efforts should be expanded to grocery stores, churches, and the farmer's markets at the local level or trade associations at the national level.

COMMUNITY NUTRITION PROFESSIONALS IN ACTION

- List the one Healthy People 2000 objective for adults that has been met and the eight objectives where progress has been made. Give examples of interventions used in your community to contribute toward these accomplishments.
- Many people believe weight gain is a fact of growing older. What physiological and lifestyle changes occur that contribute to weight gain? How might individuals help maintain body weight throughout the lifespan?
- Identify the major risk factors for women in CVD, cancer, diabetes mellitus, osteoporosis, and obesity.
- Discuss reasons why a worksite program planned by employees might be more effective in the prevention of chronic disease in a community than a cholesterol screening at an annual health fair.

- List some subpopulations at particularly high risk for the development of chronic disease and early mortality. Discuss socioeconomic, cultural, and genetic factors that contribute to this situation.
- Little success has been demonstrated by weight maintenance programs when weight loss has been used as the measure for success. What other outcomes could be used to demonstrate effectiveness? Why might other outcomes be more indicative of improved health?
- Identify the major causes of cancer and indicate the nutrition implications of each, particularly protective foods and the issue of phytochemicals.
- What is different about interventions designed for primary prevention versus secondary and tertiary preventions?
- Keep a three-day food record and physical activity log. Ask your parent (or an adult close to your parent's age) to do the same. Describe the ease or difficulty of performing this task. Ask the same of the adult with whom you worked. Compare your nutrient intake to that of this adult. How do your intakes differ? Compare physical activity logs. What lifestyle factors influence the differences? What other lifestyle choices might contribute to the differences in health risk?
- You are developing a series of six nutrition classes for a continuing education program at your local university. The classes will be open to all members of the community (not just university students). You have complete use of all kitchen equipment. Write a lesson plan for one of these classes using strategies shown to be successful in adult education.
- Develop a presentation (forty-five minutes) on women's health issues including guidelines to minimize health risks for a group of working women who belong to your church or any community group in which you are involved.
- Develop a five-day menu that follows a Step I Diet. How would this menu need to be modified to meet Step 2 guidelines? Try following the diet. How difficult would it be for you to maintain this diet? What would be the personal benefit to you in adopting this diet?
- Divide the class into groups, and assign a popular commercial weight loss program to each group. Direct each group to analyze their diet program for nutritional adequacy and determine whether it follows established guidelines for safe weight loss. Discuss the results in class.

- Discuss your opinion about the suggestion to use a "healthier weight" goal for obesity treatment. Select an original reference from the 1996 *American Journal of Clinical Nutrition Supplement* 63 (S3):409S. Critique as to the accuracy of the interpretation made by the panel in its use to defend this suggestion.

GOING ONE STEP FURTHER

- Using the Vital Statistics report, identify a nutritional problem in your county. Develop an intervention program to address the need. Determine the theoretical basis or bases for the program. Justify why you chose this (these) theory(ies). Discuss the objectives of the intervention, staffing needs, the benefits your program will provide to its participants. Outline the marketing approaches, keep both cost effectiveness and past success of approaches in mind.
- As this chapter indicates, few American adults participate in regular physical activity. Develop a study proposal to determine what proportion of your community follows a regular exercise regime and to determine potentially effective strategies for an exercise promotion campaign that you would like to implement. How would you evaluate the effectiveness of such a campaign?
- Compare the body weight recommendations made by the Dietary Guidelines committee in 1990 and 1995. Which standard would you use in the assessment of weight status for adult clients? Provide references to support your argument.

ADDITIONAL INFORMATION

Professional societies develop statements, scientific status summaries, commentaries, and position papers to clarify an issue in which the particular society has expertise.

The Institute of Food Technologists (IFT) Science Communications' documents and The American Dietetic Association (ADA) position statements relevant to chapter 10 are listed below:

IFT Science Communications' Documents

1. Human obesity: scientific status summaries, June 1994 S-026 Institute of Food Technologists. Chicago, IL.

The American Dietetic Association Position Statements

1. Vegetarian diets, *J Am Diet Assoc* 93:1317, 1993.
2. Nutrition intervention in the treatment of anorexia nervosa, bulimia nervosa, and binge eating, *J Am Diet Assoc* 94:902, 1994.
3. Nutrition recommendations and principles for people with diabetes mellitus, *J Am Diet Assoc* 94:504, 1994.
4. Weight management, *J Am Diet Assoc* 97:71, 1997.
5. Nutrition aging and the continuum of care, *J Am Diet Assoc* 96:1048, 1996.
6. Nutrition for physical fitness and athletic performance for adults, *J Am Diet Assoc* 93:691, 1993.
7. Women's health and nutrition, *J Am Diet Assoc* 95:362, 1995.

The American Society for Clinical Nutrition and American Society for Nutritional Sciences Statement

1. Trans-fatty acids, *Am J Clin Nutr* 63:663, 1996.

REFERENCES

1. The Alpha-Tocopherol, Beta-Carotene Cancer Prevention Study Group: The effect of vitamin E and beta-carotene on the incidence of lung cancer and other cancers in male smokers, *New Engl J Med* 330:1029, 1994.
2. American Diabetes Association: Nutrition principles and recommendations (technical report), *Diabetes Care* 17:490–518, 1994.
3. Boyd NF, Lockwood G, Yaffe M, et al: Long term effects of a low-fat high-carbohydrate diet on radiological features of the breast (abstract), *Cancer Epidemiol Prev* 209, 1997.
4. Bureau of National Affairs: Focus on women's health, *Health Care Policy Report* 2 (suppl):53–65, 1994.
5. *Cancer facts and figures 1996,* Atlanta, GA, 1996, American Cancer Society.
6. Carroll KK: Dietary fats and cancer, *Am J Clin Nutr* 53:1064S, 1991.
7. *Diabetes 1996: vital statistics,* Alexandria, VA, 1996, American Diabetes Association.
8. *Exchange lists for diabetic diets,* Alexandria, VA, and Chicago, 1995, American Diabetes Associaton and The American Diatetic Association.
9. Federation of American Societies for Experimental Biology, Life Sciences Research Office: *Third report on nutrition monitoring in the United States: volume 1,* Prepared for the Interagency Board for Nutrition Monitoring and Related Research, Washington, DC, 1995, U.S. Government Printing Office.

10. The fifth report of the Joint National Committee on Detection, Evaluation and Treatment of High Blood Pressure (JNC V), *Arch Intern Med* 153:154, 1993.

11. Finn SC: Women in the new world order: where old values command new respect, *J Am Diet Assoc* 97:475–480, 1997.

12. Glanz K, Hewitt AM, Rudd J: Consumer behavior and nutrition education: an integrative review, *J Nutr Educ* 24:267, 1992.

13. Haines PS, Guilkey DK, Popkin BM: Trends in breakfast consumption of US adults between 1965 and 1991, *J Am Diet Assoc* 96:464, 1996.

14. Hankin JH: Role of nutrition in women's health: diet and breast cancer, *J Am Diet Assoc* 93:994–998, 1993.

15. Heaney RP: Nutrition factors in osteoporosis, *Annu Rev Nutr* 13:287–316, 1993.

16. Heaney RP: *Osteoporosis.* In Krummel DA, Kris-Etherton PM, editors: *Nutrition in women's health,* Gaithersburg, MD, 1996, Aspen, pp. 418–420.

17. *Heart and stroke facts: 1996 statistical supplement,* Dallas, TX, 1995, American Heart Association.

18. Heimandinger J, Van Duyn MA, Chapelsky D, et al: The National % A Day for Better Health Program: a large-scale nutrition intervention, *Journal of Public Health Management* 2:27–35, 1996.

19. Henderson MM, Kushi LH, Thompson DJ, et al: Feasibility of a randomized trial of a low-fat diet for the prevention of breast cancer: dietary compliance in the Women's Health Trial Vanguard Study, *Prev Med* 19:115–133, 1990.

20. Institute of Medicine: *Weighing the options: criteria for evaluating weight-management programs,* Washington, DC, 1995, National Academy Press.

21. Kannel WB, Wilson DWF: Risk factors that attenuate the female coronary disease advantage, *Arch Intern Med* 155:57–61, 1995.

22. Kris-Etherton PM, Krummel DK: Role of nutrition in the prevalence and treatment of coronary heart disease in women, *J Am Diet Assoc* 93:987–993, 1993.

23. Kris-Etherton PM, Krummel D, Chamgpagn C, et al: Cardiovascular disease and women's health, *Top Clin Nutr* 11:822, 1995.

24. Krummel DA, Kris-Etherton PM: *Nutrition in women's health,* Gaithersburg, MD, 1996, Aspen Publications, pp. 510–511.

25. Kuczmarski RJ, Flegal KG, Campbell SM, Johnson CL: Increasing prevalence of overweight among US adults, *JAMA* 272:205–211, 1994.

26. Kuhn FE, Rachley CE: Coronary artery disease in women: risk factors, evaluation, treatment and prevention, *Arch Intern Med* 153:2626–2635, 1993.

27. Kumanyika SK: Special issues regarding obesity in minority populations. *Ann Intern Med* 1993; 119:650–654.

28. Kumanyika S: Nutrition and health campaign for all women, *J Am Diet Assoc* 95:299–300, 1995.

29. Lawrence L, Weinhouse B: *Outrageous practices: the alarming truth about how medicine mistreats women,* New York, 1994, Fawcett Columbine.

30. Leaf DA: Women and coronary artery disease: gender confers no immunity, *Postgrad Med* 87:55–60, 1990.

31. Lewis CJ, Crane NT, Moore BJ, Hubbard VS: *Healthy people 2000:* report of the 1994 nutrition progress review, *Nutr Today* 29:6–14, 1994.

32. Manson JE, Colditz GA, Stamphler MJ, et al: A prospective study of obesity and risk of coronary heart disease in women, *New Engl J Med* 322:882–889, 1990.

33. Meisler JG, St. Jeor S: American Health Foundation roundtable on healthy weight, *Am J Clin Nutr* 63(3S):409S, 1996.

34. *Monthly Vital Statistics Report* 43(12):17, 1995.

35. *National cholesterol education program: Report of expert panel on population strategies for blood cholesterol reduction,* NIH Pub 90-3046, Washington, DC, 1990, NHLBI.

36. National Institute on Drug Abuse, Division of Epidemiology and Statistical Analysis, DHHS, USPHS Alcohol, Drug Abuse and Mental Health Administration: *National household survey on drug use: main findings,* Washington, DC, 1995, U.S. Government Printing Office.

37. *Nutrition and your health: dietary guidelines for Americans,* ed 4, Washington, DC, 1995, USDA and DHHS, Home and Garden Bulletin no. 232.

38. Omenn GS et al: The beta-carotene and retinol efficacy trial (CARET) for chemoprevention of lung cancer in high risk populations: smokers and asbestos-exposed workers, *Cancer Res* 54:2038S, 1994.

39. *Optimal calcium intake,* NIH Consensus Statement Series 12, Bethesda, MD, 1994, National Institutes of Health.

40. Pate RR et al: Physical activity and public health: a recommendation from the Centers for Disease Control and the American College of Sports Medicine, *JAMA* 273:402, 1995.

41. Popkins BM, Siega-Riz AM, Haines PS: A comparison of dietary trends among racial and socioeconomic groups in the United States, *New Engl J Med* 1996; 335:716–720.

42. Position of the American Dietetic Association and the Canadian Dietetic Association, Women's health and nutrition, *J Am Diet Assoc* 95:362–365, 1995.

43. Position paper on trans fatty acids; special task force report, *Am J Clin Nutr* 63:663–670, 1996.

44. Ricker AS, Preussman R: Chemical food contaminants in the initiation of cancer, *Proc Nutr Soc* 49:133, 1990.

45. Rodriquez-Tria H: Women's health, women's lives, women's rights (editorial), *Am J Public Health* 82:663–664, 1992.

46. Roe DA: *Handbook on drug and nutrient interactions: a problem oriented guide,* ed 4, Chicago, 1989, American Dietetic Association.

47. Sempos CT: Prevalence of high blood cholesterol among US adults, *JAMA* 269:3009, 1993.

48. Sigman-Grant M: Stages of change: a framework for nutrition interventions, *Nutr Today* 31:162–170, 1996.

49. St. Jeor ST, Silverstein LJ, Shane SR: *Obesity.* In Krummel DA, Kris-Etherton PM, editors: *Nutrition in women's health,* Gaithersburg, MD, 1996, Aspen, pp. 353–373.

50. Stamler J, Caggiula A, Cutler J, et al: Multiple risk factor intervention trial, *Am J Clin Nutr* 65(suppl):183S–402S, 1997.

51. Stamler J, Stamler R, Conlon J: Blood pressure, systolic and diastolic and cardiovascular risk, *Arch Intern Med* 153:598, 1993.

52. Tinker LF: Diabetes mellitus—a priority health care issue for women, *J Am Diet Assoc* 94:976–985, 1994.

53. USDA and USDHHS: Food Guide Pyramid: a guide to daily food choices, Home and Garden Bulletin no. 252, 1992.

54. U.S. Department of Health and Human Services: *Healthy people 2000: national health promotion and disease prevention objectives, Mid Course Review,* Washington, DC, 1995, U.S. Government Printing Office.

55. Wylie Rosset J, Mossavar-Rahman Y: Diabetes and women's health, *Top Clin Nutr* 11:36–45, 1995.

CASE STUDY

A COMMUNITY-BASED INTERVENTION PROGRAM TO REDUCE THE RISK OF CARDIOVASCULAR DISEASE*

MADELEINE SIGMAN-GRANT, PHD, RD; PENNY KRIS-ETHERTON, PHD, RD; AND MARY NAGLAK, MMSC, RD

INTRODUCTION

This case study illustrates which factors to consider when implementing a community intervention program in an urban setting. Challenges facing the nutrition professional in this setting include a large minority population; the low socioeconomic status of the population; the cultural and linguistic diversity of the community; and competing problems of urban life such as crime, housing, jobs, crowded schools, and other health problems. The goal of the program was to reduce the prevalence of cardiovascular disease risk factors such as smoking, sedentary lifestyle, obesity, hypertension, and hypercholesterolemia.

The main questions raised in this case study have to do with what types of program components are successful for this population, what low-cost methods can be used to evaluate the program, and how to transfer responsibility for the program to existing community organizations. After reading the case study, students should form small groups to discuss each of the questions listed at the end.

THE CASE

The New York State Department of Health funded eight, six-year community-based cardiovascular disease prevention programs in 1988. One of these programs was the Washington Heights-Inwood Healthy Heart Program. The Washington Heights-Inwood area is a community of approximately 240,000 people in New York, with a high Latino population who have little education and a low socioeconomic status (SES). Funding was primarily allocated for implementation; less than 10 percent was allocated for evaluation of program effectiveness.

The program components were selected based on general criteria such as acceptability by the target population, the resources required and available, and the public health importance of risk factors. In addition, the experience of other programs such as the Pawtucket Heart Health Program, The Stanford Five-City Project, and the Minnesota Heart Health Program were considered. Initially, emphasis was placed on establishing program identity, increasing awareness of the program, and creating legitimacy of the program. Later, emphasis was placed on maintaining involvement in the program and how to incorporate the program into already existing programs in the community. The risk factors targeted included a high-fat diet,

*This case study is based on an actual report of the experiences of the directors of The Washington Heights-Inwood Healthy Heart Program published in the *American Journal of Public Health* 86:166–171, 1996.

sedentary lifestyle, smoking, poorly controlled hypertension, and hypercholesterolemia.

The overall program included the following six program components: a low-fat milk campaign; establishment of volunteer-led exercise clubs; development of a Spanish-language smoking cessation video; worksite-based smoking prevention activities; a cholesterol screening; a counseling, education, and referral program; and assisting community-based physicians to promote heart health in their practices. Each program component is described below.

Low-Fat Milk Campaign

Assessment of nutrient intakes and dietary behavior patterns of people in the Washington Heights-Inwood area revealed that approximately 40 percent of the saturated fat intake of this group came from whole milk and whole milk products. In addition, a separate analysis indicated that the substitution of 1 percent milk for whole milk would lower saturated fat intake to less than 10 percent of total energy, which is in compliance with current recommendations. Therefore, a multicomponent social marketing campaign was undertaken to promote the use of 1 percent milk within the community. The campaign included taste tests at local shopping establishments; low-literacy print materials; public service announcements (PSAs) on Spanish-language television; and efforts to increase the availability of low-fat milk in local restaurants, cafeterias, and community grocery stores. The PSAs and print materials provided information on both the positive and negative consequences of consuming a diet low in saturated fat. In addition, a local family-owned chain of ice cream stores took part in an annual contest allowing customers to create their own desserts using low-fat milk. Prizes (including vouchers for additional low-fat ice cream) were given for the "Best Low-Fat Desserts in Town." After the start of this campaign, there were large increases in the proportion of adults who chose low-fat milk at local restaurants and cafeterias. Consequently, there was an increase in the availability of low-fat milk in local restaurants and cafeterias.

Volunteer-Led Exercise Clubs

A needs assessment indicated very few adults took part in regular physical activity although there was an expressed interest in organized exercise programs, es-

pecially for women. Therefore, a program was developed in which volunteers went through an extensive training and certification process to conduct exercise classes that included stretching, calisthenics, and low-impact aerobics. A specific effort was made to gear the classes to people who were sedentary. In addition, the classes did not require expensive equipment or clothing. As a result of the program, fifty-six volunteers were certified. Of the thirty clubs established, twenty-one remained active for at least six months. Approximately ten to twenty people attended each club. Overall, the classes attracted more than 1,200 participants between 1992 and 1993, the majority of whom were female Latinos between eighteen and thirty-nine years of age.

Spanish-Language Smoking Cessation Video

A Spanish-language video was developed emphasizing positive messages about nonsmoking. These messages emphasized a sense of self-empowerment arising from a decision to promote one's own and one's family's health by not smoking and enhanced the value of Hispanic culture and identity in opposition to smoking. The sixteen-minute long video, entitled "Usted Puede Dejario" ("You Can Do It") included interviews with people who had successfully stopped smoking including well-known people within the community such as a local physician with a successful practice. Topics covered by the speakers in the video were reasons they quit smoking, the benefits of not smoking, how positive it made them feel to quit, and the obstacles they had to overcome. The video was distributed to a variety of locations including local physicians offices, community-based organizations, the local health departments, and the Spanish-language cable television network.

Worksite-Based Smoking Prevention Activities

This program component was conducted in conjunction with the county-run substance abuse prevention center. This agency relied on local funding for support. Various worksites throughout the community, ranging from textile manufactures to fast food establishments, participated in an annual event called "The World Without Smoke Advertising Contest." Area businesses were recruited by allowing them to promote their business at the well-publicized annual contest award ceremony. To participate in the contest, employees developed their own advertising campaign by creating posters, songs, or skits to parody cigarette advertisements that promoted smoking prevention. Prizes awarded for the contest such as gift certificates were donated by area businesses. Each year the substance abuse prevention center was given an increasing amount of responsibility for the event. After the fourth year, they agreed to take full responsibility for the event. However, at the time of the fourth contest, personnel changes and budget reductions had been made, forcing discontinuation of the contest.

Cholesterol Screening, Counseling, Education, and Referral

As part of the Washington Heights-Inwood Healthy Heart Program, cholesterol screening was identified as a high priority. Eighty-one events were scheduled at which 4,300 individuals were screened and received individualized counseling and referrals, when appropriate. The counseling and referral components involved one-on-one conversations with staff members. This component of the program gave the overall program a great deal of credibility and respect among community organizations.

Assisting Community-Based Physicians to Promote Heart Health in Their Practices

Because physicians are a respected source of health information in this community, they were approached to assist with the promotion of a heart healthy lifestyle. The following approaches were undertaken: conducting educational seminars for physicians on cholesterol management (publicized to the local medical society), sending literature from the American Heart Association to local practices, installing literature racks and frames complete with literature in twelve of the busiest practices, and distributing bilingual flyers and posters developed by the Heart Healthy Program.

PROGRAM EVALUATION

As noted, less than 10 percent of the budget was allocated to evaluate the Heart Healthy Program. The majority of these funds were used to set up procedures for monitoring and tracking the program with the help of the State Department of Health. During the first year of the program, using a random-digit dialing method, a baseline telephone survey was conducted at the state level to assess individual behavioral risk factors in the intervention communities. However, a similar follow-up survey was not conducted because of budget constraints. Some evaluation of community change was conducted, for example, evaluating changes in milk availability and consumption.

TRANSFER OF THE PROGRAM TO COMMUNITY-BASED ORGANIZATIONS

One objective of the Washington Heights-Inwood Healthy Heart Program was to transfer the program responsibilities over to existing community-based organizations so the program would continue to run once funding ceased. This transfer process was started during the fourth year of the project by discussing the program with community board members and other community leaders to get ideas about what organizations could be approached. One such organization was the Dominican Women's Development Center. Over the next two years, the center assumed complete responsibility for the program.

DISCUSSION QUESTIONS

1. What criteria might be used to assess the success of program components?

Example of appropriate criteria are:

- If the program reached a large number of people
- If the community awareness of the existence of the program increased
- If the community and individuals within understood the goals of the program
- If there was a potential established for long-term maintenance of behavioral, organizational, and social changes
- If the potential exists for other community-based organizations to assume responsibility for the program.

2. Based on these criteria, which program components do you believe would have been successful? Why?

The Low-Fat Milk Campaign

Changing to low-fat milk product was a relatively easy behavior change to make because there was no time commitment involved, the change did not affect food cost, it included interactive activities, and it emphasized positive messages and social reinforcements in campaign themes. Changes made in restaurant or cafeteria menus are likely to be maintained because there is little effort involved. The yearly contest was maintained by the local restaurant chain because it improved their business.

The Volunteer Exercise Clubs and the Smoking Cessation Video

These components each reached a large number of people and demonstrated the potential for affecting long-term changes in behavior or policy or for being effectively integrated into ongoing community organizations. Future programs might consider reserving a portion of the budget to provide "refresher" courses for volunteer exercise instructors to keep them updated and motivated.

3. Which program components would have been unsuccessful? Why?

Worksite Smoking Prevention Program

The organization chosen to keep the program within the community, the substance abuse prevention center, suffered budget cuts and therefore, the annual event, "This World Without Smoke Advertising Contest" had to be abandoned. The lesson to be learned is to choose organizations within the community that are "solidly" funded.

The Cholesterol Screening, Counseling, and Referral Program

Screening was labor intensive due to the time required by staff to provide one-on-one counseling and referrals for participants. Consequently, only a limited number of people were reached. In addition, because of the technical requirements of the program, it was not readily transferred to an existing community organization.

Assisting Community-Based Physicians to Promote Heart Health in Their Practices

There were too many other demands on the physicians' time. Physicians presently are not geared toward prevention. Therefore, even though the physicians may agree with and support the program, competing demands on their time and attention did not allow them to get involved.

4. For those program components that were unsuccessful, discuss how you would change these components of the program to improve their likelihood of success? In your discussions, consider what characteristics of the successful programs may be incorporated effectively into the unsuccessful programs.

The worksite smoking prevention program may have continued to be successful if the responsibility of the program was transferred to both the individual employers and the substance abuse prevention center right from the beginning. We can learn from this experience that all institutions are subject to budget cuts. We also must anticipate and prepare for unexpected circumstances so that as many components of a program can remain successful.

From this experience we have learned that the cholesterol screening program is very labor intensive and more technical than some other program components. Therefore, future programs should consider transferring the screening responsibility over to local health departments or HMOs early in the program. In addition, they also might consider training and certifying volunteer counselors for one-on-one counseling and referral services using a process similar to the one used for the volunteer run exercise clubs. Even if these services were performed only monthly or weekly by volunteer counselors, the program could continue to exist. Since the physicians are interested in treatment, perhaps the volunteers can create an atmosphere conducive for referrals.

5. Program evaluation was not included as a primary objective for this program. How does this limit what we are able to learn from the Washington Heights-Inwood experience?

No information is available about what influence the program had on behavior change and cardiovascular disease incidence or about the cost-effectiveness of the program. In addition, we do not know if the types of strategies and messages used in this program were effective for this population. We also can not evaluate the process taken to see what could have been done differently so that all program components could have been successful.

6. How would you propose to incorporate program evaluation into the existing program?

These are only some of the possibilities.

- Establish the importance of evaluation as a priority when writing for funding.
- Base interventions on a theory or set of theories so evaluation will be as scientifically based as measuring milk consumption or cholesterol levels.
- If funding is still limited, work with the local high schools and community colleges to establish class research projects. Use the students as researchers. Involve them with the project design. Have them collect, enter, and analyze data to reduce labor costs.
- Conduct inexpensive qualitative research using small groups at local settings (i.e., churches, etc.).

7. What factors would you need to consider when negotiating an agreement with the Dominican Women's Development Center?

- Timing of the transfer of responsibility is critical, as are other logistics such as space, personnel, protocols, and the like. They might have been more successful if they started the transfer process earlier. This would have given them the opportunity to experiment with more than one arrangement to see which was most likely to remain successful long term. This group might have had better influence on the local private physicians if they were involved earlier in the process.
- Integrate the goals of the Washington Heights-Inwood Healthy Heart Program with those of any community organization that will take responsibility for the program long term.
- Encourage the center to seek ongoing funding by collaborating with other groups in the community.

NUTRITION FOR ELDERLY ADULTS

*If I had known I was going to live so long, I would have taken
better care of myself.*
—GEORGE BURNS

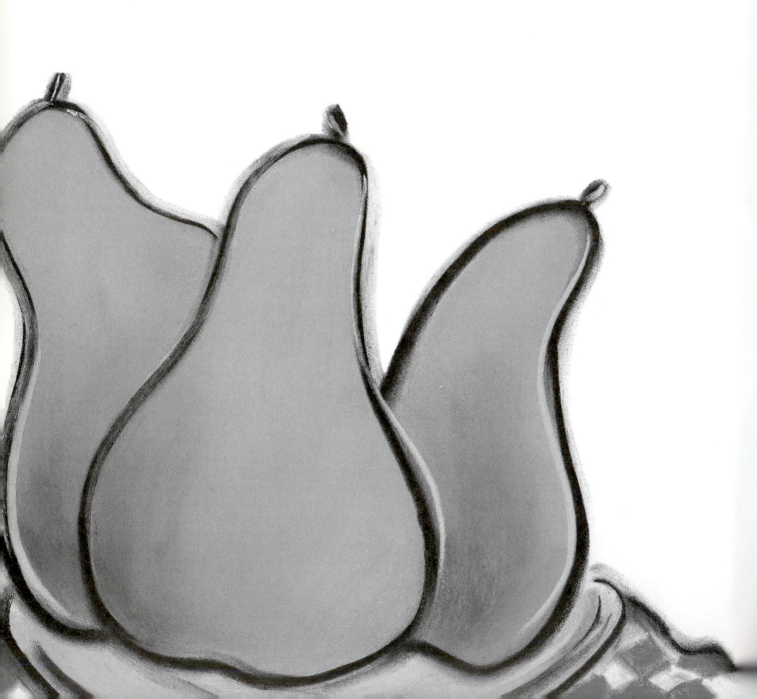

Core Concepts

A significant proportion of individuals who reach age sixty-five to seventy years are healthy and independent as are some eighty- to ninety-year-olds in the community. These elderly experience what is called "successful" aging as opposed to "usual" aging. This distinguishes between healthful aging and the effects of disease and other disabilities that may be associated with aging but that are not age-dependent.

This chapter defines characteristics of the elderly and discusses known nutritional needs of people aged sixty-five years and older. The process for screening elderly living in the community for nutritional deficiencies and components necessary for in-depth individualized assessments are described. Elements for successful nutrition interventions and expected outcomes are highlighted. Community nutrition professionals working with elderly clients must recognize the diversity of this age group and be able to integrate and effectively communicate access to nutritional and health care services.

Objectives

When you finish chapter eleven, you should be able to:

~ Define elderly adults and aged, young-old, and oldest-old.

~ Cite Healthy People 2000 objectives for elderly adults.

~ List the major risk factors for nutrition-related disease of elderly adults.

~ Identify screening characteristics within the risk factors that are useful to identify risk of malnutrition and/or poor general health.

~ Describe the continuum of care process for promoting independence and lessening disability from acute or chronic diseases.

~ Name the three nutrition intervention categories and give an example of a program within each category.

Key Words

WHO ARE AGING ADULTS?

In 1995, it was estimated that 33.6 million Americans were sixty-five or more years old (approximately 13 percent of the population).[45] Future predictions for the middle of the twenty-first century estimate this number will increase to nearly 80 million Americans (or about 20 percent of the population). Of those, 70 percent will be more than seventy-five years of age. In 1995, 3.6 million Americans were eighty-five years of age and older. By the middle of the twenty-first century, it is estimated this number will be 17.7 million people.[49] The increased number of elderly presents great challenges for community nutrition. Community nutrition professionals must be resourceful to plan and deliver cost-effective services and programs to address the needs of growing numbers of aging adults.

Aging is a process that occurs in an environmental context where human biology, lifestyle, and health care systems interact to produce "health" (see figure 11.1). Although they unfold together, aging and the physiologic effects of disease and other disabilities cannot be concluded to occur at a specific chronological age. Adults entering the age of sixty-five years and older can either age "successfully" or age "as usual." **Successful aging** represents living the best quality of life an individual can hope to achieve. **Aging "as usual"** results when the effects of lifestyle factors such as smoking, inactivity, and poor eating habits have taken their toll.[23] Therefore, although common terminology defining the elderly is done by age categories where the age subgroups are the **young-old** (sixty-five to seventy-four-year-olds); the **old** (seventy-five- to eighty-four-year-olds); and the **oldest-old** (those eighty-five years and older), the goal is for the aging process to occur successfully.

Chronological aging produces some physiological changes in cells, organs, and organ systems. As an example, consider the changes that may occur in the gastroenteric tract with aging. Gut motility may decrease, which slows transit time and potentially increases the risk of constipation. Production of acid and intrinsic factor in the stomach decreases, and pancreatic secretions also decline, in some respects, altering digestion of large loads of macronutrients (carbohydrates, protein, and fats). This alters absorption and utilization of nutrients. These changes occur at different rates in different people. Furthermore, within individuals, changes occur at different rates within cells and organ systems.

Physiologic alterations due to acquired diseases are of great importance for persons after the age of sixty-five years. The top three causes of death in the elderly are heart disease, cancer, and stroke, and these diseases can involve modifiable, nutrition-related lifestyle and environmental factors. For example, adherence to a low-sodium diet may benefit those persons with high blood pressure who are sodium-sensitive. There is some debate on the extent to which better outcomes are achieved for persons aged seventy-five years and older. If a person has lived a happy, productive, and seemingly "healthy" life for eighty or more years, should major efforts be made to have him or her modify the diet because calcium intake is "low" or blood cholesterol is "elevated"? Individualized evaluation and chronological age considerations are important when assessing potential outcomes.

Considerations about quality of life and interventions that help individuals live with chronic illness and disabilities are important. Chronic conditions among the elderly that impact daily living are arthritis, hypertension, visual and hearing impairments, **dementia,** diabetes, **osteoporosis,** and depression. At a certain point in their lives, many people reach a state where they need some support to remain on their own, which they can do only if certain needs are met. "They are in a precarious balance between the assets they posses (such as some functional capacity and a strong desire to remain at home in the community), and deficits they are burdened with (such as chronic health problems leading to a disability and being dependent on a caregiver for some daily activities)."[21] This group deserves special considerations in designing community, public health, and health care measures in nutrition to keep the balance in favor of the assets.

Another characteristic expanding in this population is ethnic diversity. In 1990, the minority elderly population was 14 percent of the population aged sixty-five years and older. By the year 2040, 32 percent of the elderly will be members of ethnic minorities. Although the percentage of elderly White individuals remains the majority of the elderly population, the overall White population percentage will decrease. In contrast, the ethnic groups of Blacks and Hispanics are predicted to increase. The combined ethnic minority percentage will increase from approximately 14 percent in 1990 to 25 percent by the year 2050. Sensitivity to minority elders' food preferences, cultural beliefs, lifestyles, and socioeconomic conditions will remain important when community nutrition professionals plan community interventions.

The economic status of the elderly also needs to be viewed as diverse, not simple. It is misleading to summarize the economic status of the "total elderly population"

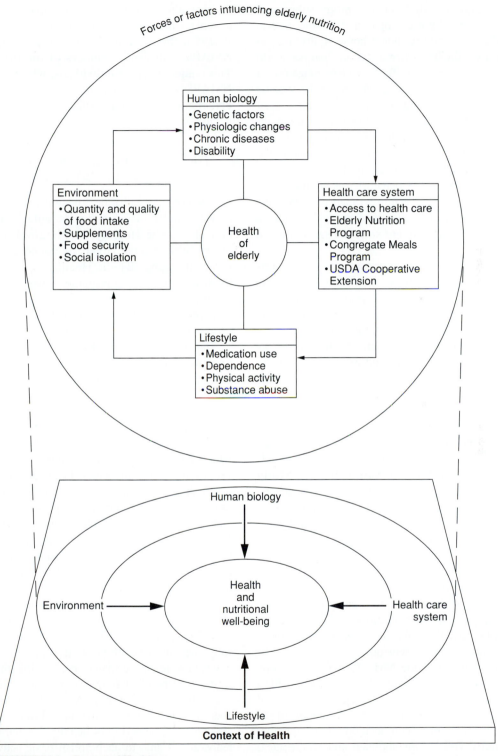

FIGURE 11.1 Context of Health
Influences on nutrition of the elderly.

because of significant differences among subgroups within this category.[50] For example, in 1990 the median net worth of the elderly (excluding home equity) ranged from $3,536 to $208,789, whereas the median net worth of persons aged forty-five to fifty-four years ranged from $897 to $45,799.[49] Not everyone shared in the income gains. Those elderly married-couple families fared best. Elderly who lived alone were more likely to have low incomes in 1990. Black women living in poverty have not improved their status over the past ten years. Among the elderly aged seventy-five and older, the 1990 poverty rate for Black, aged women (38 percent) was slightly more than double that for aged White women (17 percent). Overall, examination of detailed age groups provides a more comprehensive **assessment** since the aged are not a homogenous group.

Gender is also an important consideration when targeting the elderly. Currently, women represent 61 percent of all people aged sixty-five years and older; for the category of persons more than seventy-five years, women represent 70 percent. Adding the socioeconomic concerns that older women are three times as likely as men to be widowed, and eight of ten of the community-dwelling older persons who live alone are women dictates that a community nutrition professional planning any programs targeting the oldest-old will address concerns of elderly women.

Throughout this chapter, reference is made to a longitudinal study of healthy elderly people in Albuquerque.[18] This study, the **New Mexico Aging Process Study** (NMAPS), was initiated in 1980 with 304 participants. To become a participant in the NMAPS individuals sixty-five years of age or older had to be healthy: no overt clinical conditions such as coronary heart disease, insulin-dependent diabetes, significant peripheral vascular disease or liver disease, including negative tests for hepatitis; no history of internal cancer requiring surgery, x-ray irradiation, or chemotherapy in the past ten years; and not taking prescription medications with the following exceptions: thyroid replacement or medications to control mild-moderate hypertension.

The primary focus of the NMAPS was to examine the role of nutrition and changes in body composition and organ function in relation to the aging process and health status of the elderly. In-depth information of dietary habits, lifestyle, body composition, organ function, cognitive status, vitamin metabolism, and biochemical measures of nutritional status have been obtained annually since 1980.

Beginning in 1985, new participants were recruited to replace those who died or dropped out of the study. In 1996, there were 371 active participants in the NMAPS; 136 were members of the original cohort. This unique group of individuals, who at entry into the NMAPS were free of major risk factors, provides an opportunity to examine "successful" aging as opposed to "usual" aging.

HEALTHY PEOPLE 2000 OBJECTIVES FOR ELDERLY ADULTS

Selected objectives for health status, risk reduction, and services and protection for the elderly are shown in table 11.1. The Healthy People 2000 objectives for older adults promote targets to extend years of healthy life while aging. By the Healthy People 2000 objectives, successful aging promotes independent living, appropriate body weight, physical activity, good dental care, prevention of injury from falls, and prevention of further disability among persons with chronic diseases.

The Health Status and Risk Reduction objectives outlined for healthy, middle-aged adults (see table 10.1 on p. 271) also refer to older adults up to the age of seventy-four years. Thus, nutrition interventions planned for middle-aged adults can support achievement of Healthy People 2000 objectives for elderly adults up to age seventy-four years. There is some debate on the extent to which better outcomes are achieved for people aged seventy-five years and older. For example, would nutrition intervention help achieve the reduction of coronary heart disease deaths among old persons and reverse the rise in cancer deaths to achieve a rate of no more than 120 per 100,000 people? This is an area where population recommendations must consider the science of healthy physiological aging and how chronic illnesses unfold together for the oldest-old.

The overall goal is to prevent older adults from becoming disabled, preserve function among those with disabilities, or prevent further declines. More specifically, the aim of health promotion in the elderly population is to increase the span of healthy life; that is, life that permits independent function, not just a longer life. At age sixty-five years today, Americans have on average about 16.4 years of life remaining. Twelve of these years are likely to be a period of healthy life, during which the individual is able to accomplish basic activities associated with daily living. This is particularly true of people who enter this period of life in good health.[18] Increasing

TABLE 11.1
Healthy People 2000 Objectives for Older Adults

Objectives	Baseline prevalence (year)	Current prevalence (year)
Health status		
Reduce to no more than 90/1,000 people the proportion of all people aged sixty-five and over who have difficulty in performing two or more personal care activities,* thereby preserving independence	111/1,000 (1984–85)	
Special population targets		
People aged eighty-five and over	371/1,000 (1984–85)	325/1,000 (2000)†
Blacks aged sixty-five and over	112/1,000 (1984–85)	98/1,000 (2000)†
Increase years of healthy life for people aged sixty-five and over	11.9 years (1990)	14 years (2000)†
Reduce overweight to no more than 20 percent of the proportion of people aged sixty-five to seventy-four years	25 percent (1980)	43 percent (1991)
Reduce overweight to no more than 20 percent of the proportion of people aged seventy-five years and older	NA (1980)	26 percent (1991)
Reduce to no more than 15 percent the proportion of people aged sixty-five and over who engage in no leisure time physical activity	43 percent (1985)	22 percent (2000)†
Reduce to no more than 20 percent the proportion of people aged sixty-five and over who have lost all their natural teeth	36 percent (1986)	
Reduce hip fractures among people aged sixty-five and over so that hospitalizations for this condition are no more than 607/100,000	714/100,000 (1988)	841/100,000 (1993)
Special target populations		
White females aged eighty-five and over	2,721/100,000 (1988)	2,177/100,000 (2000)†
Reduce deaths from falls and fall-related injuries		
Special target populations		
People aged sixty-five to eighty-four	18.1/1,000 (1987)	14.4/1,000 (2000)†
People aged eighty-five and over	133/1,000 (1987)	105/1,000 (2000)†
Risk reductions		
Increase to at least 50 percent the proportion of people with hypertension whose blood pressure is under control		
Special target populations		
Women aged seventy and over	19 percent (1991)	
Services and protection		
Increase to at least 80 percent the receipt of home food services by people aged sixty-five and over who have difficulty in preparing their own meals or are otherwise in need of home-delivered meals	70 percent (1991)	
Increase to at least 70 percent the proportion of people aged sixty-five and over using oral health care system during each year	42 percent (1986)	51 percent (1993); 60 percent (2000)
Extend to all long-term nursing homes the requirement that oral examinations and services be provided no later than ninety days after entry into the facilities	Required (1990)‡	

*Personal care activities are bathing, dressing, using the toilet, getting in and out of bed, and eating
†New goals in 1995.
‡In nursing facilities receiving Medicaid or Medicare reimbursement.

the span of healthy life involves decreasing the number of days of restricted activity older people experience. This is accomplished by addressing a variety of preventable or treatable conditions of old age, many of which have nutritional implications. The *service objective* to increase delivery of home food services to those who have difficulty preparing their own meals is a direct nutrition service that supports those individuals who have lost food accessibility, yet still allows participants to remain in their homes (independent).

The objective to reduce the percentage of older adults being overweight to no more than 20 percent is one objective where nutrition interventions can have a positive impact. To promote weight loss, lowering dietary fat to 30 percent of calories and saturated fat to no more than 10 percent of calories while increasing physical activity is recommended. In addition, elderly adults are encouraged to increase their intake of complex carbohydrates–containing foods by consuming five or more servings of fruits and vegetables and six or more servings of grain products. One survey found that the vast majority of older adults failed to consume the minimum number of fruits and vegetables daily.[34] Such intake patterns increase risks for consuming limited vitamins and minerals as well as dietary fiber. **Obesity** is more prevalent among some population groups, such as Black and Hispanic females, low-income women, and individuals who have high blood pressure. Achieving weight loss among these high-risk groups can promote more successful aging and increase the period of independence.

Among *risk reduction* objectives for older adults, one objective is for at least 30 percent of older adults to engage in regular (preferably daily) light to moderate physical activity for at least a half hour per day. Light to moderate activity includes rapid walking, swimming, cycling, dancing, gardening, and yard work. In addition, the goal is for at least 20 percent of older adults to engage in vigorous physical activities for at least twenty minutes three times a week. Vigorous physical activities include activities that increase the heart rate to about 60 percent of its maximum. Another exercise-related objective is to decrease to no more than 22 percent of the people ages sixty-five years and older who engage in no leisure activity. Today 43 percent of persons aged sixty-five years or older do *not* engage in leisure activity. It is recommended that at least 35 percent of elderly regularly perform physical activities to

enhance and maintain muscular strength, muscular endurance, and flexibility. These types of physical activities pertain directly to functional status.

Reduction of hip fractures among those at highest risk, White females aged eighty-five years, is extremely difficult considering that osteopenia (i.e., a generalized reduction in bone mass and skeletal radiographic examination appears "demineralized" or "washed out") is often far advanced by old age. Nonetheless, keeping calcium intakes at high levels and maintaining regular physical activity especially can slow the loss of bone to some extent. It remains to be seen if such measures can lower the prevalence of falls and fractures, which inhibit independent living for many older Americans.

From middle-aged adults to persons up to age seventy-four years (see chapter 10), salt and sodium intakes are to be decreased so that at least 65 percent of home meal preparers do not add salt; at least 80 percent of individuals avoid using salt at the table, and at least 40 percent of adults regularly purchase foods modified or lower in sodium. Controversy exists whether this will support the *risk reduction* objective to increase to at least 50 percent of the proportion of people who have hypertension and have their blood pressure under control.

Overall, the Healthy People 2000 objectives targeted for older adults offer goals for achieving health and preventing mortality and morbidity from diseases. In view of the expanding numbers of elderly and resource limitations, community nutrition professionals will need to focus interventions on modifiable behaviors of elderly groups that are lagging behind in their health status due to personal habits that affect health. Several of the objectives for maintaining vitality and independence in older people are particularly relevant with respect to nutrition.

RECOMMENDED DIETARY ALLOWANCES

The 1989 recommended dietary allowances (RDAs) did not provide separate recommendations for older adults, that is, those sixty-five years of age and older. This was not because such recommendations were not desirable or necessary, but rather because there were few data on which to base them. There are now studies on several nutrients to define RDAs for older adults. Table 11.2 shows the recommended levels for individual intake of nutrients for adults 50 years of age and older.

TABLE 11.2

Recommended Levels for Individual Intake of Nutrients

	Males		Females	
Energy and Nutrients	**51–70 yrs**	**>70 yrs**	**51–70 yrs**	**>70 yrs**
Energy (kcal/kg)	30	30	30	30
Protein (g/kg)	0.8	0.8	0.8	0.8
Vitamin A (µg RE)	1,000	1,000	800	800
Vitamin D (µg)	10	15	10	15
Vitamin E (mg TE)	10	10	8	9
Vitamin K (µg)	80	80	65	65
Vitamin C (mg)	60	60	60	60
Thiamin (mg)	1.2	1.2	1.1	1.1
Riboflavin (mg)	1.3	1.3	1.1	1.1
Vitamin B_6 (mg)	1.7	1.7	1.5	1.5
Niacin (mg NE)	16	16	14	14
Folate (µg)	400	400	400	400
Calcium (mg)	1,200	1,200	1,200	1,200
Phosphorus (mg)	700	700	700	700
Magnesium (mg)	420	420	320	320
Iron (mg)	10	10	10	10
Iodine (µg)	150	150	150	150
Zinc (mg)	15	15	12	12
Selenium (µg)	70	70	55	55

RE, retinal equivalents; TE, tocopherol equivalents; NE, niacin equivalents

Sources: Data from National Research Council, *Recommended dietary allowances,* ed. 10, Washington, DC, 1989, National Academy Press, and for selected nutrients: Data from Institute of Medicine: *Dietary reference intakes for calcium, phosphorus, magnesium, vitamin D, and fluoride,* Washington, DC, 1997, National Academy Press; and, Food and Nutrition Board, National Academy of Sciences—Institute of Medicine: *Recommended levels for individual intake of B vitamins and choline,* Washington, DC, 1998, National Academy Press. (See discussion in chapter 2.)

Note: There are differences between the 1989 RDAs and the 1997/1998 recommended levels for individual intake of nutrients with respect to methods of derivation and age-groupings. However, space does not allow separate tables for the 1997/1998 recommended levels for individual intake of nutrients. Accordingly, the authors devised this table to summarize currently available data. It is not an official document developed or approved by the Food and Nutrition Board, Institute of Medicine, National Research Council, National Academy of Sciences.

Energy

The 1989 RDA energy recommendations are 15 to 20 percent lower for older adults than those for adults aged nineteen to fifty years. The lower energy recommendations are based on expected decreases in lean body mass and in physical activity among older adults. It is not certain that these decreases are an inevitable part of growing older.

In a national survey conducted in the summer of 1990, mean energy intake of men aged sixty-five to seventy-four years was 1,955 kcal/day and that of men aged more than seventy-four years was 1,812 kcal/day.[43] Intakes for women were 1,426 and 1,395 kcal/day for the same two age groups. In 1981, some 270 healthy elderly adults (mean age = seventy-one years) participating in the NMAPS were examined with

respect to dietary intakes.[18] The average energy intake of 125 men was 2,171 kcal/day and that of 145 women was 1,635 kcal/day. Nine years later, sixty-five men and ninety-two women (mean age = eighty years) from the original cohort were found to have energy intakes of 2,004 and 1,533 kcal/day, respectively.[16] This amounts to decreases of approximately 21.4 kcal/day per year and 5.3 kcal/day per year for men and women, respectively. When energy intakes were expressed in relation to body weight per day (kcal/kg per day), the changes were marginally significant for men (–0.21 kcal/kg per year) but not for women (–0.12 kcal/kg per year). Therefore, energy intake expressed in relation to body weight does not change significantly between the ages sixty-five and eighty years.

Protein

Dietary protein recommendations for adults fifty-one and older are also similar to those for younger adults. Among older people who have no debilitating disease, good health can be maintained on protein intakes of 0.8 gm/kg per day. This equates to an average of 63 g of protein per day for reference males and 50 g day for reference females.[14] Recommendations have been made for the elderly to consume 1.0 to 1.25 g of protein/kg body weight per day to prevent malnutrition.[6]

Vitamins

Those vitamins at risk for being low in diets of the elderly are vitamins A, B_6, B_{12}, riboflavin, and vitamin D. Within the aging population, however, intakes of vitamins are more variable. For example, vitamin intakes may be dangerously low among the very old and frail and whoever suffers from any diseases and uses many medications. In contrast, healthy, physically active elderly with well-balanced food intakes and who also use vitamin supplements could have excessive vitamin intakes.

Gastric mucosal atrophy increases with age and may cause malabsorption of vitamin B_{12} found in foods. Thus, the prevalence of vitamin B_{12} deficiency increases with age.[27] If a high folate intake is superimposed on vitamin B_{12} deficiency, there is a potential to mask the development of pernicious anemia. A delay in diagnosis and treatment of vitamin B_{12} deficiency can cause irreversible neurologic damage. The recommended intake [41] of both folate and vitamin B_{12} have been increased. Elderly shut-ins or those who live in inclement climates have had marginal vitamin D status.[20] Older persons' lower vitamin D status have also been related to poor diet and decreased absorption. Over time, vitamin D deficiency in the elderly may contribute to softening of bones and to osteoporosis through its effects on increasing bone loss and discouraging bone displacement.[5,57]

Minerals

Mineral needs of aging individuals are being actively investigated. There is evidence that in women some, but not all, of the calcium loss from bone that occurs with aging can be stopped by providing somewhat larger amounts of calcium (1200 mg) than the 1989 RDA (800 mg) and by estrogen replacement therapy.[5,23] Those women with low calcium intakes and with low bone density benefit the most. The National Institutes of Health Consensus Development Conference on Optimal Calcium Intake emphasized that high calcium intakes are important, but that they are not substitutes for estrogen therapy in blunting calcium losses after menopause.[33]

Iron deficiency anemia caused by inadequate iron intake is relatively rare among older people. In contrast, iron deficiency anemia secondary to unrecognized (occult) blood loss is common. Healthy elderly people are able to serve as blood donors if attention is paid to the frequency (and amount) of blood donated as well as to iron intake.[17]

In summary, RDAs specific for the elderly can now be advocated. Consideration is needed regarding how health status and normal aging affects dietary intake, digestion, absorption, and excretion of the variety of nutrients. Requirements for some other nutrients will most likely increase for healthy elderly to prevent incidence of diseases and for frail elderly due to higher needs. Medication usage and vitamin and mineral supplementation also influence nutrient requirements for older adults.

SCREENING AND ASSESSMENT FOR NUTRITION-RELATED PROBLEMS IN THE ELDERLY

The Nutrition Screening Initiative established a broad-based approach to nutrition screening, which starts in the community and the proceeds, if necessary, into the health services system.[56] Figure 11.2 arranges the levels from the initiative and outlined a sequence of activities that follow communitywide screening. The subsequent phases include nutrition assessment to further define associated causes for health decline, development of an age- and disease-appropriate intervention plan, and monitoring outcomes of the intervention.

Nutrition Checklist

The process begins with stimulating greater nutrition awareness among older people in a variety of community settings. Each day, older adults come together and maintain social support and friendship in nonmedical settings. The **DETERMINE Checklist** (figure 11.3) was designed to create awareness about warning signs of potential nutrition problems and to serve as a tool to

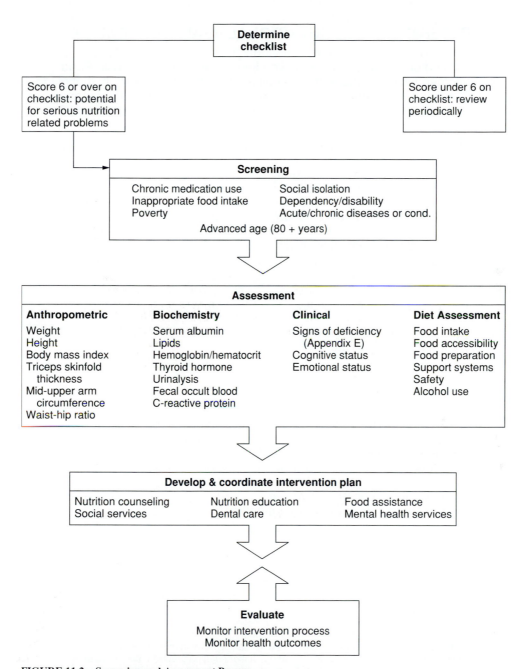

FIGURE 11.2　Screening and Assessment Process
(*Source:* Reprinted with permission by the Nutrition Screening Initiative, a project of the American Academy of Family Physicians, the American Dietetic Association and the National Council on Aging, Inc., and funded in part by a grant from Ross Products Division, Abbott Laboratories.)

DETERMINE YOUR NUTRITIONAL HEALTH CHECKLIST

The warning signs of poor nutritional health are often overlooked. Use this check to find out if you (or someone you know) are at nutritional risk. Read the statements below. Check the Yes column for those statements that apply to you. Check the No column if the statements do not apply. Circle the number in the Scoring column IF the statements ☐ applied to you and you checked YES.

Statement	No	Yes	Scoring
1. I have illness or condition that made me change the kind/or amount of food I eat	☐	☐	2
2. I eat fewer than two meals each day.	☐	☐	3
3. I eat few fruits or vegetables or milk products.	☐	☐	2
4. I have three or more drinks of beer, liquor, or wine almost every day.	☐	☐	2
5. I have tooth or mouth problems that make it hard for me to eat.	☐	☐	2
6. I don't always have enough money to buy the food I need.	☐	☐	4
7. I eat alone most of the time.	☐	☐	1
8. I take three or more different prescribed or over-the-counter medicines a day.	☐	☐	1
9. Without wanting to do so, I have lost or gained 10 pounds in the last six months.	☐	☐	2
10. I am not always physically able to shop, cook, and/or feed myself.	☐	☐	2

- -

Total the circled numbers: Total: ____

If the total is:

0–2 **Good!** Recheck your nutritional score in six months.

3–5 **You are at moderate nutritional risk.** See what can be done to improve your eating habits and lifestyle. Your office on aging, senior nutrition program, senior citizens center, or health department can help. Recheck your nutritional score in three months.

6 or more **You are at high nutritional risk.** Bring this checklist the next time you see your doctor, dietitian, or other qualified health or social service professional. Talk with them about any problems you may have. Ask for help to improve your nutritional health.

FIGURE 11.3 DETERMINE Checklist

(*Source:* Adapted with permission by the Nutrition Screening Initiative, a project of the American Academy of Family Physicians, the American Dietetic Association, and the National Council on the Aging, Inc., and funded in part by a grant from Ross Products Division, Abbott Laboratories.)

identify those with these signs. The checklist uses simple yes/no statements that can be answered by elderly persons or from a caregiver. Professionals, paraprofessionals, and the lay public can use the tool.

The DETERMINE checklist is scored by totaling the numbers for yes responses. If the total is six or greater, that individual is identified as at nutritional risk and is encouraged to see a professional. This professional can be a social service worker or a health care professional.

SCREENING

An efficient and effective approach to identifying nutritional and health problems in elderly involves **nutrition screening** and referral in primary care and community settings. Screening is used to identify individuals who may be at nutritional risk and guide them toward appropriate health care or other services to correct deficits. Screening is a cost-effective strategy because it identifies potential nutrition health problems early when they can be treated to prevent the development of a disease that is more serious or added complications. Unrecognized and untreated nutrition-related problems in the elderly cause significant disruption to normal function. Nutrition screening can and should be conducted in many settings such as elderly feeding programs, physician visits, and home care.

Nutrition screening tools search for many aspects of both nutritional and general health. They identify individuals who have deficits in any area that potentially places them at risk. Screening tools are important because they are developed to highlight problems that can be prevented or ameliorated when they are identified early and when they identify individuals who otherwise would not be recognized as suffering from a disease or disability. Screening tools are simple enough to apply in community settings in which older Americans live as well as in health care settings and should take a short amount of time to complete to be cost-effective.

The Nutrition Screening Initiative proposes a Level I Screen. At this screening level, a health professional is needed to review the major factors known to increase risk of poor nutritional status in older adults. Seven areas would trigger referral to a community nutrition professional, physician, or social service program.

- Inappropriate food intake
- Poverty
- Social isolation

- Disability and dependency
- Acute and chronic diseases or conditions
- Chronic use of medications
- Advanced age

Inappropriate Food and Fluid Intake

Food and fluid choices are integral to older adults' lifestyle choices, and environmental factors will change eating habits of older adults. Studies show life events and experiences are important factors affecting food choices of the elderly.[11] Those that most significantly affect food choices occurred either during childhood or in later years in association with significant role changes such as retirement or death of spouse. Widowed women who are skilled cooks may lose the motivation to prepare meals. Frail elderly may see cooking as a daunting challenge. The values most often negotiated when making food choices are social context, sensory perception, monetary considerations, convenience, and physical well-being.[40]

Screening areas for inadequate or inappropriate food are shown in box 11.1. Chronic inadequate or inappropriate food intake leads to abnormalities of body weight and includes being underweight or overweight. Weight changes

BOX 11.1

SIGNS OF INADEQUATE OR INAPPROPRIATE FOOD INTAKE

- Does not have enough food each day.
- Has several days each month without any food.
- Has poor appetite.
- Alcohol use is excessive.
- Daily intakes are less than recommended number of servings.
- Individual has special dietary practices, is on a special diet (either physician or self-prescribed) or complains about problems with meeting special dietary needs; individual has multiple diet prescriptions or has unusual dietary practices.
- Goes six to eight hours or longer during day without food or liquids.
- Eats one meal a day or less.
- Eats the same foods every day.

associated with nutrition-related health risks are discussed in the acute and chronic disease or condition screening area (see pp. 320–326).

It is important to realize that food and fluid intake are fundamentally related to weight. Weight and weight changes reflect altered nutritional and hydration status and are related to inappropriate food and fluid intake. The elderly are at greater risk of developing alcohol-related problems because of decreased social interaction with increasing age and increasing use of medications, potentially changing liver metabolism. Screening for alcohol abuse as a chronic condition is important.[1]

Poverty

Some screening clues to see if poverty may be a factor in nutrition and health risks are shown in box 11.2. In 1990, nearly one in five family households with an elderly head had annual incomes less than $15,000 and persons living alone or with nonrelatives had even lower incomes, with 42 percent reporting less than $10,000. For ethnic categories, the median income in 1994 for Black persons living alone or with nonrelatives was $7,557 and for Hispanics, $7,345. The percentage of persons living below the poverty threshold increases with age and is also related to ethnic status.[49] In general, the oldest-old, members of ethnic minority groups, women, elderly persons living alone, and those with disabilities are at the greatest risk for poverty.

"People who are poor are those who are likely to be hungry."[55] Individuals who are poor and who do not receive supportive services have an increased risk of undernutrition. An unknown number of them may actually be suffering from chronic malnutrition. For an elderly person, the cycle of malnutrition can begin with being acutely or chronically ill and is followed by eating less food. Alternatively, it can begin by decreasing food intake (for a variety of reasons) and then becoming ill.

Social Isolation

Social isolation, defined as having no one to help in case of illness, increases the likelihood of poor nutritional status in older adults. Eating and appetite are strongly influenced by social factors and elderly are more at risk than others. Bereavement over loss of a spouse can lead to decreased appetite and poorer caloric intake. Another factor is the distance from children who have not remained in the communities where parents live. This distance from family or other concerned individuals contributes to social isolation.

BOX 11.2

SIGNS THAT POVERTY IS A FACTOR IN NUTRITION AND HEALTH

- Income is less than $6,000 per year.
- Less than $35 per week is spent on food.
- Person is unable to buy needed food.
- "Prefers" not to spend money on food.
- Individual refuses to participate in income assistance programs in spite of need.

In addition, there are the psychological factors (such as depression) that cause individuals to decrease social contacts and not seek help or reject help if it is offered.

Social isolation can be caused by lack of transportation when the individual has physical or psychological disabilities. Currently only about one fifth of the elderly use community services.[55] Increased social interaction has positive impacts on food intake as well as the perception of general health and well-being.[44] Some indicators of possible social isolation as a factor in health and nutrition are summarized in box 11.3.

Dependence and Disability

Disorders such as arthritis of the hips, knees, and hands can cause **disability** and losses in everyday personal functions, including eating. The ability to perform self-care activities, especially those involving behaviors critical to obtaining and preparing food and the ability to feed oneself can be indirectly assessed by using a functional status screening tool. Examples include the activities of daily living and the instrumental activities of daily living (see tables 11.3 and 11.4).[26] These measures evaluate major activities like ability to feed self, walking, purchasing supplies, and handling money. The loss of ability to perform activities of daily living is an important warning sign of getting and preparing food and potential loss of independence. Of particular importance is a report that the individual has trouble self-feeding, cooking, getting to the grocery store, or shopping for food. Without intervention, these problems quickly lead to declining nutritional status. Disabling conditions, especially those that limit manual dexterity or make it necessary to use assistive devices to eat also increases the risk of malnutrition. Sensory impairments, such as blindness or cataracts, can make getting food and eating more difficult, particularly if persons have not adapted to their lost or limited sight. Deafness and hearing loss may also increase risks of poor nutritional status because it may contribute to social isolation and make use of devices such as the telephone more difficult.

BOX 11.3

SIGNS THAT SOCIAL ISOLATION IS A FACTOR IN NUTRITION AND HEALTH

- Lives alone, exhibits concern about home security, rejects help
- Is housebound
- Lost a spouse or other loved one in the last year
- Has contact with family or friends less than once a week
- Usually eats alone

The need for assistive devices such as walkers, wheelchairs, and modified dishes or utensils for preparing or consuming food is associated with increased nutritional risk because they mean that preparing and consuming food are more cumbersome. Almost 20 percent of older adults living at home have difficulties in walking or doing heavy housework; 10 percent have trouble shopping, preparing meals, or doing light housework; 5 percent have difficulties using the telephone and managing money; and 2 percent have trouble eating unassisted—all important tasks for assuring good food intakes.[49]

Cognitive or emotional impairments also affect the nutritional status of many elderly people. After eighty years of age, approximately 20 percent of all people suffer from some type of dementia. These rates rise steadily over age eighty-five.[25] Low body mass is quite common in demented elderly people, even after taking other illnesses into account.[3] In nursing homes, the prevalence is even higher. Depressive disorders can alter appetite and weight. The inability to read or write in any language, especially in English, makes communicating needs difficult and can increase dependency on

TABLE 11.3
Katz Index of Activities of Daily Living

- Bathing (sponge, shower, or tub)
  I: receives no assistance (gets in and out of tub, if tub is the usual means of bathing)
  A: receives assistance in bathing only one part of the body (such as the back or leg)
  D: receives assistance in bathing more than one part of the body (or not bathed)

- Dressing
  I: gets clothes and gets completely dressed without assistance
  A: get clothes and gets dressed without assistance except in tying shoes
  D: receives assistance in getting clothes or in getting dressed or stays partly or completely undressed

- Toileting
  U: goes to "toilet room," cleans self, and arranges clothes without assistance (may use object for support such as cane, walker, or wheelchair and may manage night bedpan or commode, emptying it in the morning)
  A: receives assistance in going to "toilet room" or in cleansing self or in arranging clothes after elimination or in use of night bedpan or commode

D: doesn't go to room termed "toilet" for the elimination process

- Transfer
  I: moves in and out of bed as well as in and out of chair without assistance (may be using object for support such as cane or walker)
  A: moves in and out of bed or chair with assistance
  D: doesn't get out of bed

- Continence
  I: controls urination and bowel movements completely by self
  A: has occasional "accidents"
  D: supervision helps keep urinary and/or bowel control; catheter is used; or is incontinent

- Feeding
  I: feeds self without assistance
  A: feeds self except for getting assistance in cutting meat or buttering bread
  D: receives assistance in feeding or is fed partly or completely using enteral tubes or intravenous fluids.

Abbreviations: I, independent; A, assistance; D, dependent.
Source: Adapted from Journal of the American Medical Association, 185:915, 1963. Copyright 1963, American Medical Association. Used with permission.

T A B L E   1 1 . 4

Instrumental Activities of Daily Living

- Telephone
   I: able to look up numbers, dial, receive, and make calls without help
   A: able to answer phone or dial operator in an emergency but needs special phone or help in getting number or dialing
   D: unable to use the telephone

- Traveling
   I: able to drive car or travel alone on bus or in taxi
   A: able to travel but not alone
   D: unable to travel

- Shopping
   I: able to take care of all shopping with transportation provided
   A: able to shop but not alone
   D: unable to shop

- Preparing meals
   I: able to plan and cook full meals

A: able to prepare light foods but unable to cook full meals alone
D: unable to prepare any meals

- Housework
   I: able to do heavy housework (like scrubbing floors)
   A: able to do light housework, but needs help with heavy tasks
   D: unable to do any housework

- Medication
   I: able to take medications in the right dose at the right time
   A: able to take medications but needs reminding or someone to prepare it
   D: unable to take medications

- Money
   I: able to manage buying needs, write checks, pay bills
   A: able to manage daily buying needs, but needs help managing checkbook, paying bills
   D: unable to manage money

Abbreviations: I, independent; A, assistance; D, dependent.
Source: Adapted from Multidimensional functional assessment questionnaire, ed. 2, Durham, NC, 1978, Duke University Center for the Study of Aging and Human Development, p. 169–170. Used with permission.

others and isolating the older person in social settings. As shown in box 11.4, there are screening clues that functional problems are a factor in nutrition and health.

Acute and Chronic Diseases or Conditions

Acute and chronic diseases, including multiple illnesses and related hospitalizations, are prevalent among older Americans, particularly those in their late seventies and eighties. Heart disease is the leading cause of death among the elderly. For those aged eighty-five years and older, heart disease was the cause of 44 percent of deaths. Influenza and pneumonia are also important causes of death after age eighty-five. Adequate nutritional status improves outcomes for those elderly with chronic diseases such as hypertension, heart disease, diabetes mellitus, and arteriosclerosis. Nutrition also plays an important role in preventing risks associated with fractures due to osteoporosis.

Five of the ten leading causes of death in our country (coronary artery disease, some types of cancer, stroke, non-insulin-dependent diabetes mellitus, and atherosclerosis) are diet related and are worsened by obesity. Elderly individuals who are overweight and experiencing symptoms of altered blood glucose levels, high blood pressure, and pain in weight-bearing joints may find relatively modest weight losses (e.g., 5 to 10 lb) helpful in managing the disability.

BOX 11.4

SIGNS THAT FUNCTIONAL PROBLEMS ARE A FACTOR IN NUTRITION AND HEALTH

- A change from independence to dependence on two of the activities of daily living (table 11.3), or
- A change in one of the nutritionally relevant skills in the instrumental activities of daily living (table 11.4)

Any unplanned gain or loss of weight as well as the presence of obesity or underweight predict increased risks of both illness and death. Older people who are extremely overweight or underweight have higher death rates; underweight is particularly highly associated with mortality in the very old.[47] Risks of pressure sore ulcers and systemic infections are also elevated among those who are underweight.[37]

The causes of involuntary and unexplained weight loss in the elderly vary. Weight loss due to a preceding or accompanying disease can be divided into four categories: increased energy needs, anorexia, altered metabolism, and poor oral health. Individuals with a cognitive impairment or who are agitated may have increased energy needs.[15] Some persons with Alzheimer's disease develop increased "wandering," which provides excessive physical activity and increases calorie expenditure. Increased energy needs are also associated with movement disorders, such as Parkinson's disease and tardive dyskinesia. These are cases where increased muscular activity due to the disease or side effects of medications leads to increased metabolism. Persons with any type of infection and who develop fevers or hyperthyroidism will have higher energy expenditures. Depression, on the other hand, causes a decreased appetite and subsequently leads to decreased energy intakes. Altered taste and small secondary to medications or reactions to medication can cause anorexia.[48] Involuntary losses of weight may indicate an undiagnosed disease (such as cancer or depression) or other adverse life events that need remediation and should not be automatically regarded as good in overweight persons. Protein-energy malnutrition (PEM) commonly coexists with chronic illness, which may alter absorption or metabolism of protein and other nutrients precipitating PEM. Smaller scale surveys suggest relatively high prevalence rates of PEM among dependent, homebound, elderly persons and among subgroups such as those with dementia, chronic illness, or multiple other illnesses who are found in nursing homes and acute care hospitals.

Oral health affects chewing, swallowing, and the type of diet that can be eaten. At the very least, oral health problems detract from the joy of eating and may also cause pain. Chewing problems are the result of tooth loss, mouth pain, and other oral health problems and they are common in the elderly.[19] By age fifty, many Americans have lost their teeth, while those who still have them often have one or more missing teeth, and significant proportions have untreated root caries, gingivitis, and periodontitis. After age eighty-five years, the majority of individuals are totally edentulous, and many, perhaps the majority, have denture-related problems.

Box 11.5 identifies the chronic diseases and associated risk factors that would trigger further assessment. Other screening areas (such as inadequate food intake and chronic medication usage) combined with a screen for acute and chronic conditions assist community nutrition professionals to identify elderly persons needing further assessment.

Chronic Medication Usage

Among the elderly living in the community, the majority are taking more than one medication and almost one

BOX 11.5

RISK FACTORS THAT SHOULD TRIGGER FURTHER ASSESSMENT

- Chronic diseases, especially those involving dietary modifications
- Involuntary loss or gain in weight; losses or gains of more than 4 kg (10 lb) in six months, reported weight 20 percent over or under best or desirable weight
- Tooth loss or mouth pain; missing, loose, or badly decayed teeth; dentures that don't fit properly; mouth sores that do not heal; bleeding or sore gums; more than a year since the last dental visit
- Sadness and depression, with little interest in shopping, cooking, or eating
- Problems with memory loss, making it difficult to shop, cook, or eat.
- Hospitalization or surgery in the past six months

fourth take at least five medications.[28] The proportions increase to 90 percent taking more than one medication and 35 percent taking five or more medications if people are receiving services in the homes.[35] The proportion of persons taking five or more medications increases to nearly half for long-term care residents. Virtually all medications (prescribed or over-the-counter) are capable of affecting nutritional status. There are a number of different mechanisms by which this may occur.

- Effects on food intake
    Appetite suppression
    Loss of taste sensation
    Oral lesions
    Nausea and vomiting
- Effects on digestion and absorption
- Effects on metabolism

The name, form, dosage, frequency, and duration of use of all medications should be recorded and appropriately evaluated.[38]

Nutritional quackery and overuse of vitamin, minerals, and other nutritional supplements are thought to be common among older Americans.[30] Some preparations, such as very large doses of vitamin A and vitamin D can cause toxicity. Use of some food supplements or unproved nutritional remedies may not cause direct harm but is often associated with delays in seeking medical help for health problems. Box 11.6 outlines some areas to explore for possible problems related to use of medications or "special" products.

Advancing Age

A person who is chronologically over the age of eighty years may be frail, needy, and dependent. However, many eighty- and ninety-year-olds are still physically and mentally active. The generalization that can be made is that vulnerability increases with advancing age. Coordinated health services that reduce the vulnerability of the oldest-old can foster continued independence and support successful aging and satisfactory quality of life. Caregivers must be alert to nutritional risks, including all those discussed above, among the oldest-old who may have diminished ability to recognize and communicate needs or who may hide needs in fear of being judged incapable of continued independent living.

ASSESSMENT

The role of assessment is to perform a comprehensive evaluation of elderly adults to identify causal problems so that the most cost-effective intervention can be selected. There are four major areas where assessment information is collected and evaluated: anthropometric, biochemical, clinical, and dietary. Assessments are best done in a health care setting where professionally trained staff has access to the medical history records of patients' health and nutritional status.

Anthropometric

Actual anthropometric measurements, rather than reports, are mandatory for sound nutritional assessment. All patients who are seen in health care settings should be weighed and have height measured on a regular basis. Scales should be calibrated frequently, and the procedures for weighing persons should be standardized. If not taken correctly, these measurements are highly unreliable and minimally useful.

There is still a good deal of dispute about the most appropriate weight goals for older Americans. For example, aging causes significant changes in size, shape, and composition of the body. Height decreases (at a rate of approximately 1 cm per decade after the age of thirty years), fat is redistributed from the extremities to the trunk, and muscle tone and mass decrease. Ethnicity

---

BOX 11.6

SIGNS THAT MEDICATIONS MAY BE PROBLEMATIC

- Use of three or more prescribed medications daily
- Use of over-the-counter vitamin or mineral supplements daily; especially if more than three of these are used
- Excessive preoccupation with and use of unproved nutritional or other remedies

---

and differences of gender may also change expectations for weight goals.[18] After age eighty, because of losses of bone, water, and lean body mass, generalization about appropriate weight goals is difficult, and indications for weight reduction must be evaluated on an individual basis. Figure 11.4 presents body mass indexes (BMIs) of healthy elderly participating in NMAPS.

Obesity is very prevalent in older Americans, regardless of what standards are used. If a BMI of about 27 is considered as obese, then more than one third of all older men and women are obese. If older adults who have a BMI of 30 or greater are considered morbidly obese, 10 percent of all men and perhaps 15 percent of all women are at significant risk. Note in figure 11.4 that some 15 percent of women more than seventy years of age have had a BMI greater than 30.[18] Body fat distribution can also measure adiposity. Central adiposity (waist-to-hip ratio over 1.0 in males and 0.8 in females) increases risk for many chronic degenerative diseases associated with obesity.

Significant weight loss over time is an indicator of poor nutritional status. Loss of more than 4.5 kg (10 lb) or loss of more than 5 percent of previous body weight in a month, 7.5 percent in three months, or 10 percent or more in six months constitutes significant weight loss. Midarm muscle below 10 percent of desirable levels are suggestive of muscle wasting.

Biochemical

Laboratory and diagnostic tests recommended for instituting prevention measures for older adults in primary health care settings include total serum cholesterol, urinalysis, and periodic tests of thyroid function and fecal occult blood. Laboratory tests that may be helpful for confirming the presence of malnutrition include re-

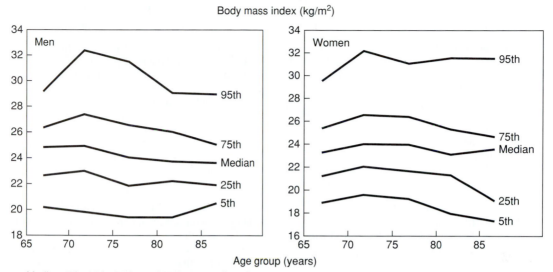

Body mass index (kg/m²)

Age group (years)

Median, 5th, 25th, 75th, and 95th percentile values

FIGURE 11.4   Body Mass Index (BMI) of Healthy Elderly
(*Source:* From Garry PJ, Owen GM, Eldridge TO: *The New Mexico Aging Process Study,* Albuquerque, 1997, University of New Mexico Press. Reprinted with permission.)

duced serum albumin or other serum proteins with shorter half-lives, such as prealbumin and transferrin.

A significant biochemical indicator of poor nutritional status is a serum albumin concentration below 3.5 gm/dl. Similarly, a serum total cholesterol below 160 mg/dl is often present in malnutrition. Reduced lymphocyte counts and delayed hypersensitivy skin tests are often seen in patients with poor nutritional status. Iron deficiency anemia and folic acid deficiencies are also determined using biochemical tests.

Clinical

Clinical signs of nutrient deficiency are outlined in appendix E. Signs of malnutrition to look for during a clinical examination of the elderly include angular stomatitis of the mouth, poorly healing wounds, an evident loss of subcutaneous fat and muscle, and fluid retention. Pressure sores are also signs of increased nutritional risk because their presence is often associated with poor nutritional status.[4] These signs may indicate primary malnutrition or may be secondary to acute or chronic disease. Signs of dehydration include decreased skin turgor, dry mouth, and mucous membranes that are not easily explained by other factors.

Physical examinations should include an oral health examination. Dental disabilities include total lack of

teeth; poorly fitting dentures; periodontal disease; decayed, missing, and filled teeth; dry mouth; facial pain; and difficulties with chewing.

Any signs of physical abuse and neglect are important in a clinical assessment and must be reported. A community nutrition professional must also remain alert for emotional symptoms of depression, abnormal bereavement, and changes in cognitive function. Screening and assessment tools are available to measure cognitive and emotional status (see tables 11.5 and 11.6). Referrals to appropriate social service and mental health professionals are essential.

Dietary Assessment

At a screening level, an insufficient food intake is defined as consuming less than the recommended minimum from one or more of the five food groups (i.e., two servings of milk or milk products, two servings of meat or meat alternates, two servings of fruits, three servings of vegetables, and six servings of breads and cereals). A more extensive probe regarding food and fluid intake is required in the assessment phase. Refer to chapter 3 for descriptions of the ranges of tools and approaches available for dietary assessment. The goal for the community nutrition professional is to identify specific nutrients at risk for imbalances.

TABLE 11.5
Cognitive Capacity Screen

- What day of the week is this?
- What month?
- What day of the month?
- What year?
- What place is this?
- Repeat the numbers 872.
- Say them backwards.
- Repeat the numbers: 6371.
- Listen to these numbers: 8143. Count 1 through 10 out loud, then repeat 694. (Help if needed. Then use numbers 573.)
- Beginning with Sunday, say the days of the week backward.
- 9 plus 3 is?
- Add 6 to the previous answer (or "to 12").
- Take away 5 (from "18").
- Repeat these words after me and remember them: I will ask for them later: HAT, CAR, TREE, TWENTY.
- The opposite of fast is slow. The opposite of up is _____.
- The opposite of large is _____.
- The opposite of hard is _____.
- An orange and a banana are both fruits. Red and blue are both _____.
- A penny and a dime are both _____.
- What were those words I asked you to remember? (HAT)
- (CAR)
- (TREE)
- (TWENTY)
- Take 7 away from a 100, then take 7 away from what is left and keep going: 100 minus 7 is _____.
- Minus 7 _____.
- Minus 7 _____. (Write down answers; check correct subtraction of 7)
- Minus 7 _____.
- Minus 7 _____.
- Minus 7 _____.
- Minus 7 _____.

Total correct (maximum score: 30) _____. (Patients with scores less than 20 are more likely to meet clinical criteria for dementia)

Source: From Jacobs J et al.: Screening for organic mental syndromes in the medically ill, *Annals of Internal Medicine,* 86:40–46, 1977. Copyright 1977, American College of Physicians. Reprinted with permission.

TABLE 11.6
Geriatric Depression Scale

- Are you basically satisfied with your life? (no)
- Have you dropped many of your activities and interests? (yes)
- Do you feel that your life is empty? (yes)
- Do you often get bored? (yes)
- Are you hopeful about the future? (no)
- Are you bothered by thoughts that you just cannot get out of your head? (yes)
- Are you in good spirits most of the time? (no)
- Are you afraid that something bad is going to happen to you? (yes)
- Do you feel happy most of the time? (no)
- Do you often feel helpless? (yes)
- Do you often get restless and fidgety? (yes)
- Do you prefer to stay at home at night, rather than to go out and do new things? (yes)
- Do you frequently worry about the future? (yes)
- Do you feel that you have more problems with memory than most? (yes)
- Do you think it is wonderful to be alive now? (no)
- Do you often feel downhearted and blue? (yes)
- Do you feel pretty worthless the way you are now? (yes)
- Do you worry a lot about the past? (yes)
- Do you find life very exciting? (no)
- Is it hard for you to get started on new projects? (yes)
- Do you feel full of energy? (no)
- Do you feel that your situation is hopeless? (yes)
- Do you think that most persons are better off then you are? (yes)
- Do you frequently get upset over little things? (yes)
- Do you frequently feel like crying? (yes)
- Do you have trouble concentrating? (yes)
- Do you enjoy getting up in the morning? (no)
- Do you prefer to avoid social gatherings? (yes)
- Is it easy for you to make decisions? (no)
- Is your mind as clear as it used to be? (no)

Score one point for each response that matches the yes or no answer after the question. (A score of 10 or 11 is usually used as the threshold to separate clients into depressed and nondepressed groups.)

Source: From Gallo JJ, Reichel W, Anderson LM: *Handbook of geriatric assessment,* ed. 2, Gaithersburg, MD 1995, Aspen Publishers, p. 78.

The nutrition interview should also probe for risks of poor nutrition due to the living environment. Absence of a stove or refrigerator, inadequate heating or cooling, nonuse of food programs if income is very limited, and concerns about home security and safety may indicate that food is difficult to obtain or prepare. The problems the individual has with availability of food and obtaining food; the social circumstances of eating, appetite, and in meeting special dietary needs; and types of unusual dietary practices need documentation.

Water is a nutrient that is often forgotten but that is extremely important in older adults. Thirst is not always a good indicator of adequate hydration in the elderly. Histories of decreased fluid intake, fever, vomiting, diarrhea, diabetes, chronic renal disease, and use of diuretics often place older people at risk of dehydration. Inadequate fluid intake can also lead to constipation. This is often not mentioned unless probed for directly. Probing for use of laxatives and fluid and fiber intake can help identify causes of constipation, which can be ameliorated with increased fluid and fiber intake, more physical activity, and regular meals. A daily intake of more than 26 g of alcohol (approximately two 12-oz cans of beer, one glass of wine, or one shot of 86 proof whiskey) by women or more than 52 g alcohol (approximately four cans of beer, two glasses of wine, or two shots of 86 proof whiskey) by men is also a cause for concern. On the other hand, if elderly people consume alcohol in moderation, they appear to tolerate it and perhaps benefit from its use. In the NMAPS,[18] there was no relation between current or earlier alcohol intake and vitamin status. There was a strong positive correlation between alcohol intake and serum high-density lipoprotein (HDL) cholesterol.

A Valid Nutrition Assessment Tool

The Mini-Nutritional Assessment (MNA) was developed for use with elderly people who are either free-living in the community or are in long-term settings.[22] It has been cross-validated in three studies involving more than 600 elderly individuals in Europe and the United States. The MNA is comprised of a series of short questions and simple measurements and can be completed in fifteen to twenty minutes. An MNA form is shown in figure 11.5. There are four components:

- Anthropometric measurements (weight, height, arm and calf circumference)
- General assessment (six questions related to lifestyle, medications, physiological status, and mobility)
- Dietary questionnaire (six questions related to number of meals, food and fluid intake, and autonomy of feeding)
- Subjective assessment (self-perception of health and nutrition)

If necessary, biological markers (biochemical indices such as serum albumin, C-reactive protein, cholesterol, and lymphocyte count) can be ordered to further classify the elderly at risk.

Age-specific standards for nutrition assessments are available to evaluate changes in body composition and dietary intake. Tools to assess environmental and social changes are also useful and available. Careful assessment by physicians and other health care personnel who are knowledgeable in geriatric medicine and gerontology is important to accurate assessment and interpretation. Accurate nutrition assessments provide information related to problems posing risks for a decline in

health and independence. This leads to better selection of and utilization of the intervention services and programs available.

DEVELOP AND COORDINATE INTERVENTION PLAN

Screening and assessment of nutritional status are useful only when they are coupled with interventions to address identified nutritional problems. A range of health and social programs are available in most communities to address nutrition-related problems of older Americans. Different programs and services are designed to meet differing needs as elderly shift along the continuum of health and independence to becoming frail and dependent. These ranges from social support and interaction to clinical care for the control or amelioration of diseases and conditions to hospice care for terminally ill. Figure 11.6 outlines the **continuum of care** necessary for older adults to prevent risk of malnutrition and improve the potential for independent living. Services and programs to ensure adequate intakes of protective nutrients, to avoid imbalances and excesses, and to manage chronic degenerative diseases affected by dietary practices should at a minimum, be available.

The goal of nutrition intervention is to improve or maintain the overall good health and functional status of the elderly population. Nutrition intervention can contribute toward successful aging. Important factors that contribute to motivating elderly persons to make dietary changes are personal characteristics such as intelligence, motivation, curiosity, religious or philosophical convictions, social characteristics (such as maintaining an active social life) responsibility for others, family integrity, intimacy, financial independence, and age-adaptable living arrangements in the physical environment.[40] With considerations of factors that impact outcomes, nutrition interventions for older people generally fall into three categories: nutrition **counseling, nutrition education,** and nutrition support.[56]

Counseling

An effective array of nutrition interventions must recognize the diversity and impact of lifelong food choices. This is accomplished in part by the intervention on the factors that are controllable. Changing poor lifetime nutritional habits to promote maintaining healthy weights, prudence in dietary intakes, and avoidance of substance

Last name _____ First name _____ M.I. _____ Sex ____ Date _____

Age _____ Weight (kg) _____ Height (cm) _____ MAC (cm) _____ CC (cm) _____

Complete the form by writing the numbers in the boxes. Add the numbers in the boxes and compare the total assessment to the Malnutrition Indicator Score.

Anthropometric assessment

	Points

1. Body mass index (BMI) (weight in kg)/(height in m)
  a. BMI < 19   = 0 points
  b. BMI 19 to < 21 = 1 point
  c. BMI 21 to < 23 = 2 points
  d. BMI ≥ 23   = 3 points
	☐

2. Mid-arm circumference (MAC) in cm
  a. MAC < 21   = 0.0 points
  b. MAC 21 ≤ 22 = 0.5 points
  c. MAC > 22   = 1.0 points
	☐.☐

3. Calf circumference (CC) in cm a. CC < 31 = 0 points b. CC ≥ 31 = 1 point	☐

4. Weight loss during last three months
  a. weight loss greater than 3 kg (6.6 lb) = 0 points
  b. does not know   = 1 point
  c. weight loss between 1 and 3 kg
     (2.2 and 6.6 lb)   = 2 points
  d. no weight loss   = 3 points
	☐

General assessment

5. Lives independently (not in a nursing home or hospital)   a. no = 0 points   b. yes = 1 point ☐
6. Takes more than three prescription drugs per day   a. yes = 0 points   b. no = 1 point ☐
7. Has suffered psychological stress or acute disease in the past three months   a. yes = 0 points   b. no = 2 points ☐

8. Mobility
  a. bed or chair bound   = 0 points
  b. able to get out of bed/chair but does
     not go out   = 1 point
  c. goes out   = 2 points ☐

9. Neuropsychological problems
  a. severe dementia or depression = 0 points
  b. mild dementia   = 1 point
  c. no psychological problems = 2 points ☐

10. Pressure sores or skin ulcers   a. yes = 0 points   b. no = 1 point ☐

Dietary assessment

11. How many full meals does the patient eat daily?
  a. 1 meal = 0 points
  b. 2 meals = 1 point
  c. 3 meals = 2 points ☐

	Points

12. Selected consumption markers for protein intake
 • At least one serving of dairy products (milk, cheese,
  yogurt) per day?   yes ☐ no ☐
 • Two or more servings of legumes or eggs per week?
          yes ☐ no ☐
 • Meat, fish, or poultry every day? yes ☐ no ☐
  a. if 0 or 1 yes = 0.0 points
  b. if 2   yes = 0.5 points
  c. if 3   yes = 1.0 points
	☐.☐

13. Consumes two or more servings of fruits or vegetables per day? a. no = 0 points b. yes = 1 point	☐

14. Has food intake declined over the past three months due to loss of appetite, digestive problems, chewing or swallowing difficulties?
  a. severe loss of appetite   = 0 points
  b. moderate loss of appetite = 1 point
  c. no loss of appetite   = 2 points
	☐

15. How much fluid (water, juice, coffee, tea, milk...) is consumed per day? (1 cup = 8 oz.)
  a. less than 3 cups = 0.0 points
  b. 3 to 5 cups   = 0.5 points
  c. more than 5 cups = 1.0 points
	☐.☐

16. Mode of feeding
  a. unable to eat without assistance = 0 points
  b. self-fed with some difficulty   = 1 point
  c. self-fed without any problem = 2 points
	☐

Self-assessment

17. Do they view themselves as having nutritional problems?
  a. major malnutrition   = 0 points
  b. does not know or moderate malnutrition = 1 point
  c. no nutritional problem   = 2 points ☐

18. In comparison with other people of the same age, how do they consider their health status?
  a. not as good   = 0.0 points
  b. does not know = 0.5 points
  c. as good   = 1.0 point
  d. better   = 2.0 points ☐.☐

Assessment total (max 30 points) ☐☐.☐

Malnutrition Indicator Score		
≥ 24 points	well nourished	☐
17 to 23.5 points	at risk of malnutrition	☐
< 17 points	malnourished	☐

FIGURE 11.5 Mini-Nutritional Assessment Form
(*Source:* From Guigoz Y, Vellas B, Garry PJ: Mini-nutritional assessment: a practical assessment tool for grading nutritional status of elderly patients, *Facts and Research in Gerontology,* 4(suppl 2):15–59, 1994.)

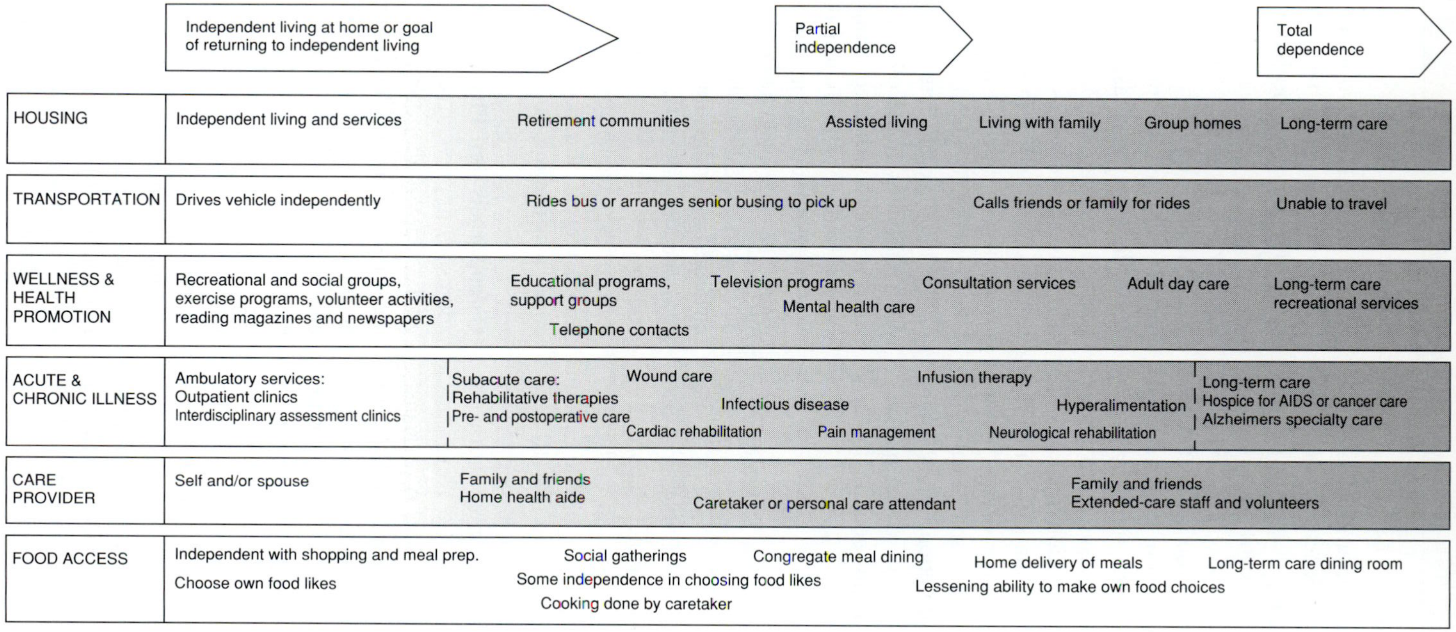

Independent living at home or goal of returning to independent living →

Partial independence →

Total dependence →

	Independent living / returning				Total dependence
HOUSING	Independent living and services	Retirement communities	Assisted living	Living with family	Group homes	Long-term care
TRANSPORTATION	Drives vehicle independently	Rides bus or arranges senior busing to pick up	Calls friends or family for rides			Unable to travel
WELLNESS & HEALTH PROMOTION	Recreational and social groups, exercise programs, volunteer activities, reading magazines and newspapers	Educational programs, support groups; Telephone contacts	Television programs; Mental health care	Consultation services	Adult day care	Long-term care recreational services
ACUTE & CHRONIC ILLNESS	Ambulatory services: Outpatient clinics; Interdisciplinary assessment clinics	Subacute care: Rehabilitative therapies; Pre- and postoperative care; Wound care; Cardiac rehabilitation	Infectious disease; Pain management	Infusion therapy; Neurological rehabilitation	Hyperalimentation	Long-term care; Hospice for AIDS or cancer care; Alzheimers specialty care
CARE PROVIDER	Self and/or spouse	Family and friends; Home health aide	Caretaker or personal care attendant			Family and friends; Extended-care staff and volunteers
FOOD ACCESS	Independent with shopping and meal prep.; Choose own food likes	Social gatherings; Some independence in choosing food likes; Cooking done by caretaker	Congregate meal dining	Home delivery of meals; Lessening ability to make own food choices		Long-term care dining room

FIGURE 11.6 Continuum of Care and Services to Promote Successful Aging

(*Source:* From Robinson, G: The continuum: long term care in transition, *Nutrition across the continuum: linking home and community nutrition care and services to promote successful aging*, Miami, FL, 1995, National Policy and Resource Center.)

abuse are examples where education and counseling positively impact better outcomes. Genetic factors and weakening organ systems after many years of working well are not altered by nutrition interventions.

The U.S. Preventive Health Services Task Force's recommendations[51] for the content of routine visits with primary physicians include counseling of a general nature on diet and exercise, substance use, injury prevention, and other primary prevention measures. Particular attention is suggested to ensure moderation in intakes of fat (especially saturated fat) and sodium. Encouraging healthy elderly to substitute complex carbohydrate foods (like low-fat, higher fiber breads and cereals) for higher fat foods reduces fat consumption, offers better nutrient density, and lowers risk of constipation. Weight loss is possible, although not necessarily expected, in these cases.

Examples of Common Nutrition-Related Problems Requiring Counseling

Hypercholesterolemia   The National Cholesterol Education Program's Population Based Panel Report provides dietary advice for older adults similar to that for younger adults. Namely, it recommends limiting total fat to 30 percent of calories, with no more than 10 percent of calories from saturated or polyunsaturated fats and the remaining 10 percent from monounsaturated fats. These and the Dietary Guidelines for Americans represent reasonable dietary goals for older Americans. However, the knowledge base is still incomplete and these recommendations must be interpreted in the light of the person's entire health profile. The atherosclerotic process takes decades rather than years to develop to the point where health is clinically impaired, and multiple nutritional and lifestyle factors are involved. The usefulness of diet-related preventive measure undertaken late in life has been debated.

Active medical management of high serum cholesterol levels is usually restricted to individuals who are most likely to benefit from long-term therapy.[8] Both older men and postmenopausal women who are healthy and have active lifestyles and a good prognosis for an extended lifetime are good candidates for preventive and therapeutic efforts. In contrast, very old, frail, debilitated older adults suffering from dementia, arthritis, osteoporosis, malignancy, or already very severe coronary disease need to be considered on an individual basis. Individualized, age- and condition-specific guidance is needed. Appropriate prevention and therapy focus on the problem that is most likely to affect quality of life, function, and morbidity.

Obesity   Another topic to address with nutrition counseling is with obesity and weight loss. Among older people who are extremely sedentary, high-fat, calorie-dense diets may increase risks of excessive calorie intakes and hence risks of obesity and associated diseases (such as non-insulin-dependent diabetes, high blood pressure, and gallstones). There is little evidence that moderate decreases in dietary fat intakes from current levels are dangerous to older people up to a certain age or "health" level if diets remain adequate in energy and other nutrients. If the older individual is not suffering from obesity-associated symptoms, the benefits of restricting calories simply to reduce weight to some theoretical ideal level are in question. Moreover, after age eighty, because of losses of bone, water, and lean body mass, generalization about appropriate weight goals is difficult, and indications for weight reduction must be evaluated on an individual basis. For those who are confined to their homes or to an institution because of infirmities, a worthwhile goal may be simply to cap any future weight and prevent worsening of the medical conditions making care more difficult.

Osteoporosis and Physical Inactivity   Another topic addressed in preventive counseling is adequate calcium intake. Factors that contribute to calcium deficiency in older persons are inadequate dietary calcium intake, inactivity, medications, and estrogen deficiency. These are factors that can be modified through behavior changes. The primary physician can also address alcohol and other drug use needs and make suggestions to reduce use or change medications if intakes are inappropriate or excessive.

More than half of all Americans over sixty-five years of age and at least one third of those aged forty-five to sixty-four years are currently less active than the levels experts consider appropriate. Regular exercise and physically active lifestyles are associated with improved function and lessened symptoms of some of the chronic degenerative diseases, and may also decrease mortality.[46] Also, immobility is associated with increased risk of institutionalization. Moreover, the maintenance of skeletal muscle is important to help the elderly avoid falls and subsequent trauma, particularly bone fractures. Skeletal muscle is responsive to strengthening exercises and elderly people should be encouraged to do strength-training activities.[10] Improvements in functional capacity through appropriate choices of physical activity and exercise are important in addition to dietary measures in improving quality of life among the elderly.

Selecting appropriate forms of physical activity for older adults requires special care because they vary even more than younger persons in exercise tolerance and health status. Guides are available for doing this.[31] Older adults should be urged to engage in light to moderate physical activity for at least thirty minutes a day. They should all engage in some leisure activity. Individualized exercise and physical activity programs are needed.

Dysphagia   **Dysphagia,** the inability to swallow, requires a team counseling effort. A physician, registered dietitian, registered nurse, and speech language pathologist trained in swallowing disorders provide for the best outcomes. Diet texture and consistency are important considerations. A standardized nationwide dysphagia diet is being developed and reviewed to provide accurate, consistent recommendations.[12]

Nutrition Education

In evaluation of the types of services needed and the health problems with nutritional implications in this population, there are significant health benefits to be gained from nutrition education targeted at different levels. Nutrition education for older Americans promotes better decision-making skills and enhances motivation to make behavior modifications to provide optimum nutrient components to support health.

Dietary messages must be reality-based and tailored to the needs of older people. After a review of the literature, Maloney and White[31] identified elements of successful nutrition education in older adults (see box 11.7).

Caution is needed in interpreting whether older adults are less likely to be motivated to change. For example, older adults can have the motivation to learn and make changes but may have more difficulty expressing what they are learning.[32] Examples of barriers include education, personality, kind and degree of chronic illness, fatigue, motivation, or cultural appropriateness. Thus, keeping sessions short and simple eliminates confusion and reduces fatigue. Important adult learning components especially applicable to the elderly adult learner are to repeat information in various ways and

BOX 11.7

ELEMENTS OF SUCCESSFUL NUTRITION EDUCATION IN OLDER ADULTS

- Use audience-centered planning approaches.
- Use personalized approaches to support generalized messages.
- Use known motivators.
- Encourage older adults to be active learners.
- Identify and target subgroups of older adults.
- Continue to reinforce changes.
- Be sensitive to age-related changes.

allow the older person to state, restate, and demonstrate information on the skills being taught.

Information can be presented in a variety of formats—auditory, written, and graphics—keeping in mind concern for any physical limitations such as visual impairment. In recognizing these limitations, use large, bold print in a clear and simple format. Visuals should be in primary colors and should use bold print with well-spaced letters (36-point) letters. Blues, greens, and purple colors should not be placed side-by-side on visual aids and posters. Nutrition educators are testing creative ways of delivering nutrition education to healthy, older adults. Elderly are interested in both nutrition information and the social interaction. Nutrition education programs must appeal to the interests of elderly and be convenient. Supermarket tours and cooking demonstrations appeal to those who have health problems that require special dietary management. Opportunities to discuss nutrition topics that are currently being discussed in the mass media and explanations of policy changes and means of obtaining access to **food assistance** programs or other services for elders also interest certain groups within the elderly.[40] Innovative approaches can also be targeted to well elderly persons who are financially secure. A program entitled Caring about Seniors' Health (CASH) was implemented by Westchester County Office for the Aging. Workshops were developed in four main areas, anatomy and physiology for seniors, stress and health—the secret connection, healthful food for fun and fitness, and keeping the body fit through exercise. The program helped seniors receive more information on how the body works and make appropriate lifestyle changes to promote health and prevent disease.[54]

Collaborations with community businesses provide an intergenerational opportunity to interact with elders in familiar settings. For example, community nutrition professionals have developed a partnership with a Children's Museum to promote nutrition activities at the museum for children and their families.[53] This participative, hands-on activity creatively interfaces grandparents and their grandchildren with a desirable motivator: a desire to learn about and change eating habits in order to remain healthy and participate in grandchildren's activities. In addition, this activity meets six of the seven nutrition education strategies listed in box 11.7. The USDA Cooperative Extension Service has also successfully developed programs for altering diet and physical activities in more healthful directions from the standpoint of cardiovascular health.[24] The American Association for Retired Persons (AARP) has developed a series of useful programs in such topics as eating healthful foods, making living and food preparation arrangements suitable and safe, and how to find resources to obtain assistive devices to help with food preparation and eating. It also has an active program for helping older people recognize and avoid quackery and fraud, including nutrition-related quackery. The Elder Hostel program combines travel and attendance at short-course classes in special sessions at various colleges in this country and abroad. Some of the courses are on nutrition topics. "Retirement courses" that focus on the foodways of older adults and assistance with special nutrition-related questions and problems are increasing in popularity. Many older people change their food purchasing, preparation, and consumption habits in the years after they retire, and they are often ready for advice about nutrition at that time.

Levitan and Johnson[29] describe another application that shows promise with some seniors. The NICE (Nutrition Information for Consumer Education) system is an interactive, touch-screen nutrition education system that was pilot-tested in supermarkets to encourage changes in purchasing behavior. Five software modules offered consumers information about nutrition and comparison of foods, calculated daily nutritional allowances, made suggestions for healthy eating, explained how to read a food label, and provided over 175 recipes, cross-indexed for nutritional benefits. To access the five modules, consumers touched the appropriate area or icon on the Main Menu screen of the computer screen. Fewer adults age sixty-six years and older used the system compared to other groups. However, of those who tried using the computer screen, older adults more often repeated using the system.

One department store chain has developed a "department" that is actually a health promotion club for older Americans. Membership fees are low. In addition to having a place to meet, a variety of social and educational programs are provided, including programs on nutrition education.

Wellness programs in which nutrition education and exercise are combined are also popular. These programs provide for social activities which promote health. In many parts of the country, walking clubs for older people are now popular. In some places, local parks and recreation departments have cooperated and plotted out an appropriate measured walking course. Mall walking is another activity that is gaining in popularity. Many malls have established hours, before the stores open, when the facility is totally available to walkers. In some communities, fitness classes for older people are available with various types and levels for those at different fitness levels.

For those elderly using nutrition support programs at a congregate meal site, a slightly different approach to nutrition education is needed. Excellent guides are now available for menu planning and incorporating innovative educational programs into such settings.[39] The American Association of Retired Persons (AARP) has produced several slide-tape programs, complete with notes, and useful materials for such presentations. Under the Older Americans' Act of 1965, two nutrition education sessions are required per year to program participants in congregate meals and home-delivered meals.

Hospital discharge planners are beginning to be more sophisticated in understanding elderly persons' educational needs for nutritional services after discharge. In some hospitals, dietitians and nutritionist function on the social service staff as discharge planners. They help to inform older persons regarding the entire range of services available in the community and provide links to those most appropriate.

Nutrition Support

Food assistance programs (described in chapters 5 and 10) provide resources for the elderly to purchase food and overcome hunger. These programs include the Food Stamp Program and the commodity food distribution programs. Six percent of the elderly population used the Food Stamp Program.[49]

Also, privately supported community programs provide food assistance. One such example is the "Seniors' Outreach to Seniors-Winning the war on hunger and isolation."[2] Tenant leaders (who are seniors) brought information and services to their neighbors. The services were offered in a location familiar and accessible to the clients (apartment building, church, etc.). The facilitator was a peer whenever possible. The peer leaders participated in planning, implementation and evaluation of the program. Other community-sponsored programs have encouraged restaurants to provide low-priced meals that permit elders to dine out in the afternoon and early evening at reduced cost.

Elderly people may also need referrals to community nutrition programs, such as the **Elderly Nutrition Program** (ENP). ENP is administered by the DHHS Administration on Aging (AOA) and gives grants to state units to provide meals and related services in congregate (group) or home (individual) settings to people aged sixty years and older. Currently ENP meals (congregate and home-delivered) provide between 33 and 40 percent of RDAs for calories, vitamin B_6, and zinc and between 45 and 58 percent of the RDA for calcium. This program is called the Title III-C program or Title VI when serving the Native-American population. These services target older people with the greatest economic and social need. Also included in this program are school-based meals for volunteer older individuals and multigenerational programs. In 1992, the Older American's Act was amended (Title III-F) to provide additional funding for health promotion and disease prevention programs, which also includes nutrition education.

From a socioeconomic perspective, ENP participants are more likely to be older, have incomes below the poverty threshold, and be female compared with the overall elderly population. With respect to the Title III Congregate meal program in 1994, 12 percent of minority participants were Black and 12 percent were Hispanic. For the Title III Home-delivered meal program, approximately 18 percent of meals were served to Blacks and approximately 5 percent were served to elderly Hispanics.[36] Low income, low education, limited English abilities, and high levels of functional disability constitute significant barriers to use of formal in-home services by elderly Hispanics.[52] Both Title III and Title VI participants in ENP have significant numbers of health problems and functional impairments that place them at nutritional risk (see table 11.7).

For those elderly living in a skilled, long-term care facility, nutritious, well-balanced meals and social opportunities are provided. These individuals are especially challenging because their health and functional statuses are much poorer than those of older people living in the community. Intakes of energy and other nutrients are sometimes low among residents of nursing homes and long-term care facilities, although sufficient food is provided. Among the causes of low intakes are the presence of disease, untreated dehydration, poor oral health, low physical activity, unsuitable meal environments, and variability in the amount and type of feeding assistance needed. Allowing an individual to feed his- or herself independently preserves dignity and respect for elderly. However, feeding assistance may be needed to encourage adequate intake. Even when feeding assistance is given, frail elderly should be encouraged to participate in drinking beverages or eating finger foods independently to maintain functional ability.

Another determinant of how much feeding assistance is needed for residents with progressive diseases (such as dementia) is the time of day. Residents may be able to

TABLE 11.7
Health and Functional Status of ENP Participants

	Title III		Title VI	
	Congregate	Home-delivered	Congregate	Home-delivered
Average number of diagnosed chronic health conditions	2.4	3.0	2.8	2.9
Hospital/Nursing Home stay in previous year (%)	26	43	30	37
Weight outside of healthy range (%)	61	64	65	69
Difficulty doing one or more everyday tasks (%)	23	77	23	44
Unable to or have difficulty preparing meals (%)	8	41	8	26
Moderate to high nutritional risk (%)	64	88	80	78
Instances of food insecurity in past month (%)	10	16	17	15

feed themselves in the morning but by late afternoon, there is more confusion, agitation increases, and partial to total assistance is needed. Staff and volunteer training and communication build skills of awareness to the varying degrees of assistance needed by each resident at meals.

Caretakers of frail, dependent elderly should be reminded to include flowers, colorful tablecloths and napkins to make mealtime visually stimulating and promote better appetites. Herb and low-salt flavor enhancers may help boost flavors in food.

Another component important to community nutrition professionals is to prevent food-borne disease outbreaks secondary to unsanitary food handling, preparation and storage. Infection control programs for dietary staff and volunteers are important in preventing serious morbidity from food-borne illnesses in high-risk elderly. Specific regulations outline the sanitation policies and procedures to prevent food-borne disease outbreaks.

SERVICES COMBINING COUNSELING, EDUCATION, AND FOOD ASSISTANCE

As the length of hospital stay declines and the aging adult population increases, sicker older adults are discharged to home. Any long-term care service network in the home must address the values of independence, dignity, privacy, and choice through the transitions. Those who are frail—impaired in their abilities to perform the activities of daily living without considerable help or afflicted with diseases and conditions that make usual ambulatory care inappropriate—require interventions to support semi-independent living. This assistance can be coordinated through federal, state, and local agencies. Churches, community businesses, or voluntary groups also perform special roles to support living at home. Community nutrition professionals can play an important role in assisting elderly with transitions from one level of care to another by providing supportive direct personal care and community-wide services.

A **home health agency** is defined as a public agency, private organization, or a subdivision that provides skilled nursing and at least one other service in the home. There are six main categories of home health services: home health agencies, home health aide organizations, hospices, staffing agencies and nursing registries, home infusion therapy companies, and home medical equipment companies.[7] Medicare, the health insurance for older adults (sixty-five years and older), covers hospice care and some skilled home health care services. Of the elderly seen in home care, many will be on special diets or weakened with limited functional capability. Some of these may be diagnosed with a terminal illness. Several home care services now include a full-time nutrition professional whose role is to assess, evaluate nutritional needs, and coordinate social service programs as well as function as a quality control expert. Educating the individual and his or her caregiver regarding the networking of services, adequate food intake, and self-care needs are an essential component of this service.

Homemaker and chore services provide reliable individuals who can assist the elderly living at home with meal planning, shopping, and other necessary tasks to maintain independence. The expected outcome of this intervention is to maintain some level of independence for the frail elderly and persons with physical disabilities by offering services in their own homes so institutionalization can be delayed or avoided.

Many communities have sheltered housing and community homes that permit the older person to live independently, while providing some nursing, congregate meals, and other assistance services on site. Adult day care is another program for providing supervision, activities, and one or more meals a day while caregivers go to work or have a respite from care responsibilities.

Hospice programs provide palliative care for patients in the final stages (usually the last six months or less) of a terminal illness. As the older population increases in number, community nutrition professionals concerns will include the nutritional status of the elderly and the quality of life of family caregivers. Respite care services provide temporary support of elderly persons living at home when their usual caretakers are unable to perform their usual functions owing to special circumstances or to emotional stress and fatigue.

EVALUATION

Nutrition-related problems can interfere with successful aging. Personal health habits, access to preventive and curative health services, and aging itself are partly responsible for them. Environment, social and economic factors also modify outcomes. The outcomes associated with improved nutrition aim for the best health and functional independence in elderly even though outcomes are influenced by physiological changes that occur in organs and systems as individuals age.[13] Effective interventions by community nutrition professionals can lead to a number of important outcomes. Optimum nutritional status in the elderly prevents or delays the onset of disease, aids in recovery from illness and trauma, preserves function, and prevents further disability. These outcomes can reduce the need for expensive health care services and reduce or prevent hospitalization. In addition, aging successfully with the aid of good nutrition can help avoid nursing home placement. Evaluation requires standardized documentation and systems to track outcomes and analyze results (see chapter 10). New systems are being developed to evaluate the outcomes of nutrition services for the elderly (see the Expert Speaks).

IMPLICATIONS FOR COMMUNITY NUTRITION PROFESSIONALS

The goal of all preventive, curative, rehabilitative, and palliative care among aging adults is to extend the years of healthy life and support independence as long as possible. Older Americans must be intimately involved in these efforts. A good continuum of care plan develops the most appropriate level of care to promote independence according to individual needs and preferences. "Respect for quality life allows elderly to remain in the community ['aging in place'] rather than a movement through various living arrangements; all of which have a great financial and emotional cost with each change."[9]

The model of community nutrition based solely on providing primary prevention services to the elderly is outdated. Nutritional problems elderly face range from preventive nutrition to management and amelioration of disease-related disabilities. Collaborations and integration of health services, government programs, mass media, the food industry, and private sectors will provide cost-effective interventions that will change elderly dietary intakes and behaviors. Community nutrition professionals must take an active role in designing new systems of care in intervention.

The Healthy People 2000 goals will best be accomplished by giving attention to the entire process: screening to identify risks for nutrition, health, social, and economic problems that threaten functional independence and pose nutrition risk; in-depth, timely assessment to determine the causes of problems; and implementing necessary interventions with a well-coordinated and communicated plan that acknowledges all the preventive and curative health services. The aging population will be the principal evaluators of the outcomes. Community nutrition professionals who have improved older adults' access to health care and services, increased independence and choices for the elderly, and improved their nutritional status will also be contributors to achieving the goals for healthy, successful aging in the twenty-first century.

COMMUNITY NUTRITION PROFESSIONALS IN ACTION

- Identify three foods targeted for the elderly. What foods are being promoted? Evaluate these foods for age-appropriateness, that is, what is the cost? Would you be able to open the food package with arthritic hands? Is the food easy to chew? Would it provide health benefits by being low in fat? reduced sodium? high fiber? What is the print size on the label? Are the preparation instructions easy to use? Are there an appropriate number of servings in the package?

- Visit a fast food restaurant and observe how many elderly persons visit in a two-hour time frame. Record some general observations on the restaurant's layout and sensitivity to frail elderly who may have decreased mobility. What kind of socialization needs are met for elderly eating in fast food places? If you were a nutritionist asked to make recommendations to the aging population about fast food establishments, what would you recommend to promote health and wellness?

- Visit a congregate meal dining site and observe how elderly persons participate. Record some general observations on the facility's layout and sensitivity to frail elderly who may have decreased mobility. What kind of socialization needs are met for elderly eating at the congregate dining site? Compare these observations to those made regarding the setting in the previous question.

- Complete a nutrition screen and assessment (see page 320) on an older family member, friend, relative, or neighbor. Report the results.

- Evaluate a magazine advertisement touting "better health, longer life span" with its use. (e.g., coenzyme Q10, superoxide dismutase, dehydroepiandrosterone [DHEA]). Develop a scientific basis to support or discredit its use.

- Review three issues of *Modern Maturity* magazine. What topics are important to older Americans? How are health and nutrition issues addressed?

GOING ONE STEP FURTHER

- Identify a special population group within the elderly that your organization serves. How well do materials and programs used to serve this group meet the adult education needs discussed in this chapter?
- You are hired as a consultant to the director of a community clinic designed to provide medical outpatient care for Southeast Asians. The clinic is a general medical outpatient facility with 20,000 visits per year, half of them by Southeast Asians. What nutrition programs would be appropriate for the Southeast Asian elderly visiting this clinic? What are the differences in food habits (purchases, preparation, meal patterns, food avoidance, and supplement use) in the community? What is the extent of differences in intake of foods, energy, protein, and micronutrients of elderly people living in these ethnic communities?
- You have been selected as a resource for a home health care agency serving an elderly population. Develop a screening tool and write procedures for referrals needed for those at high risk. Recommend nutrition monitoring indicators to provide a cost-effective, quality-assured intervention program.
- Design health promotion activities to meet specific needs of a targeted elderly population in your community. Identify topics covered and specific education concerns due to disabilities in this population group.

ADDITIONAL INFORMATION

Professional societies develop statements, scientific status summaries, commentaries, and position papers to clarify an issue in which the particular society has expertise. The American Dietetic Association (ADA) position statements relevant to chapter 11 are listed below:

1. Nutrition recommendations and principles for people with diabetes mellitus, *J Am Diet Assoc* 94:504, 1994.
2. Nutrition monitoring of the home parenteral and enteral patient, *J Am Diet Assoc* 94:664, 1994.
3. Women's health and nutrition, *J Am Diet Assoc* 95:362, 1995.
4. Weight management, *J Am Diet Assoc* 97:71, 1997.

REFERENCES

1. Adams WL, Garry PJ, Rhyne R, et al: Alcohol intake in the healthy elderly: changes with age in a cross-sectional and longitudinal study, *J Am Geriatr Soc* 38:211–216, 1990.
2. Belle S: Seniors' outreach to seniors winning the war on hunger and isolation, *J Am Diet Assoc* 9:A-19, 1993.
3. Berlinger WG, Potter JF: Low body mass index in demented outpatients, *J Am Geriatr Soc* 39:973–978, 1991.
4. Brandeis GH, Morris JN, Nash DJ, Lipschitz LA: The epidemiology and natural history of pressure ulcers in elderly nursing home residents, *JAMA* 264:2905–2909, 1990.
5. Bronner F: Calcium and osteoporosis, *Am J Clin Nutr* 60:831–836, 1994.
6. Campbell WW, Crim MC, Dallal GE, et al: Increased protein requirement in elderly people: new data and retrospective reassessments, *Am J Clin Nutr* 60:501–519, 1994.
7. Consultant Dietitians in Health Care Facilities, The American Dietetic Association: A practice guide for nutrition in home care, 1995, Chicago, IL.
8. Denke MA, Grundy SM: Hypercholesterolemia in elderly persons: resolving the treatment dilemma, *Ann Intern Med* 112:780–792, 1990.
9. Dietsche S: Oregon's long term care system—from nursing facility care to community-based care: an evolution, *Nutr Rev* 54:S48–S50, 1996.
10. Evans WJ: Exercise, nutrition and aging, *Clin Geriatr Med* 11:725–734, 1995.
11. Falk LW, Bisogni CA, Sobal J: Food choices of older adults: a qualitative investigation, *J Nutr Educ* 28:257–265, 1996.
12. Feldt P, Growen M, Tymchuk D: The national dysphagia diet, presented at Annual Meeting of the American Dietetic Association, October 1997.
13. Fernando M, Torres G: *Nutr Rev* 54(1):1996, International Life Sciences Institute, Lawrence, KS.
14. Food and Nutrition Board, Subcommittee on the 10th Edition of the RDA: *Recommended dietary allowances,* Washington, DC, 1989, National Academy Press.
15. Franklin CA, Karkech J: Weight loss and senile dementia in institutionalized elderly population, *J Am Diet Assoc* 89:790–792, 1989.
16. Garry PJ, Hunt WC, Koehler KM, et al: Longitudinal study of dietary intakes in plasma lipids in healthy elderly men and women, *Am J Clin Nutr* 55:682–688, 1992.
17. Garry PJ, Koehler KM, Simon TL: Iron stores and iron absorption: effects of repeated blood donations, *Am J Clin Nutr* 62:611–620, 1995.
18. Garry PJ, Owen GM, Eldridge TO: *The New Mexico Aging Process Study,* Albuquerque, 1997, University of New Mexico Press.
19. Gift HC: Issues of aging and oral health promotion, *Gerodontics* 4:194–206, 1988.
20. Gloth FM, Grundberg CM, Hollis BW, et al: Vitamin D deficiency in home-bound elderly persons, *JAMA* 274:1683–1686, 1994.
21. Gray-Donald K: The frail elderly. Meeting the nutritional challenges, *J Am Diet Assoc* 95:538–540, 1995.

22. Guigoz Y, Vellas B, Garry PJ: Mini-nutritional assessment: a practical assessment tool for grading the nutritional status of elderly patients, *Facts and Research in Gerontology* 4 (suppl 2):15–59, 1994.

23. Heaney RP: Age considerations in nutrient needs for bone health: older adults, *J Am Coll Nutr* 15:575–578, 1996.

24. Herman JR, Kopel BH, McCrory ML, et al: Effect of a cooperative extension nutrition and exercise program for older adults on nutrition knowledge, dietary intake, anthropometric measurements and serum lipids, *J Nutr Educ* 22:271–274, 1990.

25. Institute of Medicine: *Depression.* In Berg RL, Cassells JS, editors: *The second fifty years: promoting health and preventing disability,* Washington, DC, 1990, National Academy Press.

26. Katz S, Stroud MW: Functional assessment in geriatrics: a review of progress and directions, *J Am Geriatr Soc* 37:267–271, 1989.

27. Koehler KM, Pareo-Tubbeth SL, Romero LJ, et al: Folate nutrition and older adults: challenges and opportunities, *J Am Diet Assoc* 97:167–173, 1997.

28. Lamy PP, Michocki RJ: Medication management, *Clin Geriatr Med* 4:623–638, 1988.

29. Levithan K, Johnson E: Interactive, touch screen nutrition education system, *Am J Health Promotion* 7:87–89, 145, 1992.

30. Levy AS, Schucker RE: Patterns of nutrient intake among dietary supplement users; attitudinal and behavioral components, *J Am Diet Assoc* 87:754–760, 1987.

31. Maloney S, White S: *Nutrition education for older adults,* Alexandria, VA, 1994, USDA Food & Nutrition Service.

32. Oldaker S: Live & learn: patient education for the elderly, *Orthopaedic Nursing* 11:51–56, 1992.

33. Optimal calcium intake, NIH Consensus Statement, 12(4): June 6–8, 1–31, 1994.

34. Patterson BH, Block G, Rosenberger WF, et al: Fruits and vegetables in the American diet: data from the NHANES III survey, *Am J Public Health* 80:1443–1449, 1990.

35. Payette H, Gray-Donald K, Cyr R, Boutier V: Predictors of dietary intake in a functionally-dependent elderly population in the community, *Am J Public Health* 85:677–683, 1995.

36. Ponza M, Ohls JC, Millen BE: *Serving elders at risk: the Older Americans Act nutrition programs. National evaluation of the Elderly Nutrition Program, 1993–1995,* Princeton, NJ, 1996, Mathematica Policy Research.

37. Potter JF, Schaefer DF, Bohi RL: In hospital mortality as a function of body mass index: an age-dependent variable, *J Gerontol* 43:M59–M63, 1988.

38. Pronsky Z: *Food medication interactions,* ed 9, Food Medication Interactions, Inc., Pootstown, PA, 1995.

39. Rhodes SS, editor, and Gerontological Nutritionists: *Effective menu planning for the elderly nutrition program,* Chicago, 1991, The American Dietetic Association.

40. Roe D: *The elderly in our society.* In Roe D, editor: *Geriatric nutrition,* ed 3, Englewood Cliffs, NJ, 1992, Prentice-Hall.

41. Russell R: New views on the RDA's for older adults, *J Am Diet Assoc* 97:575–578, 1997.

42. Russell RM, Suter PM: Vitamin requirements of elderly people: an update, *Am J Clin Nutr* 58:4–14, 1993.

43. Ryan AS, Craig LD, Finn SC: Nutrient intakes and dietary patterns of older Americans: a national study, *J Gerontol* 47:M145–M150, 1992.

44. Ryan VC, Bower ME: Relationship of socioeconomic status and living arrangements to nutritional intake of the older person, *J Am Diet Assoc* 89:1805–1807, 1989.

45. Satcher D: The aging of America, *J Health Care Poor Underserved* 7:179–182, 1996.

46. Shepherd RJ: The scientific basis of exercise prescribing for the very old, *J Am Bar Soc* 38:62, 1990.

47. Tayback M, Kumanyika S, Chee L: Body weight as a risk factor in the elderly, *Arch Intern Med* 150:1065–1072, 1990.

48. Thompson MP, Morris LK: Unexplained weight loss in the ambulatory elderly, *J Am Gerontol Soc* 39:497–500, 1991.

49. U.S. Bureau of the Census: *Current population reports, special studies, P23–178RV. Sixty-five plus in America,* Washington, DC, 1992, U.S. Government Printing Office.

50. U.S. Department of Health and Human Services: *Studies in income distribution. An assessment of the economic status of the aged,* Washington, DC, 1993, U.S. Government Printing Office.

51. U.S. Preventive Services Task Force: *Guide to clinical preventive services,* ed 2, Baltimore, 1996, Williams & Wilkins.

52. Wallace SP, Campbell K, Lew-Ting C-Y: Structural barriers to the use of formal in-home services by elderly Latinos, *J Gerontol Social Services* 49:S253–S263, 1994.

53. Washington JL: Kids are cooking at the children's museum, *J Am Diet Assoc* 9:A104, 1996.

54. Westchester County Office for the Aging: Caring about seniors health (CASH) *J Am Diet Assoc* 94:A-49, 1994.

55. *What governments can do. Hunger, 1997,* Silver Springs, MD, 1996, Bread for the World Institute.

56. White JV, Dwyer JT, Posner BM, et al: Nutrition screening initiative: development and implementation of the public awareness checklist and screening tools, *J Am Diet Assoc* 92:163–167, 1992.

57. Wood RJ, Suter PM, Russell RM: Mineral requirements of elderly people, *Am J Clin Nutr* 62:493–505, 1995.

NUTRITION FOR ELDERLY ADULTS

ELSA RAMIREZ BRISSON, MPH, RD

SUPERVISING PUBLIC HEALTH NUTRITIONIST, MONTEREY COUNTY AREA
AGENCY OF AGING, SALINAS, CALIFORNIA

Aging—everybody's doing it! And doing it longer and healthier. The average age of elderly nutrition program participants in this country is seventy-seven years with the largest group served between the ages of seventy-five and eighty-five years. The media and advertisers depict younger seniors and my experience is those seniors are still working. Our participants are the old (seventy-five to eighty-four years) and the oldest old (over eighty-five years).

The Administration on Aging (AOA), area agencies on aging (AAA), state agencies on aging (SAA), and the Elderly Nutrition Program (ENP) providers form a network across the United States with a commitment of meeting the nutritional needs of the elderly. Each state has a designated SAA that works with the regional AAA throughout the state. The AAAs in turn work with local providers of congregate dining and home-delivered meals. This commentary discusses how one AAA translates the Older Americans Act into action at the local level. For more detailed information about the other 654 AAAs and over 4,000 nutrition providers, visit the AOA home page at http://www.aoa.gov/.

Nutrition is the key service that makes up the Older American's Act and it has not changed since the original legislation was passed. Jean Lloyd, MS, RD, nutrition officer for the DHHS, office of the Secretary on Aging in Washington, D.C. has worked at various levels of this program. She enthusiastically states that "the Elderly Nutrition Programs are models of public/private partnerships that take into consideration small business, communities and volunteers. The nutrition program is the foundation of the Older Americans Act and is integral to home and community-based services." I work at the AAA that was once described by Jean Lloyd as the place where the rubber meets the road. The AAA's mission is to coordinate comprehensive service through cooperative arrangements. avoid duplication, and facilitate accessibility to services in the area.

Four original purposes of the program remain unchanged. Many elderly persons do not eat because:

- They cannot afford to do so.
- They lack the skills to select foods and prepare nourishing and well-balanced meals.
- They have limited mobility, which may impair their capacity to shop and cook for themselves.
- They have feelings of rejection and loneliness, which obliterate the incentive necessary to prepare and eat a meal alone.

What has changed is how, at the local level, we ensure that the services will address the four barriers and reach the greatest numbers of eligible seniors in need of nutritious and safe food while keeping check on their progress.

We keep hearing that we must work smarter, not harder, and nowhere is this more applicable than in the ENP. The funding for nutrition in our local area has not changed significantly since the area agency received its first grant in 1980. (See the National Evaluation and the 1995 State Program Report for Title III and Title VI of the Older Americans Act for the AOA for trends and statistics in your state.) What had to change to accommodate the growing number of elderly in need of the program was how we monitor trends in congregate and home-delivered meals locally and plan accordingly. Based on data, we make changes in the local allocations to ensure the funds are spent in the most needed areas. In 1994, we adopted performance-based contracting for meals and we separated the nutrition monitoring, education, and counseling components from the meal components. At the same time we dismantled the centralized congregate program. Decentralization allowed us to maximize community involvement at the local senior centers. School districts in small rural communities came forward to provide the meal service. Now, three of the five meal providers are school districts. The other two are a recreation district and a traditional nonprofit agency serving seniors.

Two of the area providers of home-delivered meals predate the local AAA. Meals on Wheels of Salinas and of the Monterey Peninsula both began in 1972. A group of community minded and caring women started packaging meals in a church hall for a handful of deliveries to homebound seniors. Today, between the two agencies, over 400 frail, homebound persons, including elderly persons, receive a two-meal package that is delivered by more than fifty volunteer drivers each day.

These agencies and the others form the regional Senior Nutrition Program Network. This network, along with the Department of Social Services, first assembled as a team in 1987 to work on a project to reduce duplication of services. The project was funded by the California Department of Aging. Since then, the two Meals on Wheels programs have developed a marketing video and done fund-raising together. If federal funding disappeared tomorrow, it would hurt the local senior nutrition network, but based on the commitment and energy of community volunteers and agencies, nutrition services would continue, albeit a little scaled down.

The Older Americans Act provides seniors, particularly those with low incomes, with low-cost nutritionally sound meals served at strategically located centers or in their homes. The program was intended to and has promoted better health among the older segment of our population through improved nutrition and by reducing the isolation of old age while offering older Americans an opportunity to live their remaining years in dignity. The greatest indicator of possible nutrition risk is *living alone,* followed by low income. We know that older individuals who live alone and eat alone consume fewer calories than individuals eating in social situations.

In an effort to objectively measure the outcomes and successes of the ENP, the project nutritionists embraced the Nutrition Screening Initiative's program of nutrition screening, risk profile assessment and follow-up nutrition education. We have used the DETERMINE Checklist, described in this chapter, on a voluntary basis for four years. Now the checklist has been incorporated into the intake and reassessment surveys completed by all Older Americans Act funded programs nationwide. This massive national effort to collect data is called National Aging Program Information System (NAPIS).

We all knew for years that nutrition programs made a difference in people's lives, but we only had anecdotal information. By standardizing the data collection, we can maintain accurate and ongoing outcome data and profiles of the clients served. The locally collected data have given us some insights that we use in the planning process.

The focus of nutrition in the popular press is to discuss individual nutrients such as fat, vitamins, and minerals. With many individuals (young and old) the big picture of nutrition is missed, such as getting enough calories and water and protein. Through the ENP and other community nutrition programs such as food banks and community centers, the focus is *food* as the source of all nutrients and fiber in a warm and friendly place away from home.

It has been important to me to keep our program goals a priority as we move into exciting new areas and it is rewarding to look back at how we evolved. Ten years ago, the state and federal guidelines for the ENP did not follow the American Heart Association's recommendations for fat nor the American Cancer Society's recommendations for fiber and cruciferous vegetables. The fact that "nutrition" is in the title of the program demanded that we aim for lower fat content of the meals. In the 1992 amendment of the 1965 Older Americans Act, compliance with the U.S. Dietary Goals is required. Today the fat is down and fiber up in all eight menus, which are analyzed monthly.

I continued my predecessor's project to have one nutrition consultant full time for all the ENP sites instead of each program contracting with different consultants for a few hours a month. When we separated the nutrition monitoring, education and counseling components, it was accomplished. Tracy Olsen, RD, RN, the lead program nutritionist, works with two other part-time RDs and an assistant we share. She spends most of her time at the various sites throughout the county giving in-services and nutrition education presentations and doing home visits to clients at high risk for malnutrition or with nutrition-related diseases. We have gone from developing our own materials to using professionally produced materials we purchase or that are available free. We do translate materials as needed or reformat text into larger type for ease of readability. Nutritionists serving the elderly are nutrition case managers, we look at each client as a whole person with a lost of past.

It is important in the network to stay abreast of legislative activities and to be involved in funding allocation decisions. For our local network, that is one of my responsibilities. I do it along with many of the providers. Through close communication with the California Department of Aging Nutrition Section Consultants, I can bring back to our AAA information from other AAAs in the state and in other states. Dalna McKeon, MS, RD, nutrition consultant with the California Department of Aging, stated, "she likes the statewide overview and objectivity one has at the state level and sharing the best practices with the AAA nutritionist network. In California, we are blessed with a rich variety of AAAs (33 to be exact) and providers (more than 300) from which to exchange information and share ideas."

Two myths about the ENP we can't seem to shake are, first, that it is a program for persons on welfare, and, second, that it is a program that leads to institutionalization for sick and dying individuals.

- Addressing myth 1: The ENP was originally funded to alleviate malnutrition in the elderly. Malnourished individuals are more susceptible to infection, when hospitalized they stay longer, and they heal more slowly than well-nourished individuals. The ENP does not have any set income guidelines and many participants make voluntary contributions. These donations generate one third of the funding for the program locally and one fifth nationally.
- Addressing myth 2: By facilitating access to nutritious, wholesome food daily, the ENP, especially the home-delivered meals, has done much for rehabilitation of seniors and nonseniors after a hospitalization, and this is done at a very nominal cost. Data collected from Meals on Wheels of Salinas shows that the most frequent reason to discontinue services is the client got better and was able to resume shopping and cooking and returned to senior centers and other activities in the community. Institutionalization and death were low on the list of reasons for discontinuing participation.

With a strong network of programs serving the community the next step is to make the heaps of paper work disappear or be easier to manage. The nutrition services we provide are spread out among fifteen sites and 3,300 square miles. The program planning and analysis that is required to carry out a project like this is not easy. My goal is to have a paperless office and on-line communication. Without this dream, I wouldn't have gotten this far. We have a technology plan with four levels.

- Level one is to improve the speed and accuracy of data collection and claims processing.
- Level two is to connect all service providers and all sites with on-line communication for an interagency network.
- Level three is having quick access for grant information, networking with other areas of the country, and the latest research on healthy aging by using computers on our desks or laps.
- Level four is having quick access for grant information, networking with other areas of the country, and the latest research in healthy aging by using computers on our desks or laps.

Our present countywide goal is to have all providers on-line by the end of 1997. The Internet and e-mail has broken down the barrier we had in communicating among all the programs by computer. As more and more agencies embrace technology, achieving my dream seems possible.

Serving the elderly can be challenging and rewarding. It offers the creative and motivated community nutrition professional wonderful professional and personal opportunities. For me it is more than a job and the team we have formed is more like a supportive family. The wisdom and caring the staff receive daily from program participants, volunteers, and the community makes each year special.

For updates to our local program visit us at http://www.408meal.org

CHAPTER TWELVE

CLIENTS WITH SPECIAL NEEDS

*I'm personally proudest of the things I've done for children with
handicaps. We've started a new system of family-centered,
community-based, comprehensive care for kids with special
needs. We've had workshops all over the country to adopt
a new approach to understanding kids with handicaps,
to learn how they should be cared for, and to include their
families as part of the treatment.*

— C. Everett Koop, MD

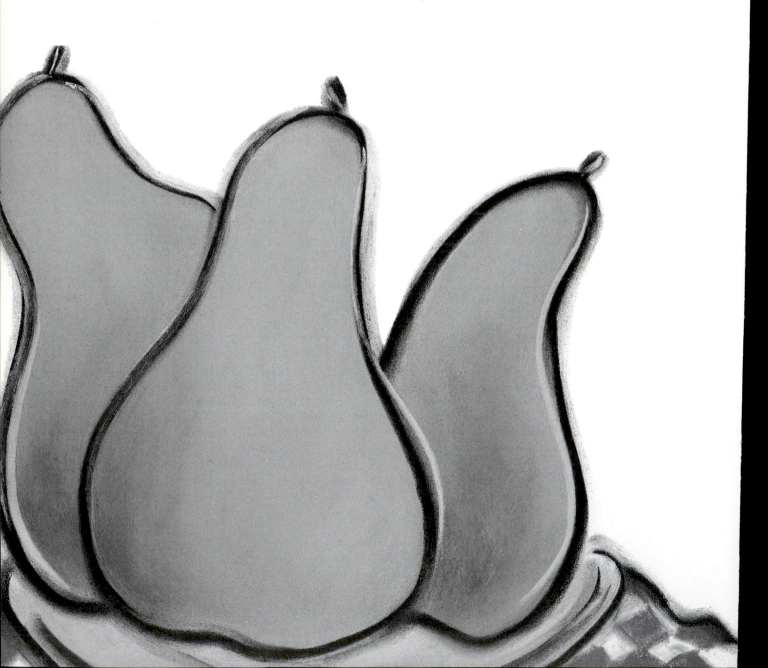

Core Concepts

Many individuals in the community have special needs beyond the normal needs for their age. Special needs populations include children and adults with physical, mental or, other impairments that limit their ability to function normally. This includes limitations due to inborn errors of metabolism, developmental disabilities, mental retardation, psychiatric disorders, and infectious diseases such as HIV/AIDS and tuberculosis as well as socioeconomic difficulties that produce homelessness, food insecurity, and low literacy. Many individuals with special needs require carefully tailored nutrition intervention strategies planned by professionals with advanced training. Community nutrition professionals must be alert to the presence of individuals with special needs in the community; represent and advocate for them, if they cannot do so for themselves; and be prepared to play a role in overseeing and coordinating nutrition and food services to meet their unique needs.

Objectives

When you finish chapter twelve, you should be able to:

~ Categorize the altered nutritional needs of children with special needs due to developmental disabilities.

~ Outline essential areas of nutrition assessment for persons with special needs.

~ Summarize the types of programs and services that exist to address special population needs.

~ Identify the role of nutrition in the prevention of developmental disabilities and other handicapping conditions.

~ Discuss ways the community nutrition professional can be involved in addressing food insecurity and homelessness in the community.

Key Words

Word	Page Mentioned
Journey to inclusion	346
Developmental disabilities	348
Mental retardation	348
Inborn errors of metabolism	348
Feeding team	356
Feeding problem	356
Oral-motor problems	356
Early intervention	359
Hunger	362
Food insecurity	363
Homeless	364
Literacy	368

I. CHILDREN AND OTHERS WITH SPECIAL HEALTH CARE NEEDS

The role of nutrition is to support growth in children, regulate biochemical processes, establish an adequate immune system, and provide sufficient energy to meet activity needs. Yet a number of unique conditions can place individuals in an extremely vulnerable position where daily attention to highly specialized feeding regimens is necessary to assure health and well-being. It has been estimated that 10 to 15 percent of the children in the United States have special health care needs and that 5 percent of the population is developmentally disabled.[1] Community nutrition professionals can play a very significant role in being advocates for these community members because the children and adults with the special conditions described in this chapter are often medically fragile, socially isolated, and economically vulnerable. In addition, recent surveys have also indicated that approximately 50 percent of these populations have a nutrition-related problem. In the context of defining the variation in health, figure 12.1 summarizes the key issues when serving persons with special needs. The community nutrition professional's responsibility is to include this context of health when optimizing the nutritional status of *all* society's members.

HISTORY AND CHANGES IN INSTITUTIONAL CARE AND NUTRITIONAL SERVICES

The structure of today's public health efforts for children, adolescents, and adults with special needs varies greatly among communities and states. Efforts range from monitoring the state of children's health to immunization programs, lead abatement, efforts to improve birth outcomes, and programs for children with special health needs.[14] The American Dietetic Association's position is that "Nutrition services are an essential component of comprehensive cares for children with special health needs [and that] these nutrition services should be provided within a system of coordinated interdisciplinary services in a manner that is preventive, family-centered, community-based and culturally competent."[19]

Nonetheless, systems of care for children and adults with special needs have not always had a family-centered approach and did not always include nutrition as a provided service. In the United States, the first institution for the individuals with mental illness and retardation was built in 1766 in the Virginia colony.[26] Historically, individuals with developmental disabilities were cared for in institutions that, during the nineteenth century, were described as, "wholly inadequate and brutal."[5] Malnutrition was commonly found among those clients in institutional care. In addition, throughout the nineteenth century, institutions were built in increasing numbers. During the period of 1950 to 1979, resident populations of state-administered programs increased from 127,425 to 186,743. Staff-to-client ratios were large and food service was rarely individualized.[26]

Dramatic changes have taken place in the treatment of individuals with handicapping conditions.[5] This change, referred to as the normalization of care, directs movement away from institutionalization and toward inclusion and integration into the community. The election of John F. Kennedy as president in 1961 and subsequent appointment of the President's Commission on Mental Retardation initiated the early thrust for change. The commission made 112 recommendations, which included research related to causes of mental retardation, methods of care, rehabilitation and learning, preventive health measures, strengthened maternal and infant care, educational programs, comprehensive clinical and social services, proven methods and facilities for care, legal rights, increased training of professional manpower, and public education related to mental retardation.[5]

In addition, as a result of a landmark class action suit (entitled the Wyatt-Stickney case) brought against the Alabama Department of Mental Hygiene, the size of institutions began to decrease in the 1970s.[26] The court imposed treatment standards because of this lawsuit and included important ratios and nutrition standards for meals served. Deinstitutionalization became a primary objective at this time, and President Richard Nixon set a national goal of reducing the institutional populations by 30 percent before the year 2000.

Nationally, the average size of residential settings has dropped from 22.5 persons per residence in 1977 to 4.9 in 1994. Almost every state has reduced the population of its large public institutions over the past twenty-five years. Only 65,745 individuals were housed in state facilities in 1994, and in four states (New Hampshire, Rhode Island, Vermont, and the District of Columbia) all state facilities were closed.

Closing and downsizing institutions is evidence of the transformation of national policy affecting people with developmental disabilities over the past twenty-five years, representing one of the great social reform movements of our time. It has been called the "**journey to inclusion**,"[17]

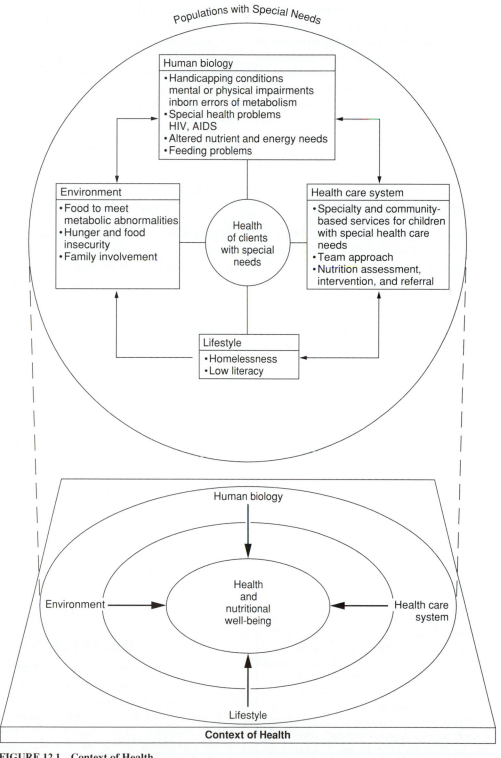

FIGURE 12.1   Context of Health
Influences on the health of clients with special needs.

thus making an important role for the community nutrition professionals to link clients with needed services and, in some cases, to play an active role in the provision of specialized services. It is predicted that future health care systems for children and adults with special health care needs will require access to regional care that links high-quality specialized tertiary care services with community-based primary care services. This approach to care will link the broad array of multidisciplinary services at the community level, and will especially link health and education services for the child.[23]

DEFINING SPECIAL NEEDS

The federal definition of **developmental disabilities** includes children and adults with a wide range of diagnoses including **mental retardation,** but also chronic health problems, cerebral palsy, autism, spinal cord injury, and severe head injury, so long as the condition began before age twenty-two and therefore affected the person's development (see box 12.1). The definition of mental retardation is somewhat different from that of developmental disabilities (see box 12.2). The current definition was as set forward in 1992 by the American Association on Mental Retardation. Mental retardation is manifest before age eighteen.

DEFINITION

Developmental disability: a severe chronic disability of an individual 5 years of age or older that is attributable to a mental or physical impairment (or, a combination of mental or physical impairment) that is manifested before the individual attains age 22; is likely to continue indefinitely; results in substantial functional limitations in three or more of the following areas of major life activity: self-care, receptive and expressive language, learning, mobility, self-direction, capacity for independent living, economic self-sufficiency; and reflects the individuals need for a combination and sequence of special, interdisciplinary or generic services, supports or other assistance that is of lifelong or extended duration. . . . [This service] is individually planned and coordinated. . . . [An exception] is that such term, when applied to infants and young children (individuals from birth to age 5, inclusive) means the probability of resulting in developmental disabilities if services are not provided.[8]

There was a time when mental retardation was defined strictly in terms of an individual's score on a standardized intelligence measure (IQ). The current definition used by the American Psychological Association categorizes individuals having mental retardation if their IQ is below approximately seventy and if they have significant deficits or impairments in adaptive behavior for their age. With standard error or measurement, a diagnosis of mental retardation is possible through an IQ of seventy-five.[22]

THE ROLE OF NUTRITION IN PERSONS WITH SPECIAL NEEDS

Individualization of nutritional care is paramount for special needs cases. Table 12.1 defines selected cases and describes potential nutrient modifications. Table 12.2 identifies nutritional risk factors associated with disorders that alter growth or food components in the diet or influence medical conditions.

Inborn errors of metabolism are inherited disorders, are genetically transmitted in an autosomal method of inheritance, and involve several characteristics in common.[28] Treatment involves lowering the amount of nutrient whose metabolic function is impaired or supplementation with another nutrient involved in the metabolic cycle. Although inborn errors of metabolism currently number in the thousands, treatment is available for approximately seventy-four.[11]

For individuals with chromosomal aberrations, syndromes, and neurological disorders, nutritional needs may differ from the norm and modifications are needed.[28] An example is related to individuals with cerebral palsy. It is generally assumed that individuals with cerebral palsy have energy needs that are greater than those of normal children. Recent studies on adults

DEFINITION

Mental retardation: substantial limitation in present functioning. It is characterized by significantly subaverage intellectual function, existing concurrently with related limitations in two or more areas: communication, self-care, home living, social skills, community use, self-direction, health and safety, functional academics, leisure, and work.

TABLE 12.1
Defining Special Needs and Nutritional Implications

Condition	Definition	Nutrition considerations
Inborn errors of metabolism	Inherited characteristics genetically transmitted	Lower the nutrient whose metabolism function is impaired and supplement with other affected nutrients
Protein dysfunction		
Phenylketonuria (PKU)	Inability to metabolize phenylalanine due to lack of an enzyme	Choose foods low in phenylalanine; optimal growth
Maple syrup urine disease (MSUD)	Inability to metabolize the three branched-chain amino acids: leucine, isoleucine, and valine	Choose foods low in branched-chain amino acids
Homocystinuria	Inability to metabolize hemocystine, a sulfur-containing amino acid in the blood due to lack of an enzyme	A low protein, low methionine diet; formula allowance of cystine
Urea cycle dysfunction	Inability to form urea, the final product of protein metabolism	
Arginosuccinicaciduria	Inability to metabolize arginosuccinic acid due to lack of the enzyme arginosuccinase	Low protein diet/formula limited to the amount required for growth; certain amino acids may need supplementation
Citrullinemia	Inability to metabolize citrulline due to lack of the enzyme citrullinase	
Carbohydrate dysfunction		
Fructose intolerance	Inability to metabolize fructose due to an absence or deficiency of enzyme aldolase	Exclude all foods containing fructose, which is present in fruits, sugar cane, sucrose and sorbitol; vitamin C supplementation
Glycogen storage disease	Inability to convert blood glucose to the storage form of carbohydrate in the body due to an enzyme deficiency	Special diet; frequent feedings of complex carbohydrates; possibly eliminate lactose, fructose, sucrose; tubefeeding; administer raw cornstarch
Galactosemia	Inability to metabolize galactose and lactose due to lack of an enzyme	Exclude foods containing galactose and lactose
Fat dysfunction		
Abetalipoproteinemia/ hypobetalipoproteinemia	Failure of normal lipid absorption or metabolism	Restrict long-chain fatty acids; adequate essential fatty acids; supplement fat-soluble vitamins, particularly vitamin E
Cholesterol acyltransferase deficiency/type I hyperlipoproteinemia		
Chromosomal aberrations		
Down syndrome	Persons with an extra chromosome, usually chromosomes 21 or 22	Lowered energy needs, low muscle tone; limited growth rate; low resting metabolism rate
Prader-Willi syndrome	A chromosomal disorder involving fifteenth chromosome	Infancy is marked by failure-to-thrive; hypotonic suck; at 15–24 months the toddler manifests unusual hunger leading to excessive weight gain.
Turner's syndrome	Girls born with 45 chromosomes; the second X chromosome absent	Lowered energy needs; limited growth rate
Acrodermatitis enteropathica	A rare disorder with onset between 3 weeks and 18 months with symptoms of failure to thrive, diarrhea, and lesions around body openings	Zinc supplementation
Wilson's disease	A recessive trait where accumulation of copper occurs in brain, liver, and kidney due to lack of enzyme to bind copper in the tissues	Special diet limiting copper to 1 mg/day; use of D-pencillamine; zinc and pyrodoxine supplementation
Medical aberrations		
Cerebral palsy	Bilateral, symmetrical, nonprogressive paralysis or uncontrolled movements	Variable energy requirements due to uncontrolled movements
Pulmonary dysfunction		
Bronchopulmonary dysplasia	Abnormal development of bronchi and lungs	Increased energy needs due to increased work of breathing
Cystic fibrosis	A disease of exocrine glands affecting the pancreas, respiratory system, and sweat glands	Increased energy needs; insufficient pancreatic enzymes must be replaced to prevent malabsorption
Spina bifida/occulta	Congenital defect causing failure of the spinal column to close	Decreased energy needs due to low ambulation
Renal disease	Variability in the kidney's ability to perform essential functions	Special diet: low calcium, low phosphorus; fluid, potassium and protein may be monitored; vitamin D supplementation; medications need consideration
Acquired	Originated after birth	
Congenital	Present at birth	
Congenital heart disease	Heart disease present at birth	Poor growth and development; increased energy needs; water balance is of concern; low sodium diet may be indicated

TABLE 12.2
Examples of Nutritional Risk Factors Associated with Selected Disorders

	Growth					Diet			Medical	
	Underweight	Overweight	Short Stature	Low Energy Needs	High Energy Needs	Feeding Problem	Special Diet	Constipation	Chronic Medication	Diarrhea
Chromosomal aberrations										
Down syndrome		✓		✓		✓				
Prader-Willi syndrome		✓	✓	✓						
Turner's Syndrome		✓	✓	✓						
Inborn errors of metabolism										
Phenylketonuria (PKU)							✓			✓
Maple syrup urine disorders							✓			✓
Homocystinuria			✓					✓		✓
Urea cycle dysfunction							✓			✓
Fructose intolerance							✓			✓
Glycogen storage disease							✓			✓
Fat metabolism dysfunction							✓			
Cerebral palsy	✓	✓	✓	✓	✓	✓		✓	✓	
Bronchopulmonary dysplasia	✓				✓				✓	
Cystic fibrosis	✓	✓	✓		✓					
Spina bifida	✓		✓	✓				✓	✓	
Renal disease							✓		✓	
Congenital heart disease	✓				✓		✓		✓	✓
HIV/AIDS	✓				✓				✓	
Fetal alcohol syndrome	✓		✓	✓		✓				
Wilson's disease	✓			✓					✓	

Source: Adapted from Baer MT, Harris AB: Pediatric nutrition assessment: identifying children at risk. *J Amer Diet Assoc.* 97:10 supp 2, S107–S115, 1997.

with cerebral palsy showed they had a higher resting metabolic rate, 1,742 kcal compared to 1,534 kcal for controls.[18] However, a previous study by Bandini[2] found the resting energy expenditure of a small group of adolescents with cerebral palsy to be lower than in adolescent control subjects. Thus, nutrition care and intervention for the individual with cerebral palsy must be individualized and account for the person's ambulating and feeding capabilities as well as uncontrolled movement (athetosis) of arms and legs.

There are times when a medical condition may be associated with a chromosomal aberration and both conditions affect nutrition approaches to promote growth. For example, a child with Down syndrome usually has lowered calorie needs. However, a child with Down syndrome who is also born with a congenital heart defect[21] will require *increased* calories to have a successful growth pattern. Often surgical repair of the heart defect is needed, bringing about a dramatic improvement in growth and a return to lowered caloric intakes.

Unfortunately, research to establish the nutritional needs in these special conditions has been limited, and the reader is challenged to continuously review the literature for new answers to many questions regarding this population.

Other children with special health care needs require additional types of nutritional management depending on which stage of the process of nutrition and human physiologies are affected: food intake, digestion, absorption, or elimination. These conditions include chronic renal disease, seizure disorders, heart disease, and disorders involving the gastrointestinal tract. Identification and treatment of gastrointestinal disorders is an important component of care in children or adults with special needs. The major symptoms include vomiting, diarrhea, constipation, dysphagia, jaundice, abdominal pain, and distention.

Gastroesophageal reflux is a condition frequently found in infants and young children that often results in a condition known as failure to thrive. Symptoms include crying and discomfort following a feeding and copious "spitting up" or vomiting.[3] Identification following parental reports of this problem may require the use of a special test such as barium swallow. Treatment may vary from positioning, thickening of feeding, medication, or surgical treatment if other treatment fails. Surgical treatment may involve placement of a gastrostomy tube as a temporary or permanent measure.[3]

Diarrhea may be chronic or acute. Either type can result in dehydration and electrolyte imbalance. The cause of diarrhea may be infections, food intolerance (e.g., gluten sensitivity or lactose intolerance), and congenital enzyme deficiency.

Constipation is found when muscle tone is low or in structural anomalies such as Hirschprung's disease. Constipation may also reflect lack of fiber in the diet and inadequate fluid intake in some individuals. Treatment includes use of a high-fiber diet, adequate water intake, and increased intake of sucrose and dextri-maltose.

Chronic use of medications is another risk factor requiring interventions for individuals and adults with special needs. Many of the drugs involved affect nutritional status negatively because they alter appetite and absorption of vitamins and minerals. They may also cause gastrointestinal side effects, drowsiness, and decreased activity. The types of drugs used for the clients with special needs include anticonvulsants, anti-infection agents, amphetamines, psychotropic agents, and diuretics. Sources exist for the student to further explore the medications or drugs commonly prescribed for individuals with special health care needs and their nutritional implications.[25]

An important resource for community nutrition professionals to better understand developmental disabilities is Isaacs et al.[16] Understanding the nutrition risks associated with infants, children, and adults with special needs advocates for the importance of adequate screening procedures.

SCREENING FOR SPECIAL NEEDS AND NUTRITION-RELATED PROBLEMS

Screening programs for identification of disorders caused by an inborn error of metabolism began in the United States in the 1960s.[12] These screenings are usually done shortly after birth when feeding has been initiated. The most usual disorders identified in statewide screening programs include phenylketonuria (PKU), galactosemia, maple syrup urine disease, homocystinuria, and hypothyroidism. The most frequently used screening test is called the Guthrie test, name for Dr. Robert Guthrie, who developed the test utilizing microbiological assay methodologies on treated filter paper.[12] Treatment outcomes are varied, depending on how early treatment is started.

Since persons with special health needs receive their health care in a variety of places, it is important to have proper screening methods in place to identify clients at greatest nutritional risk. Without specific screening programs, the nutrition needs of many clients could go undetected. In a screening program held in North Carolina, at least 50 percent of the children screened required a referral to an agency where more assessment and intervention could be provided.[15]

Screening may consist of a questionnaire with questions related to usual eating habits, dietary restrictions, food allergies or intolerance, nutritional supplements, gastrointestinal disturbances, special formulas or diets, changes in appetite or intake, anthropometric measures, recent weight loss, and previous hospitalizations or major surgeries. During hospital stays, blood is usually drawn at admission for a complete blood cell count (CBC). Growth parameters should always be taken for infants, children, and adolescents and plotted on appropriate growth grids.

It is important to have screening procedures in place so the nutrition consultant can be contacted for a more in-depth assessment if necessary.[20] Various criteria for nutrition referrals have been established in centers for developmental disorders.[10,20] An example of a criteria set follows:

- All children younger than three years
- Height and weight below the tenth percentile
- Certain conditions such as allergy, chronic diarrhea, food faddism
- Family income less than $12,500 for four people
- Teenage mother
- Postmenarcheal adolescent

An example of a nutrition screening form is displayed in figure 12.2.

NUTRITION ASSESSMENT

Once screening has resulted in a nutrition referral, an assessment will be made by a registered dietitian or qualified nutrition professional and should be tailored for the individual's diagnosis.[27] Areas that should be completed are *a*nthropometric and *b*iochemical measures, *c*linical signs, *d*ietary history, and feeding skills (ABCDs). In addition, the process requires a thorough review including information related to age, education of parents or caregiver, income, housing, activity level, and medications. Nutrition assessment guidelines for national use were developed by a conference of nutrition professionals working in university-affiliated programs with individuals with development disabilities. These guidelines are presented in table 12.3. Some dis-

cussion is warranted to help the reader understand information related to completing an assessment.

Anthropometric Assessment

Anthropometric measures include height, weight, head circumference, arm circumference, triceps skinfold measures, and mid–upper arm circumference. Consistency is extremely important in the way measurements are taken. Consideration should be given to selecting equipment that accommodates handicapping conditions. Chair scales are indicated for clients unable to stand, and in some instances, bed scales are indicated. Well-calibrated balance scales or electronic digital scales are now available.[27]

Recumbent length is an important measurement for all children up to age three. In addition, many older retarded individuals will be unable to stand and should be measured in the recumbent position. If an individual is able to stand, a measuring device should be fastened to a vertical surface such as the wall to which is attached a movable head board. For physically handicapped individuals, alternative methods have been suggested: arm span, ankle-to-knee height, or sitting height.[27]

Head circumference can be taken on children up to age six. In addition to head circumference, arm circumference and triceps skinfolds measurements are frequently taken and contribute to a more complete assessment of body composition.

Body mass index (BMI) is a clinically convenient indicator used to express body weight corrected for height. This indicator correlates well with more complex measurements in determination of fatness. Although the standards have not been developed specifically for conditions found in individuals with developmental disabilities, the index can be used to monitor changes over time.[10]

Anthropometric standards for infants, children, and adolescents up to age eighteen are provided by the National Center for Health Statistics Growth Charts.[13] Charts have also been developed that are specific for special needs: Down syndrome,[7] constitutional short stature and thyroid dysfunction, Marfan syndrome, sickle-cell disease, Prader-Willi syndrome, and William's and Turner's syndromes. Adults with developmental disabilities need anthropometric assessment for determination and maintenance of appropriate weight-for-height status. The Metropolitan Life Insurance Height-Weight Tables are applicable standards for comparison unless heights are extremely low. Skinfold standards are not developed

**A look at nutrition
(Nutrition screening)**

Child's name: _____ Today's date: _____

Address: _____

Phone: (_____) _____

Birthdate: _____ /_____ /_____   Birth weight: _____ pounds _____ ounces
         month day   year

Was your child premature (born early)?   ☐ Yes   ☐ No   Sex: ☐ Male ☐ Female
If yes, how many weeks was he/she born early?_____ weeks

The following questions will help us learn more about your child's nutritional health. Please answer each of the following questions.

1. How does your child appear to you?   ☐ Overweight ☐ Underweight ☐ Just right   ☐ Short

2. Is your child *now* on a special diet?   ☐ Yes   ☐ No
    If Yes, what kind? _____

3. Is your child *now* allergic to, or intolerant of, any foods? ☐ Yes   ☐ No
    If Yes, what foods?_____

4. Is your child *now* a picky eater?   ☐ Yes   ☐ No
    If Yes, check all that apply:
        ☐ Refuses many foods   ☐ Drinks more than 40 oz. milk per day
        ☐ Refuses solid foods   ☐ Has a poor appetite   ☐ Other _____

5. Does your child *now* take medications?   ☐ Yes   ☐ No
    If Yes, what medications and for how long? _____

6. Does your child *now* take vitamins/minerals?   ☐ Yes   ☐ No
    If Yes, name supplement(s): _____

7. Does your child *now* regularly have diarrhea?   ☐ Yes   ☐ No

8. Does your child *now* regularly have constipation? ☐ Yes   ☐ No

9. Does your child *now* regularly vomit?   ☐ Yes   ☐ No

10. Does your child *now* have a feeding tube?   ☐ Yes   ☐ No

11. Does your child *now* have dental problems?   ☐ Yes   ☐ No

12. In the past six months, was your child   ☐ Yes   ☐ No
    found to be anemic (low blood iron)?

13. Does your child *now* have any feeding   ☐ Yes   ☐ No
    or eating problems?
      If Yes, check any of the following which apply:
      ☐ Difficulty sucking   ☐ Difficulty feeding self   ☐ Chokes on solids
      ☐ Difficulty chewing foods   ☐ Chokes on liquids   ☐ Loses food from mouth
      ☐ Using bottle after age 2 years ☐ Difficulty drinking from cup
      ☐ Other: _____

14. What is your child's activity level *now*?
      ☐ Walks independently   ☐ Needs help walking (braces/walker)
      ☐ Does not walk   ☐ Not old enough to walk

15. Does your child participate in any of the following programs? (Check all which may apply *now*)
      ☐ WIC   ☐ CHDP/EPSDT   ☐ MediCal/Medicaid   ☐ Infant stimulation or
      ☐ SSI   ☐ Head Start   ☐ Special education   early intervention
      ☐ AFDC   ☐ State DD program   ☐ Private therapy   ☐ Other: _____
      ☐ CCS   ☐ Food stamps   ☐ Private insurance

16. Would you like to talk with a nutritionist about
    your child?   ☐ Yes   ☐ No

17. Do you have additional concerns about your child's growth, nutrition, or eating?

FIGURE 12.2   Nutrition Screening Form

(*Source:* This form was developed under SPRANS CE Grant MCJ-009076 and MCHIP Grant MCJ-065057. For further information on its use contact: Marion Taylor Baer, PhD, RD, or Cary Bujold, MPH, RD, University Affiliated Program/USC, Children's Hospital. (213) 699-2500. November 1994.)

(*continued*)

Child's ethnicity (Check major one)	Child's medical diagnosis (Check any which apply *now*)	
Caucasian	Asthma/pulmonary disease	HIV/AIDS
Hispanic	Autism	Mental retardation
Native American	Bronchopulmonary dysplasia (BPD)	Metabolic/endocrine disorders
African American/Black	Cancer	Muscular distrophy
Southeast Asian	Cardiac (heart) disease	Neurological disorder
Asian	Cerebral palsy	Orthopedic problems
Pacific Islander	Chromosome disorder (ex. Down syndrome)	Renal (kidney) disease
Native Hawaiian	Craniofacial (ex. cleft lip/palate)	Sensory impairment (blind, deaf)
Unknown	Cystic fibrosis	Spina bifida
Other: _____	Developmental delay	High-risk infant/child
_____	Epilepsy/seizures	Unknown diagnosis
_____	Gastrointestinal disorder (GI)	Other: _____

For office use only

Person filling out this form: _____
- ☐ Parent or caregiver   ☐ Case manager
- ☐ Educator/teacher   ☐ Health professional (OT, MD, RN, SW, PT)
- ☐ Nutritionist   ☐ Intake worker

Height/weight:
Weight:_____ lb./or _____ kg   Length/height: _____ in./or _____ cm
Head circumference: _____ in./or _____ cm
Wt./age percentile: _____   Ht./age percentile: _____   Wt./Ht. percentile: _____

Above measurements obtained from: check *one* of the following (please list the date of measurement):
- ☐ Measured by clinic staff at this visit, date_____
- ☐ Stated by caregiver, date _____
- ☐ Record (medical), date _____

					Other lab values		
Biochemical values:	Value	Date		Value	Date	Name	Value	Date
Serum iron	_____	_____	MCV	_____	_____	_____	_____	_____
Albumin	_____	_____	Hgb.	_____	_____	_____	_____	_____

Action taken:
- ☐ No referral needed
- ☐ Referral for nutritionist, Name: _____ Date: _____
- ☐ Previously seen by nutritionist, Location: _____ Date: _____
- ☐ Currently receiving nutrition services, specify: _____
- ☐ Referral for other services, specify: _____ Date: _____

FIGURE 12.2   Continued

for specific syndromes but, within limits, the Frisancho standards can be used clinically.[27]

rant further laboratory studies to complete an in-depth nutrition assessment.[27]

Biochemical Measures

Laboratory tests can be an important component of the "in-depth" nutrition assessment of clients with special needs. In persons with developmental disabilities, lack of general nutrition (i.e., calories) may be the most frequent finding; however, there is a greater chance for depletion of certain nutrients in clients who are chronically medicated. Readers are encouraged to review drug-nutrient interactions and identify those that war-

Clinical Signs

In any nutrition assessment, past history and current clinical observations are included to record signs indicative of disease and poor nutritional status. Initially, the nutrition professional should review past and present records of medical and dental examinations for signs of poor nutritional status. To obtain more information, the nutrition professional should obtain information related to prenatal experience, including weight gain, maternal alcohol or

TABLE 12.3

Guides for Nutrition Assessment of Individuals with Mental Retardation and Developmental Disabilities

Assessment component	Minimal recommendation	In-depth recommendation (in addition to minimal)
Anthropometric	Weight (no shoes, light clothing); height, length (recumbent up to 3 yr); head circumference (up to 6 yr); *Standard:* National Center for Health Statistics Growth Charts	Skinfold, triceps and subscapular; *Standard:* Foman Arm circumference; *Standard:* Frisancho

Biochemical	Complete blood count, urinalysis, amino acid screening	Serum total protein and albumin levels, fasting blood glucose level, serum urea nitrogen level, transferrin saturation, quantitative urinary and amino acid screening
		Other tests to respond to problems:
		  Anticonvulsants: folic acid, ascorbic acid, calcium, vitamin D, alkaline phosphatase, phosphorus, B vitamins
		  Prader-Willi syndrome: glucose tolerance test
		  Pica: lead, hemoglobin

Clinical	Review of past and present records of medical and dental examinations for signs of poor nutritional status	Health history to include prenatal weight gain; postnatal client or family history of diabetes, cardiac disease, infections, anemia, constipation, diarrhea, hyperactivity, food intolerances, pica, inborn errors of metabolism, malabsorption syndromes Observation to assess general appearance, speech, and oral hygiene
Dietary	Twenty-four hour recall; feeding history questionnaire	Three-day dietary record kept by caregiver, activity record (as needed), pertinent historical information related to feeding, present influences on dietary intake Other: certain conditions may require further dietary investigation and data that are more detailed
Behavioral and feeding skill development	Parental perception of feeding skills and behavior Professional perception of feeding skills and behavior	Interview to determine feeding skill development and present level of functioning Observation of oral structure and function including primitive reflexes, sucking, swallowing, biting, occlusion, and caries Observation of neuromuscular development including gross and fine motor skills, head and trunk control, eye-hand coordination, and position for feeding Observation of parent-child interaction, reinforcement patterns, environmental influences, child-examiner interaction

drug consumption, and complications of the pregnancy. Additional information would include family history of disease, feeding problems during infancy, current dental condition, food intolerance, pica, inborn errors of metabolism, constipation, and diarrhea.[27]

An important clinical indicator of individuals with developmental disabilities that impacts nutritional status is extensive dental caries and inflamed and diseased appearance of the gingival tissue (gums). Lack of dental hygiene, coupled with the medication prescribed, is an important contributor to dental problems. One medication used in seizure control (Dilantin, or phenytoin sodium) causes hyperplasia of the gums if used for a prolonged period of time. This can lead to serious chewing problems when the gums cover the teeth. Other indicators of poor nutritional status may be noted in the condition of the hair, skin, skeleton, lips, and eyes. Hair could be easily removed (plucked) indicating protein malnutrition, but this should be coupled with laboratory evaluation of total serum protein and albumin.

Dietary Assessment

Food intake of clients with special needs may also be impaired because of socioeconomic limitations and cultural characteristics of the family. Obtaining accurate, meaningful information is a difficult task for the nutrition professional for a variety of reasons. In today's world, many individuals have multiple caregivers and communication related to dietary intake is not shared freely.

Dietary assessment for this population will encompass three things: what the individuals eat, how much, and how often. The best results are obtained when a variety of methods of data collection are employed. This may involve assessment of usual food intake (twenty-four-hour dietary recall), obtaining actual food intake (using food records or food frequency), and a complete diet history. It is useful to use food models, commonly used serving spoons, flatware, cups, bowls, and measuring spoons. Once the food intake is estimated as accurately as possible, computerized dietary analysis programs exist for calculating nutrient intake.

Actual food intake should be observed whenever possible for the dietary and feeding skills evaluation. This provides realistic information related to actual food intake, what is provided, and feeding skills (discussed later) of the client or caregiver. Sometimes parents or caregivers may report excellent intake, but when observed, feeding skills are limited, oral-motor problems exist that were not addressed, and intake was much less than reported in the interview. This type of observation should then lead to a meeting with individuals from various disciplines that make up the "**feeding team,**" which could include an occupational therapist, speech pathologist, physical therapist, and the nutrition professional. During the dietary assessment, it may be reported by the parent or caregiver that the child or client refuses to eat a variety of foods, is resistant to texture changes, and may demonstrate tantrums during meal time. This kind of report reflects behavioral problems, which may be addressed by the feeding team with the addition of a psychologist or behavioral specialist. The impact of behavior will often have a strong influence on dietary intake.

Feeding Skills

Feeding problems in individuals with cerebral palsy, cleft palate, many chromosomal disorders such as Down syndrome and Prader-Willi syndrome, seizure disorders, prematurity, and hypotonia may lead to nutrition problems. A **feeding problem** is defined as an inability or refusal to eat certain foods because of neuromotor dysfunction, obstructive lesions, and/or psychological factors.[4] Problems are classified as oral-motor, positioning, and behavioral. Nutrititional consequences of these problems may include slow growth in children, inadequate weight gain, dental caries, anemia, vitamin and mineral deficiencies, developmental delays, and behavioral problems.

Oral-Motor Problems   Problems of this nature have been described as an exaggeration of normal neuromotor mechanism leading to a disruption of rhythm and organization of oral-motor patterns and interference in the feeding process. To identify **oral-motor problems** and provide appropriate counselng and intervention, the nutrition professional must first understand the oral structure, feeding development from infancy until childhood, and cultural influences on feeding from the family standpoint. Interdisciplinary teams are very effective in identifying and intervening in treatment of feeding problems. The team may consist of a nurse, physical therapist, occupational therapist, speech therapist, nutritionist, and psychologist.[4]

Oral structures are necessary for sucking, suckling and biting, and chewing and swallowing. The oral structure consists of the mandible, maxilia, upper and lower lips, cheeks, tongue, teeth, floor of the mouth, hard and soft palates, uvula, and anterior and posterior facial arches. Structures involved in swallowing include pharyngeal structures and the larynx. Pharyngeal structures function as a valve at the top of the esophagus. The larynx functions to keep food from entering the airway. The esophagus, a final component of the oral-motor system, is a hollow tube and is closed by a sphincter at each end. It is made up of a combination of smooth and striated muscles that together create the peristaltic action that directs food into the stomach.[4]

For the normal infant, the oral-motor process follows a developmental pathway that consists of suckling, sucking, swallowing, munching, chewing, tongue elevation and lateralization, and the beginning stages of self-feeding. In addition, the gag reflex contributes to proper feeding abilities. Children with special health needs such as developmental disabilities often show developmental delays in feeding in infancy (see table 12.4). When undetected or ignored, the problems persist

TABLE 12.4
Common Oral-Motor Feeding Problems

Problem	Description
Tonic bite reflex	Strong jaw closure when teeth and gums are stimulated
Tongue thrust	Forceful and often repetitive protrusion of tongue in response to oral stimulation
Jaw thrust	Forceful opening of the jaw during eating, drinking, attempts to speak, or general excitement
Tongue retraction	Pulling back of the tongue within the oral cavity at the presentation of food, spoon, or cup
Lip retraction	Pulling back the lips in a tight smilelike pattern at the approach of the spoon or cup toward the face
Sensory defensiveness	Strong adverse reaction to sensory input

and increase, thereby interfering with speech development and motor development.[4]

Positioning Problems Positioning is an important consideration in working with children with oral-motor and self-feeding problems. It provides stability to the child and increases a comfort level necessary for feeding intervention. To provide intervention for the child with a feeding problem, the appropriate professional practitioner must assess positioning needs. In most areas, this individual will be an occupational or physical therapist. In any case, the nutrition professional should be knowledgeable about positioning that occurs during feeding. This entails observing head control, trunk control, foot stability, placement of the hip and pelvis, shoulder girdle, knee flexion, and sitting base. Appropriate positioning varies, depending on the problem identified, and could include reclining on the stomach, side lying, sitting, or standing. There are many types of therapeutic positioning devices available today that provide adequate trunk supports, place the hips and pelvis in a stable position, prevent shoulder retraction, and promote head control. Proper positioning also improves visual control by the child, which will improve food intake since the child may better see the food being offered, thereby enhancing his or her ability to self-feed. Where possible, either in a clinic setting or when going into the home, it is important for the nutrition professional to observe the feeding that occurs be-

tween the mother or caretaker and the child. Good and inappropriate positioning are depicted in figure 12.3.

Behavioral and Environmental Problems The third component of feeding consists of the impact of the child's behavior on feeding or the behavioral problems caused by a feeding problem.[4] Often parents misinterpret the child's oral-motor problem as bad behavior or lack of appetite. One parent I worked with had a child with failure to thrive. Because his mother interpreted a tonic bite reflex as displaying dislike for certain foods, he received very few foods other than fluids from his bottle.

Consideration should be given to the timing of meals and distractions provided during mealtime such as noise, television, large numbers of individuals in the room, and radios playing loud music. For the child with a small appetite and a history of food refusal, it is important to provide small servings, bright colors, and foods that are separated and not mixed. For visually impaired children, the feeding area must be well illuminated and the parents or caregivers must name the food being fed. Young children respond best to mild temperatures and bland flavors, but sharper spicier flavors can be introduced as the child grows older.[4]

Another behavioral issue that the nutrition professional should evaluate is the child's manipulation of the family. Children notice very quickly the anxious concern of parents or caregivers about their food intake. A parental reaction to food avoidance may be to follow the child throughout the day and to offer food at frequent intervals. The intervention for such a behavior is to develop a schedule in which food is provided at well-timed intervals, while counseling the parent that such a program is not punishing the child.

NUTRITION INTERVENTION AND SERVICES

Following the establishment of the Children's Bureau in 1912, a number of programs were initiated that dealt with nutrition for all children. Nutrition services in the community for individuals with special needs first received attention in the 1920s with the passage of the Maternity and Infant Act. In 1935, Title V of the Social Security Act was passed, providing for three programs. Maternal and Child Health, Crippled Children's Service, and Child Welfare. By 1950, some Title V funds were earmarked for demonstration clinical programs for children with mental retardation. Workshops on nutrition and diet in relation to mental retardation were developed

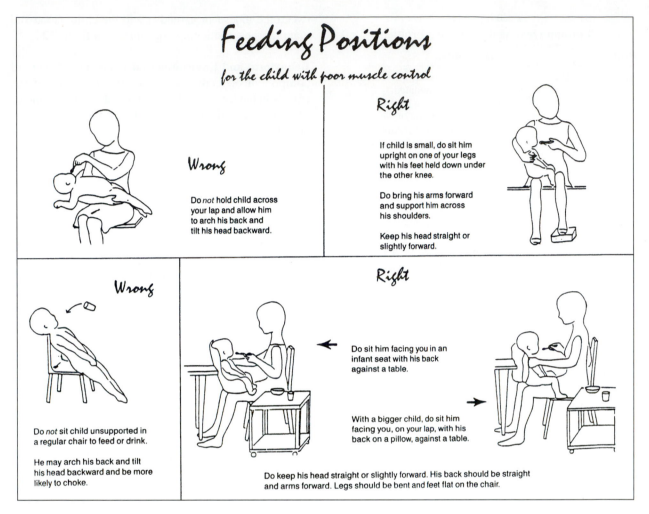

FIGURE 12.3   Good and Appropriate Positioning for Feeding
(*Source:* From *Nutrition screening for children with special needs*, 198?, New Mexico Health & Environment Department. Reprinted with permission from New Mexico Health & Environment Department.)

to update the knowledge and skills of nutrition personnel in this area and to begin planning and developing nutrition services for children with mental retardation.[9]

During the 1960s, significant legislation directly or indirectly influenced community services for children with developmental disabilities and mental retardation. Part of the legislation created the Maternity and Infant Care Projects, which were important in promoting healthy pregnancies that would prevent mental retardation and developmental disabilities; the Children and Youth Projects; and the University Affiliated Programs designed to train manpower in an interdisciplinary manner to work with individuals with mental retardation

and developmental disabilities. Later, Head Start was established with a mandate that 10 percent of the population it would serve must be handicapped.[17]

Following all of this important legislation, the passage of the Child Nutrition Act in 1966 and the Supplemental Food Programs for low-income groups vulnerable to malnutrition brought nutrition assistance to all children including those with special needs. The most important piece of legislation targeting children with special needs was passed in 1975, the Education of All Handicapped Children Act (PL 94-142).[5] This law brought children with handicapping conditions (the terminology of the 1970s) into the public school system and was the stepping stone to the current policies of inclusion. Nutrition services were not listed among services provided by PL 94-142, but ten years later when an amendment (PL 99-457) expanded education to the preschool years and to infancy, it included nutrition as an **early intervention** service. Under this law, referred to as Early Intervention (EI), the Surgeon General directed that all programs must be family-centered, community-based, comprehensive, and culturally sensitive. In 1993, PL 94-142 was renamed IDEA (the Individuals with Disabilities Education Act) and now encompasses all education for individuals with disabilities including the Early Intervention Programs.

As mentioned earlier in this chapter, the thrust for services for individuals with developmental disabilities is inclusion. This has led the movement away from institutions to the use of small residential facilities, group homes, and independent living in apartments and single homes. Many of the smaller residential facilities are regulated by standards for Intermediate Care Facilities for Persons with Mental Retardation (ICF/MR). These regulations mandate nutrition services; however, in smaller group homes, nutrition services may not be provided.

Agency management of the total care of these individuals is also changing from government agencies at the state and local level to private companies. Information on the kind of nutrition services offered from these is sparse. Some opportunities exist for the community nutrition professional to offer menu planning and education on food preparation and food buying. There is concern that often the newly noninstitutionalized individual will have his or her nutritional needs and concerns overlooked. Thus, it is important for the community nutrition professional to become aware of special population needs; to plan and advocate for necessary specialized services; and be prepared to collaborate and coordinate with a wide range of providers in many different programs and settings.

Program Planning

Planning for intervention is complex because of the many factors that influence the nutritional status of individuals with special needs. They require an approach to care that incorporates information and assistance from several disciplines. In addition, nutrition services for children and adults with special needs are provided in a variety of health care settings, including hospitals, ambulatory care, home health care, developmental centers, early intervention programs, residential facilities and schools, public health clinics, WIC programs, and Head Start. A plan should be developed that fosters optimum nutritional intake and the development of appropriate feeding skills, and coordinates interventions from all providers.[23] The nutrition professional's role thus encompasses more than simply providing dietary guidance to the individual.

For example, in recent years more and more children and adults with handicapping conditions are being fed by tube.[15] Although this process requires a surgical procedure to begin, it does not irritate the oral and nasal mucosa as does the nasogastric tube. Research has indicated that although parents view tube-feeding as the last resort, and aberrant to the usual type of feeding, it does result in weight gain and improved nutritional status.[15] For some individuals, the tube will be a temporary measure and for others a permanent method of feeding. When it is a temporary measure, the feeding therapist should be treating the underlying oral-motor, positioning, or behavioral problem that may still exist when the tube is removed.

Intervention for many individuals with special needs will also require multiple visits for change to occur. In early intervention programs serving infants and toddlers up to age three years, nutrition problems and goals should be written into the Interdisciplinary Family Service Plan (IFSP). When this plan is completed, the recommendations of each discipline are translated into measurable goals, with the participation of the family in setting those goals.

Utilizing school food service in program planning for children through adolescence has not reached its full potential, although legislation has existed since 1973. The legislation that ensures the provision of the appropriate meal for a child with handicapping conditions was Section 504 of the 1973 Rehabilitation Act. This was followed by a number of regulations written by the USDA following passage of the Education of All Handicapped Children Act (PL 94-142), now entitled the Individuals with Disabilities Act (PL 102-119). These regulations enable clinicians who see individuals with nutrition problems to request that schools modify breakfasts, snacks, or lunches at no extra charge to the student to meet the nutritional needs of their patients.

By integrating nutrition support service into a coordinated system with other health education, and social services working in partnership with families, mutual reinforcement and support can be achieved across disciplines, and services to children and their families can be strengthened.[6] Practice guidelines used in planning for nutrition assessment and intervention and designed to assist the nutrition professional with various developmental disorders have been published.[24,29] These guidelines are used in quality assurance and quality improvement programs.

Resources

Resources for clients with special needs include financial support for supplemental feedings, tube-feedings, metabolic formulas, self-help feeding devices, and educational materials for the nutrition professional on feeding and nutrition protocols for various conditions. Clients and their families should be informed about agencies such as developmental centers, cerebral palsy centers, rehabilitation services, and mental health centers in the community.

Formula procurement can be a major problem because of the high cost of these special products and because of the variability in provision protocols from state to state. For low-income infants and children up to age five, the WIC program provides formulas and food vouchers for supplemental feedings, tube-feedings, and special formulas devised for individuals with inborn errors of metabolism. After age five, state programs allocate Maternal Child Health Block Grant funds to assist children with formula procurement. In some states, Children's Rehabilitative Services provide formulas for clients that they serve. Policies vary from state to state, making it necessary for the nutrition professional to investigate what is covered by their health department and rehabilitative services. Private foundations, along with church groups and civic organizations, have been effective in some cities and states in providing materials for families. Special metabolic formulas are covered partially by private insurance companies on an individual basis. In some states, there is Medicaid coverage for supplemental beverages, tube-feedings, and metabolic formulas.

One special resource that should be shared with the family is a parent support group. Many syndrome-related parent groups exist for information and support. Examples include the Down Syndrome Association, the Prader-Willi Association, the United Cerebral Palsy, and the Association for Retarded Citizens. Providing this information to clients and the family is an important role of the nutrition professional.

An additional resource for enabling a nutrition intervention program involves use of the school food service. Often a child consumes at least two meals plus snacks at school and may require a modification of the school menu. This can be accomplished by use of a meal prescription, which is signed by the physician and a recognized medical authority.[5]

A resource to provide nutrition training to nutrition professionals and practitioners in other disciplines who work with children with special needs is available from the Maternal and Child Health Bureau as well as the Agency for Children and Youth. Demonstration projects have been funded in many states, collaborating with universities to develop new programs for improving nutrition services to children with special needs. Information about the availability of the programs is located in the *Federal Register* and through federal agency Web pages.

Inborn Error of Metabolism: An Individualized Intervention Example

PKU was discovered in Norway in 1934 by Folling, who had witnessed infants who appeared normal at birth but developed slowly and showed severe mental retardation. A distinguishing characteristic of the children was a peculiar odor to their urine, which was described "as the odor of sweaty tennis shoes." Folling tested the urine with ferrous chloride and identified the breakdown products of phenylalanine in the urine.[11]

Current treatment requires use of a formula low in phenylalanine but adequate in protein, fat, carbohydrate, vitamins, and minerals. There are formulas available for use today. The community nutrition professional's role would be to educate and assist the family that qualifies for the WIC program to procure this special formula through the program. Or, alternatively, the nutrition professional would know of or find out about any special grants and/or legislative mandates for insurance coverage of the special formula and be able to assist families in accessing these programs.

Education of the parents in the selection of foods low in phenylalanine is essential as soon as the infant starts to receive foods other than formula. Foods that can be consumed by individuals with PKU include fruits, vegetables, breads, cereals, and fats. In educating the family, the nutrition professional must outline the total diet, showing the amount of formula and the number of servings of the foods low in phenylalanine. Foods high in protein are omitted from the diet. Many families find the exclusion of meat, fish, poultry, milk, eggs, milk products, peanut butter, and cheese troubling. Foods low in protein such as pastas, breads, and cookies increase the variety of the diet available.

Ongoing treatment and monitoring of PKU is required and, in many states, is provided in tertiary centers specializing in genetic disorders. Ideal management of PKU will last *throughout* life, a concept that was not thought necessary in the early days of treatment. Treatment results have been studied extensively and conclusions show that when dietary treatment is started early in life (before three weeks of age) and there is adherence to a low-phenylalanine diet, the child with PKU should have a normal intelligence.[12] The community nutrition professional can be an important team member throughout growth and development of individuals with PKU and can provide interventions that promote positive health outcomes.

Treatment of children with metabolic and/or medical aberrations begin in a tertiary hospital or community medical center, but ongoing care will be in the community through public health programs or the primary care physician's office. As with all children who require special formulas and foods, providing the family with a guide to available resources is extremely important.

PREVENTION CONSIDERATIONS

From a Public Health standpoint, reaching and educating the public in lifestyles that promote health and prevent disease has long-range effects for society. Adequate nutrition during the fetal period is an important prevention that will lower the incidence of handicapping conditions and improve the chances of intervention for those already affected.

Prepregnancy Genetic Counseling

Increasing numbers of women contemplating pregnancy are encouraged to seek counseling from a genetic counselor related to the possibility of having an infant with a developmental disability. Inborn errors of metabolism are transmitted through the autosomal recessive mode of inheritance with a one-in-four chance that each pregnancy outcome could be a child with an inborn error of metabolism. This applies to phenylketonuria, galactosemia, maple syrup urine disease, and many others.

Counseling is available for individuals who have had children with Down syndrome, spina bifida, and Prader-Willi syndrome related to the possibility of a second child with these disorders. Many states have a genetics department within their health department where counseling can be arranged.

Prenatal Care

Adequate care during pregnancy is among the maternal/child health objectives for Healthy Children 2000.[23] Maternal characteristics associated with receiving late or no prenatal care include low income, less than a high school education, teenage pregnancy, and a large number of children. The goal for receiving care is that 90 percent of all pregnant women receive care in the first trimester.[23] Nutrition counseling for the intake of an adequate diet leading to an appropriate weight gain is discussed in chapter 8.

Alcohol consumption during pregnancy is known to cause alcohol-related defects described in the literature as "fetal alcohol syndrome." Infants with this syndrome can be growth retarded and have facial malformations and central nervous system dysfunction including mental retardation. A goal of reducing the incidence of fetal alcohol syndrome by 50 percent was set by clinics serving the prenatal population. Legislation was enacted in 1989 requiring state health departments to begin annual reporting of the incidence of fetal alcohol syndrome as part of their responsibilities under the Maternal Child Health Block Grants.[14]

Prevention and Treatment of Low Birthweight

A number of risk factors for low birthweight have been identified, including younger and older maternal age, high parity, poor reproductive history, low socioeconomic status, low level of education, low pregnancy weight gain and/or low prepregnancy weight, smoking, and substance abuse. Smoking, alcohol consumption, and illicit drug use are all associated with low birthweight and one of the contributing factors to this etiology is the low intake of foods and the subsequent nutritional inadequacy of the diet during pregnancy.

Low birthweight is defined as an infant born weighing less than 2,500 g. Very low birthweight is defined as an infant weighing less than 1,500 g. Many of these babies are also classified as premature (less than 37 weeks gestation). Increasing numbers of very low birthweight infants and extremely low birthweight infants (< 1,000 g) are surviving and are at risk for developmental disabilities, pulmonary disorders, and other morbidity.[14]

Adequate and appropriate nutrition is an extremely important component of the care of low-birthweight infants. Frequently, the low-birthweight infant is hospitalized for a long period. The parent is unable to effectively bond with the infant in the nursery and needs a great deal of support and instruction before taking the baby home. Adequate weight gain for the premature infant has been difficult to achieve on discharge when the parent has been inadequately instructed on feeding the baby who should be fed according to the corrected age, rather than the chronological age. This factor continues until the child reaches ages two or three.

Where substance abuse has been involved, it is possible the infant will be placed in a foster home. The foster parent needs instruction on feeding, involving appropriate formulas, positioning, and when to add solid food, just as the natural parent would.

Adequate Nutrition and Supplemental Feeding

The importance of adequate nutrition during pregnancy, infancy and childhood has been addressed in other parts of this text. Its importance is reiterated in Healthy Children 2000[14] and for low-income clients. The presence of WIC for maintaining the adequacy of the diet of children with special needs is extremely important.[23]

An additional nutrition consideration is the prevention of neural tube defects, which has received a lot of attention for several years following the early studies of Smithells identifying folic acid deficiency as a causative factor. Smithells studies indicated that low-income women in England and other parts of the British Isles benefited from the addition of the vitamin folic acid to their diet. Further work in the United States has confirmed these findings. Folic acid supplementation of 4 mg daily is a recommended procedure from prior to conception and through the first trimester of pregnancy to prevent neural tube defects.

Environmental Considerations

The presence of lead in the blood in children ages six months through five years is the most prevalent environmental threat to the health of children in the United States. High levels of lead in the blood can cause coma, convulsions, profound irreversible mental retardation, seizures, and death. Even low levels can result in persistent impairments in central nervous system function, including delayed cognitive development, reduced IQ

scores, impaired hearing; adverse impacts on blood production and vitamin D and calcium metabolism; and growth deficits. In adults, lead in the blood may interfere with hearing; increase blood pressure; and, at high levels, cause kidney damage and anemia.

The goal for prevention of lead toxicity by the year 2000 is to reduce the prevalence of blood lead levels exceeding 15 µg/dl and 25 µg/dl to no more than 500,000 and 0, respectively. Baseline data indicated in 1984 that some 3 million children had levels exceeding 15 µg/dl and 234,000 had levels exceeding 25 µg/dl.[23]

Sources of lead include paint, dust, and soil in inner-city urban areas. Food can play an important role in lead toxicity. Sources of lead ingestion include food served in lead-glazed ceramic dishes, cups, and pots; acidic drinks (like fruit juice) stored in leaded glass; and leafy or root vegetables grown in lead-contaminated soil. By making sure the child has three or more meals or feedings a day, absorption of lead is deterred; particularly if the diet is high in iron, calcium, and vitamin C and fat intake is limited. Fats and oils increase the absorption of lead. In areas where old water pipes exist, families are also instructed to let tap water run for several minutes before collecting the water to make infant formula and to practice handwashing for both the person preparing a meal and the child before eating the meal.

II. OTHER SPECIAL POPULATIONS

FOOD INSECURITY

In addition to the individuals with developmental disabilities, mental retardation, and the special health care needs previously discussed, there are other groups in the population who present special problems in health care. These include those who are hungry, poor, homeless, illiterate, and suffering from substance abuse and tuberculosis.

Hunger and Food Insecurity

Hunger has significant underlying socioeconomic and political causes. Approximately 39 million Americans live in poverty (annual income under $15,600 for a family of four) in 1996. Factors related to hunger include unemployment, underemployment, homelessness, low literacy, economic displacement, marital breakup, and wage and other discrimination based on gender, race, and physical and mental conditions.

Based on data from the USDA's 1989 to 1991 Continuing Survey of Food Intakes by Individuals (CSFII), about 2.5 percent of households in the United States report not getting enough to eat. Other studies during the same period found hunger rates of 11 to 13 percent.[25a] Measuring hunger has been difficult because hunger is defined in various ways. Common medical and social definitions of hunger are shown in the box 12.3. Standard questions are being developed to use in national nutrition monitoring efforts to better track hunger trends and pinpoint high-risk groups and locations. However, a drawback of federal nutrition monitoring surveys is that they do not sample the homeless, migrant families, American Indians living on reservations, or persons living in institutions.

Impacts of Hunger

Children, minorities, and households headed by a single female are disproportionately affected by poverty. Low-income families pay a higher proportion of their income for shelter and have less to spend on food. Even carefully managed resources can fail to provide sufficient food for low-income families. Families cope in many ways including participating in food assistance programs, limiting consumption by some family members, skipping meals, sending children to neighbor's or relative's homes to eat, borrowing money for food, or eating at "soup kitchens" (community meals programs).

Undernutrition, an outcome of hunger, is of special concern for infants, children, pregnant women, the elderly, and those not physically or mentally capable of taking care of themselves. Chronic undernutrition, from food consumption of insufficient quantity or inadequate quality, has serious and complex effects. Undernourished individuals have growth retardation or weight loss, reduced activity, excessive irritability or apathy, and lack of response to social situations. Cognitive development is also affected. Iron deficiency with and without anemia is associated with deficits in attention and difficulty learning new concepts. In pregnancy, undernutrition contributes to low weight gain, prematurity, delivery of low birthweight infants, and infant mortality. At all ages undernutrition reduces resistance to infection, which is linked to loss of appetite, higher energy reqirements, increased nutrient losses, and reduced immune response.

Hunger can also be periodic or transient, taking the form of empty cupboards at the end of the month or no breakfast for a school-age child. Studies have shown significant effects of transient hunger due to breakfast skipping on the attention span and problem-solving ability of school children.

Hunger is often a silent or hidden malady because many of those who experience it do not show obvious clinical signs associated with severe malnutrition. Worrying about procuring food, experiencing hunger, and developing the medical results of food insufficiency form a continuum that seriously detracts from the health, productivity, and general well-being of many Americans. Researchers have found respondents' reports of "not getting enough to eat" to be associated with poorer health status and less success performing normal social roles (such as maintaining employment and parenting).

Addressing Food Insecurity

A broad term that reflects public health and public policy concerns when households are caught in circumstances in which some members do not get enough to eat as a result of insufficient resources is **food insecurity.** In contrast,

---

BOX 12.3

DEFINITIONS OF HUNGER AND FOOD INSECURITY

Common definitions of hunger: A situation in which someone cannot obtain an adequate amount of food, even if the shortage is not prolonged enough to cause health problems. The experience of being unsatisfied, of not getting enough to eat.

Medical definition of hunger: Chronic underconsumption of adequate nutrients for growth and proper maintenance of health; clinical signs indicated longstanding malnutrition such as wasting, stunting, or anemia.[18a]

Socially based definitions of hunger: The mental and physical condition that comes from not eating enough food due to insufficient economic, family, or community resources. The inability to acquire or consume an adequate quality or sufficient quantity of food in socially acceptable ways or uncertainty that one will be able to do so.

Food insecurity: Uncertain ability to acquire enough food that is nutritionally adequate, safe, and acceptable.

food security is defined as "access by all people at all times to enough food for an active healthy, life and includes at a minimum: (a) the ready availability of nutritionally adequate and safe food, and (b) the assured ability to acquire acceptable foods in socially acceptable ways."[23a] Food insecurity or insufficiency exists when these conditions are limited or uncertain. Hunger and malnutrition are potential, although not necessarily, consequences of food insecurity.

A review of numerous community and state hunger studies conducted in the 1980s resulted in seven broad conclusions:

- Food insecurity has become a chronic problem in the United States.
- Food insecurity is not due to food shortages, it results from unequal distribution of economic resources— poverty.
- People who lack access to a variety of resources—not just food—are most at risk of food insecurity.
- The federal poverty level is an inappropriate index of hunger.
- The U.S. social welfare system does not provide an adequate safety net.
- Private charity cannot solve the hunger problem.
- Hunger is inextricably linked to poverty, which is inextricably linked to underemployment and the cost of housing and other basic needs.[23a]

These conclusions underscore the economic causes of hunger, show its link to politics and policy, and reveal the complexity of potential solutions. The situation described for the 1980s remains true in the 1990s. The active welfare reform agenda may address some of the issues, however, the impact on food security is uncertain at this time.

Many nutritionists predict welfare reform will produce declining economic conditions for some low income households, change the funding and organization of client services, and result in greater difficulties reaching some high risk clients.

Community nutrition professionals will need to draw on their advocacy, community empowerment, and collaboration and communication skills to address the nutritional needs of low income groups.[23a] These strategies are evidenced in the successful approach initiated by nutrition professionals in the state of Montana to address hunger issues.[23b] Advocating for food security and proactively addressing issues underlying hunger is being realized through the collaborative and synergistic efforts of the Montana Hunger Coalition and the Montana State Advisory Council

on Food and Nutrition (MSACFN). The MSACFN, with legislatively mandated responsibility, is powerfully positioned to assess, recommend, and help assure positive policy changes. In addition, the state's Community Nutrition Coalition has a broad-based ability to create stronger communities, to provide more relevant community input to state organizations, and to mobilize resources at the local level where the greatest impact is felt.[23b]

Homelessness

The **homeless** are a growing heterogeneous population including runaway youth, adult "street people," and young families with a wide range of unique circumstances, problems, and needs. Estimates of the homeless population range from 200,000 to 2 million, and families with children are the fastest growing segment, representing 34 percent of homeless in 1990.[27b] A large core homeless population lives in self-constructed shelters under bridges and in abandoned buildings. Others move from place to place along city streets. Many communities provide emergency and transitional shelter for homeless individuals and families. Emergency shelters provide a cot and sometimes a shower and a hot meal. Occasionally, group kitchens or a hot plate and refrigerator are available. The allowed stay may be one night or a few days. Some shelter programs provide a voucher for a hotel room and a food allowance (such as $4 per day per person) to purchase food at designated grocery stores or restaurants. At shelters for battered women and their children, food may be provided and women prepare meals cooperatively in a shared kitchen or individually in separate apartments. Transitional housing programs, which are available in some cities, offer families apartments for one to two years while they complete school or job training.

Several studies have investigated the health and nutritional needs of homeless groups. Not surprisingly, the consumption of fruits, vegetables, milk, and grains was much lower than the recommended levels. There also tends to be a high consumption of low-nutrient-density foods including soft drinks and sweetened beverages and high-sugar snacks. Dental problems, infectious diseases, drug abuse, and untreated medical and mental health conditions are common.[27a]

Intervention Programs

The direct provision of food and vouchers for food represent an immediate action to protect and support persons in need, and two levels of programs exist to provide food to hungry or homeless individuals and families. The first level is the private, voluntary level with businesses, community groups, churches, and others in the private and nonprofit sectors responding to the resurgence of hunger in America. The second level is government-sponsored programs (discussed in more detail in chapter 5). Current evidence suggests voluntary and government-funded food assistance programs will continue to be an essential part of the human services landscape.

Voluntary and charitable food assistance through the private nonprofit sector takes many forms. Examples include collections of food products and money donations for distribution to centralized food banks or local community food pantries or food shelves where individuals and families come or are sent by referral agencies to request food; food-rescue programs that collect excess prepared, perishable food from restaurants, corporate dining rooms, hotels, and convention centers for prompt distribution to soup kitchens, shelters, day-care centers, and service organizations; and preparation and service of hot noon and evening meals in soup kitchens or Loaves and Fishes programs. Another example is the delivery of holiday food baskets or meals at churches and community centers.

A goal of these programs should be to provide the most safe, nutritious, and appealing meals possible within the constraints of the emergency feeding situation. Constraints include limited food budgets, unpredictable donations, staff with limited food service training, and a cadre of volunteers that changes daily. Community nutrition professionals play an important role as consultants to these programs. They can identify opportunities for nutrition education of participants and staff and offer materials and services to promote the nutrition and health of homeless clients. Shelters and emergency feeding sites also offer the opportunity for linking homeless persons to health and social service programs and government-sponsored food assistance programs (such as Food Stamps and WIC). Community nutrition professionals have valuable skills and knowledge to bring to community-based feeding programs including safe food handling practices to maintain the quality of the food and prevent food-borne illness and meal planning and budgeting skills. They also can monitor sites so that they meet city and county codes for food preparation and service facilities. Unique roles include the ability to design comfortable shelter eating environments.

As in the planning and operation of any program, it is important to consider participants' needs, wants, and perceptions. Women with families living in emergency shelters or transitional housing in Baltimore were interviewed about participation in food assistance programs, problems in feeding their children, and interest in nutrition education.[27a] The results reveal many educational opportunities for intervention by community nutrition professionals and others. For example, although many mothers were aware of the basic food groups, only 34 to 43 percent could correctly name the food groups and greater than two thirds were interested in learning more about nutrition. Mothers in transitional housing indicated a need for transportation to stores. In North Carolina, a number of focus groups were conducted with participants of private nonprofit agencies providing assistance to poor families. The participants provided many insights about their experiences and suggested ways to reform existing programs to better serve clients' needs. Figure 12.4 summarized their perceived barriers to participation in public and/or private assistance programs and suggestions for improvement.[8a] They report that rules are limiting and discouraging. For example, homeless people are unable to participate in programs that require evidence of a mailing address.

A lesson from listening to clients is the importance of considering the environment of emergency feeding programs to reduce dehumanizing aspects that often characterize these programs such as long lines, noise, confusion, impersonal service, and discouraging rules. Increasing opportunities for participants to be involved in menu planning and food preparation can improve mealtime comfort and affirm the worth of individuals and families who are facing economic and personal crises.

Understanding how to help clients access programs available to them is an important role for the nutrition professional. Many clients become frustrated at the complexities of the system and need the support of a professional counselor in accessing food assistance and other needed services.[8a]

AIDS AND HIV

The first reported case of acquired immunodeficiency syndrome (AIDS) occurred in 1981. From that time through December 1995, there have been 513,486 persons with AIDS among all age groups according to the Centers for Disease Control. AIDS is the second leading cause of death among men twenty-five to forty-four years of age and is one of the leading causes of death among women fifteen to forty-four years of age in the

Barriers	Suggestions
Program policies Discouraging rules • Eligibility criteria • Income calculations • Overwhelming application process	Encouraging rules • Develop work transition period • Change in benefit distribution schedule • Use real net income
Program benefits Marginal value • Benefits unrealistic for needs • Benefits offset by time required • Poor quality food provided	Client independence • Offer budgeting/nutrition classes to parents through schools • Provide training and job placement
Program procedures Stigma and low morale • Poverty stigma • Treatment by staff • Agency hours of operation • Efficiency of program staff	User friendly • Train agency staff in customer service • Provide transportation alternatives • Extend service hours • Advertise services

FIGURE 12.4   Perceived Barriers to Participation in Public/Private Assistance Programs and Suggestions for Improvement
(*Source:* From Dodds JM, Ahluwalia I, Baligh M: Experiences of families using food assistance and welfare programs in North Carolina: perceived barriers and recommendations for improvement. *J Nutr Educ;* 28:101–108, 1996. Reprinted with permission.)

United States.[11a] Human immunodeficiency virus (HIV) is transmitted from infected individuals to others through blood transfusions, sharing needles used for injecting drugs, and sexual contacts.

AIDS is the most serious clinical consequence of HIV infection. From a simplistic standpoint, the HIV virion infects cells of the immune system, especially the T helper cells. When these cells are infected they can't respond normally to infectious agents and people become sick. AIDS affects all population groups and is an emerging problem in children born to mothers who are infected with HIV. An HIV-infected woman can transmit HIV to the infant in utero, during labor through secretions in the birth canal, or after birth during breastfeeding (the last method of transmission is rare).

Management of the disease requires antiviral therapy, treatment of complications, prevention of secondary infections, immunologic enhancement, nutritional support, and psychosocial support. In most clinical practices, women with HIV infection are advised to bottle-feed rather than breast-feed their infants; however, there has been recent research disputing the danger of breast-feeding.[2a] For the infant, the appearance of symptoms such as failure to thrive, repeated infections, and chronic diarrhea should be considered clinical indicators of HIV infection.

In both children and adults with HIV/AIDS, malnutrition can occur due to inadequate nutrient intake or utilization to meet physiologic requirements for the maintenance of life and the growth and repair of tissue. Weight gain becomes difficult to achieve in infants and weight loss a problem in adults. Weight loss can be profound and accompanied by chronic diarrhea or chronic weakness and fever.

Treatment programs are aimed at nutrition assessment and intervention for the nutritional problems identified. Some of the usual problems that can be found in individuals with AIDS are loss of appetite, malabsorption, and increased losses of nutrients caused by diarrhea, vomiting, gastrointestinal bleeding, increased resting energy expenditure, and protein-losing enteropathy. Finding the best treatment is difficult when anorexia is present and severe. Appetite enhancers may be used along with supplemental feedings, and sometimes parenteral nutrition and medications to reduce stool loss. It naturally follows that the physical and emotional needs of the infected child or adult and other family members require continuous support. Sanitation is also considered important in the nutritional management of an individual with AIDS to prevent infection from foodborne illnesses. Additional Meals on Wheels programs have been initiated in at least seventeen cities in the

BOX 12.4

NUTRITION CARE IN HIV/AIDS

HIV AND AIDS—WITHOUT ACTIVE INTERCURRENT INFECTIONS

- Complete a nutrition assessment and repeat every three months.
- Monitor calorie and protein consumption; adjust eating pattern to improve intake, if needed.
- Educate about nutritional needs and safe food handling and preparation to avoid food-borne illness.
- Supplement vitamin and mineral intake.
- Monitor weight (or lean body mass) monthly. Respond aggressively to any weight loss; address anorexia and consider food supplements and appetite stimulants.
- Follow albumin and triglyceride levels at each medical visit or lab draw (at a minimum, every three months).

AIDS—PRESENCE OF WASTING NOTED

- Closely monitor weight and lean body mass.
- Follow albumin and triglycerides. Consider testing prealbumin, transferrin, or total iron binding capacity, to monitor immediate status during periods of active wasting.

- Address anorexia aggressively, using appetite stimulants and medical foods as supplements. Provide assistance if food or money is not available.
- Provide nutritional guidelines to assist with control of mouth, throat, or abdominal pain, and to control diarrhea.
- Consider malabsorption as a contributing factor to diarrhea; if present, counter with special medical foods designed for such cases. Start early; don't wait for wasting to progress.
- If wasting does not respond to oral supplements, consider a course of total parenteral nutrition (TPN) until the underlying cause of wasting can be found and treated.
- Maintain some oral intake whenever possible, even if TPN is provided, to help preserve gut wall integrity.
- Supplement vitamin and mineral intake.
- Monitor for B_{12}, folate, and magnesium deficiency; supplement if needed.

Source: Adapted from Romeyn M: *Nutrition and HIV: a new model for treatment,* San Francisco, 1995, Jossey-Bass.

United States to deliver nutritious meals that are appropriate in calories and meet food safety standards. Psychological support must prepare the individual and family for death. Box 12.4 outlines the nutrition care of individuals with HIV/AIDS.

TUBERCULOUS

Tuberculosis (TB) although once thought to be headed for elimination in the United States, has surged back in a new and more dangerous form. The return of this historically debilitating disease has been accelerated by homelessness and the spread of HIV; the overlap in epidemics had greatly complicated efforts to control both diseases. New strains of tuberculosis are resistant to many drugs, which complicates treatment.

The main reason that drug-resistant strains develop is that patients fail to complete full treatment. Organisms that survived the initial doses then proliferate in the body and, in turn, infect others. Such failures are understandable. Clients with TB must take three or four drugs daily or twice a week for nine months or

more, long after they are feeling well and have little incentive to continue. Educating the client to the necessity of continuing to take the medication for a long period of time can be difficult since often the client is very low income, homeless, mentally ill, or addicted to drugs.

Tuberculosis has been exacerbated by HIV, because of the weakened immune system in HIV-infected people. In New York City, reportedly 25 to 50 percent of all individuals with TB were infected with the HIV virus, and drug-resistant strains are heavily concentrated in the AIDS population.

In *Healthy People 2000,* the goal is set to increase to at least 90 percent the proportion of local health departments that have ongoing programs for actively identifying cases of tuberculosis and latent infection in populations at high risk.[14] People at high risk include recent contacts of infectious cases, foreign-born persons from high-prevalence areas, high-risk minority populations, migrant workers, and people in nursing homes and correctional institutions in addition to individuals with AIDS and the homeless.

LITERACY

Consideration of an individual's ability to read is extremely important. Reaching some of the special populations this chapter and other chapters have discussed requires consideration of their level of **literacy.** Nutrition education is challenging because approximately 20 percent of the U.S. population read at the fifth-grade level or lower. Increasing numbers of non-English-speaking persons are being served in public health programs and require bilingual staff who can translate information into their clients' languages.

Some of the clues that an individual can't read or write include excuses that glasses are broken, complaining of their hand being hurt, never offering anything in writing, and never referring to written notes or writing them. There are many other clues, but nutrition professionals who work with low-income families should always be sensitive to the possibility of illiteracy. This, of course, means that education materials should be developed so that a reader can grasp a concept in one glance and visuals must accompany the written material. The wording next to the visual should also be readable. Additional educational tools that can be used with individuals with limited reading abilities are videotapes or audiotapes, followed by one-on-one counseling and education using food models and demonstration. Although some educators have used games, in a study recently completed in California, none of the participants in the focus groups named games as an activity they liked.[13a]

IMPLICATIONS FOR COMMUNITY NUTRITION PROFESSIONALS

Increasing numbers of clients with special needs are an important subpopulation in the community. Because some are hidden or silent and generally lack resources and ability to voice their needs and seek service, the community nutrition professional must be alert to their presence. Although numbers of this subpopulation were once cared for in institutions, residential facilities, and hospitals, the service philosophy for today and into the next century is family-centered, community-based, coordinated, and culturally competent. As a result, public health programs will be challenged to become players in providing coordinated nutrition and health care services and case management at the community level. Whether she or he is in a public health department, a Title V agency, or a home health agency, this collaboration with other professionals as team members or consultants increases the

community nutrition professional's responsibility. Communication should utilize all available technology, and specialized training is available through centers in the United States funded by the Maternal and Child Health Bureau and the Administration on Developmental Disabilities. Community nutrition professionals are challenged to determine the availability and adequacy of services in the community for clients with special needs, including those individuals with AIDS, tuberculosis, and substance abuse and those suffering from poverty, hunger, and homelessness. The major responsibility now and in the future is for the community nutrition professional to be an advocate for special needs populations.

COMMUNITY NUTRITION PROFESSIONALS IN ACTION

- In September you receive an urgent call from the school food service director. She says she has a new student in school who has PKU. As the nutritionist at the local health department, what advice will you give her?
- Visit an Early Intervention program serving infants and young children with special needs. Observe staff interactions with children and families. Interview staff about their training and work. What evidence do you see of family-centered, community-based, culturally competent services? What kinds of knowledge and skills are needed to work effectively with special needs children and their families?
- Attend a team meeting where the individualized plan of a client is being established or updated. Who are all the people present at the team meeting? What parts of the plan involve coordination with services or providers in the community? To what degree do nutrition issues receive attention?
- Volunteer to work at a meals program or shelter for the homeless. Visit with clients. In what ways are they like you? How are they different?
- Create a directory of services for families experiencing food insecurity.

GOING ONE STEP FURTHER

- Survey all Early Intervention (EI) programs in your community. Collect copies of screening and assessment tools used. What criteria are used to identify children who should be referred to a nutritionist? Determine the availability of direct nutrition services or consultation. (To obtain a list of EI programs, contact the education or public health agency in your community designated as a part H provider of PL 99-457.)

- Compare and contrast the systems for providing nutrition services to children with special health care needs in at least three states. Explore historical, political, funding, and other reasons for the development of different systems of care for special populations.
- How would you investigate the extent of hunger in your community? What different methods could be used to measure reduced diet quality, adaptive food-management coping behaviors, and the actual hunger of children and adults?
- Determine the prevalence and incidence of HIV/AIDS by age group in your community. Are appropriate nutrition education and counseling services available to this population?

ADDITIONAL INFORMATION

A reference guide for assessment, intervention, and management of nutrition care for children with special health care needs is available.

Isaacs JS, Cialone J, Horsley JW, Holland M, Murray P, Nardella M: Children with special health care needs: A community nutrition pocket guide. Chicago: Dietetics in Developmental and Psychiatric Disorders and the Pediatric Nutrition Practice Group of The American Dietetic Associaton and Ross Products Division Abbott Laboratories, August, 1997.

The American Dietetic Association has a number of position papers related to the topics of this chapter. These include

1. Nutrition services for children with special health care needs, *J Am Diet Assoc* 95:809, 1995.
2. Nutrition in comprehensive program planning for persons with developmental disabilities, *J Am Diet Assoc* 97:189, 1997.
3. Domestic food and nutrition security, *J Am Diet Assoc* 98:337, 1998.
4. Nutrition intervention in the care of persons with human immunodeficiency virus infection, *J Am Diet Assoc* 94:1042, 1994.

For current information on food security and the assessment of hunger contact:
The Center on Hunger, Poverty & Nutrition Policy
Tufts University School of Nutrition
11 Curtis Avenue
Medford, MA 02155

REFERENCES

1. Baer MT, Farnan S, Mauer AM: *Children with special health care needs.* In: Sharbaugh CO, editor: *Call to action: better nutrition for mothers, children and families,* Washington, DC, 1991, National Center for Education in Maternal and Child Health, pp. 191–208.
2. Bandini LG, Schneller DA, Fukagana NK, Wykes L, Dietz WH: Body composition and energy expenditures in adolescents with cerebral palsy or myelodysplasia, *Pediatr Res* 29:70, 1991.
2a. Black RF: The transmission of HIV-1 in the breast feeding process, *J Am Diet Assoc* 96:267, 1996.
3. Boyne LJ, Heitlinger LA: *Gastrointestinal disorders.* In Queen PM, Lang C, editors: *Handbook of pediatric nutrition,* Gaithersburg, MD, 1993, Aspen.
4. Cloud H: *Feeding problems for children with developmental disorders.* In Ekvall SW, editor: *Pediatric nutrition for chronic disease & developmental disabilities,* New York, 1993, Oxford Press.
5. Cloud HH: Impact of legislation on nutrition services for individuals with developmental disabilities, *Top Clin Nutr* 8(4):1–4, 1993.
6. Cloud HH: Position paper on nutrition in comprehensive program planning for persons with developmental disabilities, *J Am Diet Assoc* 97:189, 1997.
7. Cronk C et al: Growth charts for children with Down syndrome, 1 month to 18 years, *Pediatrics* 81:102, 1988.
8. Developmental Disabilities Assistance and Bill of Rights Act, PL 95-602, 1978, No. 503, No. 102.
8a. Dodds JM, Ahluwalia I, Baligh M: Experiences of families using food assistance and welfare programs in North Carolina: perceived barriers and recommendations for improvement, *J Nutr Educ* 28:101–108, 1996.
9. Egan M: *Nutrition services in the Maternal & Child Health programs: a historical perspective.* In Sharbough CO, editor: *Call to action: better nutrition for mothers, children & families,* 1991, Washington, DC, National Center for Maternal & Child Health.
10. Ekvall SW, Ekvall VK, Frazier T: Dealing with nutrition problems of children with developmental disorders, *Top Clin Nutr* 8:50, 1993.
11. Elsas LJ, Acosta PB: *Nutrition support of inherited metabolic disease.* In Shils M, Young V, editors: *Modern nutrition in health & disease,* ed 7, Philadelphia, 1988, Lea & Febiger.
11a. Gallagher LM, Evans S, Swaba ME: *Pediatric acquired immune deficiency syndrome.* In Queen PM, Lang C, editors: *Handbook of pediatric nutrition,* Gaithersburg, MD, 1993, Aspen.
12. Guthrie R, Susi A: A simple phenylalanine method for detecting phenylketonuria in large populations of newborn infants, *Pediatrics* 32:333, 1963.

13. Hamill PV, Drizd TA, Johnson CL: Physical growth: National Center for Health Statistics percentiles, *Am J Clin Nutr* 32:607, 1979.

13a. Hartmann TJ, McCarthy PR, Park RJ, Schuster E, Kushi LH: Focus group responses to potential participants in nutrition education program for individuals with limited literacy skills, *J Am Diet Assoc* 94:749, 1994.

14. *Healthy Children 2000,* DHHS Pub. No. HRSA-M-CH 91-2, Washington, DC, 1991, U.S. Department of Health and Human Services, Public Health Service, Health Resources and Services Administration, Maternal and Child Health Bureau.

15. Isaacs J: Nutritional care for the gastrostomy fed child with neurological impairments, *Top Clin Nutr* 8:24, 1993.

16. Isaacs J, Cialone J, Horsely J, Hollan M, Murray P, Nardella M: *Children with special health care needs: a community nutrition pocket guide,* Chicago, 1997, Developmental Disabilities and Psychiatric Disorders Practice Group and Pediatric Nutrition Practice Group of the American Dietetic Association.

17. Jaskuluski TM, Lakin KC, Zierman SA: *The journey to inclusion. A resource guide for state policymakers,* President's Committee on Mental Retardation, Administration for Children and Families, Washington, DC, 1995, U.S. Department of Health and Human Services.

18. Johnson RK, Goran MI, Ferrara MS, Poehlman ET: Athetosis increases resting metabolic rate in adults with cerebral palsy, *J Am Diet Assoc* 96:145, 1996.

18a. Kaufman M: *Reaching out to those in highest risk.* In Kaufman M, editor: *Handbook for public health nutrition,* Gaithersburg, MD, 1990, Aspen.

19. Kowzlowski BW, Powell JA: Position of the American Dietetic Association, nutrition services for children with special health care needs, *J Am Diet Assoc* 95:809, 1995.

20. Lichtenwalter L, Freeman R, Lee M, Cialone J: Providing nutrition services to children with special needs in a community setting, *Top Clin Nutr* 8:75, 1993.

21. Luke A, Rozier JN, Sutton M, Schoeller DA: Energy expenditure in children with Down syndrome. Correcting metabolic rate for movement, *J Pediatr* 125:829, 1994.

22. *Mental retardation, definition, classification & systems of supports,* ed 9, Washington, DC, 1992, American Association of Mental Retardation.

23. *National agenda for children with special health care needs: achieving the year 2000,* Washington, DC, 1995, U.S. Department of Health and Human Services, Public Health Service, Maternal and Child Health Bureau.

23a. Nestle M, Guttmacher S: Hunger in the United States: rationale, methods and policy implications of state hunger surveys, *J Nutr Educ* 24(Suppl 1):18S–22S, 1992.

23b. Paul LC: Impact of nutrition-related coalitions on welfare reform and food security in a rural state, *J Nutr Educ* 28(2):119–122, 1996.

24. Posthauer ME et al, editors: *Critical criteria and indicators for nutrition services in developmental disabilities, psychiatric disorders and substance abuse,* Chicago, 1993, American Dietetic Association.

25. Roe D: *Handbook of drug nutrient interaction* 4, Chicago, 1989, The American Dietetic Association.

25a. Rose D, Basiotis PP, Klein BW: Improving federal efforts to assess hunger and food insecurity, *Food Review* 18(1):18–23, 1995.

26. Scherenberger RD: *Formative years.* In *A history of mental retardation,* Baltimore, MD, 1983, Paul Brookes Publishing.

27. Smith MH: Nutrition assessment for persons with developmental disorders, *Top Clin Nutr* 8:7, 1993.

27a. Taylor ML, Koblinsky SA: Food composition and eating behavior of homeless preschool children, *J Nutr Educ* 26(1):20–25, 1994.

27b. U.S. Conference of Mayors: *A status survey on hunger and homelessness in America's cities: 1990. A 30 city survey,* Washington, DC, 1990, Conference of Mayors.

28. Woolridge N: *Pulmonary diseases.* In Queen PM, Lang CE, editors: *Handbook of pediatric nutrition,* Gaithersburg, MD, 1993, Aspen.

29. Woolridge NH, et al, editors: *Quality assurance criteria for pediatric nutrition conditions: a model,* Chicago, 1993, American Dietetic Association.

CASE STUDY

GOING THE DISTANCE—LINKING THE SPECIALTY CLINIC WITH COMMUNITY-BASED SERVICES

This case study described a small boy with a rare inborn error of metabolism who lives in a small town in Alabama. The family involved is Hispanic, low income, and non-English speaking. Although the family is enrolled in the WIC program, the case study illustrates the need for coordination of follow-up and location of services in the community.

TEACHING OBJECTIVES

The main questions raised in this case study have to do with understanding the metabolic disorder, the linkages between the specialty center and the community, and the special formula needed. The case study also raises the question of how to communicate with a non-English-speaking family on food selection and meal planning for a protein-restricted diet.

This material can be used for class discussion or a homework assignment and can include the literacy issues of translating the foods allowed on the diet into Spanish or finding and using pictures or food models.

THE CASE

F.M. is a seventeen-month-old male child born in California after his parents emigrated from Mexico. The family moved from California to a small Alabama town, 150 miles from Birmingham, where they had relatives and job possibilities. At fifteen months of age he was diagnosed with citrullinemia, an inborn error of metabolism that involves the urea cycle.

Dietary management of citrullinemia requires that the child replace milk with a special formula, lower in protein then regular formula or cow's milk, eat a low-protein diet, and be supplemented with arginine and butyrate. The formula chosen was Cyclinex, providing 8.5 g of protein with the remainder of his protein coming from food, for a total of 18 g of protein, and 1,500 calories. His treatment was started in the Children's Hospital in Birmingham, Alabama, and the parents were instructed using a translator.

F.M. received his formula through the WIC program and his medication from Medicaid. The nutrition professional at the Decatur Health Department was contacted prior to his discharge from the hospital. She, in turn, located a Spanish-speaking person to serve as a translator for the family. The hospital social worker contacted the Department of Human Resources to provide home visits related to financial problems. With her help, the family obtained Food Stamps, and eventually the father found employment in a poultry processing plant.

F.M. was also referred to the Inborn Errors Clinic at Sparks Clinic in Birmingham. Sparks is a training center for graduate students in the field of neurodevelopmental disorders and houses the inborn errors clinic. He was to be followed on a monthly basis until his condition was stable and then every six months. Transportation has been a problem for this family, so efforts were made to have his dietary management monitored in the public health clinic enabling the frequency of visits to Birmingham to be decreased. Because both parents will eventually need to work, efforts are being made to identify a day-care center that can serve a low-protein diet and communicate with the parents in Spanish.

QUESTIONS

1. Identify the nutritional risk factors that may be associated with F.M.'s disorder.
2. As a community nutrition professional, what would be the minimal nutrition assessment components you would request to monitor F.M.'s nutritional status in the public health clinic?
3. Who would be the members of the "team" in the community? (That is, along with all other challenges, how could the language and communication problems be addressed?)
4. As the nutrition professional at the Decatur Health Department, what resources would you be able to contact to provide you with assistance?
5. Identify the services needed to handle such a complex case in a community-based program near the family.

PART THREE

CREATING THE FUTURE OF COMMUNITY NUTRITION
MANAGING TO MAKE A DIFFERENCE

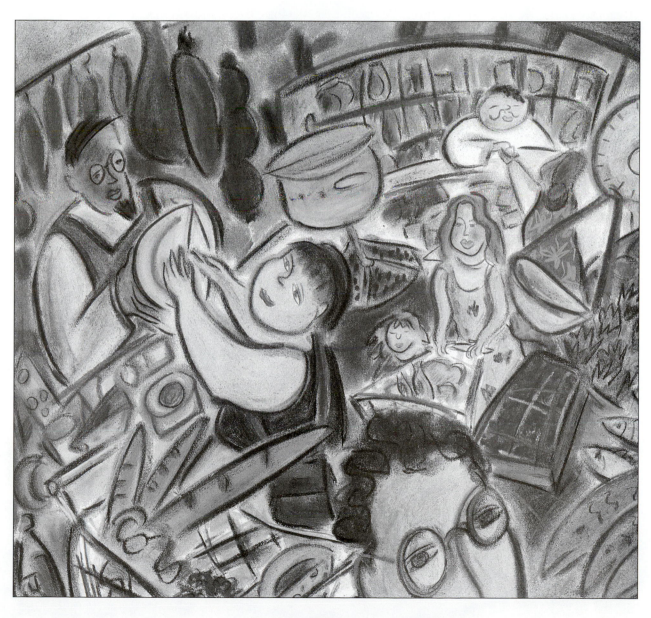

CHAPTER THIRTEEN

CREATING THE FUTURE THROUGH PLANNING

*The ultimate test of practical leadership is the realization
of intended, real change that meets people's enduring needs.*
—JAMES MACGREGOR BURNS

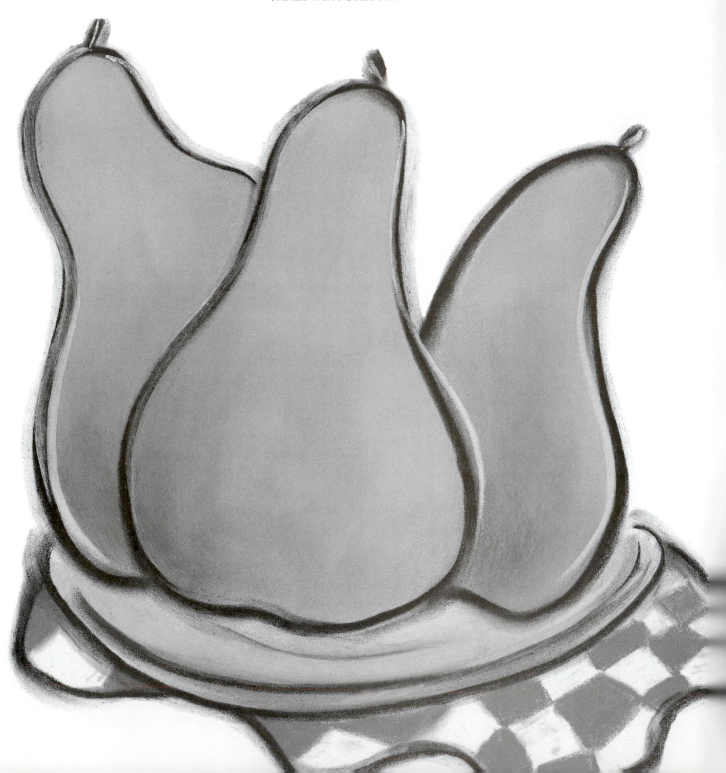

Core Concepts

Planning is a forward-looking process through which the uncertainty about the future is reduced and orderly action toward results is initiated. Planning occurs at all levels of the organization and includes strategic, program, and operational planning. Information from an environmental audit or a comprehensive community nutrition needs assessment guides strategic and program planning, respectively. Needs assessment is fundamental to comprehensive community nutrition planning. It provides information about the health and nutrition problems of the community, environmental and lifestyle factors, community values, and available resources in the organization and the rest of the community to meet nutrition needs. Complex, multifaceted problems require a systematic decision-making process for defining problems, determining priorities, setting criteria for a good decision, generating creative alternatives, and selecting alternatives using an evaluative process. Decisions about community problems are best made by those who are involved, including community members and program staff and collaborators. Goals and objectives give direction and set performance standards. Community nutrition professionals must exercise managerial and leadership roles and skills to successfully plan and direct programs that meet the nutritional needs of the community.

Objectives

When you finish chapter thirteen, you should be able to:

~ Describe the management process.

~ Differentiate between strategic planning, program planning, and operational planning.

~ Identify five areas essential to community needs assessment.

~ Define the steps of decision making.

~ Develop goals and objectives for a nutrition program.

~ Discuss management roles and skills.

~ Distinguish between the terms *leader* and *manager*.

Key Words

Word	Page Mentioned
Management	376
Management functions	377
Planning	377
Implementation	377
Evaluation	377
Strategic thinking	378
Mission	378
Strategic planning	378
Program planning	378
Operations planning	378
Strategic plan	379
Program plans	380
Planning process	382
Time horizon	382
Stakeholders	383
Environmental audit	383
SWOT analysis	383
Community nutrition needs assessment	384
Felt needs	385
Prescribed needs	385
Triangulation	385
Nominal group process	388
Inventory of resources	390
Prioritization	390
Decision-making process	391
Goal	396
Objectives	396
Process	397
Outcome	397
Structure	397
Manager	398
Leader	398

To promote optimum nutrition for all members of a community, community nutrition professionals must assure that comprehensive, community-based nutrition services are available and utilized. This requires knowledge of management processes as well as skill and confidence in applying those processes. A well-managed and coordinated system of effective nutrition services can produce a measurable impact on the health and well-being of the community. Figure 13.1 illustrates the functions of management and the types of planning that create and support an efficient and effective system of nutrition services.

THE MANAGEMENT PROCESS

Management has been called "the art of getting things done through people."[21] When community nutrition professionals plan and organize work and coordinate and direct the actions of others so that organizational

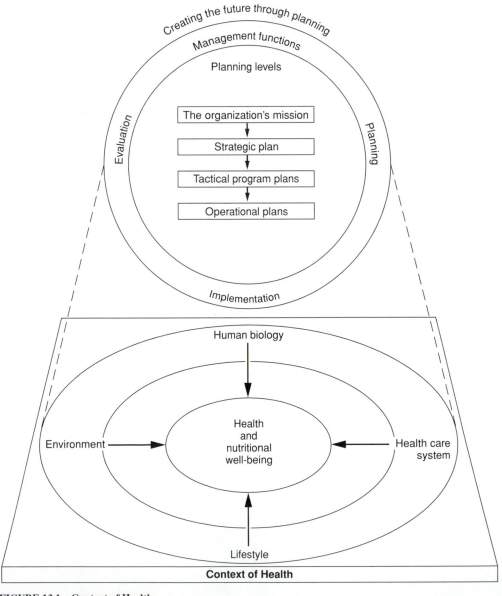

FIGURE 13.1   Context of Health
Planning to improve health and nutritional well-being.

and program goals and objectives can be accomplished, they are being managers.

Traditionally, **management functions** have been described as planning, organizing, directing, and controlling.[28] Through planning the overall purpose or mission is clarified and goals and objectives are specified. In the planning phase decisions are made about "what to do." Organizing involves defining "how" the goals and objectives will be accomplished by dividing work into particular jobs, defining relationships among workers, and assigning activities (expanded in chapter 14). Organizing also includes determining necessary resources and budgeting (described in chapter 16). The directing function includes the range of interpersonal activities ("people skills") used to lead, motivate, and facilitate productive work by all those associated with the program. In today's environment, where multiple agencies and organizations work together on nutrition interventions, a community nutrition manager frequently does not have direct authority over the work of other collaborators; thus skills of facilitation and collaboration are needed. These collaboration skills are described in the next chapter. The last function of management is control, or more commonly, evaluation. This function reflects the managers responsibility for monitoring "how well" work is being accomplished and then taking corrective action as needed. Control is accomplished by setting performance standards and routinely monitoring activities so that deviations can be detected quickly and continuous improvements made. Evaluation is addressed in chapter 15. These management functions assure high-quality, efficient program operations that lead to accomplishment of organizational and program goals and objectives and ultimately to positive impact on the nutritional well-being and health of people.

The management functions are frequently condensed into **planning, implementation, and evaluation**—decide what to do, do it in ways that meet the needs of clients and the capacity your staff and other collaborators, and monitor progress and outcomes. Budgeting and funding issues are integral throughout. All of these processes overlap and interact. The chapters of this section of the text explore these topics as they relate to the management of community nutrition services.

Management in Community Nutrition

In chapter 2, assessment, policy development, and assurance were defined as the major functions of public health.[14] A close look at these terms reveals major management responsibilities.

1. *Assessment:* collect and interpret data on problems and causes, forecast trends, evaluate outcomes
2. *Policy development:* set priorities, provide policy leadership and advocacy, mobilize resources, build constituencies
3. *Assurance:* assure necessary personnel, educational, or environmental health services to reach set goals by encouraging or requiring action by other entities or by provision of services directly, and guarantee a minimum set of essential, high-priority health services

To achieve these functions community nutrition professionals must be actively engaged in a range of management-related activities listed in box 13.1. By carrying out these responsibilities, community nutrition professionals will contribute to the mission of health: "The fulfillment of society's interests in assuring the conditions in which people can be healthy."[14]

This chapter and the following ones provide guidance to community nutrition professionals in their roles as strategic thinkers, planners of community nutrition programs, implementers, and evaluators. Community nutrition professionals must be able to create a vision of an ideal system of comprehensive nutrition services for all community members. They must bring this vision of a desired future to reality through the design and implementation of innovative community programs and interventions that address important and priority nutrition problems. Plans should define the roadmap for making a significant impact on modifiable nutrition risk factors and specify monitoring points for assessing achievement. Planning should lead to efficient, effective, and culturally- and age-appropriate nutrition programs. Finally, planning should stimulate coordination and collaboration across the food and nutrition and health care systems with a goal of efficient and effective nutrition programming.

This chapter presents the managerial and leadership roles of community nutrition professionals and elaborates the planning function. Planning levels are described and information-gathering approaches are presented followed by specific techniques used to prioritize problems and intervention alternatives. The chapter ends with a discussion of management and leadership.

PLANNING

Planning is an iterative process of forward-looking activities through which the uncertainty about the future is reduced and orderly action toward results is initiated. Planning is often the starting point in the management process. It results in a vision of the future, a mission, goals and objectives, and program action plans to reach the desired future. Planning establishes commitments, focuses and directs effort, relates resources to desired goals, and sets benchmarks or performance indicators in the form of measurable objectives for evaluation. Good planning produces programs that are aligned with community values and needs and with the organization's mission and mandates.

Strategic Thinking

Strategic thinking is a future-oriented and action-oriented process through which change is anticipated and initiated. Good planners are strategic thinkers. They can see the big picture and turn the organization in the direction where it can make important contributions. Successful strategists consider a range of internal and external issues, trends and opportunities; create a vision of a desirable future state; and establish a commitment to a course of action to bring their vision to reality. This requires information about patterns, relationships, and linkages and leads to a plan for how to achieve the vision over a period of time. A well-formulated strategy builds on an organization's distinctive competence and guides the organization into the future. Strategic thinking is a necessary ingredient in planning for community nutrition efforts.

Levels of Planning

Plans are made at many times for many purposes and all levels of the organization are involved. At the top level of the organization, an overall **mission** is determined that provides a framework for all programs and initiatives for three to five or more years. Programs and departments also periodically do comprehensive planning to spell out major strategies for a number of years into the future. These are examples of **strategic planning.** Once overall mission and strategy have been determined more specific plans are developed for separate programs, projects, and initiatives. This is called tactical or **program planning.** Strategic and program planning are discussed in this chapter. **Operations planning,** that focuses on details within projects and day-to-day activities, leads to *operational plans* or *action steps.* Specific action steps are important to successful implementation, which is discussed in the next chapter. Figure 13.2 illustrates the levels of planning

BOX 13.1

ACTIVITIES ESSENTIAL FOR DEVELOPMENT OF COMPREHENSIVE, COMMUNITY-BASED NUTRITION SERVICES

- Assess the nutritional status of specific populations
- Initiate and participate in nutrition data collection
- Identify target populations that may be at nutrition risk
- Provide leadership in the development of and planning for health and nutrition policies and programs
- Recommend and provide specific training and programs to meet identified nutrition needs
- Raise awareness among key policy makers of the potential impact of nutrition services, regulations, and budget decisions on the health of the community
- Act as an advocate for target populations on food and nutrition issues
- Plan for nutrition services in conjunction with other health services, based on information obtained from an adequate and on-going database focused on health outcomes
- Identify and assist in development of accurate, up-to-date nutrition education materials and resources
- Ensure the availability of quality nutrition services to target populations, including nutrition screening, assessment, education, counseling, referral for food assistance and other services, and follow-up
- Provide community health promotion and disease prevention activities that are population based
- Participate in demonstration and evaluation projects and nutrition research
- Provide expert consultation to community groups
- Provide quality assurance guidelines for practitioners who conduct nutrition services and deal with food and nutrition issues
- Facilitate coordination with other providers of health and nutrition services within the community
- Evaluate the impact of nutrition services on the health status of populations who receive community nutrition services

---

Source: Adapted from Probert.[25]

and table 13.1 gives examples of types of mission, goal, or objective statements established at each level of planning. These statements express commitment to achieve certain results at some point in the future. Goals and objectives, discussed later in this chapter, set specific performance targets.

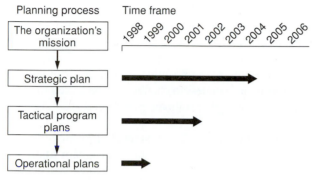

FIGURE 13.2   Planning Levels and Time Horizon

Strategic Planning   Strategic planning is "a disciplined effort to produce fundamental decisions and actions that shape and guide what and organizations (or other entity) is, what it does, and why it does it."[2] Strategic planning is the primary concern of the highest levels of the organization. It takes the long-term view and considers the entire organization and its relationship with the external environment including trends, customers, and competitors. Strategic planning requires internal and external information; and it requires introspection, courage, and risk-taking on the part of members of the organization. The essence of strategic planning is effectively relating the organization to its environment to ensure success. The process of strategic planning identifies strategic issues facing the organization and produces answers to the questions in box 13.2. After the organization as a whole has conducted strategic planning, major units within the organization build from this with a **strategic plan** for their department (e.g., a nutrition unit strategic plan). Through the strategic planning process organizations

TABLE 13.1
Levels of Planning and Examples of Mission, Goal, and Objectives

	Strategic planning
Vision	The nutrition unit will be recognized in the community and across the state for its leadership in addressing important food and nutrition issues that impact the quality of life of people in this region.
Strategy	The nutrition unit will keep food and nutrition issues before the public and propose innovative solutions to improve the health and nutritional well-being of all citizens by partnering with other agencies or providing programs directly.
Mission	The nutrition unit will assure the provision of high-quality food and nutrition services and programs that achieve and maintain optimal nutritional status for all members of the population through the development of a comprehensive, accessible, community-based system of nutrition-related services in collaboration with other providers in the community.

	Program planning
Problem priority	The nutrition unit should initiate and take leadership in a program of coordinated activities to assure availability of adequate health-promoting foods to homeless children.
Goal statement	To assure all children residing in temporary shelters have access to foods consistent with their nutritional and developmental needs.
Shelter project objective	By 2000, all temporary shelters housing children will, on a daily basis, serve foods that are consistent with children's nutritional and developmental needs.
Outcome objective	By 2000, 100% of children staying in temporary shelters will have access to meals and snacks consistent with their nutritional and developmental needs.
Process objective	By the end of the first project year, health department personnel will provide training and technical assistance about low-cost foods to meet children's nutritional and developmental needs to 100% of the temporary shelters housing children (up from 40% in 1996).
Structure objective	By eighteen months into the project, the four temporary shelters that house children and currently do not have hot meal service will install facilities for food storage, preparation, and service that meet city codes.
Intermediate objective	By 1999, 80% (up from 40% in 1997) of the temporary shelters housing children will serve hot or cold meals consistent with the children's nutritional and developmental needs.

BOX 13.2

QUESTIONS TO BE ANSWERED IN STRATEGIC PLANNING

MISSION

What business are we in?

What is our fundamental purpose or reason for being?

What types of products and services do we provide?

How do we define the customers we serve?

What unique value do we bring to our customers?

Do the answers help us understand *why* we do what we do?

STRATEGY

What will be the basic approach to achieving the mission?

What is the distinct competence or competitive advantage that will characterize our organizational or program success?

CULTURE

What should be the hallmarks of our organizational culture?

How should we treat each other and how should we work together?

What do we stand for?

What values do we hold dear?

In what ways is our organization a great place to work?

Source: Adapted from Lipton.[20]

- Examine the environment in which they operate
- Explore the factors and trends that affect the way they do business and carry out their roles
- Seek to meet their mandates and fulfill their mission
- Determine the strategic issues they must address
- Find ways to address these issues by reexamining and reworking organizational mandates and mission, strategies, culture, products, or services and cost and financing
- Create their own future[3]

Strategic planning is influenced by the internal culture and capabilities of the organization. It is also influenced by the public agenda, by the state of scientific knowledge, by the wants and needs of consumers, by the expectations of stakeholders, and by official posi-

tions of experts and professional groups. Hence, a challenge for community nutrition professionals in doing strategic planning is to balance objectivity and creativity while accommodating a wide range of competing interests.

Strategic planning leads to establishment, revision, or reaffirmation of the organization's mission, which guides action for a relatively long period. A strategic plan provides the basic framework or boundaries within which the organization operates. It includes specific strategies that define major priorities and give direction to program initiatives for a period of years. To be effective, strategic planning must be action-oriented, be done with an openness to change, and be linked to tactical (program) and operational planning.

Program Planning   The next level of planning is program planning or tactical planning. **Program plans** are for an intermediate time frame, two to three years. They follow from the strategic plan and incorporate the overall mission and strategy of the organization, but focus on a more narrowly defined area in greater detail.

Comprehensive nutrition program plans direct efforts to address priority nutrition-related problems or their causal factors using deliberate tactics. Nutrition program plans outline program initiatives that generally are maintained over a number of years; however, short-term demonstration projects or one-time programs may also be part of the overall nutrition program plan.

Nutrition program planning serves many purposes. It produces a statement of needs and nutrition-related priorities, identifies program priorities for greatest impact on important problems, describes programs and initiatives to be undertaken, outlines methods to be used, identifies target date for performance, assigns responsibility, and indicates resources available to conduct the program. The outcomes of planning include a sound justification for program decisions, coordinated efforts across programs, and program descriptions for fund raising.

Program plans address where, when, how, by whom, and with what resources. Table 13.2 illustrates a typical program planning worksheet. Planning teams for each program (e.g., WIC, health promotion, home health, etc.) in the nutrition unit complete these worksheets using input from evaluations and needs assessments. Then the worksheets are pulled together and coordinated to develop a comprehensive nutrition program plan.

TABLE 13.2
Program Planning Worksheet

Goal statement:

Program/project/initiative:

Objective (structure, process, outcome objectives)	Action/methods/activity	Timeline		Assigned responsibility or group	Evaluation	Resources needed
		Begin	End			

Program planning is usually tied to the budget cycle of the organization or funding source. Prior preparation is a must to assure necessary and sufficient information is available to enable good decisions about program methods and budget needs for the future period.

Operational Planning   Operational plans or action plans are narrowly focused and have a relatively short time horizon and involve personnel at the direct delivery level. These plans have a high degree of detail and guide day-to-day operations of nutrition programs and services. They address specifics such as nutrition assessment procedures, protocols for care delivery, or clinic staffing patterns. Operational plans are important to assure consistency and quality during implementation. They define and communicate performance expectations. Action plans are discussed further in the next chapter on implementation.

Planning Process

A number of resources are available to assist organizations with planning processes.[1,5,7,22,30] No matter what level planning is, the **planning process** includes a series of steps (box 13.3). The steps of the planning process are not necessarily conducted in a linear fashion. Cycling back as more information and insights are gained leads to greater exploration of issues and alternatives, and ultimately to a better plan.

Anticipating Barriers   Planning does not unfold smoothly and systematically. A number of potential barriers should be recognized and addressed to enable effective planning.[2,11] The rapid pace of environmental and organizational change including health and social policy reform, reengineering, technological developments, and competition makes forecasting the future difficult. Many players in the planning effort and the organization may be reluctant to establish specific goals and objectives for themselves and their area of responsibility, or they may lack the ability or information to set reasonable goals. Another common barrier is resistance to change. Since planning usually leads to change, fear of the unknown can be a barrier. A number of constraints such as lack of trained personnel, financial resources, physical facilities, government regulations, and relevant information limit what an organization can feasibly do. Because good planning is time consuming, it may be inappropriately delayed while waiting for the time and resources to do it properly.

STEPS OF A PLANNING PROCESS

1. Define the planning task: level and purpose of the planning effort; who to involve on the planning team.
2. Gather relevant information for planning:
   a. Identify internal and external stakeholders and their expectations of the organization or program.
   b. Clarify mandates—compile a list of formal and informal mandates and values, review the existing mission.
   c. Collect new information:
      Strategic planning—carry out an environmental audit.
      Program planning—conduct a community needs assessment.
      Intervention planning—do market research.
3. Identify key issues, needs, and opportunities based on information.
4. Determine which issues are within your scope and responsibility to address; and which ones you have to work around.
5. Identify strategy, goals, objectives, and/or action alternatives.
6. Evaluate alternatives and select.
7. Write and communicate the plan.

These barriers can be overcome by starting at the top of the organization to get support for planning efforts, recognizing the limits to planning and keeping the planning task within a reasonable scope, and accepting that planning is an iterative process that is begun and refined in successive planning cycles. Open communication and involvement of key players in the planning process assures good input and reduces fears about the process and its outcomes. When uncertainty about future conditions is high, a short-term contingency planning can be used to prepare for unusual events, a turn of circumstances, or as a transition into larger changes later.

Community nutrition professionals must treat planning as a critical priority and devote requisite time, attention, and resources to planning efforts at all levels.

Defining the Planning Task   The planning task is determined by the organizational level of the planning effort, time horizon, and nature of the commitment. **Time horizon** is the period allowed for impact of the plan to be felt. Commitment is the description of the product of the planning effort. The definition of the commitment is related to the time horizon and is derived from a relevant information base. For example, organizational goals express long-term commitments that are within the boundaries defined by the mission statement. These goals subsequently provide direction for intermediate and short-term programs and interventions. Thus, shorter-term plans evolve from longer-term commitments. (Note how this was illustrated in figure 13.2 and table 13.1.)

Different information is needed at each planning level and depends on the purpose of the planning effort. Many approaches for gathering and interpreting information for planning purposes exist. Two approaches presented in this chapter are the environmental audit and the community nutrition needs assessment. Market research was mentioned in chapter 7 and is further described in chapter 14.

Who to Involve in the Planning Process   Planning is a responsibility that goes beyond administrators and program managers. The planning process is strengthened by involving others, especially those who will be responsible for implementation and those who will receive the program.[10] Open planning processes help to accommodate different interests and values, foster informed decision making, and enable development of realistic goals and objectives and feasible implementation plans.

Planning bound by the old rules cannot yield new strategy. New strategy requires imagination.[13] To accomplish this Hamel recommends opening up discussion of strategy to many people, especially those that are younger and older and are not bound by the status quo. In determining the planning task, planners should make conscious decisions about what internal and external constituencies (e.g., stakeholders) to involve at each stage of the process. Involvement of a wide range of people in the planning process opens the process up to creative ideas that break from the status quo.

Involvement in planning also provides valuable opportunities for professional growth and team building. Through an open planning process, the organization can produce successful plans that respond to the changing environment while effectively building a functioning team. Planning for high-priority nutrition problems can also be improved by forming alliances with related constituencies in the service network. Collaborative planning by providers, advocates, and adversarial groups helps to assure that limited resources will be used efficiently. The topic of collaboration is expanded in chapter 14.

INFORMATION FOR PLANNING

Although there is great overlap in the types of information and methods of data gathering used at each level of planning, in general, strategic planners conduct an environmental audit and program planners conduct a community needs assessment. However, most planning begins with a review of mandates and an analysis of **stakeholders.** In stakeholder analysis, all persons and organizations who have a stake or interest in the operation and outcomes of your organization or program are identified including supporters, critics, customers and clients, collaborators, regulators, funders, and the like. After the list is generated, their values, perceptions and expectations are identified.

Environmental Audit

The **environmental audit** involves a comprehensive examination of trends and forces in the environment and consideration of their possible effects on the organization or program. A method for doing this is the **SWOT analysis** in which information about internal *strengths* and *weaknesses* and external *opportunities* and *threats* is gathered and interpreted. The internal assessment objectively evaluates resources (people, facilities, etc.), competencies, and culture of the organization; the effectiveness of the current mission and strategy; and indicators of past performance. The external assessment includes exploration of political, economic, social, educational, and technological forces and trends, along with demographic and epidemiological data. It also considers expectations of key resource controllers such as funders, clients, and regulators, and competitive and collaborative forces in the environment. New data is gathered and existing reports and data sources are reviewed. The planning team organizes and interprets the information using a system such as that illustrated in table 13.3. The interpretation of all the data results in a list of important trends and issues and their implications for the organization. From this planners determine major strategies to achieve their desired future. Note that the environmental audit includes nutrition and health issues but it goes well beyond to explore unfolding political, social and technological and other forces that could influence the mission, strategy, goals, and operations of the organization in the future. Throughout and by the end of the strategic planning process, the answers should be determined to the list of questions in box 13.2.

Planning at all levels is strengthened and informed by good strategic planning. All units of the organization can refer to elements of the environmental audit and the resulting strategic plan for guidance in program-level planning.

Community Needs Assessment

The next level of planning is program planning. It draws on information from the environmental audit but focuses on issues and trends that impact nutrition-related factors. In general, a community needs assessment guides program development. A comprehensive **community nutrition needs assessment** is a sophisticated type of needs assessment used by major nutrition units to understand the nutrition needs of the community, prioritize them, and then target efforts accordingly.

Nutrition problems originate from complex interrelationships between lifestyle, environment, human biology, and health and nutrition services. To develop comprehensive nutrition plans, it is necessary to fully understand the interplay of these factors with the community's values and perceived needs. The goal of a community nutrition needs assessment is to obtain quantitative and qualitative information to identify nutrition-related problems, their causal factors, and opportunities for reducing those problems and factors. A thorough needs assessment requires interaction with the community and target groups to understand their values and behaviors, their perception of needs, and their feelings about acceptable interventions. From this vantage point, an interpretation or "diagnosis" of the nutrition problems can be made, and community interest and support can be fostered to engage the community's involvement in efforts to address the problems. But first, the community must be identified.

Most public health professionals understand the term *community* as a group of individuals or families living together within a defined geographic boundary. Community can also be defined as a political entity (city), a service area (multicounty community health services area), an organization (university community), a common interest (medical community), or an ethnic or cultural background (Hmong community). A needs assess-

TABLE 13.3
Environmental Audit: SWOT Worksheet

Fact, issue, trend, force	Strength/weakness/opportunity/threat	Implications for us
Internal assessment Consider resources (personnel, facilities, etc.), competencies, culture, effectiveness of current mission and strategy, and past performance		
External assessment Consider political, economic, social, educational, technological, and other trends and forces; demographics and epidemiological data; expectations		

Summary of major trends, issues or needs to be addressed now and in the future

Our strategy and goals for the next time period

ment may cover the entire community defined in any of these ways, or, in some situations, the needs assessment may be narrowed to a specific target group within the community, such as the elderly or children with special health care needs.

The result of a comprehensive community nutrition needs assessment is a report that

1. Describes nutrition-related problems that exist in a defined community
2. Indicates the perceived or **felt needs** of the community and its desire for a solution
3. Identifies resources available to deal with nutrition-related problems
4. Establishes priorities for nutrition programming

The needs assessment report customarily starts with demographic and socioeconomic data to describe the community and its subpopulations, followed by epidemiological data to describe indicators of health status. Indicators specific to nutritional or health status (e.g., low birthweight rate) are compared to an ideal, such as state or national objectives for health; and discrepancies are identified. Contributing conditions such as lifestyle factors or living situation are also identified as they provide important insight to opportunities for intervention.

Nutrition problems, however, cannot be solely described from the point of view of experts ("**prescribed needs**"). As illustrated in figure 13.3, professionals and community members have different perceptions of needs and solutions. The assessment must result in understanding of the community's perception of their needs and problem ("felt needs") as well as what they consider acceptable approaches to addressing the problems.

The report also enumerates available public and private programs and services and describes deficiencies and excesses in the capacity of the service system to address identified problems. Nutrition-related problems and service gaps are listed as priorities for action. The resulting priority areas should be consistent with the community's felt needs and address important public health problems.

Five Areas of a Community Nutrition Needs Assessment

A broad base of information is essential for comprehensive community nutrition planning. Five areas of information provide a foundation for determining nutrition-related health problems (see box 13.4). For each of the five areas of essential information, it is necessary to make choices on what types of information (data elements) to gather and the best methods to use. Common methods are listed in table 13.4.

Note the advantages and disadvantages of needs assessment methods listed in table 13.4. No single method or type of information will work in every situation. A range of information-gathering methods is used to discover and understand the nutrition problems and their causes and to discover the most acceptable and effective intervention options. Experts recommend **triangulation** of needs assessment methods and information sources, or getting more than one type of information to shed light on the factors related to problems and people's perceived needs. Triangulation is illustrated in figure 13.4. Using a range of methods leads to better understanding of the problem and potential ways to address the problem and its causes.

Assess the Mission and Capacity of Your Organization The focus of the nutrition needs assessment should be within the scope of the mission of

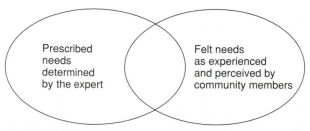

FIGURE 13.3
Two Views of the Problem: Prescribed Needs versus Felt Needs

BOX 13.4

FIVE AREAS OF INFORMATION ESSENTIAL FOR COMMUNITY NUTRITION NEEDS ASSESSMENT

1. Internal organizational mission and capacity and competency to address community needs
2. Community characteristics related to the nutrition and health status
3. Lifestyle and environmental factors
4. Community values and health expectations
5. Availability and appropriateness of health resources and food assistance and nutrition programs

TABLE 13.4

Methods of Collecting Needs Assessment Information

Approach	Description	Strengths	Limitations	Applications
Demographic inventory (census data)	Standard SES data	By census tract	Major census once in ten years	Characteristics of population
Vital health statistics (birth, death)	Standard health data at county or city level	Compare across time and locale	Two years old when available	Planning and evaluation
Health surveillance data (pregnancy and pediatric)	Regular monitoring of client population reports from CDC	Trends over time by clinic site	Questionable quality of submitted data, not representative of whole population	On-going monitoring
Nutrition status measures Growth (height, weight) Hemoglobin Serum cholesterol	Objective data from participants	Baseline and future outcome measures	Must be accurately collected and documented	Planning and evaluation
Dietary intake Food frequency questionnaire One-, three-, seven-day food record Twenty-four hour recall (in person or telephone) Food group checklist	Specific methods to determine quantity and quality of total diet, food group or nutrient intake	Data on nutrient shortfall or excess	Method used appropriately, time to analyze data	Identify specific dietary problems and practices
Survey (all types) Mailed Telephone	Standardized questions Written questionnaire Questions asked orally	Usually is quantified Reach many at once Informal, confidential, literacy not required	Can be costly to develop and analyze Costly, access to mailing list Reaches only people who have phones	Interests, values; current behaviors; consumer satisfaction
In person: at home, at program	Written or oral	Doesn't require literacy	Program survey misses views of unsatisfied clients	
National Nutrition Monitoring System	National data	National trends	Questionable application to local population	Identify potential risk areas
Review of literature Published program reports Scientific studies	Reported experience of others	Draws on proven approaches	Studied population may be different from yours	Apply scientific findings in design of programs
Interview/discussion (all types)	Qualitative data	Broad, rich views	Time consuming	Expand understanding of issues and values
Key informant interviews	Structure and/or open-ended, twenty to sixty minutes	In-depth understanding, build relationship	Can be biased if you include only those "friendly" to your cause	Community values and priorities
Focus group discussion	One to two hours, invited individuals, skilled moderator	Wide range of ideas and reactions	Time consuming to transcribe data; responses may be influenced by other group members	Designing new or revising programs, materials, or approaches
Community leadership analysis	Interview identified "leaders"	Learn power structure of community	Scheduling time with important people	Use when external support is important to success
Community Advisory Board	Ongoing group or purposefully selected representatives	They have understanding of program goals and community needs	May have own agenda	Wide range of input over time
Participant observation	Observe as member of community	Reality based	Observer must be culturally aware	Understand community practices
Inventory of resources	Directory of all nutrition-related services	Recognize referral network and partners to share challenges	May not address effectiveness or appropriate access	Identify service gaps and redundancy

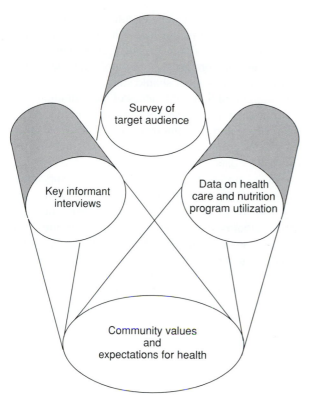

FIGURE 13.4   Triangulation of Data Sources to Understand Community Values and Expectations for Health

the sponsoring organization. Awareness of the mission and strategic directions of the organization helps to define the nutrition needs assessment and select relevant collaborators at the beginning. Then after nutrition-related problems are identified, an internal assessment should be completed to explore the capabilities, resources, expertise, and willingness that exist (or are needed) within the agency to deal with the problems and potential solutions. Thus assessment of your organization is both a first step and a final step of data gathering.

Identify Community Characteristics Related to Nutrition and Health Status   Community nutrition professionals must have a good understanding of the characteristics represented by the people in the community and how the population is changing over time. This includes demographic, socioeconomic, geographic, and nutrition and health status data. Common indicators are outlined in box 13.5.

The U.S. Census tabulations are good source documents for demographic and socioeconomic data. Cen-

BOX 13.5

DATA USED TO DESCRIBE THE COMMUNITY AND ITS NEEDS

Demographic composition: total population, categorized by age, sex, racial/ethnic group, distribution, immigration, and emigration

Socioeconomic status indicators: per capita and household income, poverty rate, education, literacy, employment status, and occupation by racial and/or ethnic group and location; major employers, public assistance, and poverty pockets

Natality statistics: number of births by racial and/or ethnic group, age, and marital status

Health status indicators: mortality rates, disability rates, incidence and prevalence of specific diseases, and morbidity rates

Nutrition status indicators: obesity, growth failure, food and nutrient intake, nutrition practices, knowledge and beliefs about food, iron status, cholesterol level, and food insecurity

Lifestyle data: nutrition, exercise, smoking, alcohol, drugs, and safety practices

Environmental data: air, water, soil, and housing quality, occupational health, recreation and leisure facilities, and transportation

Health system: health services availability and utilization and barriers to health care

Nutrition programs and services: availability and utilization of food assistance programs, resources for medical nutrition therapy, nutrition education programs, and intervention projects, and numbers and types of nutrition personnel

Food system: location and types of grocery stores and farmers markets and kinds of food available in school and worksite cafeterias, trends in restaurant and take-out food items

sus information is available from the Office of the State Demographer within state planning agencies or at libraries designated as census depository libraries or by internet. Several key determinants useful for predicting health status come from census data.

Age: Many disease conditions are age related.

Gender: Disease conditions or injuries can affect males and females differently. Life expectancy is longer for females.

Race and ethnicity: Race and ethnicity have been related to health problems. However, factors other than race may affect these outcomes more (e.g., differences in income, education, and occupations).

Residence and location: Where people live can influence their health status and access to health care services. Location determines exposure to certain environmental risks.

Family or household size: The association of family size with health status is complex and varies by target group.

Household income and educational level of head of household: Higher household income and educational levels are generally associated with higher levels of health status. Behavioral risk factors for chronic disease (such as tobacco use, poor eating habits, and lack of physical activity) are associated with lower income and education levels.

Occupational level of head of household: Blue-collar workers tend to experience a lower health status than white-collar workers. Some of this experience is related to risk-taking behaviors such as alcohol misuse or abuse and poor eating habits.

Classical measures of nutritional status are discussed in chapter 3; and the life cycle chapters in Part Two provide additional details about methods for screening, assessment, and surveillance. These methods help quantify nutrition problems and their impact on health status among target populations in the community. In addition, food consumption and nutrition status data can be extrapolated from national surveys.

Nutritional status is both a cause and an outcome of health impairments. Thus health statistics are examined. Important data elements include top causes of mortality (death) and morbidity (illness and injury); low birthweight rate by race/ethnicity; and prevalence by age, gender, race/ethnicity, and socioeconomic group for heart disease, cancer, diabetes, hypertension, anemia, dental caries, obesity, and growth impairments. Nutrition and health data are examined in relation to nutrition problems and demographic characteristics to understand where the greatest risk occurs and to prioritize targets for intervention.

Observe and Record Lifestyle and Environmental Factors   Each community is unique in terms of its cultural traditions, lifestyle, and environmental factors. These factors can either protect people from or contribute to nutrition-related health problems.

Knowledge of the social and cultural factors impinging on eating patterns and health habits are crucial to the community nutrition assessment. Although some of these cultural factors are difficult to define and isolate, a community assessment should summarize the identifiable cultural traditions and values of the community.[10]

Techniques of community organization and market research including community forums, surveys, interviews, focus group discussions, observation, and analysis of secondary data, as described in chapters 7 and 14, can be used to gain information about lifestyle factors and to gain an understanding of how community members perceive their own needs. Seeking input from community members themselves through community forums, surveys, interviews, or group techniques such as the **nominal group process** (box 13.6) focus group discussion (page 525 chapter 17) and informal discussion is crucial.

Many states have data about lifestyles collected by telephone interview for the Behavioral Risk Factor Surveillance System. Behavioral data elements include smoking, alcohol use, weight-control practices, preventable health problems, pregnancy, cancer and cholesterol screening, and food consumption. Assessment of the local marketplaces, supermarkets, small grocery stores, food cooperatives, delicatessens, health food stores, and other food outlets provides information related to food availability and purchasing behaviors. Private organizations such as the Food Marketing Institute and government agencies also monitor food purchasing and food consumption trends.

Information from community members, combined with experts' opinions and statistical data, will best guide the planning process to assure the development of programs that will be utilized by the target audience.

Identify Community Values and Expectations for Health   Many organizations are clear about the needs they would like to serve but they don't understand these needs from the perspective of their potential clients. For services to be acceptable and utilized by the target group, the services must be attuned to the values and expectations of the people to be served.[17] Market research techniques can be used to understand the community's view of nutrition-related problems and what program approaches the community likes and dislikes. A beginning step is simply visiting with individuals and groups from the community, including formal and informal leaders. Understanding the community's values, priorities, and expectations for health and health behavior is essential to planning effective programs that will be utilized.

BOX 13.6

NOMINAL GROUP PROCESS

The nominal group process (NGP) is a structured process for generating and prioritizing a larger number of issues or alternatives. It is a good group method to use when participants are new to each other, are of unequal status, or have different expertise and experience. The NGP is also good to use when the topic has controversial or political aspects. It is called "nominal," because the process does not use the normal interaction and dynamics of a group.

The steps of the NGP are

1. *Introduce the task:* Define the task in the form of an open-ended question (e.g., What are the barriers to using WIC services by low-income families in the community?) and mention the procedures to be used in the process.
2. *Silent brainstorming:* Participants individually write a list of ideas on paper. Allow five or more minutes so they search beyond the most conspicuous points. After several minutes, remind participants to "consider all angles of the question; be creative and get beyond obvious points."
3. *Round robin listing of ideas:* Go around the group and have each person mention a point from his or her list. Usually the response is a one- to five-word descriptor or phrase. The recorder writes it on a flip chart. Continue circling until all ideas have been listed or about thirty minutes has past. Tape pages up around the room as they are filled.

4. *Clarification and evaluation:* Ask "Does anyone have a question about any ideas listed?" Unclear points are discussed and clarified, and if relevant, expanded or condensed. Then each listed idea and its merits and importance is discussed. Similar points can be grouped together; new points can be added. After discussion all remaining ideas are sequentially numbered (1, 2, 3, . . .).
5. *Voting:* Ask participants to choose their top five ideas from those listed and write the number and phrase on five separate pieces of paper. Then each participant ranks the five and assigns preference score to each idea (most important = 5, next important = 4, to least important = 1) writing it at the top of the paper.
6. *Tally scores:* Write the preference score given by participants beside each item on the posted flip chart pages. Tally up scores to get a total for each item. Copy the items with the highest total scores to a clean flip chart page.
7. *Discuss the resulting priorities.*

This structured approach fosters equal involvement of all members. Through the NGP, planners and participants develop a much greater appreciation for the various aspects of the problem and the breadth of views held by people. Participants usually leave the session better informed.

In our society, health is viewed as a resource that gives people the ability to manage and change their surroundings. This view of health as a resource gives individuals the freedom to decide what behaviors to follow. Some decisions promote health; other decisions put health status at risk. Because values and behaviors are influenced by cultural traditions, belief systems, and social and physical environments, the value placed on health-promoting behaviors by community members may be in conflict with the values held by health professionals.

Joint value determination by professionals and the public should be used to create the objectives and acceptable methods of public service programs. As Drucker advises, "Non-profit people must respect their customers and their donors enough to listen to their values and understand their satisfactions. They do not impose the organization's own views and egos on those they serve."[8] This message is especially important now, when there is renewed appreciation for diversity. Many members of ethnic and racial groups desire to retain their individuality rather than being assimilated into the

dominate culture. Recognition of differing values for health and health behaviors and program and intervention alternatives is essential before establishing program and intervention priorities.[10] Planners must listen to the community to understand their values. Methods such as the "slip" or "snow card" method can facilitate discussion among community groups (see box 13.7).

Inventory Health and Nutrition Service Resources An inventory of health and nutrition resources (listing agency and type and volume of services provided) is critical to an understanding of nutrition-related services and referral systems in the community. All health, human service, education, and voluntary programs involved in the provision of food or nutrition services should be included. They may provide preventive, curative, rehabilitative, or palliation services. From the perspective of the consumer, these services might provide a basic need (such as housing or food), information and referral, outreach, advocacy, counseling, or individual treatment and

BOX 13.7

SLIP METHOD OR
SNOW CARD METHOD

Participants write thoughts, ideas, or information points on small pieces of paper such as Post-it notes. Participants stick slips on the wall randomly or in general categories. Then as discussion unfolds, slips can be ordered, regrouped, or removed to priority or "back burner" categories. New slips of paper with new points can be added. This technique captures big and small ideas and serves as an external memory as discussion and deliberation continues. The posted slips prevent important ideas from being lost when more conspicuous ideas or issues represented by a strong voice in the group get heard.

The working group experiences a sense of accomplishment as a wide range of ideas are explored and order comes to disparate views.[26]

Source: Adapted from Bryson J: *Strategic planning for nonprofit organizations,* San Francisco, 1995, Jossey Bass; Scholtes P: *The team handbook: how to use teams to improve quality,* Madison, WI, 1996, Joiner Associates Inc.

case management. Also important in this age of managed health care are the affiliations, formal and informal, for medical nutrition therapy referrals and their reimbursement.

Data, usually collected by survey, should ideally include types of services, numbers and types of clients, numbers of visits, budget allocation to specific services, types and numbers of personnel, and underutilized capacity or unmet demands. However, the latter pieces of information are more difficult to access. During this phase, a thorough internal assessment is conducted of your own organization's services, clients, past impact, and future capabilities.

The goal for community nutrition is to have an effective service management system, which is defined by Kanter as "an integrated set of activities, methods, and technologies which maximize all available and potential resources to serve the population and subpopulations within the community."[15] To positively impact the nutrition outcomes in the community, a system of coordinated health facilities, services, programs, or personnel is required. A successful **inventory of resources** should discover what is available and used to capacity, what is available but inappropriate or underutilized, and what

gaps for nutrition-related services exist. Then planners can work in concert with the community to fill unmet nutrition service needs. By involving all nutrition service providers in the assessment, there is wider recognition of nutrition-related problems and better solutions put forth to address service gaps.

As data from all five areas are collected and examined, patterns suggesting pressing or emerging problems begin to unfold. When the data are organized, interrelated, and interpreted, it becomes useful information for problem solving. Box 13.8 illustrates a way of summarizing and interpreting data.

Prioritizing the Problems

Data collection and its interpretation results in considerable understanding of problems; however, the essence of planning is **prioritization** of needs and action alternatives in the face of constraints and uncertainties. Prioritization is an important step in selecting a manageable number of problems to address. Methods for prioritization must be fair and objective and reflect community values. Methods such as the nominal group process that involve constituencies affected by the results have the added benefit of serving as a learning process for participants (see box 13.6).

Four criteria for priority determination are widely used:

1. *Size:* uses incidence or prevalence rates or proportion of population with risk factor to compare number affected by each problem
2. *Seriousness:* considers what happens if nothing is done based on urgency, severity, economic loss to family and society, and potential for affecting others
3. *Effectiveness of intervention:* estimates of the probability of preventing or reducing the problem based on what is known about the efficacy of available interventions
4. *Political support:* considers propriety, economics, acceptability, resources, and legality.[27]

Setting priorities, according to Drucker, is the true test of leadership because doing so means abandoning some problems to focus resources on solving another, more important and pressing problem.[8] Formulating nutrition priorities is not implementing programs; rather, it is focusing attention and effort on priorities the community nutrition professional can defend in public health terms. Prioritization determines why the problems identified should or should not be addressed.

BOX 13.8

NUTRITION ISSUES IN THE COMMUNITY		
Key nutrition issue	*Population group of concern*	*Possible underlying causes*
Poor-quality diet	Frail, home-bound elderly	Chronic disease, lack of social contacts and caretaker, transportation difficulties
Childhood obesity	Low-income preschoolers	Lack of activity, lack of access to safe play areas, intake of high-carbohydrate and high-fat snack foods, caretaker knowledge of child's nutritional needs is inadequate

Before proceeding to program development and implementation, however, consider whether it is appropriate for your organization to be addressing a specific problem. Do the highest-priority problems (identified by the prioritization process) fall within the boundaries specified by your organization's strategy and mission statement? If yes, then proceed to decisions about appropriate programs and interventions to address problems.

PROBLEM SOLVING AND DECISION MAKING

The Decision-Making Process

The planning process involves decision making at every juncture. Sound decisions emerge from an objective **decision-making process,** which involves five distinct steps:

1. State the problem or situation requiring a decision.
2. Define criteria relevant to a "good" choice in the decision situation.
3. Generate alternative solutions.
4. Assess each alternative against established criteria.
5. Select the most suitable alternative based on the objective assessment carried out at step 4.

These steps are followed by two more: implementing the solution and evaluating the results.

The combination of a defined problem and creatively generated alternatives assessed against clearly defined criteria leads to high-quality decisions. Through this process, those involved in decision making become aware of the strengths and limitations of various alternatives as judged against criteria relevant to the decision situation. Although no one best solution is possible, the process reveals the preferred solutions. Decision makers, then, have rational information to justify choices and can communicate the rationale for decisions to others. A concrete decision-making process

avoids the pitfall of basing decisions on emotional reactions, past biases, and hunches. It also prevents powerful opinion leaders from dictating the decision process.

Who Makes the Decision?

Group or participatory decision making is the preferred approach when a high level of involvement and commitment by members will be needed to implement the decision.[9] Participatory decision making takes more time; but a shared understanding of the problem, generation of creative alternative solutions, open consideration of the strengths and limitations of alternatives, and commitment to the final solutions are valuable payoffs.

In some situations, the decisions are made unilaterally by the supervisor, nutrition director, manager, or health director. Unilateral decisions can be more efficient and even necessary in an emergency, when confidentiality is imperative, or when the support of others is not necessary to implement a solution. However, unilateral decisions often suffer from lack of information.

Decisions can also be made by consultation. The decision maker asks for others' opinions: "I'm thinking about doing it this way. What's your reaction?" In this consultative approach, the decision maker may or may not use the advice given in the final decision. Each of these approaches to decision making is appropriate for certain situations.

To structure and simplify problem solving and decision making, planners may fix some aspects of the process so that they are effectively removed from constant deliberations. For example, the forms illustrated in this chapter guide definition of decisions to be made and some elements or criteria used in decision making (see pages 380 [questions for strategic planning], 390 [public health criteria for prioritization], 394 [levels of prevention and intervention], and 393 [decision matrix]).

Criteria

A group of individuals facing complex but important decisions often disagree. Decisions are multifaceted, and there is no single right answer. It is critical to understand that opposition will exist and that the process of exploring and discussing opposing points of view usually improves the final decision. Using the decision-making process with specific criteria structures the discussion around important and relevant factors. An objective process leads to a defensible decision rather than one based on preconceived ideas and power tactics.

Great attention must be given to defining the criteria relevant to a "good" choice. Some criteria mentioned earlier in this chapter included number affected, severity, and public perception. Community nutrition professionals must be able to define relevant criteria for the decision situation. Criteria should be clearly stated, understood, and agreed upon by those involved in the decision-making process. Criteria reduce the complexity and subjectivity of the decision by separating complex factors into single characteristics that can be assessed independently. Criteria assure that each alternative is assessed consistently. For example, criteria for selecting among intervention alternatives could include:

Available resources (personnel, money, equipment, knowledge, skill, and time)

Political feasibility

Community acceptability

Reputation or credibility of the organization that is to address a problem

Potential or available energy within the organization to address a problem

Legal mandates requiring an organization to address a problem

These criteria are shown in figure 13.5, which is a decision matrix for selecting interventions based on feasibility.

The definition of decision criteria increase the objectivity of prioritization and selection procedures; however, scoring ultimately relies on the wisdom and values of the planning group. Explicit criteria and scoring are used to help raters override preconceived judgments. A number of people with a variety of skills and backgrounds are used as raters. Because ratings are based on estimates, community and professional members who have knowledge about the community, who understand the health data obtained in the needs assessment process, and who appreciate the felt needs and values of the community should be involved. It is important to consider these skills in selecting planning team members and determining the mix and size of the planning team.

Alternatives

This phase includes generating possible solutions to the problem. Alternatives can include previous strategies and new ways of doing business in the future. Community members, potential clients or customers, as well as staff should be involved in the process of generating alternatives. Involvement of people representing different perspectives expands options, helps to clarify ideas, and expands ownership of the problem and its solution. A creative, nonjudgmental approach will ensure that all possible ideas are considered. Brainstorming (see box 13.9) or the more structured nominal group technique can be used to generate alternatives. During the idea generation phase, capture all ideas on paper or computer so ideas are not forgotten.

Once all of the ideas have been recorded, sort and organize the information. The matrix of intervention alternatives shown in table 13.5 is an example of organizing to potential interventions for a specific nutrition problem. This form reminds planners to consider primary, secondary, and tertiary prevention levels as well as individual-based, community-based, and systems-based intervention types. Definitions for each prevention level and intervention type were given in chapter 2.

Assess Alternatives Against Criteria

This is the evaluation phase. Planners and decision makers use analysis to assess each alternative and determine the "best" alternative or alternatives to pursue. An example of this is the selection of specific interventions from among many alternatives generated to fill in figure 13.5. Steps at bottom of figure 13.5 walk the decision makers through the evaluation and selection process.

COMMITMENT TO ACTION

Planning Documents

A vision, strategy, or program plan is just an idea until it is communicated to others and put into action. When it is committed to writing, it serves as a resource, a set of priorities, and a roadmap for action. The written document should be concise and easy to read. It should spell out in understandable terms the desired future and how to get there.

Step 1: List the problem: _____

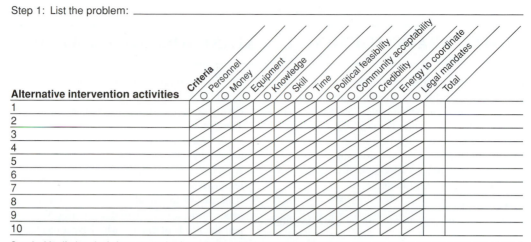

Step 2: Identify the criteria important to implementing possible interventions. (Add/delete from the criteria identified across the figure.)

Step 3: Weight the criteria on a scale of 1 to 10, where 1 is the least important criteria and 10 is the most important criteria. (Place the weighted values in the circle below the criteria.)

Step 4: Identify all possible intervention activities to address the problem. Write them in the appropriate rows.

Step 5: Based *within each criteria, rank* each intervention activity where the highest number most favorably meets the criteria and the lowest number least favorably meets criteria. Place the rank number in the upper left-hand corner of the box. Complete the rankings for each intervention activity within *each criteria* by moving vertically down the column.

Step 6: After *each* intervention activity has been ranked *within each criteria,* multiply the criteria weight (step 3) with the specific intervention ranking and place it below the diagonal line. This provides a weighting sum within each criteria.

Step 7: Sum all the criteria scores for each intervention activity obtained in step 6, by moving horizontally across each row to obtain a feasibility index. Place in the appropriate "*total*" box.

FIGURE 13.5   Decision Matrix for Selecting Interventions Based on Feasibility
(*Source:* Mullis RM, Snyder MP, Hunt MK: Developing nutrient criteria for food-specific dietary guidelines for the general public. Copyright The American Dietetic Association. Reprinted by permission from *Journal of the American Dietetic Association,* Vol. 90(46):847–851, 1990.)

A major nutrition unit of a health department or other organization would be expected to have a strategic plan that is updated every few years, a coordinated set of program plans that define specific programs and projects over a period of one to five years, and implementation or operational plans, including protocols and work schedules that detail expectations for day-to-day operations. A comprehensive nutrition plan for the unit would identify all major programs and initiatives and how they are coordinated together to meet the priority nutrition needs of the community. Comprehensive planning is updated annually in coordination with organizational budgeting activities.

Parts of a Written Plan

Like any written communication, the planning document should be designed to meet the readers' needs for information. Thus the content and layout will vary depending on the who the intended users of the planning document will be. The plan may be used by employees to implement work, it may be used as part of a grant proposal, it may be used as a public relations tool, or it may serve all three plus more purposes. As an example see table 13.6, which highlights the goals of a metropolitan city-county health department, and illustrates how plans for nutrition activities support the agency's goals. Note how the nutrition activity represents a tactic to be used by the nutrition program to have a positive impact on health.

Written plans for nutrition programs generally include the following:[25]

Description of the community

Priority needs

Goals and objectives

List of programs and planned intervention strategies

Specific policies and procedures that will guide the program and interventions

Evaluation methods to be used

Often plans identify the work unit or position category responsible for implementation and the necessary resources or budget allocation.

A comprehensive nutrition plan for a city, county, or state will also include: mission statement, values, subunit

BOX 13.9

USING BRAINSTORMING TO EXPAND IDEA GENERATION

Brainstorming is a creative, idea-generating process. It taps the right side of the brain for free-wheeling, abstract thinking. Analysis and evaluation, which come naturally to technically oriented, left-brain people, is outlawed! Sometimes it helps to have a "warm up" exercise to shift participants' thinking to the right side of the brain before the actual topic of the meeting is tackled. Pick a silly topic that moves participants out of their usual line of thinking.

SUGGEST WARM UPS
What are 101 things you can do on a rainy day? do with used auto tires?

RULES FOR BRAINSTORMING
- Everyone should participate, anyone can jump in at anytime.
- Judgment about or discussion of ideas is not allowed. (That comes later.)
- Don't hold back any ideas no matter how outrageous.
- Write all ideas on paper or a flip chart so group members can scan them.
- Hitchhiking off listed ideas (going off on tangents) is fine.

The free-form approach of brainstorming generates excitement, equalizes involvement of participants, and, if rules are followed and people "let themselves go," can produce a range of creative and innovative ideas.

SEQUENCE OF EVENTS IN BRAINSTORMING
1. State the subject of brainstorming. It is helpful to state the topic in a "why," "how," or "what" question. (What are ways to support the nutritional needs of homebound elderly?)
2. Give participants a minute of silence to think about the question.
3. Invite everyone to call out ideas. Enforce ground rules as needed ("No discussion, next idea").
4. A recorder writes quickly. Sometimes it is helpful to have two recorders at two flip charts.
5. If necessary to stimulate ideas: ask for the most outrageous ideas, ask for partial solutions ("What would support the needs of elderly who have a functioning spouse or caretaker?"), or go around the table to get everyone to offer an idea.

After brainstorming is over, move to discussion of the ideas generated. Encourage participants to keep an open mind and move toward innovative solutions. A good approach is to "PIN the ideas—not NIP them." To PIN an idea, first identify *positive* attributes of the idea, then explore *interesting* elements of the idea, and finally consider *negative* aspects of the idea. This forces consideration of the positive merits and possibilities of an idea and overcomes the natural tendency to focus on negative aspects. This discussion should lead to synthesis of new approaches drawing from the positive and interesting aspects of ideas while being mindful of, but not overly restricted by negatives. Brainstorming following an open-minded discussion leads to more effective problem solving.

TABLE 13.5

Intervention Alternatives to Address a Nutrition Problem

Step 1: State the problem: _____
           (As identified by the needs assessment)
Step 2: Identify target groups: _____
           (Those persons for whom you would like to prevent or reduce the problem)
Step 3: Identify all current and possible interventions and list them in the categories below.
           (Ideas should be concrete, focused, and specific to the problem and target groups)

Intervention type; prevention level	Primary prevention	Secondary prevention	Tertiary prevention
Individual-based: creating change in individuals			
Community-based: creating change in populations that receive some service			
Systems-based: creating change in organizations, policies, laws, and structures			

Step 4: Circle those interventions in which your agency has or could have some direct involvement or responsibility.

TABLE 13.6
Nutrition Program Plan
St. Paul–Ramsey County Nutrition Program—1996 Work Plan

Mission of the nutrition program

To assure that hunger is alleviated and the health of St. Paul and Ramsey County residents is improving by providing:

- WIC and nutrition services targeted toward achievement of the year 2000 objectives
- Assessment to identify unmet nutrition needs
- Nutrition-related health education otherwise unavailable to low-income persons
- Nutrition expertise for the life cycle
- Professional training, advocacy, and programs in the community to foster prevention of chronic disease through healthy eating

Strategies

Screening and assessment, clinical nutrition services, nutrition education/information, media, food access, and consultation

Health department priority areas with goals, and nutrition program activity
(one activity listed from many included in the plan)

I. Chronic disease

Goal: To promote early detection and prevention of cardiovascular disease and cancer for Ramsey County residents and to reduce avoidable mortality and morbidity from other noninfectious diseases.

Nutrition activity: Assess the eating behaviors/food intake of targeted groups in the West Seventh and West Side areas, using appropriate screening tools. Make referrals to needed resources, including nutrition counseling/education.

II. Infectious disease

Goal: To reduce the incidence and severity of reported cases of AIDS in specific Ramsey County populations.

Nutrition activity: Provide nutrition therapy to newly diagnosed HIV positive persons and persons with AIDS through Ramsey County Public Health/St. Paul Public Health.

III. Environmental conditions

Goal: To work collaboratively among government agencies and community-based organizations to reduce environmental health risks.

Nutrition activity: Assist the intradepartmental work group in determining methods to provide public education on foodborne illness prevention

IV. Pregnancy and birth

Goal: To promote healthy family development through improved birth outcomes.

Nutrition activity: Teach prenatal nutrition classes in the community as requested, including women's shelters, family centers, and schools

V. Child growth and development

Goal: To promote optimal growth and development among Ramsey County children through improved services to parents, children and adolescents, including those with special needs.

Nutrition activity: Produce cable TV segments on children and growth and development.

VI. Disability and decreased independence

Goal: To assist the ill, elderly, disabled, and mentally ill in maintaining independence.

Nutrition activity: Promote Food Stamp participation to suburban elderly.

VII. Mental health

Goal: To promote the development of life skills and emotional systems to protect and improve mental health.

Nutrition activity: Disseminate "Nutrition at a Glance" for chemically dependent clients.

VIII. Service delivery systems

Goal: To improve access to health care and promote healthy families through coordinated services.

Nutrition activity: Provide consultation to managed care organizations to improve nutrition education strategies for low income and ethnic populations.

Adapted with permission of J. Soecthing, St. Paul-Ramsey Nutrition Program, St. Paul, Minnesota.

strategy statements, goals and objectives and other performance measures, staffing plans, financial plans, implementation and action plans, monitoring and evaluation plans, and a plan for updating the plan. Written plans including goals and objectives provide the basis for guiding, leading, and coordinating the efforts of the organization and work groups.

ESTABLISH GOALS AND OBJECTIVES

Goals and objectives give meaning and direction to the work of the people associated with the organization. They are standards by which organizations, work groups, and constituents judge performance. Community nutrition professionals must be skilled in writing goals and objectives.

Goals state what is to be achieved and may state when results are to be accomplished, but they do not state how the results are to be achieved. Objectives are subordinate to goals and are more specific and measurable. Both goals and objectives express desired results.

A **goal** is a statement of direction, general purpose, or wide interest. Goals tend to be broad, all-encompassing ideals because they are derived from values. The formulation of general goals is essential because many of the most important human goals can adequately and meaningfully be stated only in abstract terms. Goals should be motivating and may be somewhat unreachable. An example of such a goal statement is "to increase the health status and quality of life for all citizens of this state."

Objectives are more concrete, closer in time, and more measurable than goals. Although each problem may have only one goal, each goal usually has several objectives. Objectives are specific measurable statements of what is to be accomplished by a given point in time. Objectives provide the main energizing and directive force for managerial action. Objectives are the focal point around which managers concentrate their efforts and mobilize available resources. Specific objectives serve as control points for evaluation.

Writing Goals

A goal is the "other side" of the problem. A written goal is a positive statement of what would exist if the problem was no longer there. For example, a goal might be "to reduce the number of premature deaths related to a high-fat diet." Goals should be future oriented, easily understood, and broad.

Writing Objectives

The general guideline for formulating objectives for a person, unit, section, or department is to state the objectives in terms of specific results, not in general terms. The objectives must be tangible and recognizable so they can be communicated to all those involved in planning, implementation and evaluation. They must be achievable with available resources.

Model state nutrition objectives have been developed to allow states to "identify their own target populations, focus on dietary intake and the food supply, and include objectives related to the delivery of service."[1]

Objectives contain four common elements: (1) the name or indicator of the problem being addressed, (2) a target (who or what), (3) a time frame for completion, and (4) the standard to be reached or the amount of change expected in either the indicator or the target. To be properly evaluated, an objective must be stated in numerical terms, indicate the present status of the indicator, and indicate the status to be achieved.[7]

Two formulas for writing sound objectives are:

1. To (action verb) (desired result in problem or indicator) (target) (time frame) (resource required). Examples are "To increase to 90 percent the proportion of frail elderly who are screened for nutrition risk factors no later than the second visit by home health providers using the DETERMINE checklist." "To increase the consumption of fruit and vegetables by elementary school children to four servings per day by the end of the school year through classroom, cafeteria, and family promotions."
2. By (date), the following results (numerical) on (target) will have been accomplished. Examples are "By 2000, 35 percent (up from 28 percent in 1993) of Vision City adults will engage in light to moderate physical activity for at least thirty minutes per day." "By the end of the school year, 80 percent of third-grade classroom teachers will present the lesson on fruits and vegetables."

Outcome, Process, and Structure Objectives

A common problem faced by people writing objectives is how to link what may be a long-term and rather unmeasurable goal with objectives that can be measured in a month, year, or several years. Another challenge is to write objectives that not only tell you how you are getting from one point to another but also whether you are going in the right direction. **Process, outcome,** and **structure** objectives help to meet those challenges. All three types of objectives are important to effective program planning and implementation. Intermediate or bridging objectives are also used to define intermediate performance targets.

Outcome objectives define a desired future state via a unit of measure (indicator) at some point in the future. Indicators are often morbidity or mortality or other health status indicators. Outcome objectives are not steps, processes, or actions to achieve that result. In the medical arena, outcome objectives are intended to define the desired health state. An example is "By 2003, the prevalence of modifiable nutrition-related risk factors (fat consumption, low physical activity, blood lipids, overweight) will be reduced by 30 percent among worksite employees."

Process objectives define benchmarks for how the program, intervention, or action step will be implemented. They express the "who will do what by when." Process objectives are used to guide and assess progress. Examples are "Participating worksites will offer at least three components of the Eating on the Run program to employees over a six-month period." "Health department nutritionists will provide two consultation visits to participating worksites each year."

Structure objectives define the resources necessary to achieve desired outcomes. They are expressed in terms of budget, staff, facilities and space, equipment and capabilities. An example is "By 2000, worksites employing 300 or more persons will have a health promotion director or occupational health nurse trained in the Eating on the Run program."

Intermediate objectives (or bridging objectives) are often used as measures of progress to the larger objective. They bridge the gap between the specific activities planned (process objectives) and the long-term outcomes (outcome objectives). These objectives access intermediate results that have a high probability of reducing the target health problem. They can measure the impact of a specific intervention. Intermediate objectives usually measure changes in knowledge, attitudes, beliefs, skills, behaviors, and practices or shorter-term indicators of nutritional or health status. Depending on the problem, it is often easier and less expensive to measure the intermediate outcomes in individuals than the final outcome of a health problem in the community. Examples are "By the end of the first year, 60 percent of employees who participate in two or more components of the program will shift to lower fat food choices at the workplace." "By the end of the first program year, sales of reduced fat choices in the cafeteria will increase by 15 percent "

Table 13.7 illustrates a set of objectives that are tied directly to an identified nutrition-related health problem and its risk factors and contributing factors. Note how the plan for what to do and how to accomplish it follows after the identification of problems from the needs assessment.

TABLE 13.7
Objectives Linked to the Analysis of the Health Problem

Health problem	Risk factor	Contributing factors
Cerebrovascular disease	Hypertension	1. Obesity 2. Physical inactivity

Outcome objective	Intermediate objective	Process objectives
By 2000, reduce stroke deaths to no more than 20 per 100,000 people (Baseline: 30.3 in 1987).	By 1998, increase to 90% the proportion of people who are taking action to control their blood pressure.	1.a. By December 31 (year), health care providers will refer 75% of hypertensive, overweight clients for nutrition intervention. 1.b. By December 31 (year), 80% of referred hypertensive, overweight clients will receive one or more diet and exercise sessions. 2.a. By December 31 (year), exercise facilities and programs will be identified in all inner city neighborhoods. **Structure objective** 2.b. By December 31 (year), walking paths will be constructed in six city parks.

MANAGEMENT ROLES AND RESPONSIBILITIES

Management Roles and Skills

A **manager** is someone who actively carries out the management functions of planning, implementation, and evaluation. A manager plans and makes decisions, secures and organizes resources, coordinates or directs implementation, and monitors and makes adjustments with the aim of achieving goals and objectives in an efficient and effective manner.[11]

Certain roles and skills are required of all managers. Mintzberg grouped roles that managers fill under the categories of interpersonal, informational and decisional roles.[21] The degree to which a community nutrition professional successfully carries out management roles is influenced by his or her skill. Katz identified three basic skills of managers—technical, human (or interpersonal), and conceptual.[16] The relative importance of these skills depends on the managers scope of responsibility (see figure 13.6).

Management of community nutrition programs and interventions requires technical knowledge about food and nutrition and needs across the life cycle (see chapters 8 to 12) and how to select and implement appropriate interventions. Technical knowledge of individual and community assessment (chapter 3 and earlier in this chapter); behavior change (chapter 7), and communication skills (chapter 17) are also necessary. Another type of skill needed by the community nutrition professional is interpersonal skills. Managers interact with people inside and outside the organization. The ability to communicate with, listen, understand, and motivate individuals and groups requires effective interpersonal skills. The community nutrition professional needs conceptual skill to be a good manager. This is the ability to think abstractly, to understand various cause and effect relationships, to grasp how different parts and competing forces come together, and to view situations in a holistic manner. Conceptual skill allows the community nutrition professional to think strategically and see the whole picture, and to make broad-based decisions that serve the overall organization as well as the nutrition programs and its staff, collaborators, clients, and other stakeholders. In addition, community nutrition professionals must possess diagnostic and analytical skills. As managers, they must diagnose problems and their causes and identify potential solutions by collecting information, sorting it out, and developing strategies and plans. In exercising all these roles and skills community nutrition professionals must be mindful of ethical principles and values. Ethical consideration must be integrated into policies, plans, and day-to-day operations. Ethics is discussed in detail in chapter 19.

Leaders and Managers

What is leadership? At first glance, you may think that the terms *leader* and *manager* are synonymous; however, it is important that they be seen as two essential, but distinct and complementary functions.[18] A **leader** *sets direction* by shaping both a vision and the strategies to achieve that vision. Leaders must be broad-based strategic thinkers who are also risk takers. They must excel at aligning support for their visions. This includes getting others to accept the vision and its message as well as its likelihood of its success. Leadership also includes motivating and inspiring others by appealing to their basic values and needs for achievement, self-esteem, and self-fulfillment. Leaders lead change processes and redirect people's energies and other resources. They lead transformations of products, services, technology, and organizational practices.

Managers *set a plan into action* by organizing and staffing systems so they operate efficiently. Managers are concerned with accomplishing concrete tasks and establishing control mechanisms to minimize deviations from goals and engaging in effective problem solving and decision making. Whereas leaders are engaged in motivating people to accept change and break from the status quo, managers must establish orderly systems that follow procedures and policies and meet set performance targets.

First-line management

Conceptual
Human
Technical

Middle management

Conceptual
Human
Technical

Top management

Conceptual
Human
Technical

FIGURE 13.6   Relative Skills Needed for Effective Performance at Different Levels of Management
(*Source:* Adapted and reprinted by permission of Harvard Business Review. From "Skills of an effective administrator" by Robert L. Katz, Sept/Oct 1974. Copyright © 1974 by the President and Fellows of Harvard College; all rights reserved.)

You can find leaders at all levels—a leader does not need a title to exert leadership. In contrast, managers are given titles and management responsibilities as part of their position descriptions. Druckers defines management as "doing things right" and leadership as "doing the right thing."[8] Other contrasts and similarities are shown in box 13.10.

Although effective managers must portray substantial leadership qualities to motivate people and coordinate their activities, collect information, make decisions, and influence other decision makers; in general, managers' primary responsibility is to assure the accomplishment of organization and program goals and objectives. On a personal level, this requires problem-solving skills, planning skills, assertiveness, self-knowledge, the drive for task completion, negotiation and communication skills, and other interpersonal skills. In contrast, effective leaders create and drive organizational vision. The characteristics of leaders include being visionary, influential, and persuasive; taking risks; and having passion and self-perception.

Great management, whether as a manager or as a leader, requires having imagination and integrity, being honest, keeping promises, and being willing to empower others. Great management involves respect and uses delegation to make associates and followers feel empowered, capable, and responsible. Great managers have the capacity to create excitement![29] Management is a continual exercise of learning, teaching and persuasion; it requires excellent teaching skills.

BOX 13.10

CONTRASTS AND SIMILARITIES BETWEEN MANAGERS AND LEADERS

Managers—	*Leaders—*
doing things right	*doing the right thing*
Short-term view	Long-term view
Implementation	Vision
Technical	Conceptual
Tactical plans	Strategic plans
Control mechanisms	Inspire change
Risk taking	Risk taking
Honesty	Honesty
Integrity	Integrity

Leadership

According to Kouzes and Posner leadership is a learnable set of practices, and everyone has the capacity to lead. However, the key is "having the courage and spirit to move from whatever place you're in to make a significant difference."[19] Leadership starts within a person. Community nutrition professionals develop and refine leadership abilities through experience and reflection.

Personal power is the extent to which one is able to link the outer capacity for action (external power) with the inner capacity for reflection (inner power).[12] According to Hagberg personal power develops through stages:

- Feeling powerlessness
- Learning the ropes as an apprentice
- Gaining formalized power through position and by expertise and reputation
- Having power by reflection, integrity, and mentoring
- Empowering others through vision beyond position
- Exuding power from wisdom and inner peace

Leaders at higher levels of development can champion and protect entrepreneurs and risk takers within the organization who are willing to innovate and break from the status quo.[23]

From the point of view of a model of shared leadership Chinn[5a] describes interpersonal and group process techniques that reflect respect and cooperation. Leadership is shared and all persons are expected to live their values. By merging knowing and doing and working collectively, worlds can be transformed.

Covey has popularized seven habits of highly effective people.[6] Habits are powerful factors in our lives. They are consistent, often unconscious patterns, that express character and produce effectiveness or ineffectiveness. According to Covey our habits are shaped by three central values of life: experiential (experiences we have), creative (what we bring into existence), and attitudinal (how we respond to the circumstances of life). A person's actions emerge from internalized principles and patterns of behavior that are based on knowledge (what to, why to), skill (how to), and desire (want to). The most effective people have, or consciously work on, developing the habits described in box 13.11.

Learning to Manage and Lead

Management skills are acquired through formal education and experience, continuing professional education,

BOX 13.11

SEVEN HABITS OF HIGHLY EFFECTIVE PEOPLE

1. *Be proactive:* Individuals exercise a conscious choice about the conditions around them. Proactive people listen carefully becoming more self-aware and more aware of their surroundings. They distinguish between their *circle of concern* (things they care about) and their *circle of influence* (things over which they have some control). Proactive people focus their attention on things they can do something about, whereas reactive people focus on problems and concerns and negative circumstances.
2. *Begin with the end in mind:* This habit is the ability to see the big picture, know what is most important, and have a vision for where you want to be.
3. *Put first things first:* Spend your time doing the things that really make a difference. Set priorities and organize your time to do the most important things. Focus on building and maintaining trusting relationships, living with integrity, fulfilling expectations, and keeping promises.

4. *Think win-win:* Foster high-trust relationships and work for mutual benefit in all human interactions.
5. *Seek first to understand and then to be understood:* Communication is the most important skill in personal and professional life. Listen actively to others, and openly communicate your views, needs, and perspectives.
6. *Synergize:* Bring together pieces to form a whole that is greater than the sum of its parts. Use networking, collaboration, coordination, and team building; compensate for weakness; and recognize, respect, and value differences and diversity.
7. *Sharpen the saw:* Renew the four dimensions of your nature—physical, spiritual, mental, and social-emotional. Have a commitment to continued growth and development, lifelong learning, and renewal.

Adapted from Covey SR: *The 7 habits of highly effective people.* New York, 1989, Simon & Schuster.

readings, seminars, guided work experiences and employment with increasing and varied managerial responsibilities, participation in and leadership of internal and external committees and groups, observing good role models, accepting challenging job assignments, and seeking leadership opportunities in professional associations and civic organization. Effective nutrition program managers and leaders are continually learning and integrating what they learn into programs. Effective management is a continual process of learning and developing and fostering learning and development in others.

Successful organizations are "learning organization" which are nimble in structure and process. The people in the learning organization are empowered to create and adapt to ensure short-term and long-term success. A leader works as a teacher to help people redefine reality with more accuracy and insight, and this empowers them to shape a desirable future. A true leader is a steward who serves his or her vision and the people who help to make a reality.[4]

To build strong leadership as community nutrition professionals, a multifaceted approach that spans all levels of professional activity is essential. The approach must involve changes in professional image, recruitment, and educational training to ensure a supply of leaders who can both create and assume top positions in the community. This can best be accomplished by a concerted effort of academia, employers, and professional organizations to overhaul their programs and support the movement for leadership in the nutrition profession.

Women represent the largest group in applied nutrition. If they are to use all of their management and leadership talents, community nutrition professionals must break the "glass ceiling"; community nutrition professionals must aspire, plan and act to reach their full potential.[24]

Organizations should not assume that male and female managers differ greatly in personal and management qualities. They also should make sure policies, practices, and programs minimize the creation of sex differences in managers' experiences on the job. There is little reason to believe that either women or men make superior managers or that women and men are different types of managers. Instead there are likely to be excellent, average, and poor managerial performers within each sex. Success in today's highly competitive marketplace calls for organizations to make best use of the talent available to them. To do this, the most effective managers must be consistently developed, encouraged, and promoted regardless of their gender.

To master the global challenges of today and the future, organizations and society cannot do without com-

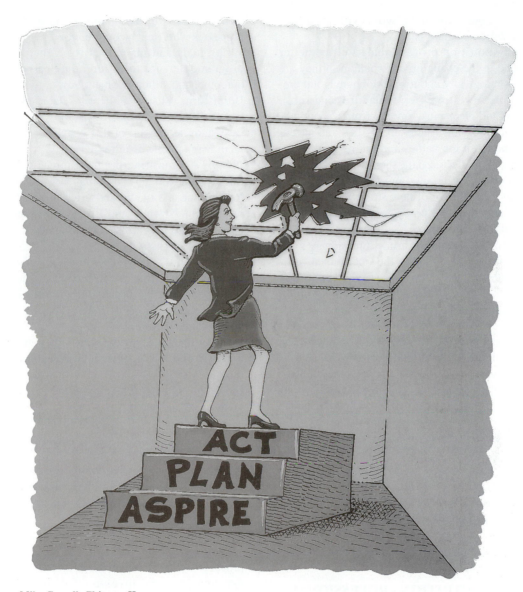

Mike Carroll, Chicago, IL.

plete and complementary aspects of the total human experience. Organizations badly need whole, that is, healthy and balanced, individuals able to draw from the richness of both male and female inheritance and experience.[24]

This is an important message for community nutrition professionals who must develop and utilize leadership and managerial roles and skills to impact the nutritional well-being of people. Flexibility and constant learning about self, about the environment, and about collaborators and clients are essential to planning and leading programs that can meet this challenge.

IMPLICATIONS FOR COMMUNITY NUTRITION PROFESSIONALS

In these times of rapid change, both inside the organization and in the external environment, community nutrition professionals must have a solid knowledge base and skills in strategic thinking, planning, community assessment, decision making, managerial roles, and leadership. Community nutrition professionals must be able to create a vision of a comprehensive system of community nutrition programs and services for all community members, and must work with others toward the realization of that vision.

Community nutrition professionals will be better able to respond to the changing environment if they are able to think strategically about nutrition needs and creatively explore new strategies for addressing those needs. Visions and plans must emerge from a sound understanding of emerging forces and issues and a genuine understanding of the values and felt needs of community members. Collected data should clarify what is good about existing programs and services and what must be abandoned in favor of new strategies and initiatives. Community nutrition professionals must be willing to abandon the status quo.

As a start, community nutrition professionals must become involved in planning at the operational, program, and strategic levels. A well-formulated nutrition plan can effectively and efficiently direct the resources of the community and the organization to prevent nutrition problems or seek permanent solutions to existing problems. It accomplishes this by addressing needs, wants, and capabilities of community members.

Planning involves decision making at every juncture. Sound decisions emerge from an objective decision-making process. Community nutrition professionals can draw on their technical knowledge base to identify relevant decision criteria, however, they must creatively generate innovative new approaches to program and intervention design.

Goals and objectives give direction to nutrition programs and activities. They are standards and challenges that guide efforts to important outcomes. Planning is just one management function. It must be linked up with implementation and evaluation to bring about results.

COMMUNITY NUTRITION PROFESSIONALS IN ACTION

- Collect examples of strategic planning or needs assessment documents. What data sources and kinds of information were used? How well did the assessment address the five areas of a community needs assessment? How did the planners prioritize the issues or problems?
- Visit a web site for planning data such as the Centers for Disease Control or the Census Bureau. Abstract data relevant to your state, city, or county.
- Practice using two or more methods to generate ideas or expand exploration of issues or alternatives—brainstorming, nominal group process, focus groups, and the snow card technique. Compare these meth-

ods. List steps in the planning and decision-making processes where each could be used.
- Write goals and objectives for a specific nutrition program. Be sure to differentiate between process, outcome, and structure objectives.
- Brainstorm a list of nutrition-related problems that would likely be found in Vision City (refer to the case study at the end of this chapter). Then prioritize them using public health criteria.
- Interview a nutrition program director. Identify the roles that person plays as a manager and as a leader.
- Review the list of the activities in box 13.1. Select one in which you would like to gain greater experience and offer to assist a community nutrition program with that activity.
- Based on your experience with an organization, write answers to the questions in box 13.2. Then interview other people in the organization to see if they have the same perceptions of the organization's mission, strategy, and culture.
- Identify instances where you have performed as a manager and as a leader. In which role do you feel most comfortable? What knowledge, skills, and experience do you need to expand your confidence in managerial and leadership roles?

GOING ONE STEP FURTHER

- As a class, group, or individual conduct a needs assessment for a community organization, agency, or program. Include all five areas of a community nutrition needs assessment.
- Participate in or facilitate a planning team effort.
- Use the problem-solving and decision-making processes to address a problem faced by a community nutrition program. Involve others in the process as appropriate.
- Examine the mission, goals, and objectives of your organization. Is the mission energizing? Are the goals challenging? Are the objectives measurable? If indicated, rewrite them to follow guidelines from this chapter.
- Write a plan for nutrition services for the next year. Base the plan on relevant strategic planning, needs assessment, or market research information.
- Determine your stage of personal power by completing the Personal Power Profile available from:
  Personal Power Products
  1735 Evergreen Lane N.
  Plymouth, MN 55441–4102 (612–551–1708)

ADDITIONAL INFORMATION

Check the business section of university and major bookstores for current books on management and leadership.

A position paper of the American Dietetic Association identified leadership and management skills as integral to health promotion and disease prevention programs. See: The role of nutrition in health promotion and disease prevention programs; J Am Diet Assoc 98:205, 1998.

REFERENCES

1. American Public Health Association: *Healthy communities 2000: model standards,* ed 3, Washington, DC, 1991, American Public Health Association.
2. Bryson JM: *Strategic planning for public and nonprofit organizations,* rev. ed., San Francisco, 1995, Jossey Bass.
3. Bryson JM, Alston FK: *Creating and implementing your strategic plan,* San Francisco, 1996, Jossey Bass.
4. Burns JM: Leadership, New York, 1978, Harper.
5. Centers for Disease Control and Prevention: *Planned approach to community health (PATCH),* Atlanta, 1993, Aspen.
5a. Chinn PC: Peace & Power: Building communities for the future, ed 4, New York, 1995, NLN Press Pub. No. 14–2697.
6. Covey SR: *The 7 habits of highly effective people: powerful lessons in personal change,* New York, 1989, Simon & Schuster.
7. Dever GA: *Community health analysis.* Gaithersberg, MD, 1991, Aspen.
8. Drucker PF: *Managing the non-profit organization,* New York, 1990, Harper Collins.
9. Fink A, Kosecoff J, Chassin M, Brook RH: Consensus methods: characteristics and guidelines for use, *Am J Public Health* 74:979, 1984.
10. Gonzalez VM, Gonzalez JT, Freeman V, Howard-Pitney B: *Health promotion in diverse cultural communities,* Palo Alto, CA, 1991, Stanford Center for Research in Disease Prevention.
11. Griffin RW: *Management,* ed 4, Boston, 1995, Houghton Mifflin.
12. Hagberg JO: *Real power: stages of personal power in organizations,* Salem, WI; 1994, Sheffield Publishing.
13. Hamel G: Strategy as revolution, *Harvard Business Review* 74(4):69–83, 1996.
14. Institute of Medicine, National Academy of Science: *The future of public health,* Washington, DC, 1988, National Academy Press.
15. Kanter RM: *The change masters: innovation and entrepreneurship in the American corporation,* New York, 1984, Simon & Schuster.
16. Katz RL: Skills of an effective administrator, *Harvard Business Review* 52:23, 1974.
17. Kotler P, Andreasen AR: *Strategic marketing for nonprofit organizations,* ed 5, Englewood Cliffs, NJ, 1995, Prentice-Hall.
18. Kotter JP: *Leading change,* Boston, 1996, Harvard Business School Press.
19. Krouzes JM, Posner BZ: *The leadership challenge,* San Francisco, 1996, Jossey-Bass.
20. Lipton M: Demystifying the development of organizational vision, *Sloan Management Review* 37(4):83–92, 1996.
21. Mintzberg H: The manager's job: folklore and fact, *Harvard Business Review* 68:163, 1990.
22. National Association of County Health Officials: *Assessment protocol for excellence in public health (APEXPH),* Washington, DC, 1991, National Association of County Health Officials.
23. Osborne D, Gaebler T: *Reinventing government: how the entrepreneural spirit is transforming the public sector,* Reading, MA, 1992, Addison-Wesley.
24. Owen Al: Women as managers, *Top Clin Nutr* 9(2):1–7, 1994.
25. Probert KL, editor: *Moving to the future: developing community-based nutrition services,* Washington, DC, 1996, Association of State and Territorial Public Health Nutrition Directors.
26. Scholtes PR: *The team handbook,* Madison, WI, 1996, Joiner Assoc.
27. Speigel AD, Hyman HH: *Basic health planning methods,* Germantown, MD, 1978, Aspen.
28. Stoner JAF: Management, ed 5, Englewood Cliffs, NJ, 1994, Prentice-Hall.
29. Teal T: The human side of management, *Harvard Business Review* 74(6):35–44, 1996.
30. Wolfe WS, Bremner B, Ferris-Morris M: *Monitoring the nutrition of your community: a "how-to" manual,* Ithaca, NY, 1992, Cornell University Press.

CASE STUDY

VISION CITY, USA

DESCRIPTION

This case study presents data on the demographic, economic, social, and health factors of a metropolitan city. It illustrates data elements commonly available in the initial stages of a community needs assessment. However, the data are incomplete. The challenge is to make reasonable decisions based on the available information, and to identify additional steps that should be taken to extend the community nutrition needs assessment of Vision City.

METHODOLOGY/TEACHING OBJECTIVES

The Vision City case study provides students with a realistic situation to explore the processes and skills essential to planning. The case can be used as a homework assignment, a classroom discussion, or as a major project. Individuals or groups of students could select or be assigned to the agencies and questions below. The case can also serve as a starting point for the development of a nutrition program plan.

THE CASE

Vision City is an urban city located in the Midwest with a temperate climate and a mean temperature of 70° F. It has four distinct seasons. Its dominant geographic feature is the Heartland River, which borders the western side of the city.

DEMOGRAPHIC CHARACTERISTICS

A distinct characteristic of Vision City is that the proportion of elderly people and middle-aged working adults has increased in recent years. In fact, the elderly population has increased faster than the total population because of movement into the city. A second significant characteristic is the number of people from culturally diverse groups. Many Southeast Asians have settled in the area, it is an urban center for American Indians, it has a large Hispanic community, and Vision City continues to receive immigrants from eastern Europe. People have stated a variety of reasons for moving into the city, but the more commonly heard reasons are access to many health services, social and cultural opportunities, availability of recreation, and lack of job opportunities in their former communities.

The employment rate of the labor force has increased recently. In some households, however, employment does not provide enough income to prevent poverty, and eligibility for welfare payments is more restrictive than in the past. A significant number of households headed by women live in poverty.

Sex and Age Distribution

The age distribution of the Vision City population is shown in table 13.A. Note the size of the baby-boom generation and the fact that there are more women ages thirty-five to fifty-four available to work than men.

Race Distribution

Vision City's racial and ethnic groups are shown in table 13.B. In the case of Hispanics, specific neighborhoods have primarily Spanish-speaking people. The median age distribution among the racial groups varies substantially.

Employment and Economic Income

In Vision City, 9 percent of the workforce is unemployed. Seventy percent of women aged fifteen to fifty-five years are employed. The median income for a family of four for the total population is $28,900. For low-income households of four persons, the median income is $15,755. Figure 13.A shows the sources of household income for the total and low-income population.

Figure 13.B identifies the types of low-income households. Of the total population in Vision City, 11 percent do not have health insurance. Of the low-income households, more than half of the adult members skipped at least one meal per month because of lack of money, and 20 percent

TABLE 13.A

Sex and Age Distribution in Vision City, USA

	Total	Male (%)	Female
All ages (years)	500,000	241,680 (48.0%)	258,320
< 5	35,893	17,049 (47.5%)	18,844
5–14	135,205	68,955 (51.0%)	66,250
15–19	26,623	14,643 (55.0%)	11,980
20–34	127,676	70,222 (55.0%)	57,454
35–54	95,473	38,189 (40.0%)	57,284
55–64	29,395	13,962 (47.5%)	15,433
65–79	41,735	15,860 (38.0%)	25,875
80+	8,000	2,800 (35.0%)	5,200

TABLE 13.B

Race and Median Age Distribution Percentage of Ethnic and Minority Groups in Vision City

Race	Percentage	N	Median age
White	60	300,000	31.9
Black	17	85,000	25.0
Asian/Pacific Islander	10	50,000	28.7
Hispanic	5	25,000	23.2
American Indian	4	20,000	28.7
Other	4	20,000	N/A
Total	100	500,000	

N/A = Not available

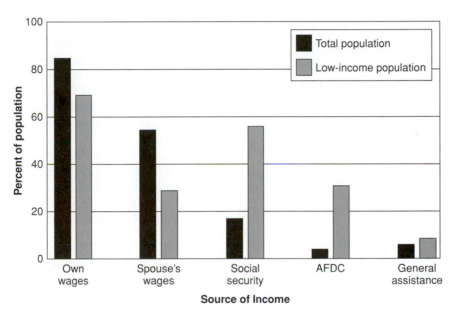

FIGURE 13.A   Sources of Household Income

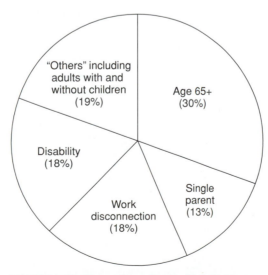

FIGURE 13.B   Types of Low Income Households

of the households with children reported their children had involuntarily missed meals. Lack of money affects finding affordable, adequate housing; paying for basic necessities; and carrying adequate medical coverage. These factors influence diet and health.

Factors affecting diet and health are complex. Low levels of educational attainment, subtle discrimination, and low income interfere with health-promoting behaviors. Table 13.C presents family size, education, and employment data for Vision City families.

VITAL HEALTH STATISTICS

The birthrate for all women in Vision City is 14 births/1,000 population. A substantial problem in Vision City is the high birthrate among teenage women (see table 13.D).

Morbidity is defined as the number of sick persons or cases of disease in relationship to a specific population. Morbidity identifies health conditions that interfere with life activities. The components of morbidity for life stages are described in table 13.E. Racial disparities exist for chronic diseases. Black residents of Vision City have greater incidence of strokes, tuberculosis, and diabetes; and overweight and diabetes are very prevalent among the Hispanic and American Indian residents.

Mortality is the number of deaths in a given population. The infant mortality rate by race in Vision City and the United States are identified in table 13.F. The top five causes of death by life stages for Vision City are outlined in table 13.G.

QUESTIONS TO BE ANSWERED

Scenario: Assume you are a community nutrition professional employed by one of the following agencies in Vision City:

- Area Agency on Aging
- Southeast Asian Community Health Clinic
- Salvation Army Food Pantry
- City Health Department

Read the Vision City Case. From the perspective of your agency what nutrition-related problems and predisposing conditions are most significant? Then respond to one or more of the following sets of questions and directions.

1. *Conducting a community needs assessment:* The data presented in the case study are incomplete. What additional information is needed for a comprehensive community nutrition needs assessment? How will you proceed with a needs assessment to gather a wider base of information for nutrition program planning? Who from your agency and collaborating groups will you involve in the needs assessment?

2. *Prioritizing needs:* Develop a set of decision criteria for determining priority needs in Vision City. Make the criteria relevant to your agency's constraints and capacity. Apply the criteria to prioritize identified problems or risk factors in Vision City.

3. *Writing goals and objectives:* Based on facts available in the case study, describe the nutrition-related health problems, potential risk factors, or predisposing conditions present in Vision City that could be within the scope of your agency's mission to address. What are the potential consequences to health and well-being if the problem, risk factor, or condition is not changed? Write a goal and process, outcome, and structure objectives to guide your agency's efforts to improve one or more of the problems.

TABLE 13.C
Family Characteristics of Vision City, USA

Characteristics	General population	Low income
Average family size	2.5	4
Educational attainment		
Completed HS or GED	91%	64%
College degree	25%	5%
Employment		
Full time	57%	26%
Part time	14%	21%
Low literacy	3%	10%

TABLE 13.D
Teenage Birthrate Among Women of Vision City

Age (years)	Birthrate/1,000 population
10–14	1.2
15–17	31.8
18–19	80.2

TABLE 13.E
Vision City Components of Morbidity by Life Stages

Infants and children	Adolescents	Adults 20–34	Mature adults 35–64	Older adults 65+
Child maltreatment	Depression	Cancer	Dental disease	Limitations in activity due to chronic conditions
Learning disorders	Teenage pregnancy	Occupational injury	Diabetes	Physical disabilities, hypertension, cancer, accidents and falls
Handicapping conditions	Sexually transmitted diseases AIDS	Diabetes	Arthritis	Perceived health status needs
Communicable diseases	Acne	Dental disease	Cancer	Social isolation
Accidents and homicide	Overweight and underweight	AIDS, infectious diseases	Circulatory diseases	Dependency
Dental disease	Accidental injury	Alcohol and drug abuse	Hypertension	Depression
Developmental delay	Handicapping conditions	Hypertension	Alcohol and drug abuse	Drug misuse
Growth failure	Dental disease	Depression	Infectious diseases	Infectious diseases
Anemia	Eating disorders Anemia	Heart disease	Obesity	Obesity
AIDS	Alcohol and drug abuse	Obesity		Inadequate nutritional intake

TABLE 13.F
Infant Mortality Rates of United States and Vision City

Population	Infant mortality rate
United States (all races)	10.2
Vision City	
White	9.4
Black	18.4
Southeast Asian	N/A
American Indian	10.0

N/A = not available

TABLE 13.G
Top Five Causes of Death by Life Stages in Vision City

Rank	Infants under 1	Children 1–14	Adolescents 15–19	Adults 20–34	Mature adults 35–64	Older adults 65–74	Older adults 75+	Total population
1	Birth-associated development problems	Accidental death by motor vehicle	Accidental death by motor vehicle	Accident	Heart disease	Heart disease	Heart disease	Heart disease
2	Congenital birth defects	Cancer	Suicide	Suicide	Cancer	Cancer	Stroke	Cancer
3	Ill-defined condition (SIDS)	Congenital birth defects	Cancer	Cancer	Accident	Stroke	Cancer	Stroke
4	Immaturity	Diseases of nervous system	Homicide	Heart disease	Diseases of digestive system	Diseases of digestive systems	Influenza and pneumonia	Accident
5	Infections and parasitic diseases	Homicide	Injuries (undetermined)	Homicide	Stroke	Influenza and pneumonia	Arteriosclerosis	Influenza and pneumonia

CHAPTER FOURTEEN

IMPLEMENTING PROGRAMS TO MEET COMMUNITY NEEDS

Above all else, our logic is not necessarily the same as the customer's logic. . . . The ability to understand the customer's needs and wants, to determine the nature of the service package, and to audit the current strategy can be summed up in a simple phrase, "Always be learning." The best service strategy is the one that is constantly being questioned, challenged, refined, and improved.

—KARL ALBRECHT AND RON ZEMKE

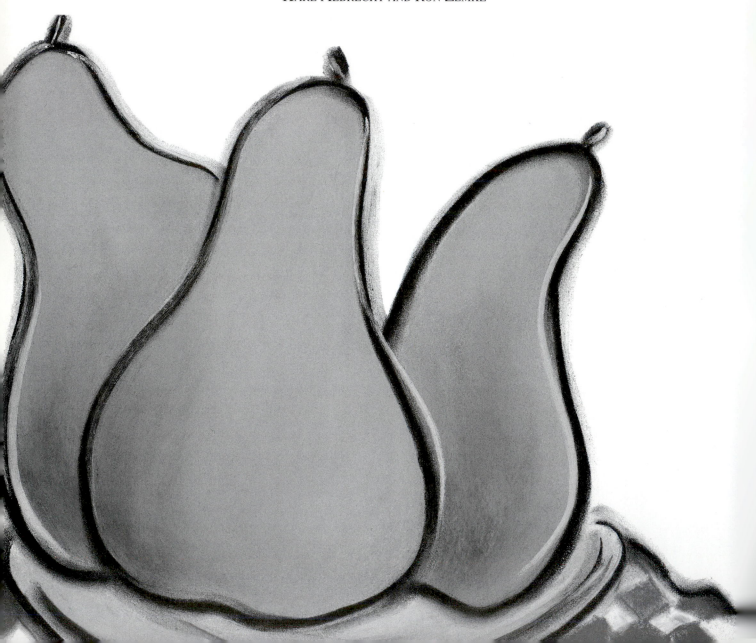

Core Concepts

Goals and program priorities are translated into action through implementation. The community nutrition professional designs the program to specifically meet the needs of the target audience within the community, and organizes activities, determines staffing requirements, and assigns responsibility for launching the program. Defined procedures and protocols assure consistency and quality throughout implementation. Management information systems are used to document and track program efforts and accomplishments. Customer-centered organizations, programs, and staff ensure the programs meet the needs and expectations of target audiences. Programs are designed, implemented, and evaluated by teams of people within the organization or brought together through interorganizational coalitions and partnerships. During implementation, community nutrition professionals use the skills of conflict management, and negotiation.

Objectives

When you finish chapter fourteen, you should be able to:

~ Apply the steps of the strategic marketing process to design a nutrition program.

~ Discuss the role of procedures, protocols, and management information systems in program implementation.

~ Describe a nutrition program in which quality customer service is the priority.

~ Determine staffing requirements for a program.

~ Participate as an effective leader and as a team member.

~ Explain the elements of principled negotiation.

~ Describe how coalitions and networking are used to more effectively address community nutrition problems.

Key Words

Word	Page Mentioned
Wants	413
Needs	413
Marketing principles	413
Customer-oriented	413
Market mix variables	413
Strategic marketing process	414
Segmentation	414
Product	416
Position	416
Action plan	416
Best practices	419
MIS	420
Quality service management	421
Staffing	422
Position description	423
Types of teams	425
Conflict	430
Negotiation	431
Cooperation	433
Coalition	433
Networking	433
Referral systems	436

The goal of community nutrition is to positively impact the health and nutritional well-being of people. Identification and prioritization of problems was addressed in the previous chapter, and other chapters of this text highlight nutritional challenges of various groups within the population. This chapter addresses how to design and deliver programs that meet the expectations of people in the community (figure 14.1). It recognizes that the expert definition of nutrition priorities and programs must be integrated with the needs, wants, and values of people.

As a starting point, consider the difference between clients and citizens, as described by Tom DeWars.[30] Clients are people who are dependent on and controlled by their helpers and leaders. They are people who understand themselves in terms of their deficiencies. Clients tend to wait for others to act on their behalf. Citizens (and customers), on the other hand, are people

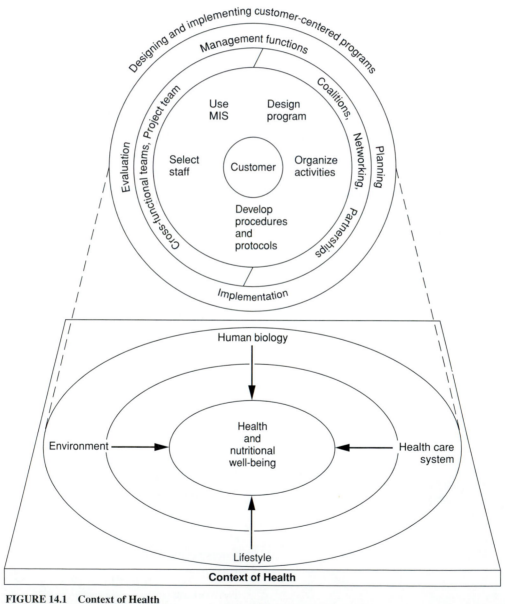

FIGURE 14.1   Context of Health
Designing and implementing customer-centered programs to meet community needs.

who understand their own problems in their own terms. They believe in the capacity to act.

Good interventions and programs continually listen to their customers and design, refine, and adjust to create programs that are responsive and empowering. This chapter addresses implementation from the perspective of being customer-centered.

DESIGNING CUSTOMER-ORIENTED PROGRAMS

In the 1990s, organizations in the public sector, as well as in the private business sector, began to realize that success comes from keeping customers foremost in mind. Businesses in the private sector know the importance of attracting and pleasing customers, whereas in the public sector, many organizations focus on pleasing policy makers and taxpayers rather than the specific customers of the program or service provided. Osborne and Gaebler provided a wake up call to public institutions with the publication of *Reinventing Government,* which showcased the dramatic improvement in accomplishments as well as cost savings when public organizations become entrepreneurial and put customers first.[30]

In success organizations, day-to-day operations reflect program and business decisions that represent a good fit between the organization's vision and goals and the **wants** and **needs** of the people who are its reason for being. Appreciation for the relationship between the provider organization and the customer is the essence of marketing and customer service.

A customer-centered organization uses strategic marketing to design their programs, products, and services to meet the needs of their customers. Staff in customer-centered organizations also tend to behave in a different way by applying the principles of quality customer service. The beginning of this chapter presents an approach to designing and implementing programs, products, and services that are customer-centered; addresses procedures and management information systems to assure quality; and then describes implementation with the customer foremost in mind—quality service management.

Strategic Marketing

Customer-centered organizations use an approach to management called strategic marketing. The principles and process of strategic marketing are presented here.

If you were to ask several people what is meant by "marketing" most would say "selling" or "advertising." They would be only partially correct. Marketing is a process of creating, building, and maintaining beneficial exchange relationships with target audiences for the purpose of influencing behavior. A marketing mind-set, according to Kottler and Andreasen,[21] begins with the consumer. Through marketing, the organization systematically studies customers' (target audience) needs, wants, perceptions, preferences, and satisfaction by using surveys, focus groups, and other means. This information is used to design services and products, to price them, to communicate (promote or advertise), and to deliver them to satisfy the target audience's needs and wants. The ultimate aim of marketing is to connect what the organization has the capacity and commitment to offer with the customers who want it. A customer-centered organization is one that makes every effort to sense, serve, and satisfy the needs and wants of its target audiences and constituencies within the constraints of its budget. For the community nutrition professional, this means program decisions are carefully crafted to match the needs of the target audience.

Marketing Principles

The **marketing principles** are

1. Marketing seeks to bring about a voluntary exchange of value. The marketer seeks to formulate enough benefit for the target audience to produce a voluntary exchange.
2. Marketing involves segmentation of the community into subgroups or target audiences.
3. Effective marketing is **customer-oriented,** not organization-oriented. Sensitivity to the target audience's needs and desires is a core component of effective marketing.
4. Marketing utilizes and blends a set of tools called the **market mix variables,** or the four P's: product, price, promotion (communication), and place (distribution).[21]

The not-for-profit sector (including government and nonprofit organizations) offers challenging settings for the application of the marketing principles. Four characteristics of not-for-profit organizations require special attention:

1. *Multiple constituencies:* Not-for-profit organizations have at least two major constituencies: their clients and their funders. The former poses the problem: how can we design a program, product, or service that offers value to clients? The latter raises the problem: how can we get sufficient resources to design it right in the first place?
2. *Multiple objectives:* Not-for-profit organizations tend to pursue several important objectives simultaneously rather than only focusing on profits.
3. *Services versus physical goods:* Not-for-profit organizations frequently produce services rather than goods. Customers of nutrition services frequently desire helpful information as well as support and understanding.[11]
4. *Public scrutiny:* Not-for-profit organizations are usually subjected to close public scrutiny because they provide needed public services, are subsidized, are tax exempt, and in many cases are mandated into existence. They experience political pressures from various constituencies and are expected to operate in the public interest.

The ultimate objective of all marketing is to stimulate a specific action in the target audience. The following examples illustrate the application of marketing principles to situations commonly experienced by community nutrition professionals: efforts to get individuals to change their food selection behaviors to reduce risk of cancer by substituting low-fat foods for those high in fat or by eating five fruits and vegetables a day; efforts to get worksite or school cafeterias to modify menus and recipes to match the Dietary Guidelines for Americans; efforts to secure funding from a foundation or payment from health plans; and efforts to enroll pregnant women in early prenatal care.

The Strategic Marketing Process

Organizations use strategic planning to adapt to the changing environment (see chapter 13). Customer-oriented organizations use strategic marketing to develop and maintain a strategic fit between the organization's goals and resources and the needs and wants of its customers or target audiences. The **strategic marketing process** is an extension of needs assessment and planning. It takes identified problems, goals, and program priority areas and moves on to the design of specific programs, products, or services for implementation. Social marketing, described in chapter 7, is a

special application of marketing that is used widely in health promotion, including nutrition interventions.

Eight steps summarized from the literature on strategic marketing are illustrated in figure 14.2 and described here.[21] Note how the goals of the nutrition program are adjusted to fit the wants of the target audience through the strategic marketing process.

Step One: Problem Definition   Based on identified health priorities and opportunities in the environment, define a potential area for change where a program, product, or service can reduce the problem and move toward the achievement of health goals. This step is accomplished through the needs assessment process described in chapter 13.

Step Two: Goal Setting   Set measurable goals for separate segments of the population. This enables program designers to determine the scope of the plan and a budget. Goals and more specific, measurable objectives establish benchmarks for success.

Step Three: Target Audience Segmentation   At this step, you select a specific segments of the population on which to focus efforts. Effectiveness is enhanced by tailoring programs to specific subgroups within the overall population. **Segmentation** is used to divide the total market or the total population into a smaller target audience or segment of people who have relatively similar wants. It can be based on any number of observable factors such as geographic location, age, risk factor or disease condition, socioeconomic status, attitudes and values, place of residence, or employment.

Step Four: Consumer Research and Analysis   This is the most crucial step. It recognizes that "one size does not fit all" and seeks to understand what would fit the needs and preferences of the targeted audience. Considerable time and resources must be allocated to the challenge of understanding the potential audience, their values and preferences, and their knowledge regarding the behavior you wish to change or the program you wish to engage them in. Market research through telephone or mailed surveys, focus groups, observation, and existing data is used to determine the interests, motivations, and values of the target audience; the characteristics of products and services they would be likely to use; their language and style preferences; and their knowledge and use of potential distribution channels.

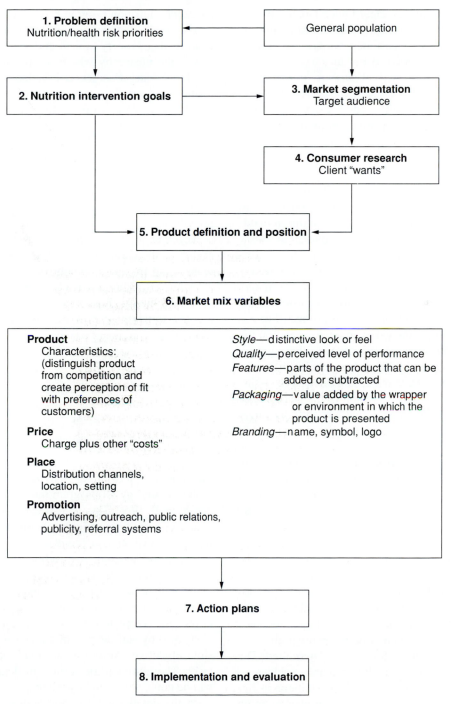

FIGURE 14.2   Strategic Marketing Applied to the Design of Nutrition Programs

This step should result in a clear understanding of target audience needs and wants. *Needs* are often not directly articulated by the consumer, but are essential to well-being and are related to the hierarchy of basic needs identified by Maslow.[23] *Wants* are an expressed desire for something; they indicate the consumer's perceived desirability or "felt needs." Customers have many needs and wants; the relative importance of these as motivators to seek a program, product, or service is tied to their values.[21]

Step Five: Product Definition and Position   Information from the previous step is carefully considered to define the product concept. In marketing terms, a **product** is anything that can be offered to a market to satisfy a need or want. It can be a physical object, service, person, program, policy, idea, or message. It is also necessary to determine the market niche or position this product will have among competitors. **Position** is the image that customers will have of the product. For example, should it be positioned as innovative and on the cutting edge, culturally specific to one ethnic group, quick and easy to use, solid and dependable, elite, economical, or upscale? Care must be exercised to define the product and its niche or position in the marketplace in a way that will be most compatible with the target audience's preferences.

Step Six: Market Mix Variables   This step is where community nutrition professionals purposefully design the product so it can be successful in its niche by making decisions about market mix variables. *Market mix variables* are factors that are directly under the control of those designing the product. They guide the development of the product and how it will be offered in the market place. The market mix variables are commonly known as the four P's—product, price, place, promotion. This step provides the strategic opportunity to create a good fit between the wants of the target audience and the goals of the community nutrition program.

At this step, each of the four P's is determined. The core *product* and its style, quality, features, packaging, and branding are determined (see the definitions in figure 14.2). The *price* is the monetary cost plus anything else that must be given up by the consumer to receive the product. The price could be a fee, but it can also include travel and waiting time, embarrassment, or inconvenience. *Place* is the distribution channel. Although clinics are traditional sites for nutrition counseling and education, nutrition programs, products, or services can be creatively distributed through schools, worksites, mass media, grocery stores, and sports clubs. *Promotion* is the means by which the product is communicated to the target audience. It includes outreach, public relations, advertising, and other promotion efforts. Referral systems and word of mouth have been a commonly used means of making people aware of community nutrition services. More formalized communication activities should be used to effectively connect the target audience with the programs, products, and services designed to meet their needs and wants.[13] Box 14.1 outlines numerous ways to promote community nutrition programs.

Together the selection of a target audience (market segment), the choice of a competitive position (market niche), and the development of the market mix variables (the four P's) to reach and serve the customers are called the "marketing strategy." Table 14.1 illustrates the development of a marketing strategy for dietary counseling of pregnant teenagers.

Step Seven: Action Plan and Budget   This step involves detailed planning of the people, tasks, and resources to implement the designed program, product, or service. Two phases are described—planning the schedule of activities and planning resource needs.

Planning and Scheduling Activities   Action planning is routinely used by all program managers to plan and organize work flow. This is also called operational planning. Community nutrition professionals must be familiar with and feel confident in their ability to create action or operational plans. Action planning is a process that determines how all activities related to implementation will be organized and conducted. According to Craig,[6] an "activity" is defined as a specific procedure or process, completed at a certain point in time, and implemented by staff as part of a plan for reaching the desired objective. Activities are made up of a series of tasks. The **action plan** defines in detailed terms what will be done, when, and by whom.

In the development of the action plan, a planning grid helps to organize all the key activities and tasks needed to reach a goal, such as designing a product and bringing it to the marketplace. Figure 14.3 provides a sample format for organizing activities and tasks, including definitions of terms and tips for its use.

BOX 14.1

PROMOTION OF COMMUNITY NUTRITION PROGRAMS

Outreach—actions to recruit the target audience to participate in the program

Contests

Free samples

Direct mailings

Designed buttons, decals, bumper stickers

Flyers placed on windshields in parking lot

Notices in church bulletins

Sidewalk sign placed outside office or program site

Brochure describing benefits of program

Public relations—actions to earn public understanding and acceptance

Demonstrations in grocery store or mall

Cable television program

Exhibits at civic and professional meetings

Presentations at civic groups

Invited tours of your organization

Sponsoring of a sports team or event

Having program profiled in newspaper

Distributing free "how-to-do-it" handout related to nutrition message

Advertising—nonpersonal forms of communication conducted through paid media under clear sponsorship

Signs on buses and in bus shelters

Cross-promotion with another group reaching out to the target audience

Radio announcements

Ads in local newspapers or newsletters read by target audience

Grocery bag labels or stuffers

Point-of-purchase display

Web page

Publicity—the planting of news about the program or product in published (newspaper), broadcast (radio and TV), or electronic media (Web) that is not paid by the sponsor

Feature story in newspaper

Ribbon cutting news coverage

Endorsements by other organizations

Being a guest speaker on a talk show

TABLE 14.1
Marketing Strategy Worksheet

Marketing process	Example
Target audience	1. Teenagers age fourteen to eighteen who become pregnant
Market mix variables	Prenatal dietary counseling offered by dietitian
Product	Message: 1. Modify snacking behavior to increase nutrient intakes of vitamins A and B_6, folic acid, calcium, and iron. 2. Gain adequate weight 3. Identify accessible food resources
Price	Miss class or afterschool activities; no monetary charge
Place	School-based health clinic
Promotion	• School newsletter • Brochure in school nurse's office • Planned Parenthood clinics • Community family planning
Competitive position	• Tailor counseling services to priorities of teens • Offer at school where pregnant students spend day • Integrate into prenatal program for academic credit

Source: Adapted from Ward M: *Marketing strategies: a resource for registered dietitians,* Binghamton City, New York, 1984, Niles and Phipps.

The steps to completing a planning grid are:[35]

1. Specify the final outcome. How will you know when this project has been successfully completed?
2. Identify the final activity and its result.
3. Identify the starting point and its result.
4. Brainstorm a list of separate, distinct activities that will take place between the starting and ending points.
5. Refine the brainstormed list: clarify what is unclear, eliminate redundancy, subdivide tasks that are too large, and combine those that are too small.
6. Prepare the grid.
7. Arrange the list of activities in sequence down the left column of the planning grid. Use of self-stick notes is recommended so that the steps can be easily rearranged until the sequence seems right.
8. Fill in the results column.
9. Enter a tentative date for each item. You need to complete this step before others because the time available for performing some activities affects the scope and nature of other activities. (Do you have

Step number	Sequential steps activities tasks	Due date	Results	Responsibility	Whom to involve/contact	Budget and cost	Other categories

Definition of terms used in the action planning grid

Step number

Simple numbering is used most frequently to indicate the sequence of events, but you may use some other code if you like.

Sequential steps/activities/tasks

Enter, in chronological order, each task that is part of this activity. For example, if the step involves "data collection," then the tasks might be (1) develop operational definitions, (2) prepare checksheets, (3) test and refine checksheets, (4) train data collectors, (5) collect data.

Result

Each discrete step produces some result; for example, a report, a tangible change, a decision, a phone call, a meeting. There is always something that indicates the completion of a step. Enter here a word or phrase describing what that completion sign is for this step.

Responsibility

Enter here the name of one or two people who are responsible for seeing that this task gets done. Note: They do not necessarily carry out the action themselves. They may just coordinate the actions of others.

Due date

The calendar date when this step should be finished.

Whom to involve/contact

If appropriate, enter here the names of people who should be part of the team working on this task, or who should at least be contacted and informed of progress or events.

Budget/cost

If funds have been allocated for this activity, or if there is a limit to expenditures, enter that figure.

Other categories

Customers

This column lets you keep track of people who are particularly interested in or concerned about the successful outcome of this step or the project as a whole. Typically, this includes people whose work depends on what is accomplished at this step.

Limitations/specifications

Enter here any constraints under which the people involved with this step must operate, such as amount of time per week they can spend on the task, how many other people they can call on for help, the maximum time they can stop a process (if at all), and so forth. Note: You may also enter time and money limits here, though the categories of "budget" and "due date" usually indicate the same thing.

Hazards/pitfalls

Past experience with this activity may lead you to expect trouble in some form. Enter here any information that will help the team avoid pitfalls.

By-products

Many times a team will be given secondary objectives: "While you're at it, see if you can do this for another purpose." Although secondary purposes should not be allowed to interfere with the primary objectives of the activities, they should be allowed if they may lead to useful results without detracting.

FIGURE 14.3   Format for the Action Planning Grid

(*Source:* From Scholtes P, et al: *The team handbook: how to use teams to improve quality,* Madison, WI, 1988, Joiner Associates Inc.)

thirty days or six months available for the product design?) Due dates also indicate when the person responsible for that item must be available. If you have an inflexible deadline, start at the end of the list and work backward. Use prior experience and any knowledge about similar activities to set realistic deadlines.

10. If necessary, revise items.

11. Complete the remaining columns described in figure 14.3.

Another common technique for scheduling activities is Gantt scheduling.[6] In Gantt scheduling (figure 14.4), a bar chart is used to indicate the start and completion dates of activities. Activities are listed in the column on the left and dates are listed across the top. To use the Gantt technique, one works from left to right, plotting activities as they must occur and establishing a completion date for the job. Horizontal dotted lines are drawn so that their lengths represent the planned duration of each activ-

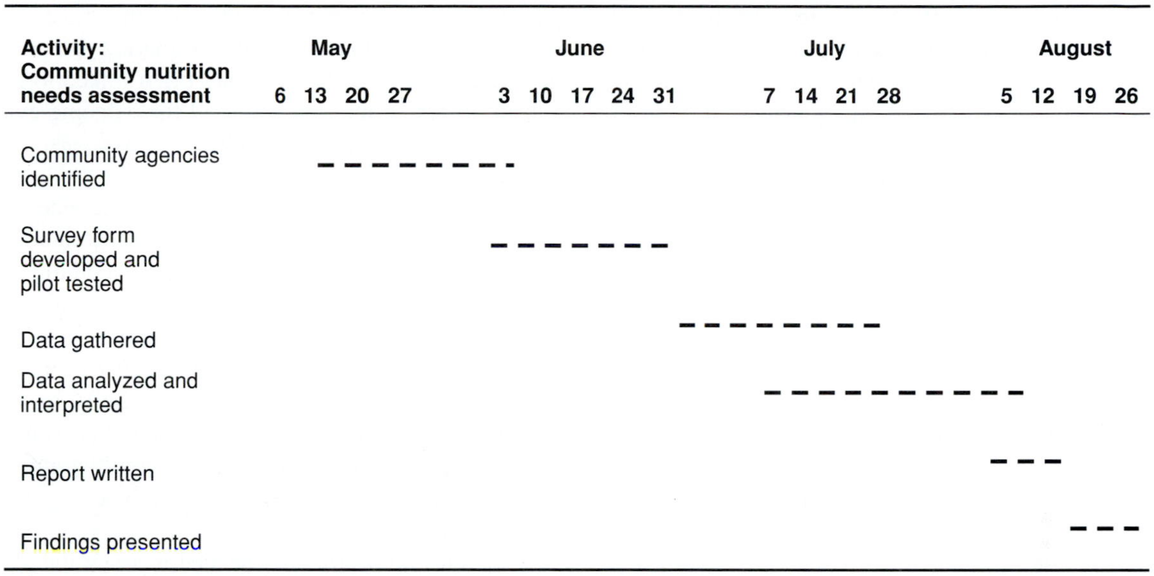

Activity: Community nutrition needs assessment	May				June					July				August			
	6	13	20	27	3	10	17	24	31	7	14	21	28	5	12	19	26
Community agencies identified	– – – – – – –																
Survey form developed and pilot tested					– – – – – –												
Data gathered									– – – – – – –								
Data analyzed and interpreted										– – – – – – – –							
Report written														– – –			
Findings presented																– – –	

FIGURE 14.4   Gnatt Scheduling of Activities Related to a Needs Assessment

ity. Progress on each activity is monitored by drawing solid lines parallel to and below the dotted lines to show actual duration for activities underway or completed.

Planning Resource Needs   The action plan must include attention to resource needs and expenditures. What resources (personnel, materials and supplies, equipment, facilities) are needed to carry out the action plan? Where will these resources come from? Will the product generate revenue? The answers to these questions define the financial picture. Money to finance community nutrition projects can come from a variety of public and private funding sources, including grants, contracts, payment from health plans, and payments for products and services. These topics of budgeting and financial management and proposal writing are discussed and illustrated in chapter 16.

Step Eight: Implementation and Evaluation   Carry out the plan, introduce the program, product or service, and evaluate. This step documents the types of measurements, controls, and review procedures that will be used (see chapter 15 for details on evaluation). It is important that the authority for evaluation, as well as decisions regarding adjustments, are clearly defined early in the implementation step. Evaluation activities should also be listed on the action plan.

In summary, this eight-step model can help community nutrition professionals design a new product venture that meets the needs and wants of the target audience. It can also be used to retool existing programs to make them more customer-centered. The customer orientation is essential to making community nutrition services relevant and accessible to members of the community.

PROCEDURES AND MANAGEMENT INFORMATION SYSTEMS

Procedures and Protocols

Getting ready for implementation requires the development of carefully defined procedures that will assure consistent quality during implementation. Successful organizations search for "**best practices**" (practices used in house or by other organizations that are judged as state-of-the-art and state-of-the-science and consistently meet customer needs and produce positive outcomes). Then the planning team customizes and innovates to define procedures that meet the requirements and constraints of the particular project and the needs of the target audience.

The aim is to develop workable processes and procedures that assure quality implementation and positive outcomes; and that are closely attuned to customers needs and wants. The amount of time allowed for this task depends on the complexity and nature of the project. For example, this activity can range from revising a set of client education materials to a comprehensive statewide campaign to modify eating behavior, as illustrated in the case study at the end of this chapter.

Most nutrition interventions require carefully defined protocols, practice guidelines, standards of performance, or quality assurance criteria that delineate appropriate intervention processes for the age group or disease or condition targeted. Sources used in the development of procedures and protocols include past experience within the organization, best practices and protocols used by similar types of programs, and quality assurance guidelines and practice guidelines from professional and scientific organizations. Many considerations and guidelines for intervention are described in Part Two of this text. When carefully developed, the protocols become the bases for performance monitoring and quality assurance, which are described in chapter 15.

Projects are most likely to succeed when launched using good operational plans, executed by highly motivated teams.[14] Team building can begin by involving staff in front-end planning. Staff who will be involved in the implementation of the program, as well as others with expertise in the project area, should participate in the development of procedures and performance standards.

In preparation for implementation, all staff should be trained in use of the procedures and protocols, and in the required documentation. Training is minimized when staff are involved in front-end development and testing of procedures.

Management Information Systems

Once the project is launched, activities must be documented and monitored. Effective management of the project requires timely information so that problems in resource availability, performance of activities, and volume of services can be identified early and adjustments made. Procedures and data systems for documenting and summarizing information about activities and programs and services delivered for management and evaluation is called management information systems (**MIS**).

Four kinds of information are generally needed for management of nutrition programs. Systems to document and monitor this information must be put in place in the design phase for the program or service and refined as necessary to secure helpful information to monitor and adjust the program.

Direct-service-type programs require a system for documenting and tracking clients through an appropriate sequence of service: screening and assessment, intervention, referral, and follow-up. *Individual client records and case management files* are maintained as paper records or computerized electronic files. Client records and case management information are used for quality assurance audits; they are often linked to financial information, and may be used for outcome evaluation and cost-effectiveness studies.

Service delivery information is used at the program level to monitor units of service against service objectives. In direct-service programs, it is based on appointment schedules and encounter records. In community or environmental interventions other strategies are used to count contacts with or exposures to the message or program. Service delivery information produces participant counts, service output reports, and descriptive measures of the population served. Service information is used to monitor performance and report to administrators and funders, and it is also of interest to advocates and the general public.

Financial information is needed to track the allocation of resources to planned programs and activities. This includes budgets, reports of expenditures and revenues, and records of billing and collections when fees are charged (see chapter 16).

Evaluation information is gathered to assess specific indicators of program performance and client outcomes compared to established external program objectives, as well as to state and national objectives.

MIS must be designed prior to implementation of the project so efficient methods for tracking program participants, program activities, costs, and outcomes are in place. Existing MIS in the organization can be used for some documentation and tracking, although most new programs require some additional documentation tailored to the specific activities and objectives of the program. By working with computer, accounting, and medical records personnel within the organization, the community nutrition professional can develop appropriate procedures and forms for tracking essential information for management purposes.

Most public health and community services have or are implementing computerized systems to document and manage data for the above purposes. Data systems should be tailored to program and organization needs, as well as to reporting requirements of funders and state and national nutrition monitoring systems.

MIS and Public Health Nutrition

Beyond uses for a specific project, the community nutrition professional should be aware of general purpose uses of MIS in public health nutrition. Standard health and nutrition status indicators that have scientific and practical significance in monitoring the public's health and the impact of nutrition programs should be incorporated into the evaluation MIS.[17] The internal MIS system may be supplemented with external data sets for overall program management purposes, including needs assessment and monitoring the program's contribution toward state and national health objectives.

In addition, the MIS of local and state public health agencies should be designed to contribute data to state and national systems that track information for a number of purposes listed below. Note how the following purposes relate to the public health responsibilities of assessment, policy development, and assurance:

1. To identify and track populations and geographic areas in need of service by poor rankings on health status indicators
2. To document types of services available and how well they are delivered
3. To determine accessibility and utilization of services by the population at risk
4. To measure intervening changes in behavior, knowledge, and risk status
5. To assess the effectiveness of existing services in improving health status.[17]

QUALITY SERVICE MANAGEMENT

Service management is the art of designing, developing, and delivering distinctive customer service.[2] Quality customer service is now excepted as an essential ingredient in public service as well as the business world.[30] Through **quality service management** organizations meet customers' needs, and therefore further the accomplishment of programs whose goals are to assist or help members of the population or target audience. In organizations where service quality is a priority, attention focuses on achieving results for the customer rather than simply counting services delivered.

One model for quality service management is the concept of the cycle of service. In this model, service is viewed as a repeatable cycle of events in which the provider attempts to meet the customer's needs and expectations. At each point of contact, the customer forms judgments about the service. If these contacts are handled in mediocre ways, the quality standard is mediocrity. Alternatively, if the points of contact are managed to ensure customer satisfaction, the standard is excellent quality. Quality control involves designing services to meet customer needs and wants and monitoring service processes using customers' criteria for satisfaction as a standard. The quality management cycle is illustrated in figure 14.5.

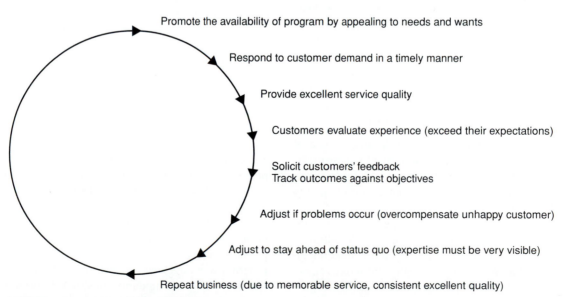

Promote the availability of program by appealing to needs and wants

Respond to customer demand in a timely manner

Provide excellent service quality

Customers evaluate experience (exceed their expectations)

Solicit customers' feedback
Track outcomes against objectives

Adjust if problems occur (overcompensate unhappy customer)

Adjust to stay ahead of status quo (expertise must be very visible)

Repeat business (due to memorable service, consistent excellent quality)

FIGURE 14.5 The Quality Management Cycle

Principles of Quality Service Management

Successful service providers operate with a high level of concern for and attention to the needs of the customer. Studies of successful service organizations have identified five operating principles that can be applied by community nutrition professionals. These principles are:

1. Listen to and understand the evolving needs and expectations of customers. Respond to what is learned with quality improvements in problematic processes or procedures, or staff behaviors.
2. Establish a clear vision of what superior service is. Communicate that vision to all persons involved in the program. Make quality customer service important to everyone in the program.
3. Define concrete standards for quality customer service (including scheduling practices, intervention procedures and protocols, etc.) and regularly measure against those standards. Quality service means 100 percent performance; anything less is not acceptable.
4. Bring in good people; train and coach them to work on behalf of customers. Empower them with the knowledge and skills to reach the performance standards and to act on behalf of customers.
5. Recognize and reward service accomplishment. Reinforce employees who go "one step beyond" for customers.[39]

These principles mean personal attention to customers and to the staff who are responsible for customer service. To meet customers' expectations the program and organization must understand the way their customers think, feel, and behave. This understanding is gained through needs assessment and market research described earlier along with a system for regular listening to the customer.

Listening to the Customer

Berry and Parasuraman emphasize the importance of systematic listening to the voice of (1) customers, (2) noncustomers, and (3) employees.[4] Multiple views and methods enable a richer understanding of quality expectations and actual delivery.

Customers' perceptions and experience are commonly measured with satisfaction surveys. In addition, systematically capturing complaints and comments allows service failures and opportunities for improvement to be identified. By surveying noncustomers you gain an understanding of how the service is perceived by nonusers and their reasons for nonuse. It also enables comparison of your service against competitors. Surveying employees identifies their perceived obstacles to improved service and tracks employee morale and attitudes. Berry and Parasuraman encourage managers to become personally involved in listening to the voice of customers, noncustomers, and employees from a variety of perspectives.[4] Peters indicates that when you listen, what you should expect to hear is "Wow!"[32] When you hear this, you can count on repeat business and word of mouth to bring others to your program.

In summary, quality customer service means meeting or exceeding the expectations of customers. To consistently do so requires vision, commitment, and a quality management process. Community nutrition professionals must ask and listen to customers, monitor quality indicators, and act on data. Staff must be given the responsibility and skills to meet customers' needs. Performance that produces and improves quality should be recognized and rewarded.

STAFFING

Staffing is the process of providing necessary human resources to the organization or program. The staffing objective of increased organizational effectiveness is achieved by bringing on board and maintaining staff with the appropriate set of expertise and skills to successfully implement the program, project, or service.

To secure appropriate nutrition staff, community nutrition professionals must work with the human resources department within their organizations. The human resources department in public health agencies and most other organizations is responsible for policies relating to recruiting, hiring, and determining compensation (salary levels) for employees. Managers in the nutrition unit or other departments initiate requisitions for new positions and work with human resources to procure staffing. However, this is just one step. Other steps and decision processes the community nutrition professional should be prepared to address in staffing a project are shown in table 14.2. In the table, words in brackets indicate terminology used by human resources personnel.

A software package to help community nutrition professionials navigate the job classification and compensation process is available[36] The SSNAPS software program was developed to aid public health nutritionists in creating and updating position descriptions, exploring appropriate salary levels to compensate nutri-

TABLE 14.2
Staffing Your Project

1. Consider the sets of activities necessary to achieve goals and objectives of the project.
2. Who is going to carry out each activity? [position titles], [series and classes] How will each task be done? [job design] What skills/knowledge/abilities are needed to do the activity? [job analysis]
3. How will staff relate to each other and to the rest of the organization? [responsibility, authority, accountability; allocation of formal power]; [organizational chart]
4. Prepare a document to communicate the duties and responsibilities to others. [position description]
5. Where will you get them? [procurement; job specifications; job requisition; recruitment, selection, orientation, training]
6. How can you assure productive contribution of all staff members to the goals and objectives of the organization/project? [performance standards and appraisal; staff development; quality assurance, continuous quality improvement]
7. Consider the role of the project director in assigning and supervising work, and guiding and coordinating individual and team performance.

---

tion employees, and recruiting and retaining qualified nutritional personnel. Readers are encouraged to refer to this excellent resource.

Position Classification for Public Health Nutrition

Surveys of public health nutrition personnel reveal great disparity and inconsistency in the assigned responsibilities and qualifications required for positions having the same job title.[18] To address this confusion *Personnel in Public Health Nutrition for the 1990s* provides a rational and consistent approach to classifying public health nutrition positions.[7] Using current terminology, the publication defines the title, major duties, functions, and knowledge, skills, and abilities of public health nutrition personnel. Benchmark position descriptions for each class are included. Positions are classified into nine classes based on their major functions and grouped into three series based on their focus (see figure 2.4, p. 31). The series are management, professional, and technical.

Careful definition of positions assures that appropriately skilled and cost-effective public health nutrition personnel are available to operate the program.[7] A position description is written for every position to classify it and assign a pay grade. The **position description** is the official record of the work assigned to an employee. It is used to establish qualifications for hiring and pro-

motion, orient new employees, develop performance standards, and determine training needs related to job functions. A sample position description for the public health nutritionist class is shown in box 14.2. The actual position description can vary from the sample to meet the specific needs of the situation.

Staffing Community Nutrition Programs

The size and complexity of the overall nutrition program, the population to be served, and the public health service delivery system all influence nutrition staffing requirements. General recommendations for staffing nutrition programs are detailed in box 14.3. Box 14.4 illustrates how to estimate staff requirements based on client contacts.

The number and position classification of nutrition personnel in an organization depends on several factors:

- Size, age distribution, health, and nutritional status of the population
- Numbers and concentration of medically, socially, and economically high-risk clients
- Mix of community- or population-focused programs versus direct client care–focused delivery services
- Availability of nutrition services provided by other health or human services agencies or related agencies in the jurisdictional area
- Number and type of related agencies
- Expectations of the public and other constituents
- Constraints imposed on service delivery by population disbursement, geographical and language barriers, and climate

Beyond the number and classification, another decision to be made is where nutrition personnel are located in the organization. Each agency must determine the placement for its nutrition personnel within its formal structure (or organizational chart). Where nutrition personnel are located depends on the basic structure of the organization, its mission, legislative mandates, funding sources, priorities, and service delivery systems, as well as the philosophy of administration regarding discipline-specific versus cross-functional teams.

Staffing patterns (position classes and numbers of personnel in each class) are generally reviewed on an annual basis as part of the program-planning and budgeting process. In addition, attention is given to staffing as each new program initiative or revision is considered. Depending on the responsibility and level of experience

BOX 14.2

POSITION DESCRIPTION: PUBLIC HEALTH NUTRITIONIST

MAJOR DUTIES

The public health nutritionist is responsible for planning, implementing, and evaluating the nutrition programs and services of the local health department. She or he advises the health director regarding the nutrition issues and problems in the community, and establishes and maintains programs and services to address priority needs. The public health nutritionist collaborates with health department staff and other organizations in the community to assure the availability of necessary nutrition programs and services.

FUNCTIONS/RESPONSIBILITIES

Planning and evaluation: Conducts community assessment of nutrition and diet-related health problems and resources to determine needs of the population and opportunities for effective intervention; solicits customer, professional, and collaborator input in the design and development of nutrition programs; develops operational plans for nutrition service delivery including timelines, evaluation standards, and budget needs; utilizes agency and client information systems to document, monitor, and evaluate nutrition program activities and outcomes; and participates in determining nutrition care and program policies for various target populations.

Education and behavior change interventions: Interprets and disseminates current scientific information regarding food, nutrition, diet, and health to professionals working in the health department, health and social service agencies, educational institutions, and to the public; plans, arranges, presents, and evaluates educational programs; disseminates information through the media including newspaper, radio, TV, and the Internet; designs intervention programs using behavior change and social marketing strategies; selects and/or develops, evaluates, and revises nutrition and health promotion materials for use in

health department programs assuring cultural, ethnic, educational, and literacy relevance to the target audience; and supervises field experiences of students.

Consultation: Provides technical assistance to health agency staff and other professionals and organizations in the community.

Supervision: Plans, assigns, directs, and evaluates the work of other nutrition staff; recruits, selects, and orients new staff; assigns work and assures staff accountability for productivity; participates in developing and reviewing standards for nutrition personnel; assesses training needs and develops and implements a plan for continuing education and career development.

Management: Compiles, analyzes, and reports county health and nutrition data to monitor quality of service, and program outcomes; and prepares monthly and annual nutrition program reports.

Budget: Prepares and justifies budget requests, oversees resource utilization in nutrition programs and takes corrective action when indicated, and identifies funding sources and writes grant proposals.

KNOWLEDGE AND SKILL REQUIREMENTS

Broad knowledge of the principles, theories and practice of public health nutrition and health promotion, and ability to translate and communicate this information to professionals and the public.

QUALIFICATIONS

Minimum education: master's degree in public health

Professional credentials: registered dietitian and licensure by state

Minimum experience: one year of public health nutrition experience after master's degree (three years experience desired)

---

needed, a position classification is determined, and depending on the volume of work the number of positions are determined. If existing staff cannot be freed from other activities to conduct the new activities, or when the type of expertise needed is not available, a job requisition is initiated and recruitment begun.

Activities relating to staffing a nutrition program should be specified in the implementation action plan. All personal must be adequately prepared for their responsibilities. Specialized projects may require inservice training and staff development, procurement

of technical assistance or consultation, or recruitment of new personnel with the needed expertise.

IMPLEMENTATION THROUGH TEAMS

Today traditional hierarchies and formal systems are being replaced with teamwork and partnering.[15] This is true within organizations as work becomes more interdependent; and it is true of the way many community nutrition problems are addressed by multiple organizations working collaboratively on shared goals as coalitions.

BOX 14.3

STAFFING RECOMMENDATIONS FOR NUTRITION PROGRAMS

- A *public health director* (*nutrition*) is recommended for the large public health agency that employs five or more nutrition personnel plus support staff.
- *One assistant public health director* (*nutrition*) in addition to a public health director (nutrition) is recommended for the nutrition program in a public health agency serving a population of over 500,000 or that offers a complex public health nutrition program comprising a multiplicity of programs and services, manages a substantial nutrition program budget, and employs a large staff.
- A *public health supervisor* (*nutrition*) is needed by health agencies that provide significant amounts of one-on-one client nutritional care planning and counseling through clinical or home health programs.
- *Public health nutrition consultants* are generalists or specialists. Generalist public health consultants are employed by many local and state health agencies. The allocation of generalist public health nutrition consultants depends on the number and complexity of agencies and nutrition programs within the geographic area. In most states, a generalist nutrition consultant should be responsible for providing technical assistance to no more than three to four densely populated counties and/or municipalities or six to eight rural counties. Specialist public health nutrition consultants are usually employed on categorical program teams in state health agencies, in large complex city or county health agencies, or by special demonstration health projects or specialized voluntary health agencies.
- The *public health nutritionist* often functions as the one nutritionist working with other members of the public health team in a local health agency. For program development implementation and evaluation with a community or population focus, one public health nutritionist per 50,000 population is generally suggested.
- The *clinical nutritionist* functions as case manager and/or care coordinator and nutrition counselor in clinical or home health programs serving large numbers of medically high-risk clients.

Staffing is based on an assessment of the size, risk level, and care needs of the target population, the amount of time required per encounter, the number of follow-up encounters required, and the amount of time required for care coordination and case management functions (see box 14.4).

- *Nutritionists* or *community dietitians* plan, manage, and coordinate the individual client's nutrition care. This care includes nutrition assessments, care planning, education and counseling, follow-up, and group education. A rule of thumb suggested by the Association of State and Territorial Public Health Nutrition Directors for staffing ambulatory or home health programs serving a target population at high nutritional risk is one nutritionist or dietitian supervising two nutrition or dietetic technicians per 1,000 registered clients. Other suggested staffing ratios vary from one direct service professional per 500 client population to one per 800 to 900 client population.
- *Nutrition technicians and nutrition assistants* from the technical support series provide services that complement the professional skills of the nutritionist and provide a cost-effective way of extending nutrition services. Staffing for technical support positions is recommended at a ratio of two nutrition technicians and/or nutrition assistants per one nutritionist in direct care services or one nutrition technician per 360 to 500 clients.
- *Clerical staff*—public health nutrition managers and professional workers will be more productive and cost-effective if sufficient clerical support is available, and if appropriate technologic support including computers, e-mail, fax machines, and telephone-answering equipment are available to all staff.

Source: Adapted from Dodds JM, Kaufman M, editors: *Personnel in public health nutrition for the 1990s,* Washington, DC, 1991, The Public Health Foundation. Used with permission.

Committees and task forces have been used for a long time, but a number of labels have evolved to describe new ways of organizing people for work: design and project teams, self-managed work teams, high-performance teams, and cross-functional or superteams. Intraorganizational teams are also common; they are referred to as coalitions, alliances, and partnerships. The latter are addressed in the last section of this chapter.

Types of Teams

A team is defined as two or more people who interact and influence each other toward a common purpose.[25] Different **types of teams** can be formally created or they can emerge informally.

Informal groups emerge whenever people interact on a regular basis. They often combine personal and social needs as well as organizational needs. For example,

BOX 14.4

A METHOD FOR ESTIMATING STAFFING NEEDS
FOR CLIENT NUTRITION CARE

STEP ONE

Establish the target populations for your agency's nutrition program and specify the type of service.

Calculate for each target population:

L = the estimated length of time for each encounter

N = the total number of encounters needed per year (number of encounters multiplied by the number of clients or clients in a group)

Target Population 1

Clients with special nutrition needs because of their health status, for example, pregnant and lactating women, infants and children with identified nutrition-related health problems (e.g., WIC program), persons requiring therapeutic diets for chronic diseases.

- Type of encounter: individual counseling
- Length of encounter: 30 minutes = $L_1 = \frac{1}{2}$ hour per client.
- Number of encounters per year = $N_1 = 2 \times$ number of clients seen in one year

Target Population 2

Persons identified at high nutritional risk through nutritional screening and assessment who are not also served as part of a high-health-risk population, for example, older children identified at high nutritional risk because of poor growth or abnormal biochemical assessment.

- Type of encounter: individual counseling
- Length of encounter: thirty minutes = $L_2 = \frac{1}{2}$ hour per client.
- Number of encounters per year = $N_2 = 2 \times$ number of clients seen in one year.

Target Population 3

Health care providers, educators, social workers, and child care staff providing nutrition care and food service to high-risk populations, for example, MCH nurses and nursing assistants.

- Type of encounter: group classes
- Length of encounter: one hour divided by fifteen participants = $L_3 = \frac{1}{15}$ hour per person
- Number of encounters per year = $N_3 = 2 \times$ number of participants in one year

Target Population 4

School children, the elderly, or the general public involved in health promotion and disease prevention programs, for example, community aggregate meal site for the elderly.

- Type of encounter: group classes
- Length of encounter: one hour divided by thirty participants = $L_4 = \frac{1}{30}$ hour per person
- Number of encounters per year = $N_4 = 2 \times$ number of participants for one year

---

women managers may meet periodically to share issues and successes and support one another. Through informal groups, members learn unwritten "rules" or norms, and they learn about and discuss matters that affect them and begin to form reactions or plans that can lead to personal or group problem solving. Informal groups offer access to information, friendship, and support and also provide status and security.

A formal team is created deliberately and charged with carrying out specific tasks to help the organization realize its goals. Formal teams include work groups, committees, task forces, cross-functional teams, and high-performance teams.

Work groups traditionally consist of a leader or manager and all staff members who report to the manager. To deemphasize the hierarchy and to accommodate the shift to participatory management terms like "coach" and "associates" are used. A work group is not neces-

sarily a team. *Team* implies commitment to a common vision, cooperation, and communication. In many settings, individuals work side by side in similar or complementary activities as "work groups," but they do not always employ the three C's of teams—commitment, cooperation, and communication.

A *committee* is a group formed for a specific purpose (e.g., quality assurance committee) that exists for a long time even as members come and go.

Temporary teams are called *task forces* or *project teams*. They are formed to deal with special tasks or problems and are disbanded when the task is complete. Members are selected based on what each person can achieve and the skills each has, rather than on the formal authority or title of the person.

Cross-functional teams, which bring together people from a number of work units and skill and expertise areas, can be created to work on important, defined pro-

BOX 14.4 (CONTINUED)

STEP TWO

Estimate K, the effective hours per worker per year available. Total hours minus annual leave (an estimated average), holidays, sick leave (estimated based on average amount used in past), travel time, continuing education, and personal time, for example.

Total available working hours per year	
(40 hr × 52 wk) =	2,080
minus annual leave (8 hr × 15 days =	− 120
	1,960
minus sick leave (8 hr × 6 day's) =	−48
	1,912
minus travel time (hr) =	−52
	1,860
minus continuing education (hr)	−16
$K =$	1,844

STEP THREE

Estimate H, the number of hours needed for adjunct activities per year, for example, planning and preparation, recording and reporting, consultation, meetings, and personal time.

STEP FOUR

Apply the formula:

$$\frac{L_1N_1 + L_2N_2 + L_3N_3 + L_4N_4 + H}{K}$$

= staff needed to serve program's target populations number of direct service nutrition

Insert your program's figures in the following blanks:

$$\frac{L_1(\ ) \times N_1(\ ) + L_2(\ ) \times N_2(\ ) + L_3(\ ) \times N_3(\ ) + L_4(\ ) \times N(\ ) + H}{K(\ )} = \underline{\quad}$$

Example: Estimating the nutrition direct care staffing needs of one county nutrition program

Target population 1:

7,000 clients at two thirty-minute individual encounters per year.

6,000 clients seen in group classes of thirty persons each class lasting thirty minutes and seen two times a year.

Target population 3:

In-service programs for nursing staff: one-hour presentation, twice a year with fifteen nurses and assistants attending each time.

K is calculated at 1,844 hours

H is estimated at 400 hours

$$\frac{\frac{1}{2} \times 14,000 + \frac{1}{60} \times 6,000 + \frac{1}{15} \times 30 + 400}{1,844}$$

$$= \frac{7,502}{1,844} = 4 \text{ direct care nutrition providers}$$

Adapted from Freeman RB, Holmes EM: *Administration of public health services.* Philadelphia, 1960, WB Saunders.

jects or to conduct routine, on-going program operations. One common example in health departments and health care is the interdisciplinary team. Cross-functional teams are the choice when there are complex problems to solve and layers of management to cut through. They are valuable for breaking down turf barriers and refocusing efforts on customers' needs. Often these teams lack authority to make commitments and decisions without consulting with their respective department heads. In the new organizational philosophy, they are given greater authority to act for the common good.

Self-managed teams and *high-performance teams* have the responsibility, authority, and accountability to manage themselves without any formal supervision. The team has responsibility for an entire scope of work and has the power and authority to determine such things as work methods, scheduling, assignment of members to different tasks, priorities, and productivity

standards. They order their own materials and supplies and have the authority to interact with customers and other teams. Within the organization, self-managed teams are compensated and given feedback according to the performance of the group as a whole.

These new models of organizing people for work move away from the traditional mind-set of managerial control and power and individual responsibility; and move toward trust and openness and shared responsibility for decisions and actions that further the organization's mission and more effectively meet the needs of customers.

Characteristics of Teams

To utilize and manage teams effectively it is important to understand their characteristics. Effective teams have leadership roles, norms, and cohesiveness.

Leadership Roles   A team begins with a formally appointed or elected leader, or as the team works together an informal leader emerges. Experts in the field of management and organizational behavior believe that by eliminating the authoritarian aspect of organizations and depending on commitment and natural leadership, teams enjoy unchecked creative power.[12,37] This fosters innovation, problem solving, commitment, and enhanced performance and productivity.

Norms   Norms are expectations about how to behave. Pressure to conform to norms is strong in most settings. Conforming to norms can be very useful because it frees members to concentrate on tasks. Conformity can be negative if it stifles initiative and innovation and restricts the group's performance.

  Norms vary across the community. The work of community nutrition professionals takes them in and out of a number of groups and teams. Each will have its norms related to dress, punctuality, value for tradition versus innovation, and the like.

Cohesiveness   Cohesiveness is the strength of the members' desire to remain in the group and their commitment to it. Cohesiveness is enhanced by competition, interpersonal attraction, expanding opportunities for interaction, and creating common goals and fates for all group members.

  Cohesiveness and cooperation within groups helps meet goals and accomplish tasks. Teams become cohesive when they face conflict with outside individuals or other teams, or pressure of an outside enemy (e.g., the challenge of the nutrition problem itself, or competition for budget allocations).

Groupthink   When groups are both conforming and cohesive a phenomenon called groupthink can occur.[12] *Groupthink* is an unexamined consensus that results in ineffective decision making and poor quality decisions. It is further described in box 14.5. Community nutrition professionals should recognize the lure of groupthink and push for higher-level analysis of issues, search for alternatives, and exploration of assumptions. Some of the group process methods for problem solving and prioritization presented in chapter 13 can be used.

Stages of Team Development

By studying the dynamics of groups, Tuchman identified five stages that teams move through: forming, storming, norming, performing, and adjourning.[38]

BOX 14.5

GROUPTHINK

SOME CAUSES OF GROUPTHINK
- High cohesion
- Insulation from outsiders
- Lack of methodical procedures for search and appraisal
- Directive leadership
- High stress with a low degree of hope of finding a better solution
- Complex/changing environment

SOME CHARACTERISTICS OF GROUPTHINK
- Failure to reexamine assumptions
- Stereotyped views of rivals or enemies
- Ethical or moral consequences of decisions are not explored
- Self-censorship in which members are not inclined to express doubts or present counterarguments
- Self-appointed mind guards protect members from adverse information

TO PREVENT GROUPTHINK
- Leader should try to remain neutral and encourage criticism and new ideas
- Use subgroups or consultants to introduce different viewpoints
- Encourage members to search for and freely present alternative ideas

---

Source: Adapted from Hellriegel D, Slocum JW, Woodman RW: *Organizational behavior,* St. Paul, MN, 1992, West Publishing Co.

Forming   This is a stage of orientation to the group and the task. Implicit and explicit ground rules emerge. Other aims of the forming stage are clarifying the team's mission, defining goals and objectives, and establishing procedures for getting the work done.

Storming   Conflict over roles and leadership sometimes emerges. Members must resolve personal versus team goals and sort out commitment to the task. Continued conflict may be an indication that the charge to the group is unclear.

Norming   Group identity emerges as members establish common goals, norms, and ground rules. Members more freely voice opinions. Trust and solidarity emerge.

Performing Roles differentiate and members take initiative for completing tasks. The structure of the group now supports and eases group dynamics and performance. To operate at a high level at this stage, members need to receive feedback, to challenge assumptions, and to exercise creative problem solving.

At times team performance begins to level off or deteriorate. This may happen if members become complacent, burned out, or defensive. If these symptoms are present, the team needs refocusing and revitalization, or if the essential task had been accomplished, they are ready for the next stage.

Adjourning Temporary groups such as task forces or project teams complete their charge. For some projects, closure means transferring responsibility for ongoing activities to a specific person, department, or organization. With disbandment in mind, the group's focus shifts away from high task performance to closure. Members may feel pride and excitement or a sense of loss.

Teams spend different amounts of time in each stage, but in general if they move to performing without clarifying roles and expectations they have less success. Beck and Yaeger[3] indicate that the storming state is not inevitable. If teams know their mission, goals, and management expectations, they move more quickly to the performing stage. People who are experienced in team work and team members who have worked together before also move more quickly to the performing stage.

When Teams Meet

Meetings are a tool of communication and planning; but team work does not happen because people come together in one room. Team performance requires an orchestrated effort to achieve effective group dynamics and translate a group effort into individual accountabilities.[3] This is launched and nourished in a series of meetings.

Rules for Making Teams and Meetings Work

- Clearly define, preferably in writing, the *goals* and *charter*.
- Specify the team's *authority*. Do they investigate, advise, recommend, decide, implement?
- Match the *size* of the group to the task and the situation.
- Select a *chairperson* based on ability to run an efficient meeting, encourage participation of all members, and see that paperwork is done.
- Distribute an *agenda* and *supporting material* to all members before meetings to permit them to prepare

in advance. This enables members to be ready with informed contributions and keeps them focused.
- Start and end meetings *on time* as announced at the outset.[37]

The optimal size of teams is an unresolved issue. Size varies according to circumstances such as the scope of the charter and the range of expert resources to address the charter. Research suggests that with less than five members, the advantages of the group are diminished because creativity and ideation are minimized. Potential resources increase as the size increases. With more than ten to fifteen members, a team becomes unwieldy, and it is difficult for each member to influence the work of the team and therefore feel a part of it. In other situations, thirty may be the size needed to involve all parties who have valuable know how and resources. Larger teams can be divided into subgroups to address parts of the charter or complete a related series of tasks.

Effective Teams

Early research on group dynamics and effectiveness found effective teams were usually quite small consisting of six to seven members, and that smaller groups are more durable.[24,37] Box 14.6 outlines characteristics of effective teams. In today's settings with complex issues and a dynamic environment, the basic building blocks of commitment, accountability, and skills are required of all team members. According to Katzenbach and Smith,[16] when these building blocks are present the result is high performance and personal growth.

Independent Work Is a Part of Team Work

The most important work of teams does not happen in meetings; it happens where the members do significant amounts of work to deliver on the commitments made to the team.

Managers create effective teams by first of all giving the team a charter (also called a challenge, task, charge, or assignment). The charter should have a clear goal and an achievable set of objectives.

The members of the team then decide how to achieve the goal. They deliberate how much task interdependence their work requires. Then the work is broken down and assigned to subgroups and individuals. Work assignments should address specific and concrete issues rather than broad or abstract ideas. Each team member has to do roughly the same amount of work, or there will be differing commitments to the outcomes.

BOX 14.6

CHARACTERISTICS OF AN EFFECTIVE TEAM

1. The team members share a sense of purpose or common goals, and each team member is willing to work toward achieving these goals.
2. The team is aware of and interested in its own processes and examines norms operating within the team.
3. The team identifies its own resources and uses them, depending on its needs. The team willingly accepts the influence and leadership of the members whose resources are relevant to the immediate task.
4. The team members continually try to listen to and clarify what is being said and show interest in what others say and feel.
5. Differences of opinion are encouraged and freely expressed. The team does not demand narrow conformity or adherence to formats that inhibit freedom of movement and expression.
6. The team is willing to surface conflict and focus on it until it is resolved or managed in a way that does not reduce the effectiveness of those involved.
7. The team exerts energy toward problem solving rather than allowing it to be drained by interpersonal issues or competitive struggles.

8. Roles are balanced and shared to facilitate both the accomplishment of tasks and feelings of team cohesion and morale.
9. To encourage risk taking and creativity, mistakes are treated as sources of learning rather than reasons for punishment.
10. The team is responsive to the changing needs of its members and to the external environments to which it is related.
11. Team members are committed to periodically evaluating the team's performance.
12. The team is attractive to its members, who identify with it and consider it a source of both professional and personal growth.
13. Developing a climate of trust is recognized as the crucial element for facilitating all of the above elements.

Source: From Hanson PH, Lupin B: Team building as group development. *Organizational Development Journal,* 1986. Used with permission. For information contact Dr. Donald W. Cole, RODC, The OD Institute, 11234 Walnut Ridge Rd, Chesterland, OH 44026.

Team members should meet periodically to share progress, update changes, identify and solve problems, and capitalize on discovered opportunities. Without regular meetings, team members are likely to redirect their focus to other priorities and their team contribution may level off.

The team must feel it has sufficient resources—skills, money, and flexibility—to fulfill its charter. Multifunctional and interorganizational teams will only work if hierarchical patterns of communication are broken down. In addition, members must have a sense of outcome interdependence. They need to share a sense of common fate or they will have little sense of belonging and commitment. High-performing teams are facilitated by top management, which must foster an environment of openness, commitment, and trust.[16]

As a member or leader of a team, the community nutrition professional can practice behaviors that foster high level performance of teams (see box 14.7).

Paying Attention to Cultural Factors

Appropriate team process is influenced by culture. Some cultures value discussion more than others (e.g., American Indian talking circle in which no decision is made until everyone has had a chance to say anything they want to about the issue). In many ethnic cultures, elders' input is given great weight. Other cultures value individual decisions and initiative. A team is unlikely to be effective if it fails to recognize cultural influences of members and of the host or partner organizations participating.

MANAGING CONFLICT

Conflict is a disagreement between two or more individuals or groups arising from differences of opinion, facts, objectives, or methods. The allocation of scarce resources and disagreements about roles and responsibility for activities are common sources of conflict. Conflict is also fueled by differences in status, goals, values, knowledge, or perceptions.

Conflict is a natural part of team, organizational, and interorganizational dynamics. It is not only inevitable but it is necessary for organizations to survive. Conflict leads to a search for solutions, and thus it is an instrument of problem solving, innovation, and change. The role of the manager or leader in conflict situations is not to suppress or resolve all conflict, but to manage con-

TEAM MANAGEMENT FOR COMMUNITY NUTRITION PROFESSIONALS

1. *Orient the team:* Give them a clear direction, facilitate problem solving to focus the team members in determining the best way to accomplish the mission and goals, help everyone become clear about the goal.
2. *Plan of attack:* Help the team determine when and how it plans to accomplish the tasks. Clarify what team members need from the leader, other team members, and people or organizations outside the team to get their work done? Be sure each member knows his or her responsibility—the deliverables.
3. *The work:* Give team members the freedom and flexibility to accomplish their responsibilities. Check from time to time, listen, offer encouragement, and be responsive when support is needed.
4. *Team problem solving:* Come together at regular intervals to keep members informed of progress, to identify and solve problems and plan for next steps. Use the power of the group to focus individuals and help the organization or partners perform at a higher level and produce results.

flict so as to minimize its harmful aspects and maximize its beneficial aspects.

Conflict Management Skills

Conflict management skills are needed by community nutrition professionals in the complex and dynamic environment of community nutrition. Good communication and listening skills are needed to develop trust and cooperation when there is no way of avoiding conflict. Conflict should be recognized as an opportunity to make changes within an organization or team that may be beneficial. Community nutrition professionals need to confront conflict and respond in a manner that leads to solutions in which all parties feel like winners. Tools are available to help professionals understand and develop their conflict management behaviors.[20]

An effective manager must demonstrate the commitment to actively involve and support those affected by a conflict situation. Then, to arrive at a mutually agreed-upon decision, it is important that a manager develop an atmosphere of trust and effectively guide the group through conflict resolution. A manager needs to encour-

age active listening and open communication so that individuals' perceptions of the situation and attitudes about it are exposed for others' reactions. This reality testing moves beyond emotions to an understanding of what is actually the basis for the problem.

Negotiation

Negotiation is defined as a process in which two or more parties, having both common and conflicting goals, state and discuss proposals concerning specific terms of a possible agreement.[12]

According to Adler, Rosen, and Silverstein, planning and preparation are the best strategies for negotiation. Having clearly defined goals, substantial information, and a well-thought-out, but flexible strategy is essential to successful negotiation.[1] They have developed a checklist for preparing for a negotiation (see box 14.8).

Principled negotiation is a means toward reduced conflict. It is based on finding commonality and compatibility between the goals of each party. Principled negotiation, which was developed at the Harvard Negotiation Project,[10] is deciding the issues on their merits rather than on the power, position, or persuasion of either side. Its focus is mutual gains whenever possible, while being hard on the merits but soft on the people. Where interests conflict a fair, objective standard is sought. Principled negotiation has four elements, which are illustrated in box 14.9.

Better outcomes are achieved through negotiation when the options are expanded. Obstacles to identifying options are premature judgment, searching for a single answer, assuming a fixed pie, and thinking that "solving their problem is their problem."[10] Inventing more options can evolve from what, when, how, and where questions. For example, the amount, the timing, the methods, or the location could all have variations in the negotiation process.

Negotiators are advised to be clear about their bottom line—the point at which no agreement is possible.[1,10] Fisher and Ury suggest the definition of a BATNA, which is your "best alternative to a negotiated agreement." In the BATNA, you define both the desired goal and a bottom line at which an agreement is not acceptable. Once these are determined, there is more room for exploring options that fall between the best and the bottom. Another point of the BATNA is exploring what you will do if no agreement is reached. This step takes some of the risk out of the negotiation because you have consciously explored other alternatives and in essence have a "Plan b." The third point of the BATNA is considering the BATNA of your opponent.[10]

BOX 14.8

PLANNING FOR A NEGOTIATION

1. Identify goals and interests in priority order
   - Yours
   - Their (best guess)
2. Secure necessary information
   - Information I need from them
     Before the negotiation
     During the negotiation
     After the negotiation
   - Information I need, but can find from sources other than them
     Before the negotiation
     During the negotiation
     After the negotiation
   - Information they need from me (my best guess)
     Information I am willing to disclose—and the circumstances
     Information I am not willing to disclose
3. Invent options
   - Best alternative (mine/theirs)
   - Promising alternatives
   - Bottom line for no agreement (ours/theirs)
4. Consider negotiation strategy
   - Criteria for a negotiated agreement
   - Choices of approaches
     Hardball, conciliatory, friendly
     Unconditional constructive strategy
   - Offers
     First offer made (by me or them)
     First realistic offer (by me or them)
     Potential trade-offs and reasons I give for trade-offs
5. Ongoing assessment of negotiation
   - Points that suggest negotiation is going well
     Strategy in case negotiation is going well
   - Points that suggest negotiation is not going well
     Strategy in case negotiation is not going well
6. Documents needed
   - Documents already prepared
   - Documents that need to be prepared

Source: Adapted from Adler R, Rosen B, Silverstein E: Thrust and parry: the art of tough negotiating, *Training & Development,* March:43–48, 1996; Fisher R, Ury W: *Getting to yes,* New York, 1981, Penguin Books; and Fisher R, Brown S: *Getting together: building relationships as we negotiate,* New York, 1988, Penguin Books.

BOX 14.9

ELEMENTS OF PRINCIPLED NEGOTIATION

People: Separate the *people from the problem.*

Focus: Focus on *interests,* not positions.
Work toward *shared* goals and commitment to outcome.

Options: Generate a *variety of possibilities* before deciding.
Invent options for mutual gain.

Criteria: Insist the *result* be based on some *objective standard.*

Source: Adapted from Fisher R, Ury W: *Getting to yes.* New York, 1981, Penguin Books.

Agreements may be reached more easily if negotiators move beyond self-interest. The best way to achieve your aims may be by helping the opponent achieve their aims or by making the agreement look more attractive to them. This is the reason the preparation and planning phase includes attention to learning about the goals and interests of the opponent.

Good negotiation can build trust and establish a solid ground for future relationships. Fisher and Brown give guidelines for how to be an effective negotiator. In their view, every relationship has conflicts of interest, but every relationship has a common interest in dealing with the conflict. They recommend using an unconditional constructive strategy throughout the negotiation process[9] (see box 14.10).

The actual negotiation process can unfold over a period of time. Frequently there is a meeting at which each party presents their view of the situation and their interests. At this session you should ask and listen to gain a good understanding of your shared and differing interests, values, and goals. This meeting should also explore objective criteria for an agreement and begin generating options.

In the next session, each party presents its preferred option. You search for mutual gains, and identify possible trade-offs to achieve an agreement. The aim is to develop an agreement beneficial to all parties.

BOX 14.10

AN UNCONDITIONAL CONSTRUCTIVE STRATEGY

Do only those things that are both good for the relationship and good for us, whether or not they reciprocate.

1. *Rationality:* Even if they are acting emotionally, *balance emotions with reason.*
2. *Understanding:* Even if they misunderstand us, *try to understand them.*
3. *Communication:* Even if they are not listening, *consult them before deciding* on matters that affect them.
4. *Reliability:* Even if they are trying to deceive us, neither trust them nor deceive them; *be reliable.*

5. *Noncoercive modes of influence:* Even if they are trying to coerce us, neither yield to that coercion nor try to coerce them; *be open to persuasion and try to persuade them.*
6. *Acceptance:* Even if they reject us and our concerns as unworthy of their consideration, *accept them as worthy of our consideration, care about them, and be open to learning from them.*

Source: From *Getting Together.* Copyright © 1988 by Roger Fisher and Scott Brown. Reprinted by permission of Houghton Mifflin Company. All rights reserved.

At the final session, you secure agreement and outline plans for implementation and follow-up. This is important for assuring follow through by all parties. Celebrate common ground and shared efforts toward mutual goals.

Recognizing that conflict is inevitable, and harnessing it for constructive purposes will serve the community nutrition professional well. Using a concise step-by-step approach to coming to mutually acceptable agreements through negotiation is also an important skill. These approaches are important to keep in mind in collaborations across organizations which is the final topic of this chapter.

JOINT VENTURES: INTERORGANIZATIONAL IMPLEMENTATION

Pursuing Cooperative Ventures: Coalitions and Networking

Community nutrition professionals are involved in community-based interventions that focus on creating change in populations. Population change cannot be achieved by one agency or by several working independent of each other. Community nutrition professionals must work with other groups to develop the **cooperation** needed to solve major community nutrition/health problems.[33] Cooperation includes exchanging information, altering activities and sharing resources to achieve mutual benefits and a common purpose. To work effec-

tively with other groups, community nutrition professionals must have knowledge and understand interactions with a broad range of community groups, policy makers, health professionals, and advocates as well as the general public. Developing cooperative ventures is a strategy that will extent resources and facilitate change in the community.

Coalition Building and Networking

Coalition building is considered a formal process. Networking, by contrast, is informal. A **coalition** is described as a temporary alliance of distinct partners or persons for joint action. The terms "partnerships" and "alliances" are often used interchangeably with coalitions and thus are used the same way in this chapter. **Networking** is the exchange of information, and the sharing of ideas and resources with another person or cluster of people.[34]

Documented support for coalitions in the public health community is endorsed in the National Academy of Science "Diet and Health" report, which recommends coalitions to promote the public's health. "It is apparent to the committee and the Food and Nutrition Board that if one of our national goals is to reduce the risk of chronic disease, and if dietary modification is likely to assist in achieving this goal, then various sectors of society need to collaborate in implementing dietary recommendations of the type prepared by the committee."[5]

Major Functions of Coalitions

There are three major functions of coalitions.[33]

- Solve or monitor a problem or coordinate a special event that an individual organization might not otherwise take on because of limited resources. Coalitions offer a means of extending limited resources and of adding something important to an overburdened agenda without putting full resources behind it.
- Exchange or coordinate information. With the new health care system changing and reorganizing, it is important to keep abreast of new developments that will affect your community. For example, the seamless health care system that is supposedly developing describes a major role for health promotion, disease prevention, and primary care. Keeping informed of these developments can help provide opportunities for identifying where nutrition and health education fit into this seamless health care.
- Advocate for policy change. Include diverse groups in promoting legislation and public policy issues important to nutrition. For example, if managed care organizations including HMOs, medical associations such as AMA and AAFP all advocate for medical nutrition therapy, it has a greater chance of being accepted.

Benefits of Coalitions

Nutrition intervention coalitions benefit consumers, health group partners, and health professionals. Table 14.3 describes the benefits of coalitions and partnerships to the community, public health agencies, community partners, and the community nutrition program.[22]

Weighing Risk and Benefits of Coalitions

The benefits of forming coalitions as described in table 14.3 are substantial. However, as the benefits are weighed, recognition of potential risks is necessary.[22] It is important to take steps to minimize risks.

Potential Risks to the Agency   The agency may fear that credibility will be tarnished by associating with profit-making groups. Nutrition intervention with partners will involve negotiating and some compromises to reach mutual goals. Some find it hard to believe that the profit-makers of business partners can be compatible with the public good. In some instances, agencies have unrealistic expectations for coalitions. In the planning process, clearly stating the objectives and expected outcomes of the project will minimize this situation.

Potential Risks to the Community   There is risk of confusing or misleading the community if the intervention's integrity is not assured. Monitoring the scientific basis for the intervention and consistently applying it are quality control concerns that surface. Business partners particularly fear that confidentiality about proprietary information will not be monitored. Protecting proprietary information is essential to their competitive edge in the marketplace. Public sector partners in general may be viewed as slow-moving, red-tape-bound bureaucracies with significant decision-making barriers. Business partners often need flexibility and quick turnaround on decisions to stay competitive.

Minimize the Risk of Coalitions

There are several ways to reduce the risks of working with coalitions. Understanding the role of the agency in the coalition is key to minimize the risks. The following strategies will also help minimize the risks:

- *Credible health information source:* In coalitions, the agency's role is to be the credible health information source. The credible health information source is recognized by community residents, community partners, and other health professionals as a legitimate source of accurate health information services.
- *Nutrition criteria protect credibility:* The inherent risk to credibility in population-based strategies is minimized when food- and brand-specific nutrient criteria or standards are used to decide which food products can be identified as healthier choices and promoted in the intervention. The use of criteria protects your agency, food marketing partners, and the consumer by providing a scientifically defensible basis for decisions about which food products can be promoted and which cannot. Establishing criteria is an early and absolutely essential step in the nutrition intervention coalition process.
- *Personal credibility counts:* Coalitions are based on personal relationships. Your personal conduct can enhance the integrity of the nutrition intervention. Examples of being personally credible include following through on commitments of time and resources and maintaining the confidentiality of partners regarding their proprietary information. Speak cordially and tactfully to create an atmosphere in which partners can trust one another.[22]

TABLE 14.3
Benefits of Coalitions and Partnerships

Benefits to the community from nutrition intervention coalitions and partnerships

- Partners make it possible to communicate clear and consistent messages to improve healthy behavior.
- Consistent messages reduce the confusion created for consumers when groups with seemingly comparable goals make different recommendations.
- Potential for healthier food products appear in the marketplace.
- Potential for community to solve its own health and nutrition problems results in improved services without duplication of efforts.
- Communities are organized to provide health-promoting programs which can be the most cost-effective way to combat the high health care costs that result from chronic disease.

Benefits to public health agencies from nutrition intervention coalitions and partnerships

- Provide leverage for the agencies limited resources.
- Foster positive community image for the agency.
- Provide visibility and understanding, which can translate into more political and financial support for nutrition interventions.

Benefits to community partners from nutrition intervention coalitions and partnerships

- Partners share expertise and resources. Money, materials, and staff can be extended by working together.
- Partners gain access to important information about the community's nutrition and health needs and resources.
- Partners gain access to the community's nutrition and health professional network.
- Business partners who want to position their healthy food products with nutrition-conscious consumers gain credibility by actively associating with a health agency.
- Partners who are themselves sources of credible health information, such as local affiliates of the American Heart Association, American Cancer Society, and The American Dietetic Association benefit from sharing the visibility, resources, and credibility of the coalition.

Benefits to the community health professional from nutrition intervention coalitions and partnerships

- Community health professionals enrich their knowledge and enhance their marketable skills.
- Networking is expanded and individual effectiveness is enhanced.
- Creativity is stimulated when partners who have common goals but different expertise share their individual perspectives on issues.

Source: Adapted from Lansing D: *Nutrition intervention in chronic disease,* Atlanta, 1990, US Department of HHS, Center for Disease Control and Prevention.

Nutrition Coalitions

There are several examples of effective partnering and coalition-building in the nutrition area. These include programs at the national, state, and local level.

The National Action Plan to Improve the American Diet   The National Action Plan to Improve the American Diet was a major effort to apply the combined efforts of the government and nonprofit and food industry sectors to work together to shape food consumption in a positive way to promote health and to reduce the burden of disease among the U.S. population. More than thirty-five public- and private-sector organizations are involved in this effort. The plan defined actions to reach the dietary changes called for in *Healthy People 2000,* the nation's prevention objectives[28] (see chapter 2).

As a first project, the partnership sponsored a major national conference addressing the issue of healthy eating for America's children and youth.[26] The outcome of the conference was a strong consensus to focus on two priority objectives:

- To create demand for a healthful diet and physical activity by advancing consistent messages for children and their families
- To create environmental support to build and maintain healthful choices for both nutrition and physical activity

The project is an example of a national effort to achieve healthy eating and reduce the risk of chronic disease.

Food and Nutrition Science Alliance (FANSA)   In 1992, four major nutrition organizations joined forces to translate scientific expertise into accurate and consistent information for the public and the media. The Food and Nutrition Science Alliance (FANSA) represents more than 100,000 members from the American Dietetic Association, the American Society for Nutritional Science, the American Society for Clinical Nutrition, and the Institute of Food Technologists. The four organizations are committed to working together to disseminate one consistent message and to minimize confusion and assist consumers in developing and maintaining healthful dietary practices. FANSA operates on a set of principles that were developed by the four organizations. This partnership effort has developed periodic press releases on key nutrition topics, such as transfatty acids and the need for obesity research.[29,31]

5 a Day for Better Health Program   The 5 a Day for Better Health Program is a large public-private partnership that approaches consumers with a simple, positive message: eat five or more servings of fruits and vegetables every day. The program is jointly sponsored by the National Cancer Institute (NCI) and the Produce for Better Health Foundation (PBHF), a nonprofit consumer education foundation representing the fruit and vegetable industry.[19] The program's objectives are to

- Increase public awareness of the importance of eating at least five servings of fruit and vegetables every day for better health
- Provide consumers with specific information about how to incorporate fruits and vegetables into their daily eating patterns.

The increased consumption of fruits and vegetables is promoted within the context of low-fat, high-fiber diet.

The NCI and the PBHF grant licenses to partner organizations for the use of 5 a Day Program materials. This includes retailers, shippers, packagers, merchandisers, commodity boards, trade associations, and branded products. State and territorial health agencies coordinate 5 a Day activities at the state level. At the community level, the collaboration of industry and health licensees use statewide coalitions to plan and implement the program. Participants include individuals from state and county health agencies, state departments of education and agriculture, cooperative extension service, voluntary agencies, the food industry, hospitals and state dietetic associations. An example of an effective state and local program is described in the case study from the Arizona Department of Health Services at the end of this chapter.

The American Dietetic Association Partnerships
Recognizing the need to create relationships beyond the boundaries of the dietetic profession, the American Dietetic Association participates in more than 100 partnerships, many through its National Center for Nutrition and Dietetics. These partnerships cover a full spectrum of age groups—from the American Academy of Pediatrics to the National Council on Aging—and a variety of populations with special nutritional needs—including the Amer-

ican Heart Association, the Women's Health Initiative, and the American College of Sports Medicine, to name a few. The networks, resources, and reach provided by partnerships like these help move key health and nutrition messages to the forefront.

Networking

As the world grows more complex and health care more sophisticated, networking is one of the most important elements in communicating with the public, with fellow health care professionals and with the private sector. As John Naisbitt described in his now classic book *Megatrends,* "networkers are people talking to each other, sharing ideas, information and resources. . . . The important part is not the network, the finished product, but the process of getting there—the communication that creates linkages between people and clusters of people."[27]

Networks can move in many directions like a spider's web. Select the direction carefully and evaluate steps as you proceed. For example, as a community nutrition professional, networking with the school system including school feeding programs is important for the maternal and child health work that you are doing. Knowing the elderly feeding programs and how they are delivered in the community is vital for the other end of the life cycle.

Coordination and Referral Systems

Coordination and **referral systems** are essential to maximize the services available to the community and to provide continuity of care. For example, managed care has a strong coordination and referral or case/care management system in place. Coordination involves getting nutrition programs already in existence to work together and become familiar with each others program to avoid duplication of services and to extend services and reduce conflicting information to the public. Referral is getting recipients, clients, or patients to use all the services they need and for which they are eligible.[33]

Coordination

Probert lists the nutrition service providers and programs that should be coordinated within the community.[33]

- *Nutrition personnel of state and local health agencies and special projects such as Maternal Child Health (MCH), WIC, high-risk perinatal projects, commu-*

nity health centers, and services for children with special health care needs. Close working relationships with one another make it possible to share information and coordinate goals, objectives, program plans, standards, and criteria for service.

- *Nutritionists and other personnel in other agencies such as human service department, schools, or extension services.* Such agencies have educational or service programs that will be supportive of health plans for individuals and families in areas such as menu planning, food preparation, and home management.
- *Nutritionists and dietitians in ambulatory health programs, treatment centers, rehabilitation centers, home health programs, and other group care facilities.* Linkage with treatment centers is necessary for appropriate follow-up of clients on special dietary regimens who return home.

- *Nutritionists and other health care providers within the program.* An organized internal system of interdisciplinary referral for nutrition counseling is essential even in a small project.

Referral

The community nutrition professional is responsible for providing continuity of care. This includes the use of many agencies to provide the services needed. Table 14.4 provides a list of agencies that may be involved in a referral system. It is a referral guide for nutrition-related problems that provides information on available community resources such as health service providers, educational institutions, and community groups. Knowledge of these community resources will enhance the patient's care.

TABLE 14.4
Referral Guide for Nutrition-Related Problems

Problem	Agency	Problem	Agency
Educational	Child day-care facilities School systems Vocational training programs Department of Education Veterans Affairs Bureau of Indian Affairs Migrant opportunity programs Community action programs	Social—*continued*	Local service and religious organizations Volunteer organizations Mental health services Migrant opportunity programs Community action programs Human services
Economic	Employment services Vocational training programs Rehabilitation programs Human services, including food assistance programs Religious and other voluntary organizations Bureau of Indian Affairs Social Security	Transportation	Local service and religious organizations Volunteer organizations Migrant opportunity programs Community action programs
Medical	Hospitals Health departments—state, county, and city School nurses Local physicians Services for children with special health care conditions Veterans Affairs Hospital Indian Health Service Other local health services	Environment	State and county health departments Public service and utility companies Local government officials University cooperative extension programs
		Food	County and city human services departments, including food assistance programs Local services and religious organizations Volunteer organizations Migrant opportunities programs
Social	Child care facilities School systems Legal aid	Volunteer organizations	First Call For Help Voluntary health organizations

A standard nutrition referral form or computerized system used by all nutrition programs can help facilitate coordination of services. A nutrition referral system should include the following minimum information:

- Client identification (name, age, address, and telephone number)
- Name of referring professional and/or agency (address and telephone number)
- Diagnosis and reason for referral
- Type of service needed
- Specific diet prescription (if applicable)
- Location to which nutrition services report should be sent
- Identification of other consulting professionals currently or recently dealing with the patient

A schematic diagram (figure 14.6) illustrates the nutrition services referral system from community to family and from family to community.

Industry Partners: Benefits for the Community Nutrition Professional

Corporations, particularly those that do business within health care programs, focus much of their marketing on building relationships with health care professionals and creating programs for them. Community nutrition professionals have two kinds of opportunities in working with companies: joint ventures in marketing activities and corporate sponsorship of grants.

It is important, however, to retain perspective and to remember that no matter how public-spirited, no private concern or industry is in business to lose money. Survival dictates that all organizations must operate in the black including nonprofit organizations. Consequently, American corporations must keep their primary focus on the bottom line. The key for community nutrition professionals is to make the opportunity a win-win situation for both, a partnership in which the corporation gets sound advice and active communication, and the community nutrition professional gets visibility.[8] Obviously, as health professionals, we must know our own goals; it is important that both parties understand the needs and objectives of the proposed partners as well. Community nutrition professionals who develop and excel in understanding potential partners will make important contributions to the health and well-being of American society.

Benefits for Community Nutrition Professional

At the most basic level, partnerships strengthen the impact of good nutrition messages and enables it to be

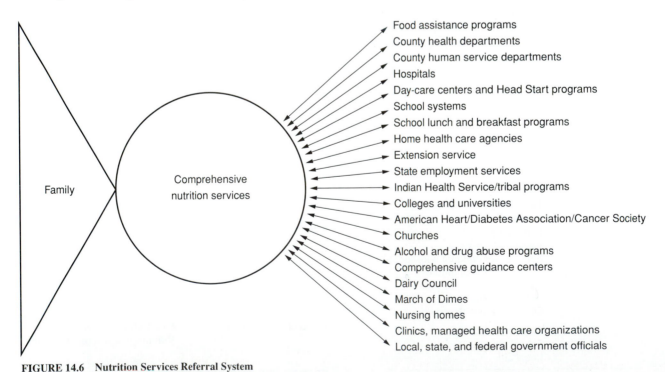

FIGURE 14.6   Nutrition Services Referral System

broadcast more widely. They permit community nutrition professionals to communicate through the mass media, thus multiplying the effect and scope of the message. An example of this approach has been developed by the American Dietetic Association (ADA) with the nutrition campaigns for Women's Health, Children's Health and Older American's Health.

With regard to Women's Health, the ADA and Ross Laboratories lead the coalition; with Children's Health, the Kellogg Company and the National Dairy Council provide the funding. Campbell Soup is the major backer of the Older Americans initiative. Industry provides resources and perspectives perhaps otherwise unavailable to the community nutrition professional. With the major changes in health care, community nutrition professionals need support from outside the profession, support that can complement their own education, expertise, and experience. The business end of the partnership should provide the vision, perspective, and business strategies that can move the health and nutrition issues to the forefront and position community nutrition professionals for a major role in present and future health care.

IMPLICATIONS FOR COMMUNITY NUTRITION PROFESSIONALS

Peters and others predict that teamwork will replace hierarchy as the dominant form of organization in the twenty-first century.[37] At the same time, there will be more interorganizational cooperation and collaboration. Downsizing, flatter organizations with fewer middle managers, has forced organizations to more fully empower its members into true teams—teams that work inside the organization and teams that cross organizational boundaries.

As was demonstrated in the examples cited in the chapter, coalitions can be valuable means to more creative, more comprehensive, and more widely distributed nutrition interventions. These new models offer great opportunities for community nutrition professionals, if they have the skills and confidence to lead, facilitate, and participate in the work of teams. A team is not like a pack of sled dogs, with one dog the leader—it's more like a flock of wild geese, where the leader is always changing but the flock stays together headed in a common direction.

Implementation includes established operational or action plans, developing procedures and protocols, securing necessary staff, and using MIS to track activities and their outcomes. When planning and implementing these operational details it is easy to be organization-focused. However, the real art and science of implementation is staying customer-focused. Implementation must include asking, listening, and adapting.

A major theme of this chapter is the importance of staying close to the customer. This is the challenge to the community nutrition professional whose goal is improving the health and nutritional well-being of the community.

COMMUNITY NUTRITION PROFESSIONALS IN ACTION

- Reflect on a current or recent experience you have had with a team? Did the team have a clear charter? Did the team go through the stages defined by Tuchman? When and how did members contribute to the team effort? Was the majority of work completed in meetings or between meetings? Did conflict emerge? If so how was it managed? How can you use the information in this chapter to enable future teams to be more effective?

- Develop a procedure or protocol for an upcoming nutrition program or project. In doing so consider the following: What sources of information do you need before you begin? Who should participate in the development? Who should review it? Does it have to be approved by anyone? If so, by whom? What are the benefits of having an appropriately detailed procedure put in writing? What are the risks or benefits of proceeding without a written procedure? How can the procedure guide the staff but still enable responsiveness to customers' needs?

- Visit a community nutrition program as a customer-participant. Be aware of each event in the cycle of service. Where did the providers meet or exceed your expectations? Where did they fall short? After the experience, analyze the cycle of service from the point of view of the provider. Where did providers "go the extra mile"? What adjustments could be made to improve the level of customer service?

- Collect position descriptions for community nutrition personnel in government, nonprofit, and for-profit organizations. Compare and contrast the titles, duties or responsibilities, and qualifications.

- Design a new nutrition product to meet the needs of college students (or another specific target audience). In great detail develop the market mix variables:

(1) the *product,* its characteristics including style, quality, features, packaging, and branding; (2) the *price* including what the user will give up in order to get and use to the product; (3) the *place* or channels through which the product will be distributed; and (4) the *promotion* plan for how you will let the target audience know about the new product.

- Volunteer to be a part of a new or existing coalition. Consider what you can bring to the team as well as how you can benefit. Be prepared to contribute to the work of the coalition.

GOING ONE STEP FURTHER

- Starting with a priority nutrition program that has been identified in your community (or in Vision City, from the chapter 13 case study), follow the eight steps of strategic marketing to design a nutrition program to address the problem.
- Analyze all the components of the management information system(s) for one nutrition program in your organization. Identify the types of data documented and tracked, and the processes used for recording, storing, summarizing, and reporting the information. Are there any redundancies or inefficiencies in the processes? How much of the collected information is actually used for management purposes? Who uses the information? When? For what purpose(s)?
- Prepare and conduct an in-service education program on quality service management.
- Assess you current networks and make a plan to expand your network in at least one direction. Initiate the plan.
- This chapter presents the strategic marketing approach to the design of a program, product, or service (i.e., an intervention to bring about a changed behavior in the target audience). Turn back to chapter 7 on behavior change strategies. How does the designer of nutrition interventions incorporate behavior change theory with the customer-centered marketing approach?

REFERENCES

1. Adler R, Rosen B, Silverstein E: Thrust and parry: the art of tough negotiating, *Training & Development* March:43–48, 1996.
2. Albrecht K, Zemke R: *Service America!* Homewood, IL; 1985, Dow-Jones Irwin.
3. Beck J, Yaeger N: Moving beyond team myths, *Training & Development* March: 51–55, 1996.
4. Berry LL, Parasuraman A: Listening to the customer—the concept of a service-quality information system, *Sloan Management Review* 38(3):65–79, 1997.
5. Committee on Diet and Health: *Diet and health implications for reducing chronic disease risk,* Washington, DC, 1991, National Academy Press.
6. Craig DP: *HIP pocket guide to planning and evaluation,* Austin, TX, 1978, Learning Concepts.
7. Dodds JM, Kaufman M, editors: *Personnel in public health nutrition for the 1990s,* Washington, DC, 1991, The Public Health Foundation.
8. Finn S: Personal communication, Ross Laboratories, Columbus, OH, February 1997.
9. Fisher R, Brown S: *Getting together: building relationships as we negotiate,* New York, 1988, Penguin Books.
10. Fisher R, Ury W: *Getting to yes,* New York, 1981, Penguin Books.
11. Hauchecorne CM, Barr SI, Sork TJ: Evaluation of nutritional counseling in clinical settings: do we make a difference? *J Am Diet Assoc* 94:437–440, 1994.
12. Hellriegel D, Slocum JW, Woodman RW: *Organizational behavior,* St. Paul, MN, 1992, West Publishing Co.
13. Helm KK, editor: *The competitive edge: advanced marketing for dietetics professionals,* Chicago, 1995, The American Dietetic Association, pp. 264–265.
14. Himmelfarb PA, Maharaj GR: Launching projects successfully with front-end project planning, *Quality Digest* May:66–68, 1996.
15. Kanter RM: *World class leaders: the power of partnering.* In Hesselbein F et al, editors: *Leaders of the future,* San Francisco, 1996, Jossey Bass.
16. Katzenback JR, Smith DK: *The wisdom of teams. Creating the high-performance organization,* Boston, 1993, Harvard Business School Press.
17. Kaufman M: *Demystifying data: data use in state and local public health nutrition programs. Measuring achievement of the 1990 Health Promotion/Disease Prevention Objectives for the Nation,* Chapel Hill, 1985, University of North Carolina.
18. Kaufman M et al: Survey of nutritionists in state and local public health agencies, *J Am Diet Assoc* 1986;86:1566.
19. *The Keystone national policy dialogue on food, nutrition and health,* Washington, DC, 1996, The Keystone Center, Keystone Co., p. 113.
20. Kilman R, Thomas K: *Thomas-Kilman conflict mode instrument,* Tuxedo, NY, 1974, Xicom Co.; and Thomas KW: *Conflict and conflict management. In MD Dunnett,* editor: Handbook of industrial and organizational psychology, Chicago, 1976, Rand McNally.
21. Kottler P, Andreasen AR: *Strategic marketing for nonprofit organizations,* ed 5, Englewood Cliffs, NJ, 1995, Prentice-Hall.

22. Lansing D: *Nutrition intervention in chronic disease,* Atlanta, GA, 1990, U.S. Public Health Service, Centers for Disease Control and Prevention.

23. Maslow AH: *Motivation and personality,* New York, 1954, Harper & Row.

24. Mears P: *Healthcare teams,* DelRay Beach, FL, 1994, St. Lucie Press.

25. Montana PJ, Nash DF: Delegation: the art of managing, *Personnel J* 60:784, 1981.

26. Mullis R, Owen AL, Blackovich L: Nutrition Action Conference on Healthy Eating for Children: a policy dialogue, *J Nutr Educ* 27:222–224, 1995.

27. Naisbitt J: *Megatrends,* New York, 1982, Warner Books, p. 215.

28. National action plan to improve the American diet: A public/private partnership, Washington, DC, 1993, Project of the Association of State and Territorial Health Officials.

29. Nettleton J: FANSA: a partnership for nutrition, *Food Technol* 48:929, 1994.

30. Osborne D, Gaebler T: *Reinventing government,* Reading, MA, 1992, Addison-Wesley.

31. Owen A: A collaborative effort for nutrition in the USA, *British Nutrition Foundation Nutr Bull* 20:171–173, 1995.

32. Peters T: *The pursuit of WOW!,* New York, 1994, Random House.

33. Probert KL, editor: *Moving to the future: developing community-based nutrition services,* Washington, DC, 1996, Association of Public Health State and Territorial Nutrition Directors.

34. Ross Professional Development Series: Linking strategies for dietitians: networking, liaison building and mentoring, Columbus, OH, 1989, Ross Laboratories.

35. Scholtes and others: *The team handbook: how to use teams to improve quality,* Madison, WI, 1996, Joiner Associates.

36. *SSNAPS software for successfully navigating the personnel system. User's guide,* Chapel Hill, 1996, Department of Nutrition, School of Public Health, University of North Carolina.

37. Stoner JRF, Freeman AE, Gilbert DA: *Management,* ed 6, Englewood Cliffs, NJ, 1994, Prentice-Hall.

38. Tuckman BW: Developmental sequence in small groups, *Psychological Bulletin* 63:384–399, 1965.

39. Zemke R: *The service edge: 101 companies that profit from customer care.* New York, 1989, Penguin Books.

CASE STUDY

USING A PUBLIC AND PRIVATE PARTNERSHIP TO MEET ARIZONA'S NUTRITION AND HEALTH NEEDS

SHARON SASS, RD, COMMUNITY NUTRITION EDUCATION CONSULTANT
AND SHERYL LEE, MPH, RD, CHIEF, OFFICE OF NUTRITION SERVICES
ARIZONA DEPARTMENT OF HEALTH SERVICES.

The program is 5 a Day for Better Health in Arizona.

DESCRIPTION

This case describes Arizona's public and private sectors working together to provide nutrition information and education on the need to consume five fruits and vegetables per day for better health. It is designed to illustrate the importance of public and private partnerships to provide accurate nutrition information to the public. It also demonstrates that a larger segment of the population can be reached with a joint effort. The case involves a partnership between public and private sectors to develop the program. Public sector partners included:

- Arizona Department of Health Services (ADHS) Office of Nutrition Services (ONS)
- National Cancer Institute (NIC)
- Arizona Department of Agriculture (ADA)
- Maricopa County Farm Bureau
- University of Arizona

Private industry partners included:

- Arizona Iceberg Lettuce Promotion Council (AILPC)
- Western Growers Association (WGA)
- Yuma Vegetable Growers Association
- BBCO, a retail grocery store
- Bashas, a retail grocery store
- Safeway, a retail grocery store
- Dairy Council of Arizona
- Arizona Beef Council

One of the major products from the program is an Arizona Grown Harvest Calendar indicating the fruits and vegetables grown in Arizona and describing the months in season and the nutrient content of the fruits and vegetables. The calendar is published on a monthly basis

on the front page of the Food Section of the *Arizona Republic* newspaper.

METHODOLOGY AND TEACHING OBJECTIVES

The goal of the 5 a Day for Better Health program is to

- Increase consumption of fruits and vegetables by increasing consumer and food industry awareness of the availability and quality of Arizona grown produce
- Provide information on the significant health benefits of fruit and vegetable consumption

THE CASE BACKGROUND

Poor diet and activity patterns contribute to five of the ten leading causes of death including heart disease, some types of cancer, stroke, non-insulin-dependent diabetes, and atherosclerosis. In 1994, these diet-related diseases represented 62.4 percent of total deaths (21,375) in Arizona. Heart disease, cancer, and stroke were the three leading causes of death in Arizona and a particularly large increase (19 percent) in the number of deaths from 1993 to 1994 were noted for diabetes. On a national level, poor diet and activity patterns cause almost as many deaths as smoking in the United States each year. In *Arizona 2000: Plan for a Healthy Tomorrow,* the ADHS identified improving dietary habits as the second highest priority health objective in the area of preventable disease related to lifestyle. The health objective receiving highest priority in this area was that of increasing physical activity.

Based on currently available national and state health and nutrition data, the significant issues regarding dietary habits and nutritional concerns for the people in Arizona include inadequate intake of fruits and vegetables, excessive fat intake, overweight, chronic diseases such as cardiovascular disease and diabetes, anemia, and food insecurity.

THE BEGINNING

The ADHS/ONS began by initiating the NCI 5 a Day for Better Health activities in 1991. At that time, meetings were held with the Arizona Department of Agriculture and vegetable growers to discuss ways to implement 5 a Day in Arizona. Including partners in the early stages of development is the best way to make the partnership successful, because everyone involved assumed ownership for the program and responsibility for its success. In 1993, the ADHS entered into an Interim Letter of Agreement along with NIC, which authorized the use of the 5 a Day for Better Health program and its logo, messages, and materials. In June 1994, the ADHS became a licensee through a Health Authority License Agreement with NCI.

Early activities of this program included the development and publication of a *5 a Day for Better Health Fruit and Vegetable Activity Book for Child Care Programs*. The book is now in its fifth printing and it also has a Spanish version.

DEVELOPMENT OF ARIZONA GROWN/ 5 A DAY FOR BETTER HEALTH

In 1992, the ADHS/ONS and the ADA collaborated to conduct the Arizona Grown/5 a Day for Better Health Program with initial funding from the AILPC. This program was an outgrowth of an already existing Arizona Grown program conducted by ADA. The goal of the Arizona Grown program was to increase consumption of foods grown in Arizona by educating consumers about the freshness, variety, availability, and quality of Arizona foods. The Arizona Grown/5 a Day for Better Health actually built the program around the already successful program of the ADA. In 1993, the Arizona Grown/5 a Day for Better Health began using the Arizona Grown logo. Arizona is the third largest producer of vegetables and citrus in the United States.

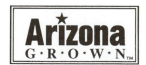

THE PROGRAM

The goal of the Arizona Grown/5 a Day for Better Health program, as stated previously, is to increase consumption of Arizona fruits and vegetables and to have greater awareness of the health benefits of fruit and vegetable consumption. The program consists of activities in media channels and retail grocery stores and statewide community education programs. The program includes an interagency agreement that provides the authority for implementation of this joint program between the ADHS and the ADA. The ADA serves as the lead agency for agricultural and retail grocery activities. The ADHS serves as the lead agency for activities in community education settings and health related organizations. Program planning, fiscal decisions, media activities, and evaluations are conducted jointly.

Media Channel

A registered dietitian (RD) is used on a consultant basis to serve as spokesperson for the program. Since the launch of the program during 5 a Day week in September 1993, she has achieved over 17 million media impressions through television, radio, and print media. Media placements have been diverse, including many business and general interest outlets due to linking of the economic aspects of agricultural information and the health messages of 5 a Day. Media efforts also include monthly distribution of a program update and harvest calendar featuring Arizona Grown fruits and vegetables (see figure 14.A) that are used in-season along with 5 a Day recipes. These updates may feature activities in the retail or community education channels. Key to the success of media efforts has been collaboration with the NCI and the Cancer Information Service. Each month, new Arizona Grown/5 a Day for Better Health materials are distributed through the 1-800-4-CANCER information line. Activities in the media channel have been evaluated with process tracking as well as outcome measurement through a telephone survey of 3,600 Arizona adults conducted in fall 1995. Preliminary results show that of those surveyed that had heard of 5 a Day, 27.5 percent indicated learning of 5 a Day through the media, whereas only 4.9 percent indicated learning of 5 a Day in a retail grocery store.

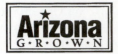

FEBRUARY

Red Fruits and Vegetables for the Month of Hearts

February is the month for hearts! Take care of yours by eating 5 or more servings of fruits and vegetables every day! Look for *Arizona Grown* Fruits and Vegetables that are red this month like beets, red cabbage, red blush grapefruit, red leaf lettuce, radishes and tomatoes. Nearly 50 different Arizona Grown fruits and vegetables are being harvested this month. Look for the ones listed below in your retail grocery store during February. It's easy to get your *5 a Day* - make it the *Arizona Grown* way!

Arizona Grown Produce	Vitamins A	Vitamins C	Fiber	Cruciferous	Arizona Grown Produce	Vitamins A	Vitamins C	Fiber	Cruciferous
Anise					Leeks		✓		
Artichokes		✓	✓		Lemons		✓		
Asparagus		✓			Lettuce, Butter	✓			
Beans, Fava		✓	✓		Lettuce, Endive				
Beets					Lettuce, Escarole	✓			
Bok Choy	✓	✓			Lettuce, Iceberg				
Broccoli		✓		✓	Lettuce, Leaf	✓			
Cabbage, Green		✓		✓	Lettuce, Romaine	✓			
Cabbage, Red		✓		✓	Napa Cabbage	✓	✓		✓
Carrots	✓		✓		Onions, Green		✓		
Cauliflower, White		✓		✓	Oranges, Mandarin		✓	✓	
Cauliflower, Green		✓		✓	Oranges, Navel		✓	✓	
Celery		✓			Oranges, Sweet		✓	✓	
Cilantro					Oranges, Temple		✓	✓	
Daikon		✓			Oranges, Valencia		✓	✓	
Dill					Parsley				
Grapefruit, Red Blush	✓	✓	✓		Radishes		✓		
Grapefruit, White		✓	✓		Rapini	✓	✓		✓
Greens, Beet	✓	✓	✓		Rutabagas		✓		✓
Greens, Collards	✓	✓		✓	Spinach	✓	✓	✓	
Greens, Kale	✓	✓		✓	Tangelos, Minneola		✓	✓	
Greens, Mustard	✓	✓		✓	Tangelos, Orlando		✓	✓	
Greens, Swiss Chard	✓	✓		✓	Tomatoes	✓	✓		
Greens, Turnip	✓	✓		✓	Turnips		✓		✓
Kohlrabi		✓	✓	✓					

✓=More than 10% Daily Value (A,C, Fiber) or is a cruciferous vegetable.

Information provided by Arizona Department of Agriculture and the Arizona Department of Health Services

FIGURE 14.A   Harvest Calendar

Retail Grocery Store Channel

The number of retail grocery store chains licensed to participate in the 5 a Day for Better Health or Arizona Grown programs has increased from three to nine chains since the launch of the Arizona Grown/5 a Day for Better Health program in September 1993. This represents 70 percent of the retail grocery stores in Arizona. Participating retailers have conducted successful activities including a coloring contest, 5 a Day Week promotions, printing of bags with 5 a Day promotions (7.5 million bags with a customized 5 a Day fitness message printed by one chain) and supermarket tours for children. Five retail grocery chains, representing 289 stores, participated in an Arizona Grown/5 a Day for Better Health promotion for National Nutrition month in March 1995. Promotional materials included

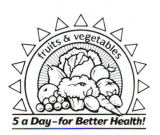

consumer posters, signs, and brochures as well as a poster for store personnel on seasonal availability of Arizona grown fruits and vegetables. A total of 157,500 consumer brochures were printed and distributed. The cost of the promotion was shared between the ADA, the ADHS, vegetable growers, and the participating retail grocery chains. In 1997, an "Eat Right—the Arizona Grown Way Recipe Contest" was conducted with three grocery store chains and industry partners.

Community Education Channel

Arizona Grown/5 a Day for Better Health community education contacts have been established in each of the fifteen counties in Arizona. Activities are conducted through collaborative, not contractual arrangements. Support for local activities has been provided through materials, technical assistance, and training. Innovative activities have been conducted in schools, seniors' centers, and community events. Ten of the local agencies conduct process and outcome evaluation of 5 a Day activities through the state-funded Nutrition Subvention program.

Linking Arizona Grown with a 5 a Day for Better Health has been successful because of excellent collaboration between state agencies with little or no difficulty

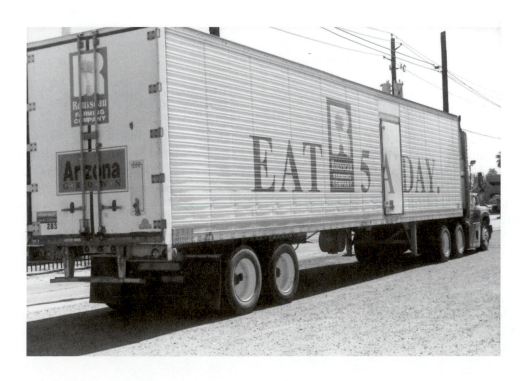

crossing agency boundaries, industry support, partnership with the University of Arizona NCI-funded research project *5 a Day: Healthier Eating for the Overlooked Worker,* and participation from public health nutritionists throughout the state.

SIGNIFICANT OUTCOMES FROM THE PROGRAM

Two significant outcomes have occurred because of the success of the program. First is the additional resources for the program obtained from the Arizona legislature, and second, they have now built linkages to the Arizona Nutrition Network.

Funds from Arizona Legislature

During the 1996 state legislative session, members of the agricultural industry were successful in obtaining an additional $25,000 of state funds to support the Arizona Grown Program. Use of the state funds requires 50:50 match with private donations. To date, $10,000 of the required match has been provided by vegetable growers in Arizona. These additional Arizona Grown funds will be used to support promotion of all types of products grown and produced in Arizona as well as the media component of the Arizona Grown/5 a Day for Better Health program. Some funding may be used to expand ADA efforts to provide nutrition education for children that links the Arizona Grown message with information on the Food Guide Pyramid.

Linkage to the Arizona Nutrition Network

The Arizona Nutrition Network was initiated in February 1996 with funding from USDA to develop a statewide network of public and private partners to initiate nutrition education activities using social marketing methods targeted to the Food Stamp eligible population in Arizona. The network is a collaborative effort of the ADHS/ONS and the Arizona Department of Economic Security (DES). The ADA has been an active partner in the network. The network recently selected the 5 a Day as the primary message for initial activities. A nutrition education plan reflecting 5 a Day as the primary message has been written and submitted to USDA for funding. Participation in the Arizona Nutrition Network is allowing the Arizona Grown/5 a Day program to expand its target audience to include lower-income individuals who are considered more difficult to reach with health education messages. The primary target audience for network activities are female heads of households and their children. Activities proposed for funding include a cookbook, a puppet show for children in grades K–3, monthly bulletins for widespread distribution, and a social marketing campaign. All activities will feature 5 a Day for Better Health messages.

SOME QUESTIONS

1. To develop a 5 a Day program in your community, what agencies would you select to begin initial discussions about the program?
2. What private sector groups would you select in the initial planning to get the program off the ground? What criteria would you use to select private sector partners?
3. How could you expand the program to reach a broader audience? How would you pursue the use of computer technology (Internet and others) to expand the program?
4. Since you will need experts in communications to develop certain aspects of the program, where would you solicit help for this activity? Could you find resources in your own agency and some in the private sector also or would you obtain pro bono (free) services from a public relations/information agency in the private sector?
5. What additional educational programs would you develop to enhance the project?
6. How can you develop the skills to achieve a successful partnership in your community?
7. At each step in the development of your 5 a Day program, what would you do to assure that emerging program components are tailored to the needs of the community? How can you reach low-income families, children, workers, and the like?
8. The NCI provides guidelines to health authorities who are licensed to use the 5 a Day for Better Health Program. What other kinds of standards and protocols would be necessary to hold the program and its many partners to high standards?
9. Your program will need a director and staff. What would the position description look like for the director and key staff?

CHAPTER FIFTEEN

EVALUATING NUTRITION PROGRAMS

If you don't measure results, you can't tell success from failure.
If you can't see success, you can't learn from it.
If you can't recognize failure, you can't learn from it.
If you can demonstrate results, you can win public support.
—DAVID OSBORNE AND TED GAEBLER

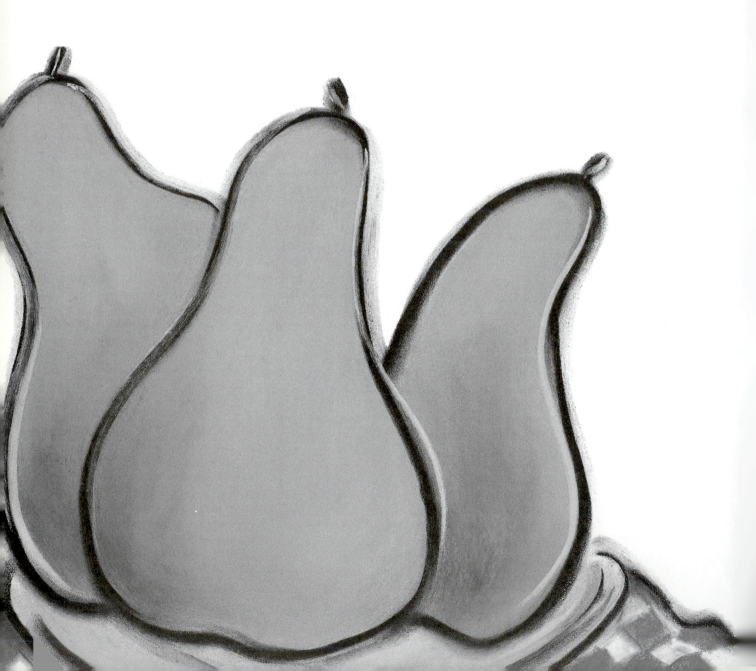

Core Concepts

Community nutrition professionals have the responsibility of assuring that nutrition programs and services are operated in an efficient manner so that program goals, objectives, and standards for performance are achieved. The evaluation function incorporates processes that define standards, measure performance, compare performance with standards, and plan adjustments to improve results. This chapter presents the concepts, principles, and processes of managerial control, quality management, program evaluation, and the more complex evaluation techniques associated with outcomes measurement, effectiveness evaluation, and cost-effectiveness and cost-benefit analyses.

Objectives

When you finish chapter fifteen, you should be able to:

~ Define the steps of the control process.

~ Discuss trends in total quality management, continuous quality improvement, and performance improvement.

~ Identify distinct types of program evaluation appropriate to each phase of the life span of a nutrition program.

~ List aspects of evaluation design that require special planning for more complex effectiveness evaluations.

~ Develop plans for conducting an evaluation.

~ Distinguish between cost-effectiveness and cost-benefit analyses, and give an example of a situation where each could be used.

Key Words

Word	Page Mentioned
Managerial control	450
Standards	450
Indicators	450
Total quality management	452
Continuous quality improvement	452
Quality assurance	454
Process	454
Outcome	454
Protocols	456
Practice guidelines	456
Outcomes measurement	457
Clinical outcomes	458
Cost outcomes	458
Patient outcomes	459
Formative evaluation	459
Demonstration project	459
Process evaluation	460
Outcome or summative evaluation	460
Goal-free evaluation	460
Variables	462
Experimental design	463
Quasi-experimental designs	463
Nonexperimental designs	464
Cost-effectiveness analysis	466
Cost-benefit analysis	466
Efficiency	466
Cost analysis	469

This chapter completes the management processes of planning, implementation, and evaluation. Together these processes enable nutrition programs to positively impact the health and nutritional well-being of the population. As shown in figure 15.1, evaluation encompasses a broad range of methods and tools for keeping the nutrition program on track and moving toward the accomplishment of goals and objectives, while operating efficiently. In management texts, this is called the control function.

Managerial control is presented as a foundation, then the chapter goes on to explore the important application of the control process to quality management, outcomes measurement, evaluation across the life span of programs, effectiveness evaluation, and cost-effectiveness and cost-benefit evaluation. Community nutrition professionals must be skilled in planning for and conducting evaluations. By measuring and then learning from successes and failures, nutrition programs and services become more effective and more cost effective.

MANAGERIAL CONTROL

The purpose of evaluation or **managerial control** is to maximize the probability that the organization will achieve its short- and long-term goals and objectives and do so through efficient use of resources. Control is a means of assessing activities to take corrective action.[13] During the execution of any plan, changes in the external environment, such as increasing unemployment or shifting political leadership and priorities, or changes inside the organization, such as staff turnover or higher risk clientele, are likely to occur. Such changes require new responses or adjustments in plans. Control systems are an intrinsic part of the management process because they help managers anticipate, monitor, and respond to changing circumstances in a timely manner. The control function enables an organization to adapt to changing conditions, limit the compounding of problems, and minimize costs.

The control process illustrated in figure 15.2 is closely linked with planning and implementation. Management sets goals and objectives and puts in place monitoring systems to detect deviations from goals and objectives and to ascertain causes of the deviations during program implementation. The control system tells the manager that things are going as anticipated (the current plan should be maintained), that things are not going as anticipated (the current plan should be modified), or that the situation has changed (a new plan should be developed).

In small organizations operating in a stable environment, monitoring systems can be simple, perhaps including weekly staffing records, monthly service counts and expenditure reports, semiannual quality assurance audits, and annual outcome evaluation and personnel performance reviews. Complex organizations with multiple goals and organizations operating in turbulent environments need more complex monitoring systems.

Areas of control include resource allocation and utilization (or costs) and program operations and goal attainment (production of results). Budgeting and financial management, which are addressed in the next chapter, deal with the control of resources.

The Control Process

The control process consists of four steps, as illustrated in figure 15.2. The first step is the establishment of standards. **Standards** are expressed in measurable terms and become the target against which subsequent performance is compared. A challenge in setting standards is deciding what behaviors or results can be observed, measured, and documented. These **indicators** of performance must be relevant to short- and long-term goals and objectives. For example, a Meals On Wheels program has a goal of providing hot, nutritious meals to homebound disabled elderly people. A measurable, relevant indicator is the temperature of the food when it is delivered. A performance standard could be that the entrée of home-delivered meals will be at or above 145° F 100 percent of the time when measured at the participant's home.

The second step is measuring performance. This is an ongoing activity that involves actual observation and documentation of relevant behaviors, actions, or results. Procedures must be developed and implemented to record and summarize indicators of performance. Client encounter records, checklists, audit forms, expense accounts, time sheets, and tickler files are examples of tools to aid documentation. Performance is commonly expressed in units of volume, quality indicators, or cost.

Objective data of actual performance are essential to the control process. Actual data fed back to employees can serve as a motivator to increase performance or correct procedures to improve quality. Data can also serve as rewards and incentives to continue high-level performance. Valid data are essential to appropriate corrective action and good managerial control.

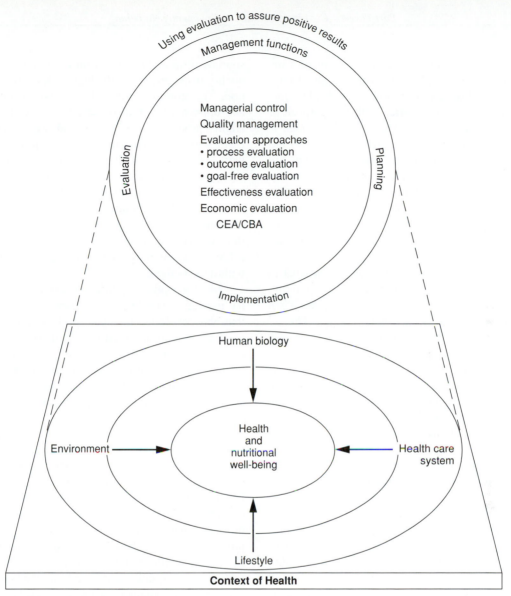

FIGURE 15.1   Context of Health
Managing the evaluation function of nutrition programs.

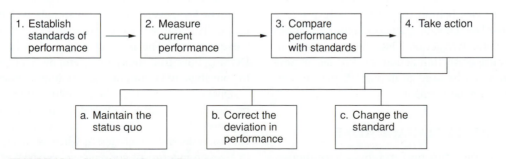

FIGURE 15.2   Steps in the Control Process
(*Source:* Griffin, Ricky W., *Management,* Third Edition. Copyright © 1990 by Houghton Mifflin Company. Adapted with permission.)

The third step involves the actual assessment. Current performance is compared with the standard on a regular basis, and a determination is made. The frequency of this assessment varies with the purpose of the standard. In the WIC program, actual caseload is compared with the agency's allocated caseload monthly. In a congregate dining program, menus are analyzed on a regular schedule to determine if they provide one third of the Recommended Dietary Allowances for major nutrients. A performance standard related to program outcome objectives, such as rates of anemia in the preschool population, may be assessed annually.

The fourth step involves the decision about what to do. Three courses of action are possible: do nothing, change the performance, or change the standard. When performance is on track, no action is required. The assessment confirms earlier decisions and serves as a motivator to continue activities as planned.

Sometimes, comparing performance to standards leads to the conclusion that the standard is too high or too low. When performance consistently exceeds the standard, the standard may be obsolete and should be upgraded. New conditions in the internal or external environment such as different skill levels of personnel; changing expectations on the part of clients, society, or professionals; and advances in knowledge and technology may stimulate the need for a change in performance level, defined as a standard.

"Benchmarking" is used by many high-performance organizations to set standards for performance. Benchmarking involves identifying the "best practices" within parts of the organization or in other organizations, and setting that level of performance as the performance standard to reach or exceed.

Deviation—falling below the standard—however, triggers required action. This should begin with examination of the causes behind the performance problem and should involve relevant staff in diagnosing causes and planning corrective action. Once the causes are understood, specific correction action must be taken. Several approaches can be used to initiate changes to correct the deviation in performance.

QUALITY MANAGEMENT

In all organizations, top performance, high-quality products and services, and efficient utilization of resources ultimately depend on a commitment to total quality management at the highest level of administration. This commitment is then translated into systems and opportunities that involve personnel at all levels. Highly productive work units and organizations result from worker involvement in decisions about their work, assessment of their performance, and plans for corrective adjustments when needed. It is the responsibility of top administrators to make training, tools, and time available to enable employees to participate in defining and implementing quality improvement plans that assure the smooth operation of programs and achievement of performance objectives while staying within the budget.

This description captures the essence of **total quality management** (TQM), a management philosophy that was developed in Japan (by U.S. consultants) and has been widely adopted by high-performing U.S. organizations. The guiding principle of TQM is that quality must start at the top and have the total and continuing commitment of management. It must permeate the whole organization and become a way of life for all employees.

TQM is often implemented in the form of **continuous quality improvement** (CQI) programs and, more recently, performance improvement and outcomes measurement.[5,9] The commitment to quality goes beyond faultfinding. Rather, as in the 3M Corporation, every problem is viewed as a treasure—a newfound opportunity for enhancement of work processes, refinement of product or service details, or improvement of relationships with suppliers and customers.

Crosby,[7] Deming,[8] and Juran[16] are the "gurus" of the quality improvement movement, which has developed over several decades and now encompasses total quality management, continuous quality improvement, and performance improvement. The relevance of quality management for government organizations was made dramatically clear with the publication of Reinventing Government.[23] The principles of quality identified by Deming hold true today (e.g., empower all employees to contribute to continuous quality improvement).[27]

Quality is defined by the constituency assessing it—provider, client, family, collaborator, payer, local community, and state. Providers define quality in terms of technical processes and effectiveness; whereas clients are likely to assess it in terms of convenience, personal satisfaction, and having perceived needs met. Collaborators may judge in terms of professional competency, and funders or payers in terms of cost-effectiveness and appropriateness.

TQM recognizes that ultimate quality is in the eyes of the consumers, and consumer satisfaction is a crucial part of performance. This had led to another trend in quality improvement, *quality service management* or quality customer service, in which the customer's needs and wants are first and foremost.[1]

Deming and others asserted that quality is 80 percent administration (leadership) and structural systems (the way people and things are organized) and 20 percent performance by employees.[8] Performance and productivity are not only employee responsibilities, they are the responsibility of managers. According to Crosby,[7] performance problems are usually not the result of lack of will or skill of employees, but rather they are related to poor job design, failure of leadership, or unclear purpose.

Community nutrition professionals must be involved in defining and assuring quality of nutrition programs and services. High-quality programs require continuous attention. Standards must be reviewed and updated regularly to reflect the current research in nutrition as well as state-of-the-art health and human service delivery systems. Monitoring and control systems should be used as resources come into the nutrition unit, throughout the processes of program implementation and operation, and at the end, when program accomplishments are reviewed and reported and plans are made for subsequent planning cycles.

Community nutrition professionals should recognize control and evaluation processes as opportunities for program enhancement. Quality management leads to greater accomplishment of goals and objectives, and higher satisfaction of consumer's needs and wants, while, at the same time, assuring resources are used judiciously and efficiently. Table 15.1 presents terms used in quality management and effectiveness evaluation.

TABLE 15.1
Glossary of Terms Used in Quality Improvement, Effectiveness, and Economic Evaluations

Term	Definition
Clinical effectiveness	A change in clinical indicators that relate to the patients' risk or disease state as a result of implementation of the intervention (nutrition care)
Cost-benefit analysis	An approach to evaluation that converts outcomes to monetary terms (dollars) so that both costs and outcomes are expressed in economic terms
Cost-effectiveness analysis	An approach to evaluation that takes into account both costs and outcomes of two or more alternative methods of intervention for a specific purpose
Effectiveness	Desired outcome is achieved when the intervention is used under ordinary conditions (real-world rather than experimental controlled conditions)
Effectiveness evaluation	A systematic process for assessing the outcomes of a health care program or protocol
Indicator/criterion	A defined, measurable dimension of the quality or appropriateness of an important aspect of patient care or other intervention; may address the structure, process, or outcome of care
Intervention	A purposefully planned action designed to achieve a defined outcome (e.g., nutrition counseling over a twelve-week period to enable the patient to decrease caloric consumption and thereby reduce weight)
Outcome	An end result of the health care process; a measurable change in the patient's state of health or functioning
Outcomes measurement	Documentation and periodic assessment of key indicators of performance
Practice guidelines	Evidence-based descriptions of clinical practices that have been established by experts and validated through field-testing
Process	An organized set of tasks related to the delivery of the intervention
Protocol	Detailed guidelines for care that are specific to the disease or condition and type of patient
Quality assessment	An act of comparing present program structure, process, and outcomes with stated criteria for performance
Quality assurance	A systematic program for assuring excellence in health care; includes definition of indicators or criteria and thresholds or standards, devising methods for determining the degree to which standards are met, and mechanisms to identify and correct deficiencies
Standard	The target against which performance is compared
Threshold	A precise specification of the level of performance that constitutes quality

QUALITY ASSURANCE, CONTINUOUS QUALITY IMPROVEMENT, AND OUTCOMES MEASUREMENT IN NUTRITION SERVICES AND PROGRAMS

In the past, **quality assurance** was focused on the **process** of care (what the provider does). Process is a fundamental element of program quality and cannot be ignored. However, there is now a shift to outcomes measurement, with attention to the results or **outcomes** of programs and services (what happens to those who experience the process). Monitoring of the processes and outcomes of nutrition intervention must be an ongoing part of nutrition program activities. By identifying strengths and weaknesses of the interventions provided by community nutrition professionals, the nutrition program can become a stronger contributor to the overall organization and the health of its clients and the community.

In quality assurance or CQI efforts, nutrition care is regularly or continuously documented and evaluated, and results are reviewed for the purpose of identifying needed action. Quality improvement should begin with high-priority areas as listed in box 15.1. When threshold standards are met and desired outcomes are achieved, providers and protocols are working, and nu-

BOX 15.1

PRIORITY AREAS FOR QUALITY IMPROVEMENT

Projects for quality improvement should be purposefully selected. Start with a smaller quality improvement project then when the team has experience move on to larger projects.

Use this checklist to select an area for improvement.

- Related to your activities
- Significant because of one or more of the following:
  - High volume
  - High importance
  - High cost
  - High visibility
- Potential for direct impact on clients' satisfaction
- Variations in process or outcome currently exist
- Improvements can raise effectiveness
- Improvements can produce dollar savings
- Managers as well as direct service providers can be expected to cooperate in the improvement effort

trition care is more likely to be effective. Data showing that outcomes are achieved consistently over time should be presented to medical directors, administrators, funders, and legislators as support for the nutrition program. Less positive results should lead to program improvement by examining potential results for failure and then introducing procedural or protocol changes into the nutrition care.[33] Subsequent assessment can verify whether the revised protocols are effective in producing desired outcomes in most clients.

Evaluating the process and outcomes of nutrition care can be simplified into five phases. These phases form a cycle that provide feedback for continuous improvement of nutrition care. Attention to these phases helps to assure quality care while documenting results. The evidence of success that is produced by such a system will provide strong justification for internal allocation of funds to support nutrition services or external payment for care delivered. Figure 15.3 illustrates the phases as a feedback loop. Note their similarity to the steps of the control process (figure 15.2) and with the mnemonic of CQI—plan, do, check, act. A discussion of each phase follows, but first look at an example in box 15.2.

Box 15.2 illustrates the integration of both process and outcome indicators in an example of quality assessment used in a community-based nutrition program for prenatal patients. Three process indicators are listed. However, the appropriate screening procedures for monitoring as well as specific guidelines regarding the content of counseling and recommendations for weight gain would be elaborated in other departmental documents defining protocols for nutrition care. Clear delineation of relevant, measurable patient outcomes focuses attention on assessing whether the process actually produces the desired outcomes. Consideration of process and outcome in tandem provides more useful data to guide future nutrition care than assessing process alone. Note in the example how current performance was compared to the performance standards (process and outcome criteria) and the conclusions led to corrective action. A second cycle of the assessment verified that the corrective action cleared up the performance discrepancy.

Five Phases of Nutrition Quality Improvement

1. Define Protocols or Practice Guidelines for Nutrition Care Clearly define the level, content, frequency, and duration of nutrition care that is appropriate for the specific disease or condition or prevention aim.

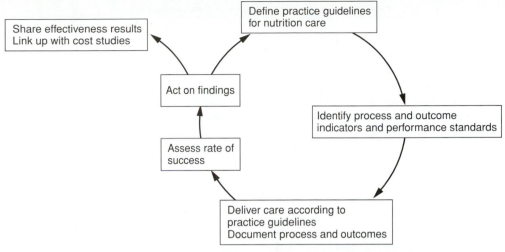

FIGURE 15.3 Feedback Loop for Evaluating the Process and Outcomes of Nutrition Care

BOX 15.2

QUALITY ASSESSMENT OF NUTRITION CARE: PROCESS AND OUTCOMES

Aspect of care: Nutrition care of prenatal patients with low weight gain.

Nutrition care indicators: Prenatal care program objective— Prenatal patients will achieve weight gain consistent with healthy outcome of pregnancy as defined by the National Academy of Sciences guidelines for weight gain (NAS, 1990).*

Process criteria
a. Community nutritionists monitor all prenatal patients to identify low weight gain; threshold 95%.
b. When low weight gain is identified the patient receives counseling on adequate dietary intake; threshold 95%.
c. A referral is made to WIC if indicated; threshold 95%.

Outcome criteria
a. Weight gain by next visit; threshold 80%
b. Improvement in dietary intake; threshold 80%.

Evaluation: Medical records of all prenatal patients who attended clinic during one month were requested and audited.

Process assessment: Of a total of 100 patients, 25 had a weight gain that fell below the recommended weight gain curve. However, nutritionists had counseled only 15 of 25 (60%) of the cases; and referrals to WIC were made for only 3 of 6 (50%) women who were low income, not currently in WIC.

Outcome assessment: Of the 15 low-weight-gain patients who were counseled, 12 (80%) achieved weight gain as demonstrated by measured weight at next visit; 13 (87%) had evidence of improved dietary intake. Outcomes could not be assessed for 2 (13%) due to transfer to another clinic for prenatal care.

Conclusions:
1. Many prenatal patients with low weight gain are not receiving adequate and appropriate nutrition care.
2. Those who receive nutrition care do achieve the established outcome criteria.

Actions: Brief interviews with staff showed a lack of knowledge about monitoring prenatal patients for low weight gain and procedures for referral to WIC. The nutrition director scheduled a mandatory staff meeting to discuss the findings of the quality assurance audit. Since process was a problem, not outcome, the protocol for monitoring weight gain of prenatal patients was reviewed and a WIC referral form was developed. A repeat audit was scheduled in three months.

Improvement/follow-up: Data collected three months later showed improvement. Of 105 total prenatals, 28 had low weight gain. All 28 were identified and received counseling by a nutritionist (100%) evidence by documentation in the medical record. Of the 10 who had low income, 5 were already on WIC and the other 5 (100%) were referred to WIC. Outcomes remained above 80% for both outcome criteria.

_____

*Subcommittee on Nutrition Status and Weight Gain During Pregnancy, Institute of Medicine. Nutrition During Pregnancy. Washington, DC: National Academy Press, 1990.

Many guidelines are available that specify appropriate nutrition care for specific diseases, conditions, or prevention aims. These guidelines may be in the form of a diet manual, quality assurance standards, practice guidelines, or detailed protocols. Examples of guidelines are cited in the life cycle chapters. In some clinical settings, guidelines for practice take the form of clinical pathways or critical care maps.

In some cases, no written guidelines exist, but providers carry in their heads a set of expectations for the type of care to be delivered to various clients under varying situations. This is not acceptable; written **protocols** or **practice guidelines** are essential. They define and guide appropriate and acceptable initial and follow-up care and help to assure consistency and quality of care across providers.[20]

Protocols or practice guidelines establish minimum care that should be provided to expect that desired outcomes can be achieved. They clarify the role of nutrition as a part of the health promotion and disease prevention aim or as a necessary aspect of medical management for specific risk conditions or diseases. Moreover, important for payment and reimbursement, written practice guidelines can be used to communicate appropriate levels of nutrition care to managed care organizations, funders, and third-party payers. In addition, protocols and practice guidelines are a basis for process and outcome criteria for quality improvement systems.

2. Identify Outcome Indicators
Specify the end result that the nutrition program or service is expected to achieve. Express it in terms of measurable outcome indicators.

Outcomes are measurable changes in the client's state of health or functioning. They may be proximal outcomes that occur in a fairly short period of time, such as caloric or nutrient intake, weight gain, and serum cholesterol level, or intermediate outcomes, such as recurrent infections or weight maintenance. Outcomes may also be measured in the population over the long term in more general terms such as disease incidence, disability, or death. Table 15.2 outlines different outcome indicators that could be assessed at different points of time.

Several considerations affect the choice of outcome indicators. Selected indicators must be practical and feasible to measure and there must be a logical link between the nutrition intervention and the outcome. For example, since nutrition is directly linked to helping

TABLE 15.2
Outcomes of Nutrition Intervention

Short-term (proximal) outcomes: knowledge improvement, behavior change, physiological indicators of risk (e.g., weight gain or loss, cholesterol reduction, anemia), other specific indicators related to life stage, risk level, or compromised health status

Intermediate outcomes: sustained changes in knowledge, behavior, physiological indicators or related consequences, improved functional status, changes in individual or organizational practices, delay or prevention of complications or deterioration, downstream health care, education, or social service utilization

Long-term (distal) outcomes: chronic disease onset in later life, associated health care costs, years added to life

prenatal patients gain appropriate weight during pregnancy, total pregnancy weight gain would be a good outcome indicator for nutrition care of prenatal clients. Because weight is routinely available, it is a practical measurement to use.

For many purposes, readily available biochemical and anthropometric measures can be identified as relevant outcome indicators of nutrition care. Indicators relevant to various stages of the life cycle were mentioned in Part 2 of this text. The definition and adoption of specific indicators is an ongoing challenge. Various practice groups of the American Dietetic Associaton have developed indicators. (Some were listed table 4.2.)

3. Deliver Care Consistently According to Protocols or Practice Guidelines, and Document the Processes and Outcomes of Care
Once practice guidelines are developed, community nutrition professionals must consistently deliver care according to those guidelines. Training may be necessary to assure that all staff understand and agree with the guidelines and charting or record keeping procedures that are necessary to verify that care was delivered.

Because of time demands, documentation is frequently a challenge. Checklists, stamps, stickers, and other memory-aiding devices can be developed to remind providers of all aspects of the care or intervention appropriate to a specific disease or condition. These devices also facilitate regular and consistent documentation. Computerized data collection forms and medical records structure documentation procedures and can improve the accuracy and consistency of documentation when used correctly.

Documentation of outcomes is generally dependent on follow-up visits or the ability to track clients over time. Follow-up visits provide an opportunity to check and support client compliance, and they make it possible to measure outcome indicators. Protocols should include follow-up visits, and clinic procedures should be structured to track and reschedule clients so that the outcomes of nutrition care can be measured and documented.

4. Assess the Rate of Success of Nutrition Services   Collect and summarize data from patient and program records and evaluate the results.

Preestablished performance standards serve as standards or thresholds for performance. Recognizing that many, but not all, clients will benefit from nutrition intervention, standards define the rate of success community nutrition professionals expect to achieve in their practice for each specific type of care. The assessment phase allows community nutrition professionals to examine their performance over a period of time. Gathering data about performance may seem threatening, but it is an invaluable means of recognizing success as well as identifying problems that can be corrected.

It is critical that time be allocated to the tasks of reviewing records and summarizing data for the assessment of nutrition care. This activity is routinely done as part of quality assurance programs in most hospitals. However, it must be expanded to ambulatory and public health clinics and managed care organizations. With the expansion of computerized record systems, some performance standards are automatically computed at the end of the day, week, or month. This makes it easy to monitor performance on a regular basis and compare trends over time.

5. Act on the Findings   Utilize the results to report effectiveness results to others and to redefine guidelines or procedures for improved outcomes in the future.

The final steps make the rest of the quality assessment process worthwhile. The ability of community nutrition professionals to review the findings objectively and use them for expansion and continuous improvement of services is key to the evaluation process. Through evaluation, community nutrition professionals not only accept accountability for the results of nutrition care but also have the information they need to justify the value of nutrition care in terms of clients' health outcomes. Further, when nutrition care is not found to be effective, data about the processes and outcomes can provide clues to corrective action.

Outcomes Measurement

The outcomes movement, which was discussed in chapter 4, involves outcomes measurement, outcomes management, and outcomes research.[30] These are the newest applications of quality control and improvement in organizations and across the health care system. The **outcomes measurement** view of quality assessment and management focuses on *effectiveness,* or how well interventions work in routine practice settings (box 15.3). Cost outcomes are also of concern, including both the costs of delivering specific interventions and costs associated with the resulting consequences. Methods of economic analysis (discussed later in this chapter) are used to identify the most efficient interventions, that is, the interventions that achieve more of the desired results for the lowest or most reasonable investment of resources.

Outcomes measurement and outcomes management are activities carried out at the organization or program level; while outcomes research may be conducted within one or across several organizations. Managed care organizations are adopting these approaches to achieve and assure high quality. Results of outcomes measurement are also used to communicate quality and value to clients and to gain a competitive advantage over other provider organizations.

Outcomes measurement involves documentation and periodic assessment of key indicators of performance. Indicators are collected within the clinic, program, or organization and compared against organizational, local, state, or federal averages or norms, or a benchmark level.

BOX 15.3

EFFICACY VERSUS EFFECTIVENESS

Efficacy reflects the level of outcome expected when the intervention is applied under ideal conditions.

Randomized clinical trials measure efficacy.

Effectiveness is the level of outcome achieved when the intervention is delivered under ordinary circumstances by average practitioners for typical clients.

Effectiveness evaluation and *outcomes research* focuses on effectiveness in real-world settings.

TABLE 15.3
How Outcomes Information Is Used

Players	Application of outcomes information
Clinicians	• Determine optimum clinical practices • Identify ways to maximize clinical and patient outcomes • Determine which procedure and therapy costs are reasonable for the outcomes they produce
Health care provider organization (hospitals and clinics)	• Establish guidelines and protocols for appropriate care • Guide continuous quality improvement projects • Establish benchmarks for measuring clinical and budgetary performance • Demonstrate quality to peers, patients, and payers
Health department	• Establish guidelines and standards for programs • Set benchmarks for monitoring performance • Allocate resources for most effective interventions
Payer/purchasers (insurance companies, Medicaid, and Medicare)	• Select the best care providers • Define covered benefits • Set reimbursement/payment levels
Managed care organization	(Similar to the provider organization *and* the payer/purchaser)
Patient/client	• Participate in decisions about intervention alternatives based on outcome expectations
Health care sector (providers, insurers, and government)	• Plan jointly across parts of the system • Determine the most cost effective settings (hospital, community, long-term care, outpatient) for care delivery of specific care for specific diseases or conditions for specific population groups
Society (taxpayers and policy makers)	• Shape judgments about the quality of health care and the value gained for resources invested • Form judgments to determine willingness to pay and to affect allocation of resources to health care

Source: Adapted from Splett PL: *Cost outcomes of nutrition intervention, part 1: outcomes research,* Evansville, IN, 1996, Mead Johnson. Reprinted with permission of Mead Johnson & Company, copyright 1996.

Outcomes management uses the results of outcomes measurement to adjust intervention processes so that outcomes and cost effectiveness can be improved. Outcomes management utilizes the process illustrated in figures 15.2 and 15.3. An outcomes management system

• Relies on protocols or practice guidelines to define the appropriate intervention
• Routinely and systematically measures clients' perceptions of function and well-being as well as clinical outcomes and cost outcomes
• Pools large amounts of data from a large series of clients
• Analyzes and disseminates results so timely action can be taken

Outcomes research is used to compare outcomes between competing intervention alternatives to determine which intervention is most effective and cost effective. Outcomes research investigates interventions as they are used in typical practice settings as opposed to strictly controlled conditions of randomized clinical trials. Data are collected and analyzed and conclusions

drawn to inform decisions about implementing or revising practice guidelines and intervention alternatives. Outcomes research also aids planning and decision making by providing data on which to base prediction of future clinical, cost, and patients outcomes if specific interventions are adopted.

Three classes of outcomes are measured: clinical outcomes, cost outcomes, and patient outcomes. **Clinical outcomes** are the health status–related outcomes and can include mortality, risk factors, signs and symptoms of disease, and complications resulting from the disease or condition or its treatment. Clinical outcomes are defined and assessed based on clinicians' and community nutrition professionals' views of what are relevant and important indicators of health or disease progress in specific life cycle stages or disease states. Definitions of outcome indicators and clinically meaningful changes in clinical outcome are based on scientific studies, expert judgment, or established norms.[18]

Cost outcomes express the monetary value of resources consumed or saved as a consequence of the intervention and its resulting clinical outcomes.[12] For example, prenatal participation in WIC has been shown to reduce the need for infant intensive care utilization because fewer low-birthweight infants are born.[4] Cost outcomes are of major importance to health care administrators and policy makers.

Patient outcomes emphasize attention to the consequences of interventions that are of concern to clients. These include symptom relief, survival, adverse side effects of the condition or its treatment, functional status, quality of life, and level of satisfaction with care.[29]

Various players in the health care arena have differing interests and needs for outcome data, and they use information from outcomes measurement and research for different purposes. Some of the uses of outcomes information used by key players are outlined in table 15.3.

EVALUATION ACROSS THE LIFE SPAN OF A PROGRAM

Evaluation is a process of formulating questions, collecting and summarizing data to address the questions, and interpreting the findings to guide decisions about action. Evaluation assesses past decisions and plans, and their execution, and informs decisions about future action plans.

Evaluations are crucial to developing and maintaining effective community nutrition programs and services that meet the community's and clients' needs. The purpose and focus of evaluation efforts change over the life span of a program. The life span of a program can be divided into four stages: the idea stage, the formative stage, the implementation and maintenance stage, and the mature stage. Evaluation is important at every stage, but different types of questions guide the selection of evaluation methods to be used at each stage.

The Idea Stage

At the idea stage, the evaluation aim is to identify the priority nutrition-related needs that should be addressed. This is accomplished through comprehensive community needs assessment or a more limited needs assessment focused on a high-risk target group or segment of the population. The needs assessment process was discussed in detail in chapter 13.

Needs assessment data at the idea stage are required to answer the question, What should we do? That is,

what program, service, or product is needed by the community at large or by a target audience within the community? The result of the evaluation at this stage is a commitment to do something in the identified area. However, exactly what to do is not yet known.

The Formative Stage

The purpose of **formative evaluation** is twofold: (1) to determine the specific features of the program, intervention, or product to be offered and (2) to develop and refine operational procedures (activities and intervention methods) for implementing it. At this formative stage, it is absolutely essential to involve potential clients. The focus is to match the clients' perceived *wants* with the priority *needs* that were defined, usually according to health criteria, by health professionals directing the needs assessment.

Market research, as described in chapters 7 and 14, is crucial in the formative stage. The methods of data collection can include focus groups, surveys, interviews, and observation.[3,17] By involving potential clients, the product, price, place, and promotion can be determined, and special features can be tailored to clients' preferences. The result of market research involving potential clientele is the design of a nutrition program that is acceptable, accessible, and culturally relevant to the target audience.

After the specific program is designed, it must be pilot tested. This small-scale preliminary trial, also called a **demonstration project,** can be used to evaluate the processes and procedures of operating the program. It allows for an evaluation of the recruitment and delivery methods and enables bugs to be worked out before full implementation. Final periods of the formative stage can also be used to measure preliminary outcomes. Often pilot studies are used as a method to evaluate the value of an idea before funds for full-scale implementation are committed. For example, the WIC program funded demonstration projects on breast-feeding promotion for several years before directly allocating extensive resources to breast-feeding promotion.

Evaluation at the formative stage answers the question, How should we do it? In this stage, the details of the intervention program are developed and the pilot is tested. The result of evaluation at the formative stage is the development of a sound program that fosters a match between clients' needs and wants and the operational capacity of the sponsoring organization.

The Implementation and Maintenance Stage

Following formative evaluation, the program is ready for the next stage: full implementation. During the early period of implementation, evaluation, and feedback systems focus on process evaluation. **Process evaluation** is important for documenting that the program is actually being implemented and delivered to the target audience as planned. It monitors the progress and quality of implementation activities by using financial and program records, quality assurance or CQI, and other reviews.[26] Process evaluation is aided by a well-designed management information system (MIS), where information is documented, stored, summarized, and reported out.

Quantitative information about participation and service delivery should be supplemented with periodic surveys of providers and clients to assess satisfaction with processes and services and to identify potential barriers to successful program operation and the eventual accomplishment of objectives. Personnel responsible for implementation of the program should review results of ongoing process evaluation and participate in decisions regarding corrective adjustments.[24]

Process evaluation questions at the implementation and maintenance stage include: Are the procedures and protocols for services being followed? Do they work smoothly? Are we reaching the desired clients? Are clients satisfied with services? Process evaluation is an essential prerequisite to outcome and effectiveness evaluation, which is examined later in the implementation phase.

At periodic points in program implementation and ongoing maintenance, evaluators take stock of performance in terms of meeting program objectives. Assessment of program objectives is called **outcome** or **summative evaluation.** Progress toward outcomes is assessed and summed up at the end of the program or at regular reporting periods, usually annually. Outcome evaluation compares the results of the program during a defined period of time with the specific, measurable outcome objectives that were established.[21,26] It answers the questions, Did we achieve what we set out to achieve? Is there evidence that clients achieve defined outcomes?

Systems of data collection must be in place throughout the year to make this possible. Outcome evaluation relies on an MIS that efficiently summarizes and organizes data regarding services delivered, clients' outcomes, and resources used. A challenge of outcome evaluation is tracking clients after their involvement with nutrition programs so that outcome indicators can be measured.

The result of process and outcome evaluation during the implementation and maintenance phase of programs is assurance that the program is doing what it was designed to do. Ongoing evaluations procedures should facilitate outcomes measurement and enable incremental adjustments in the program. This should assure efficiency and effectiveness of the program or service.

The Mature Stage

When programs have reached maturity, ongoing process and outcome evaluation continues to be necessary to prevent deterioration of performance. In addition, needs assessment and marketing information should be gathered to assess the program's current fit with and relevance to current and future needs. When evaluation results indicate that the program no longer fits with priority needs, it may be time to dismantle the program and shift resources to higher-priority areas.

Goal-free evaluation, originally described by Scriven for education programs,[28] is a comprehensive evaluation approach that is appropriate for mature programs that require a substantial commitment of resources.

Goal-free evaluation is a comprehensive examination of a program and its costs and consequences, both positive and negative, as seen by clients, providers, external stakeholders, and society. This type of evaluation is especially important for policy decisions and is often carried out by outside evaluators. It is most commonly used for mature programs when reauthorization decisions are pending and at times of agency reorganization or priority setting. Goal-free evaluation is closely aligned with policy analysis, where a broad range of criteria are examined, including ethical and equity considerations (see chapter 19).

Whereas other evaluation methods tend to accept the existence of the program as a given, goal-free evaluation asks, Is this really what we should be doing? How much of it should we be doing? How does the program impact on other aspects of the organization, providers, clients, and society?

Goal-free evaluation uses available process and outcome evaluation results, but through interviewing and other methods a much broader description of the program and its consequences is developed. Goal-free evaluation draws heavily on the view of the broad constituency to develop a picture of the program's processes and practices and its direct and indirect consequences. It forces examination of accepted assumptions about programs, opens programs to wider scrutiny and wider visibility, and facilitates access to the advice of a range of experts. This can be a beneficial process that may lead to broader program support, modernization of assumptions and intervention techniques, authorization of needed resources, or reallocation of resources to more important or more effective programs.

By using goal-free evaluation, community nutrition professionals will be better equipped to integrate nutrition priorities and programs into the existing priorities of the organization and collaborating agencies.

PLANNING MORE COMPLEX EFFECTIVENESS EVALUATIONS

In-house evaluations of the results of nutrition programs and services provide important information to improve nutrition services. They can also serve as a starting point for more elaborate effectiveness evaluations and outcomes research. With additional time allocated to evaluation, community nutrition professionals can plan and conduct these more complex evaluations. Effectiveness evaluation determines the magnitude of change that is attributable to the nutrition intervention. Outcomes research uses effectiveness evaluation and extends it to examine cost and patient outcomes. Outcomes research can include cost-effectiveness and cost-benefit analyses. Guidelines for planning studies on effectiveness, outcomes, and cost effectiveness of nutrition services and interventions have been published.[11,22,30–32] Effectiveness evaluation and outcomes research require attention to the proper design of the evaluation itself. Steps involved in effectiveness evaluations are shown in box 15.4.

In complex studies, additional steps, such as selecting comparison groups and controlling for other factors that could also influence outcomes, are necessary to show a true causal relationship between the nutrition intervention and outcomes achieved.

To strengthen the scientific validity of effectiveness or outcomes studies in routine clinical settings, and have greater confidence regarding the impact of nutrition intervention, the recommendations in box 15.5 should be considered when planning a study. In addition, the Bradford Hill criteria (see page 66 in chapter 3) are necessary

BOX 15.4

STEPS IN DETERMINING EFFECTIVENESS

- Choose disease state or condition
- Identify relevant alternatives
- Define outcomes
- Design the study
    Groups to be compared
    Sample
    Variables (and indicators) definition and timing
    Analysis plan
- Select standard measurement tools
- Collect data
    Intervention details
    Patient characteristics
    Key outcome
    Other outcomes
- Analyze data
- Use results

BOX 15.5

TIPS FOR PLANNING AN EFFECTIVENESS OR OUTCOMES STUDY

- Evaluate two or more methods of intervention at the same time to remove the possible influence of outside forces on outcomes.
- Evaluate varying aspects of the content of nutrition care and the amount of contact rather than care or no care. This gets beyond defending nutrition services (versus no nutrition care) and move the profession on to developing greater knowledge about what kind of nutrition intervention leads to the greatest effectiveness.
- Determine the level for a clinically meaningful outcome ahead of time; then use that value to calculate a sample size for the study.
- Randomly or systematically assign clients to intervention alternatives (rather than haphazard or self-selection) to prevent bias in the groups.
- Implement the study prospectively and monitor quality and completeness of data and encourage complete participation of study participants. This leads to higher-quality data, reduces attrition, and improves the generalizability of the results.
- Track other outcomes including short-term, proximal outcomes of nutrition interventions such as dietary intake, and consider measuring quality-of-life issues.
- Continue the study until a large enough sample size has been enrolled in each intervention alternative.
- Verify that study participants are a fair representation of the population to which results are to be applied. Examine the characteristics of participants in each intervention and compare those characteristics with the reference population.
- Get appropriate statistical advice to conduct statistical analysis of data and interpret findings.

before assuming a causal relationship between nutrition intervention and outcomes. The following discussion of evaluation design issues will establish why such considerations are important.

When a series of studies show similar results, a strong case is established for nutrition intervention in the disease or condition. For example, Trouba[35] illustrates the use of published reports to justify the role of nutrition education and food supplementation in prenatal care.

DESIGNING EFFECTIVENESS EVALUATIONS

In the evaluation of nutrition programs and services, the ultimate questions are, Did it work? Did the specific intervention bring about the desired effect or outcome? These are questions of causation, which can be demonstrated only with carefully planned and controlled investigations. This section presents an overview of evaluation designs and essential aspects of evaluation studies that can be used to determine whether an outcome is really achieved, the magnitude of the effect, and if it can be attributed to the nutrition intervention.

The "design" of an evaluation involves determining: (1) the groups to be compared, that is the experimental and control (or comparison) groups; (2) how the sample will be selected; (3) the definition of variables (indicators) and the methods and timing for their measurement; and (4) the plan for analyzing the data.

Sample Selection

The first point of sample selection is to study people and settings that directly match the intent of the program. The sample studied must be drawn from the target population. For example, a cholesterol screening and intervention program desires to identify and reduce the cholesterol level of young adults at risk for future cardiovascular disease. Worksites that employ young adults could be used as places to recruit and enroll subjects who represent the actual age group targeted by the cholesterol intervention program. In contrast, a shopping center cholesterol screening clinic that attracts elderly shoppers would not be a good place to sample for the study.

Adequate sample size is necessary to observe the true distribution of results within each study group. Most outcome indicators will have a range of normal variation. The challenge is to detect a meaningful change that is large enough to indicate an effect of the intervention. A hazard of small sample sizes is that an effect may not be detected even when the intervention has some effect.[6] Sample size determinations are based on normal variation of the outcome indicator, a minimum value or threshold for a clinically meaningful change, and a prediction of attrition (study dropout) rates. In practical terms, many evaluations are carried out with as few as twenty to forty in a group. In complex effectiveness evaluations, it is best to consult with a statistician regarding appropriate sample size.

Variables and Their Measurement

Variables are data elements that are documented in evaluation and research studies. Three kinds of variables are specified in effectiveness and outcomes evaluations: independent variable (exposure to the nutrition intervention), intervening or confounding variables, and the dependent variable or outcome of interest. The independent variable is simply exposure to or participation in the nutrition intervention. At times it is necessary to further define the intervention into amount, intensity level, or time period of participation. Data about the type and amount of intervention verify that the intervention was in fact delivered according to protocol, and these data also allow further investigation into the relationship between aspects of the program and the magnitude of effect produced.

Intervening or confounding variables are other factors that could influence the effect of the nutrition program on the participant. For example, men may respond differently than women, so gender would be an important variable to document. Other examples include presence of risk factors, previous experience with the problem or intervention, concomitant participation in another similar program, educational attainment, and lifestyle factors. Data on intervening or confounding variables are used in the analysis to sort out the true effects of the intervention from other factors that could interfere with or mediate effects. Consideration of these variables leads to a greater understanding of how well the program works and for whom, and it may give clues as to why or when the program does not work.

The dependent variable is the specific indicator of effectiveness of the program or intervention. It must be directly linked to the intervention and is probably specified in an outcome objective of the program. A decrease in serum cholesterol could be the dependent variable of a cholesterol program, an increase in a score on a nutrition knowledge test could be the measured outcome of a school-based nutrition education program, and an increased rate or duration of breast-feeding would be obvious indicators of success of a breast-feeding promotion and support program. Longer-term outcomes such as disease incidence or use of medical care could also be dependent variables, although there are more intervening variables between the nutrition intervention and these distal outcomes.

The next challenge is determining how to measure the variables. Each variable must be observed and recorded in a way that assures its validity, reliability, and precision. Validity is the degree to which the measure captures the essence of the phenomenon being observed. Reliability refers to the ability to obtain the same result with repeated measurement. Precision defines the extent to which the measurement can discriminate between differences in magnitude. Some variables can be determined from program records, some from special surveys or questionnaires, and others from biochemical or anthropometric techniques. Consider the challenges to measuring the following variables that could be included in the evaluation of a nutrition intervention: client's perception of body image, weight loss, knowledge of heart-healthy eating practices, percentage of budget spent on food, and duration of breast-feeding.

Once variables are defined and their means of measurement is determined, the periodicity of measurement (when the variable will be observed and recorded) must be determined; and detailed procedures must be outlined to guide data collection and assure consistency by all those involved throughout the entire study. See box 15.6 for a worksheet to aid in selecting variables and their measurement.

Groups to Be Compared

Conclusions about the effects of evaluated interventions are made by comparing one group to its prior level or to a performance standard (nonexperimental design), one group to another group (quasi-experimental design), or people randomly assigned to experimental treatment (intervention) and control (none or an alternative intervention) groups (experimental design). Types of studies in these categories are shown in box 15.7 and described in detail by Mohr.[21] Epidemiological studies, including cohort and case-control studies, as described in chapter 3,

are also relevant to understanding the effects of nutrition interventions.

Experimental Design   The classic design for evaluation is the **experimental design.** Study subjects from the target population are randomly assigned to either the group that gets the program (the experimental group) or to a control group that does not receive any intervention or receives an alternative or placebo intervention. The program is followed according to a definite protocol, and after a relevant period of time outcomes are measured. Differences between groups are computed, and the program is deemed successful if the experimental group has more of the measured outcome than the control group and if the effect is large enough to be meaningful in practical terms. Statistical techniques are usually applied to determine the statistical significance of the differences.

The classic experimental model is considered the gold standard for asserting that a nutrition intervention caused the effect; however, it is often difficult to execute. The program may serve most who are eligible, and nonparticipants are likely to be different from participants in lifestyle, age, interests, knowledge, or income and thus are not appropriate comparisons. Professional ethics also may prohibit withholding an intervention from people who need it. Another drawback of using the experimental model is its high cost.

There are ways to overcome these difficulties. When resources are scarce and some people must do without or be on a waiting list, it is possible to randomize people to either the program or to the control (no service) group. Also when new programs are introduced over time, the delayed receivers can be the controls for those who get the program early. Demonstration projects can be designed to have participants randomly assigned to the program or a control group and thus facilitate use of the experimental design for effectiveness evaluation.

Quasi-Experimental Designs   **Quasi-experimental designs** are those that do not meet the strict requirements of the classic experimental model but can produce valid results. Cook and Campbell indicate that the most basic criteria for such designs is the extent to which they protect against the effect of extraneous variables on the outcome indicators.[6] The best designs are those that control relevant outside factors and lead to valid inferences about the effects of the program.[6,21] Quasi-experimental designs are very commonly used

BOX 15.6

WORKSHEET FOR SELECTING VARIABLES
AND MEASUREMENT PROCEDURES

Objective of the evaluation:

Area of study:

Groups to be compared:

How sample will be selected (client characteristics):

Data Element Needed (variables)	Indicator (specific dimension to be measured)	Measurement Method (tools and procedures)	When will measurement be taken and recorded? (timing)
Exposure to Nutrition Intervention (type, amount)			
Intervening Variables			
Outcomes (proximal)			
(intermediate)			
(distal)			

---

for effectiveness evaluation because they test results in routine settings. See box 15.3 contrasting efficacy, which generally requires an experimental design, with effectiveness, which can be determined with carefully planned quasi-experimental designs.

Nonexperimental Designs   Sometimes it is impossible to use even a quasi-experimental design. The evaluator then has to resort to one of the three common **nonexper-**

imental designs: (1) a before-and-after study of one or more participants, (2) an after-only study of a group of program participants, or (3) an after-only study of participants and a nonrandom comparison group. The weakness of all these designs is that they fail to control for many of the *threats to validity* (see references 21 and 6). With these designs it is highly possible that some other cause could be responsible for an outcome observed in the studied individuals. However, when data

BOX 15.7

PRACTICAL EVALUATION DESIGNS FOR NUTRITION INTERVENTIONS

DESCRIPTIVE, NON-EXPERIMENTAL DESIGNS
What is happening?

A. Case study	post pre-post series	In-depth observations of individual case(s) to gain insight. Focus on relationship between services and participants. Especially useful in first-of-a-kind situations.
B. Ex post facto	retrospective self-reports for pre-post	Measure change by comparison with client's self-reported status prior to service. Used when preprogram documentation is unavailable.
C. Before and after	pre-post	Good data collection before and after intervention.

COMPARATIVE, QUASI-EXPERIMENTAL DESIGNS
Does the change follow after the nutrition intervention?

D. Staged designs (replication)	pre-post pre	Data from successive sets of participants are compared. Requires definition of outcomes and indicators and stable data collection over time.
E. Comparison group (participants/nonparticipants)	pre-post pre-post	Comparison of change experienced by participants with a similar (matched) group of people who did not participate in the program. Bias of self-selection a problem. Most popular evaluation design.

F. Program comparison
   Program A
   Program B
	
	pre-post
	pre-post
		Provides comparison of results using different methods to achieve similar objectives (e.g., videotape versus one-on-one instruction). This is the basis for cost-effectiveness analysis.

G. Time-series design	pre-123-post-123	Separates true program effects from natural history and maturation effects and can be used to determine long-term changes. Important in nutrition intervention to demonstrate maintenance or continued improvements.

EXPERIMENTAL DESIGNS
Does the nutrition intervention cause the effect?

H. Randomized clinical trials (RCTs)
   Treatment
   Alternative
	
	post
	post
		The acid test of research and evaluation. Rules out the possibility that outside factors are responsible for the changes in health outcomes. Subjects are randomized to experimental treatment and alternatives (control) that may be no treatment, standard treatment, different level of intensity, and so on.

Source: From Splett PL: *The practitioner's guide to cost-effectiveness analysis of nutrition interventions,* Arlington, VA, 1996. National Center for Education in Maternal and Child Health. Used with permission.

on carefully selected process and outcome variables are systematically collected and summarized with care, these designs can provide valuable insights. Some information is better than no information at all. Nonexperimental designs do, however, leave considerable room for differing interpretations of how much change occurred and how much of the observed change was caused by exposure to the program or intervention.

Although nonexperimental designs provide preliminary data about the possible effects of the program, they are not appropriate choices for effectiveness evaluations or outcomes research. However, they can provide useful preliminary evaluation data. For example, if a carefully planned before-and-after study finds little change in outcomes for the participants, the program, as it was delivered, is probably having little effect. It may not be worthwhile to invest in more rigorous effectiveness evaluation until the program is modified. At this point, it would be most productive to direct attention to process evaluation and to review of state-of-the-art delivery methods or "best practices" used by other successful programs.

Caution must be exercised when making claims about the effectiveness of nutrition programs and services when the programs or specific services have not been adequately evaluated with sound evaluation designs.

ECONOMIC EVALUATION: COST-EFFECTIVENESS AND COST-BENEFIT ANALYSES

Cost-effectiveness analysis (CEA) and **cost-benefit analysis** (CBA) go beyond the assessment of effectiveness to relate outcomes to costs. These economic evaluations help to address whether the magnitude of outcome is worth the investment of resources necessary to make it happen. In addition to carefully measuring outcomes, economic evaluation requires investigators to carefully determine the costs or resource requirements to deliver the nutrition services and, in the case of CBA, to estimate a monetary value for the results achieved.

The general label for these types of evaluations is *economic evaluation.* Economic evaluation is the comparative analysis of alternative courses of action in terms of both their costs and consequences.[12,14] It has two essential characteristics: it is concerned with making a choice between alternative uses of scarce resources, and it structures comparisons of both inputs (costs) and outputs (which are labeled benefits, consequences, effects, or outcomes in various applications) between alternative programs or interventions.

Economic Evaluation in Nutrition

Before 1979, economic evaluation was rare in the nutrition literature. At that time the American Dietetic Association proposed a model for estimating the economic benefits of nutrition.[19] The model, which provides a sound base for considering logical and scientifically based linkages of nutrition services and interventions to outcomes, is shown in figure 15.4.

Ten years later, Disbrow summarized data on costs, health status and economic benefits, and results of economic analysis.[10] In 1991, following a critical analysis of existing studies in four areas of practice, the American Dietetic Association (ADA) published summary documents that justify nutrition care in terms of its intermediate-term cost savings and economic gains.[31] In that publication, research designs were proposed for testing practice guidelines, evaluating the outcomes of nutrition care, and determining the cost effectiveness of nutrition care. In 1995, ADA published a position paper detailing the body of literature supporting the cost effectiveness of medical nutrition therapy.[2]

During the same time economic evaluation was increasingly used throughout health care and public health to evaluate new and old medical procedures and technology and public health interventions.[15,34]

Throughout this time, the methods of economic analysis as applied to health have been evolving. An expert panel convened by the U.S. Public Health Service recently reviewed the theory and practice of CEA and then made recommendations for standardizing cost-effectiveness analysis methodology for application in health and medicine.[12] Staff of the Centers for Disease Control and Prevention also reviewed methods and described methodology for CEA as it applies to public health intervention and prevention.[14] Current recommendations merge the theoretical base of economic analysis with its practical application in decision making.

Definitions

Cost-effectiveness analysis and cost-benefit analysis are ways to select between competing alternatives based on their **efficiency.** That is, the ratio of costs to output (or outcome). In these types of evaluation, the analyst uses carefully gathered estimates of cost and outcome for competing alternatives, which can be intervention strategies, procedures, technological choices, or program options.

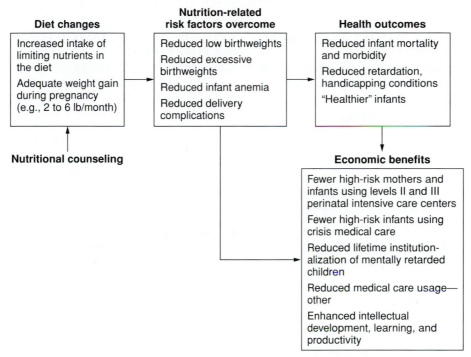

FIGURE 15.4   Potential Economic Benefits of Nutritional Counseling in Pregnancy
(*Source:* From *Costs and Benefits of Nutritional Care Phase I,* Chicago, 1979. Copyright The American Dietetic Association. Reprinted by permission.)

Many terms have distinct meanings in economic evaluation. *Effects* usually refers to the programmatic objectives of the alternative (e.g., reduced incidence of anemia or an increased nutrition knowledge score), measured in natural units (e.g., number of new cases or standardized knowledge score). The term *benefits* is usually reserved for outputs valued in monetary units (e.g., dollars of medical services avoided). Estimates of monetary benefits includes the fact that consequences can be negative as well as positive. Cost savings from improved health as well as added costs for complications or side effects of treatment that some people experience are included. *Outcomes,* defined here as anticipated and unanticipated consequences of the program and its processes, is an inclusive term for all types of outputs and is used throughout this section.

When outcomes are expressed in units natural to the objectives of the program or intervention strategy, the method is labeled "cost-effectiveness analysis." When outcomes are valued in monetary terms, the method is called "cost-benefit analysis." Examples of CEA and CBA are shown in the box 15.8.

Steps of Economic Analysis

Economic evaluation requires a systematic process of defining, measuring, and valuing the costs and outcomes of two or more competing alternatives for accomplishing something. The six steps shown in figure 15.5 are based on a synthesis of the principles and recommendations for economic analysis.

State the Objective

The first step, like the first step of any evaluation, is to clarify the purpose of the evaluation. The objective would state why you are doing the economic evaluation and what decision you expect to inform with the information collected. For example, cost-effectiveness studies could be planned for the purpose of answering these questions: What is the cost effectiveness of enhanced prenatal care compared to basic prenatal care? What is the most cost-effective alternative system of delivering nutrition services to children with special health care needs in this state? Answers to these questions could be used by community nutrition professionals, administrators, and policy makers to make decisions about the type and system of care to fund.

BOX 15.8

EXAMPLES OF CEA AND CBA

A COST-EFFECTIVENESS ANALYSIS REPORTING COST PER UNIT OF OUTCOME

Stunkard and associates* compared the cost per 1% decrease in percentage overweight for seven weight loss programs conducted in different settings.

Program setting	Cost per 1% decrease in overweight
University clinic	$108.67
Worksite program delivered by professional leaders	$33.61
Clinic using very-low-calorie diets	$28.00
Clinic using behavior therapy	$19.62
Worksite program delivered by lay leaders	$11.10
Commercial program	$7.31
Worksite program designed by the investigators	$0.92

A COST-BENEFIT ANALYSIS REPORTING NET COST SAVINGS

Brauer and associates** studied nutrition counseling for patients with Crohn's disease. The investigators reported a net savings to society of $164 per person during the study year for patients who received six monthly nutrition counseling sessions compared to patients who did not receive nutrition counseling. The economic benefits came from reduced medication use, fewer hospital days, and fewer days lost from work in the counseled group compared to persons who did not get nutrition counseling.

*Stunkard AJ, Cohen AY, Felix MR: Weight loss competitions at the worksite: how they work and how well, *Prev Med* 18:460, 1989.
**Brauer PM, Ines S, Thompson BR: Economic impact of nutrition counselling in patients with Crohn's disease in Canada, *J Can Diet Assoc* 49:236, 1988.

Step 1. State objective

Step 2. Define the framework
- Perspective
- Alternatives
- Time horizon

Step 3. Determine costs
- Define all activities
- Specify measurement
- Collect cost data
- Calculate costs
- Discount

Step 4. Determine outcomes
- Define outcomes
- Select design
- Collect data
- Analyze data
- Discount

Step 5. Relate costs to outcomes
- Ratio
- Array

Step 6. Summarize, interpret, and report findings
- Ethical implications
- Sensitivity analysis
- Usefulness to decision makers

FIGURE 15.5   Six Steps of Economic Analysis
(*Source:* Adapted from Splett, PL: *The practitioner's guide to cost-effectiveness analysis of nutrition interventions,* National Center for Education in Maternal and Child Health.)

Define the Framework of the Analysis

The framework of an economic analysis is three things: the alternative to be considered, the perspective for analysis, and the time horizon.

When selecting the alternative to be evaluated, consider the commonly used approach, lower-cost alternatives, best practices, and other approaches that are in use or have political support for adoption. To be helpful to decision making, all reasonable alternatives should be evaluated.

The perspective for analysis defines whose resources are at stake. It determines the scope of the analysis. The societal perspective includes all costs and outcomes of an intervention, no matter to whom they accrue, over as long a time as is pertinent and reasonable. In contrast, the institutional or organizational perspective is specifically focused on the costs that come out of the organization's budget and the outcomes that are directly relevant to the organization and its clients. Other perspectives are those of the payor, program, and the client and family. Economic experts recommend framing the analysis from the societal perspective; however, the program, organization, or payor perspectives usually have most relevance for making decisions about nutrition intervention alternatives.

The time horizon addresses the relevant period for the course of the nutrition intervention (i.e., one contact, three visits during the prenatal period, or semiannual contacts across a lifetime), and the period over which the outcomes are experienced. These periods may be different, as shown in figure 15.6. When planning an economic evaluation you decide the point at which outcomes will be measured even though additional outcomes continue to accumulate. For example, nutrition intervention in chronic diseases such as hypertension, diabetes, and cardiovascular disease present a dilemma as to what outcome to measure when. In contrast, the time horizon for inputs and outcomes of nutrition intervention during pregnancy is easier to define. The time horizon is the time periods you define as relevant to the measurement of the intervention and the outcomes in your specific analysis.

There is no one correct way to frame an economic evaluation. The goal and perspective for analysis determines which costs and outcomes should be included and how each is valued. Once the framework is decided it must be applied equally to all alternatives evaluated.

Determine Costs

Types of Costs Economists define costs in three categories: direct (organization and operating costs), indirect (out-of-pocket expenses borne by the participant and family, such as medication, travel, and forgone earnings), and intangible (grief, pain, and suffering).

Cost Estimation Costs of each nutrition intervention are estimated using the process of **cost analysis.** When applied in a systematic and careful manner, cost analysis provides a defensible estimate of resource consumption necessary to implement each alternative. Cost analysis must be carried out with equal precision for each alternative. Cost analysis as applied is illustrated in box 15.9. For more detail on cost analysis turn to pages 488–489 in the next chapter.

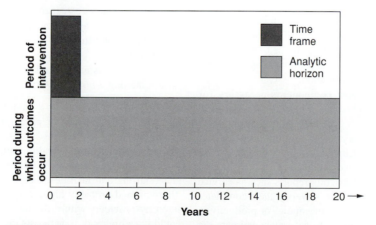

FIGURE 15.6   Time Horizon for Intervention and Outcomes
(*Source:* From Haddix AC, Teutsch SM, Shaffer PA, Dunet DO: *Prevention effectiveness: a guide to decision analysis and economic evaluation,* New York, 1996, Oxford University Press.)

The findings of the cost analysis can be summarized and reported in a number of ways, including:

Full-cost: total cost of program over a period of time (usually one year or the normal duration of a clients' participation in the program).

Average cost: cost per unit of output/outcome (e.g., cost per nutrition assessment or cost per low-birthweight infant prevented).

Incremental cost: cost for nutrition as an add-on to existing service (e.g., nutrition assessment added to an EPSDT visit).

Marginal costs: cost of doing a little more or a little less (e.g., adding a second nutrition follow-up visit for people completing a weight loss program).

Incremental or marginal costs are more relevant to economic analysis than total or average costs, because they relate to the extra cost to produce each added effect. For example, a substantial amount of resources are consumed to develop a program and system to deliver nutrition messages through local grocery stores. Once the program is developed, adding another store greatly expands the number of families reached but the "marginal" costs are considerably less than the original cost of introducing the program in the first store.

The same cost analysis process is used to estimate the monetary value of the outcomes. Costed outcomes could include home health or medical visits, laboratory tests, or medications used in the treatment of disease consequences or intervention side effects. Issues and approaches for costing outcomes are addressed in detail by Gold et al.[12] and Haddix.[14]

Determine Outcomes

Types of Outcomes   Whereas inputs are always valued in dollars, outcomes can be measured in three basic ways: (1) units natural to the program objectives measured with ad hoc numerical scales (e.g., gain in knowledge scores, pounds of weight loss, or number of cases prevented); (2) economic benefits associated with the health improvements valued in monetary terms as direct (health care resources sav-

BOX 15.9

COST ANALYSIS IN PRENATAL CARE

Here is how a community nutrition professional could determine the cost of nutrition services in prenatal care from the perspective of the public health center based on the current program year.

1. Prepare a flow chart of all activities involved in providing nutrition services to pregnant clients. Note that pre- and postservice activities are included in costs. For example, client recruitment and outreach, nutrition assessment and counseling of clients, record keeping and scheduling, client follow-up and monitoring, and program administration and evaluation.

2. Identify the principal cost components necessary for each activity. This might include nutrition and clerical personnel, fringe benefits, nutrition education materials and equipment, laboratory tests to monitor anemia, office and clinic space, nutrition reference materials, office supplies, and administrative overhead.

3. Use work schedules and existing reports such as service statistics or accounting records (verify their completeness and accuracy), conduct time studies or productivity studies, or use other methods to accurately estimate the quantity of principal cost components necessary to carry out each activity.

4. Work with accounting staff to assign a monetary value based on the actual cost to the organization for each cost component.

5. Keep track of all assumptions made along the way.

6. Calculate the total costs for prenatal nutrition services. Then divide by the number of women served to get an average or unit cost. If the cost analysis looked only at nutrition costs as a component of an existing prenatal care program, the costs would be called the incremental costs.

7. Since all costs are expended in the current time period, discounting is not necessary.

Similar steps with similar assumptions would be carried out for each alternative compared in the economic analysis.

For example, a free-standing nutrition service delivered at a location other than the health department, requiring separate staffing and facilities, would likely have significantly different, and probably higher, costs. Nutrition services offered by providers with different professional backgrounds could have higher or lower costs due to varying amounts of time spent with the client and differing salary scales. Cost analysis would reveal cost differences.

ings or losses) or indirect (out-of-pocket costs experienced by the patient); and (3) the subjective value or utility of health improvements, as the patient, family, expert, or society perceives them, measured in standard units such as satisfaction or preference score[36] or quality-adjusted life years (QALY). The concept of QALY is described in box 15.10. These ways of measuring and expressing outcomes relate to the clinical, cost, and patient outcomes addressed in outcomes measurement.

Data for Estimation of Outcomes   Economic evaluation requires sound estimation of the effectiveness of the compared alternatives. The outcomes selected as indicators of effectiveness must be clearly linked (theoretically and empirically) to the interventions (programs or activities), they must be evaluated in a time frame that has a realistic relationship to the proposed intervention, and they must be evaluated in such a way as to control for other factors that could influence outcomes.[14,26,30] Effectiveness data may come from previous epidemiological and clinical studies, or data collection for an effectiveness evaluation can be planned as a step in the economic analysis. Issues in the evaluation of effectiveness discussed earlier in this chapter are important to the quality of data used in economic analysis.

Many CEA and CBA reports rely on estimates of effectiveness derived from previous evaluations or meta-analyses. A *meta-analysis* is a specific process of reviewing and integrating the findings of all available studies on a defined topic. A meta-analysis produces a more accurate estimation of the magnitude of effect than a single study.[25] Whether effectiveness evaluation is carried out as part of an economic evaluation or previously collected data are used, the analyst must verify the quality of the methods used to determine effectiveness results. Box 15.11 outlines some questions to guide the critique of existing data on the outcomes of nutrition interventions reported in published articles, program reports, or government documents.

Relate Costs to Outcomes

This is the step where cost effectiveness or cost benefit is determined. The estimated amount of costs are related to the estimated magnitude of outcome achieved and presented in the form of a ratio, net cost or net benefit, or an array table (see box 15.12 and tables 15.4 and 15.5 for examples).

Cost-Benefit and Cost-Effectiveness Indices   The ratio is an index of *efficiency*. It relates costs to outcomes as a cost-benefit ratio or a cost-effectiveness ratio. The ratios communicate the cost for a unit of outcome and allow direct comparison between the efficiency of one alternative and the efficiency of the other alternative(s). However, when a ratio is used, it is difficult to visualize the total cost to implement the intervention, and the actual magnitude of the change is not evident.

When inputs (the intervention) and the outcome and other consequences have been costed, a net cost or cost savings can be reported. In this calculation, future health care costs and future health care savings associated with the outcomes of the intervention are summed, then this amount is subtracted from the input costs. The result is a net cost or a cost savings.

The net-cost approach recognizes that in many health care interventions, benefits do not exceed resource costs. The net-cost calculation can be related to a

---

BOX 15.10

QUALITY-ADJUSTED LIFE YEARS

Quality-adjusted life years is a universal measure of health status that expresses length of healthy life. The goal is to extend the state of good health as long as possible and minimize periods of ill health or disability.

QALY takes two things into account:

- Length of life
- Quality or state of health (well-being) during various periods of time

   Length of life comes from a life table of the population. Life tables specify the proportion of the population of people living and dying at each age interval and the average years of life remaining at the end of each age interval.

   Measures of well-being include mental, physical, and social functioning. For example, social functioning includes an individual's limitations in performing usual social roles of work, school, housework, and the like; physical functioning can be measured in terms of being confined to bed, chair, or home due to health reasons.

   Various tools have been developed to assign a quality of life or well-being score (a number from 0.0 [death] to 1.0 [optimal health] to an individual's functioning.

   The QALY is calculated by multiplying years of life times quality of life.

BOX 15.11

CHECKLIST FOR CRITIQUE OF EFFECTIVENESS REPORTS

TITLE, AUTHORS, AND SOURCE
Do authors have experience and credibility in topic area?

EVALUATION CONTEXT
- Evaluation purpose: What was the purpose (objectives, research questions, or hypothesis) of the study?
- Intervention: What was the specific intervention studied in terms of type, content, duration? What was the setting for delivery of the intervention?
- Outcomes: What outcomes of the nutrition intervention were assessed?
- Reference population: To whom can the results of the evaluation be applied?

EVALUATION, DESIGN AND DATA COLLECTION PROCEDURES (METHODOLOGY)
What evaluation design was used? Does it allow for attribution of outcomes to the nutrition intervention?

Comparisons: What groups or alternatives were compared?

Sample: How were subjects selected from the reference population? How were subjects placed in study groups? (random assignment, matching, voluntary participation, convenience)? Is the sample representative of the reference population? Was the sample large enough? What was the attrition or dropout rate? Did it differ between groups?

Variables: Were all relevant intervention, intervening, and outcomes and variables defined and tracked? Were the indicators used for measurement appropriate? What was the time horizon for evaluation of outcomes?

Instrumentation/data collection: Where, when, and how were data obtained? Were measurement instruments and procedures reliable and valid?

ANALYSIS AND PRESENTATION OF FINDINGS
What is the magnitude of change in key outcome indicators? Is it clinically meaningful? Is it statistically significant? Were appropriate statistical tests used? Are the author's conclusions objective (data-based) rather than speculative?

DISCUSSION
Are strengths and limitations of the evaluation discussed? Are findings compared to results from similar evaluations?

CONCLUSIONS AND RECOMMENDATIONS
Are conclusions and recommendations consistent with and supported by the data?

Source: From Splett PL: *The practitioner's guide to cost-effective analysis of nutrition interventions,* Arlington, VA, 1996, National Center for Education in Maternal and Child Health. Used with permission.

BOX 15.12

COST-BENEFIT RATIOS
WIC Prenatal Benefit/Cost Study*

A study was conducted in five states to determine the impact of prenatal WIC participation on Medicaid costs for women and their infants during the first sixty days after birth. Medicaid costs for the WIC women and their infants were compared to Medicaid costs for low-income women and their infants who did not participate in WIC prenatally.

To report the results, the investigators used Medicaid saving (costs for nonparticipants minus costs for WIC participants) divided by prenatal WIC participation costs. The following benefit/cost ratios express the dollar payoff of each dollar invested in prenatal WIC services for each state.

Florida	1.77
South Carolina	2.44
Texas	2.44
Minnesota	1.83
North Carolina	3.13

*Source: Mathematica Policy Research, Inc. The Savings in Medicaid Costs for Newborns and Their Mothers from Prenatal Participation in the WIC Program, October 1990.

TABLE 15.4

Costs per Work-site and per Person to Provide Cholesterol Screening and a Nutrition Education Program, in Dollars

	Cholesterol screening	Educational program	Total
Fixed costs per work-site			
Preparation[a]	158	77	235
Travel[a]	106	19	125
Mileage[b]	91	15	106
Total fixed costs per work-site	355	111	466
Variable costs per person			
Supplies	3.70	10.59	14.29
Provider salaries			
At work-sites	9.60	5.63	15.23
For follow-up	1.88	2.67	4.55
Mail and phone	0.19	0.44	0.63
Total variable costs per participant	15.37	19.33	34.70
Total costs per participant[c]	22.81	27.55	50.36

[a]Hours of preparation or travel multiplied by salary of provider.
[b]Miles to and from work-site multiplied by 27.5¢ per mile.
[c]Variable costs per participant plus fixed costs per participant.
Source: From Byers T, Mullis R, Anderson J, Dusenbury L, et al.: The costs and effects of a nutritional education program following work-site cholesterol screening, *Am J Pub Health;* 85(5):650–655, 1995. Reprinted with permission.

TABLE 15.5

Mean Cholesterol Levels at Baseline, at Six Months, and at Twelve Months, and Percentage Cholesterol Change from Baseline, by Type of Educational Program[a]

	Baseline		Six Months		Twelve Months	
	Usual program	Special program	Usual program	Special program	Usual program	Special program
Total						
Number of subjects	464	380	286	267	268	225
Mean cholesterol	229.6	230.0	228.8	226.8	222.4	225
% cholesterol change, group[b]	—	—	−0.3	−1.4	−3.1	−6.8
% cholesterol change, individuals[c]	—	—	−0.4	−1.2	−3.0	−6.5
% cholesterol change attributable						
to special program[d]			−0.8*		−3.5**	

[a]Means are adjusted for age, education, and prior awareness of elevated cholesterol.
[b]The percentage reduction from baseline in group mean cholesterol levels.
[c]The mean percentage reduction from baseline in cholesterol levels of all study subjects who were reexamined.
[d]Arithmetic difference between special and usual programs in mean cholesterol reductions from baseline for all study subjects who were reexamined.
*P = .02 for contrast of special versus usual change.
**P < .01 for contrast of special versus usual change.
Source: From Byers T, Mullis R, Anderson J, Dusenbury L, et al.: The costs and effects of a nutritional education program following work-site cholesterol screening, *Am J Pub Health;* 85(5):650–655, 1995. Reprinted with permission.

unit of a specific outcome indicator (such as case averted) or a universal unit of outcome, such as QALY. The net cost also has the advantage of allowing comparison between programs and strategies with different objectives, as long as the outcomes can be translated into the universal unit of QALY.

Interpret and Report Findings

Economic analysis is an important tool in making decisions about intervention and program alternatives, policies, and resource allocation. However, before a final conclusion can be drawn other factors must be considered.

Discounting   Discounting is a mathematical procedure used to convert future costs and future outcomes to "present value." When resources are used over a long period of time (more than one year), they must be discounted to a standard base year. Discounting is done because inflation reduces the value of money over time, and there is a tendency to prefer dollars and outcomes now, rather than in the future. In CEA and CBA, cost and outcomes are discounted using 3 or 5 percent[12] before costs are related to outcomes.

Sensitivity   Uncertainty about some assumptions used in the estimation of costs or the determination of outcomes is unavoidable. Sensitivity analysis, uses "what-if" tests to examine whether variations in assumptions affect the conclusions of an analysis. It produces best-care and worst-case scenarios. For example, Franz et al. examined the impact of different dietitian's salaries and higher and lower blood glucose changes before concluding that intensive nutrition intervention was preferred over usual nutrition care for persons with type II diabetes.[10a] Sensitivity analysis is an important part of the process of interpreting the findings from an economic evaluation.[12,14,30] When an alternative remains the preferred choice even after sensitivity analysis, that alternative is confirmed as the dominant alternative and the conclusion is considered "robust."

Ethics   Economic analysis assumes a criterion of efficiency—interventions that produce greater results, or can be conducted at a lower cost, or that are both more effective and less costly are preferred over other alternatives. However, sometimes the alternative that is preferred based on economic criteria is not preferred when other criteria are used in the decision process. For

example, it often costs more to reach and serve vulnerable populations such as frail elderly, children with special health care conditions, and low-income families. These groups may also have difficulties that interfere with the achievement of defined outcomes. Compared to competing alternatives, interventions for these vulnerable groups may be less cost efficient.

In situations such as these, social values and public health responsibilities to assure necessary services for vulnerable populations would supersede economic criteria. Thus, ethical consideration are examined during the interpretation stage of economic analysis. When certain groups, particularly vulnerable groups, are disadvantaged by the dominant alternative that should be pointed out in the report. For an expanded consideration of ethics, readers are directed to chapter 19.

Report Findings   The reporting step is very important. To impact decisions, now and in the future, findings on the costs, effectiveness, and cost effectiveness of nutrition programs and interventions must be disseminated to persons in decision-making roles. These persons include physicians and case managers, agency administrators, public health officers, managed care organizations, employee benefit managers, insurance underwriters, legislators, and policy makers. CEA and CBA studies can be reported in memos, program reports, proposals, abstracts, and articles published in professional and scientific journals. The type of report and method of communication should be tailored to the needs of the recipient.

Uses of Economic Evaluation

Getting accurate and defensible estimates of costs and outcomes for economic evaluation is challenging, but the results can aid community nutrition professionals in valuable ways. First, the steps of cost analysis and effectiveness evaluations force the community nutrition professional to examine details of existing and competing program alternatives. Greater awareness of program operations and resource requirements often leads to ideas for streamlining procedures and improving performance. Second, because resources are scarce across all of health care and human services, cost effectiveness and cost benefit are increasingly used as criteria to decide funding priorities. Nutrition programs can compete more favorably when community nutrition professionals have accurate data on costs and effects and can demonstrate the cost effectiveness or cost benefit of recommended nutrition alternatives.

IMPLICATIONS FOR COMMUNITY NUTRITION PROFESSIONALS

Evaluation is a fact of life for community nutrition professionals in all settings and at all levels. It must be a routine part of program operations from beginning to end. Those involved in direct service delivery must conscientiously observe and document program activities and client outcomes. Those in management positions must take the lead in setting standards for nutrition activities, designing evaluation studies, and analyzing results. All community nutrition professionals must be involved in interpreting findings and planning adjustments to improve effectiveness and efficiency.

As the absolute minimum, community nutrition professionals must have clear objectives and performance expectations for their programs. Evaluation procedures and systems must be in place to monitor performance. Community nutrition professionals must have actual data about the important outcomes produced by their programs; and they must know what program elements are essential for producing those outcomes. And, finally, community nutrition professionals must be prepared to use evaluation findings to defend and preserve program elements essential to effectiveness.

Evaluation and managerial control require an inquisitive mind, the ability to formulate questions, the discipline to plan and follow through in a consistent manner, and the objectivity and courage to act on the findings. These abilities enable the community nutrition professional to continuously improve performance while being mindful of resources.

COMMUNITY NUTRITION PROFESSIONALS IN ACTION

- Why is it important to build evaluation in at the very beginning of a program?
- Discuss the different emphasis of evaluation depending on the maturity of a program.
- What steps are necessary to collect evidence that a nutrition intervention is truly effective?
- Who should be involved in evaluation activities? How can you justify taking staff away from service delivery to spend time doing "paper work" for evaluation?

- What information has to be collected to do a cost-effectiveness analysis? What information has to be collected to do a cost-benefit analysis?
- Critique an article reporting the evaluation of a nutrition program or an aspect of nutrition care.
- Select a local nutrition intervention project and design an evaluation to determine if it is effective.

GOING ONE STEP FURTHER

- Develop plans to determine the cost effectiveness of an existing community nutrition program or intervention. Complete the analysis using actual data.

ADDITIONAL INFORMATION

1. Barr, JT: *Critical literature review: clinical effectiveness in allied health practices* (includes dietetics), U.S. Department of Health and Human Services, Agency for Health Care Policy and Research, AHCPR Pub. No. 94–0029, 1993.
2. Cost-effectiveness of medical nutrition therapy. Position paper of the American Dietetic Association, *J Am Diet Assoc* 95:88, 1995.
3. Gold MR, Siegel JE, Russell LB, Weinstein MC: *Cost-effectiveness in health and medicine,* New York: 1996, Oxford. (Consensus of experts on the appropriate methods for standardizing the conduct of CEAs for use in the policy arena.)

REFERENCES

1. Albrecht K: *Service America: doing business in the new economy,* Homewood, IL; 1985, Jones-Irwin.
2. American Dietetic Association: Cost-effectiveness of medical nutrition therapy. Position paper of The American Dietetic Association, *J Am Diet Assoc* 95:88, 1995.
3. Andreasen AR: *Marketing social change,* San Francisco, 1995, Jossey-Bass.
4. Averuch A, Cackley AP: Savings achieved by giving WIC benefits to women prenatally, *Public Health Reports* 110(1):27–34, 1995.
5. Berwick D: Continuous improvement as an ideal in health care, *N Engl J Med* 320:95–106, 1988.
6. Cook TD, Campbell DT: Quasi-experimentation: design and analysis issues for field settings, Boston, 1979, Houghton Mifflin.
7. Crosby PB: *Quality is free,* New York, 1990, McGraw-Hill.

8. Deming E: *Quality, productivity, and competitive position,* Cambridge, MA, 1982, Institute of Technology Center for Advanced Engineering Study.

9. Dever GE: *Quality improvement methods for public health practice,* Gaithersburg, MD, 1997, Aspen.

10. Disbrow DD: The costs and benefits of nutrition services: a literature review, *J Am Diet Assoc* 84(4):S3, 1989.

10a. Franz MJ, Splett PL, Monk A, et al.: Cost effectiveness of medical nutrition therapy provided by dietitians for persons with non-insulin dependent diabetes mellitus, *J Am Diet Assoc* 95:1018–1024, 1995.

11. Gallagher-Allred C, Voss AC: *Nutrition intervention and patient outcomes: a self-study manual,* Columbus, OH, 1995, Ross Products Division, Abbott Laboratories.

12. Gold MR, Siegel JE, Russell LB, Weinstein MC: *Cost-effectiveness in health and medicine,* New York, 1996, Oxford.

13. Griffin RW: Management, ed 4, Boston, 1995, Houghton Mifflin.

14. Haddix AC, Teutsch SM, Shaffer PA, Dunet DO: *Prevention effectiveness: a guide to decision analysis and economic evaluation,* New York, 1996, Oxford.

15. Health care cost-benefit and cost-effectiveness analysis (CBA/CEA) from 1979 to 1990: a bibliography, *Med Care* 31(7; suppl.):JS2–JS150, 1993.

16. Juran JM, Gryne FM: *Quality planning and analysis,* New York, 1980, McGraw-Hill.

17. Krueger R: *Focus groups: a practical guide for applied research,* Newbury Park, CA, 1994, Sage.

18. Kushner RF, Ayello EA, Beyer PL, Skipper A, et al.: National Coordinating Committee clinical indicators of nutrition care, *J Am Diet Assoc* 94:1169–1177, 1994.

19. Mason M, editor: *Costs and benefits of nutrition care: phase 1,* Chicago, 1979, The American Dietetic Association.

20. *Medical nutrition therapy across the continuum of care,* Chicago, 1996, The American Dietetic Association.

21. Mohr LB: *Impact analysis for program evaluation,* Newbury Park, CA, 1992, Sage.

22. Monsen E: *Research: successful approaches,* Chicago, 1992, The American Dietetic Association.

23. Osborne D, Gaebler T: *Reinventing government,* Reading, MA, 1992, Addison-Wesley.

24. Patton M: *Utilization focused evaluation,* Thousand Oaks, CA: 1996, Sage.

25. Petitti DB: *Meta-analysis, decision analysis and cost-effectiveness analysis: methods for quantitative synthesis in medicine,* New York: 1994, Oxford.

26. Rossi P, Freeman H: *Evaluation: a systematic approach,* ed 5, Newbury Park, CA, 1993, Sage.

27. Scholtes PR: *The team handbook,* Madison, WI, 1996, Joiner Associates, Inc.

28. Scriven M: *Goal-free evaluation.* In E House, editor: *School evaluation,* Berkeley, CA, 1970, McCutchan.

29. Spilker B, editor: *Quality of life and pharmacoeconomics,* ed 2, Philadelphia, 1996, Lippincott-Raven.

30. Splett PL: *Cost outcomes of nutrition intervention, part 1: outcomes research, part 2: measuring effectiveness of nutrition interventions, part 3: economic and cost analysis of nutrition interventions,* Evansville, IN, 1996, Mead Johnson.

31. Splett PL: Effectiveness and cost effectiveness of nutrition care: a critical analysis with recommendations, *J Am Diet Assoc* 91(Suppl):1–53, 1991.

32. Splett PL: *The practitioner's guide to cost-effectiveness analysis of nutrition interventions,* Arlington, VA, 1996, National Center for Education in Maternal and Child Health.

33. Splett PL, Russo PM: *Documenting the quality and effectiveness of nutrition care.* In Fox MK, editor: *Reimbursement and insurance coverage for nutrition services,* Chicago, 1991, The American Dietetic Association.

34. Tengs TO, Adams ME, Pliskin JS, Asfran DG, et al.: *Five hundred life-saving interventions and their cost effectiveness,* Boston, 1994, Harvard Center for Risk Analysis.

35. Trouba PH, Okereke N, Splett PL: Summary document of nutrition intervention in prenatal care, *J Am Diet Assoc* 91(Suppl):S21–S26, 1991.

36. Von Campen C, Sixma H, Friele RD, Kerssens JJ, Peters L: Quality of care and patient satisfaction: a review of measuring instruments, *Med Care Res Rev* 52(1):109–133, 1995.

EVALUATION EVERYDAY, NOT SOME DAY

PATRICIA L. SPLETT

DESCRIPTION

This case study illustrates evaluation issues and challenges faced by a typical public health nutritionist in everyday operation and management of a nutrition unit in a local health department. A similar range of evaluation issues could be faced in most settings where community nutrition professionals are actively connected to program, agency, and community priorities. The case points out how evaluation is closely integrated with planning and implementation, and it shows how evaluation is essential to decision making.

The case can best be used as a group assignment so students can explore and discuss the challenges presented and the range of options faced by the nutrition manager and her staff and collaborators. It should stimulate discussion about the appropriate selection and application of evaluation approaches described in the chapter. Students can, individually or as a group, plan a specific evaluation based on one or more of the issues described in the case.

In this case study, students will be challenged to think realistically about what can be accomplished through an evaluation, the value of involving others, and the importance of utilizing information that is already available from regular reports and program records.

THE CASE

The River Valley Health Department serves a county of approximately 60,000 people. Its major program areas include the WIC program, a cancer prevention program as part of health promotion and disease prevention, services for children with special health care needs through an Early Intervention (EI) program, as well as home care services, which have recently shifted to emphasize home visiting health promotion and prevention and away from sickness care, which is provided by hospital home health services. The department also has environmental health and public health nursing units.

Sue Feldby is the nutrition manager of a unit that has three major program areas and a staff of five people—three community nutrition professionals and two nutrition assistants. The program areas are:

- WIC program serving 2,200 women, infants, and children
- Community-based health promotion disease prevention activities
- Maternal and child health

The nutrition unit also serves as an informal information and referral center for nutrition questions and needs from citizens and service providers in the community. Periodic TV interviews with Sue and other nutrition staff keep the department and its nutrition services in the limelight. The nutrition unit is known for its innovative response to emerging problems; but with tight resources and sinking morale the nutrition manager is cautiously reviewing current operations and plans for the future.

WIC

The River Valley Health Department has had a WIC program since 1982. WIC has consistently been reaching its assigned caseload of 2,200 except for February, when it dropped off because of inclement weather. In the past year, WIC staff have noted increasing numbers of Laotian WIC applicants due to emigration into the area.

Monthly summary reports generated from WIC certification records show 320 individuals were certified for WIC participation in the previous month. Following is the distribution of nutrition risk factors identified during the nutrition assessment for certification:

Overweight	32	percent
Underweight	5	percent
Anemia	18	percent
Inadequate diet	41	percent
Other	4	percent

In addition, ninety-two high-risk nutrition contacts for education and counseling were completed and

364 participants received a secondary nutrition education contact during the month. These numbers are down 15 and 18 percent, respectively, from the previous month.

WIC does a quarterly client satisfaction survey. The last survey had some surprising results. Some respondents complained about the noise of the nutrition education videos being shown in the waiting room, others said they and their children enjoyed the videos and WIC should have more. On the survey, WIC participants were asked if they like the "walk-by" nutrition education exhibits and the food demos at the WIC clinics. Only a few participants were aware of them.

WIC and Family Nutrition Program staff spend a lot of time preparing "walk-by" nutrition education exhibits, which can easily be set up on a table in the waiting area. Some staff think few WIC participants pay attention to the exhibits unless food is given. Then the interest is in getting the food not the nutrition message.

Maternal and Child Health

The health department sponsors a home visitor program, which provides support to high-risk pregnant women and to families with special needs children (they have handicapping conditions or developmental delays) as part of the EI program. Thirty-five special needs children are being followed by the program, five of whom have complex nutrition needs.

All special needs children should have a nutrition assessment according to the program guidelines; however, nutrition staff have not had time to see all the children. After nurses or other EI staff people see a child with a nutrition problem, they discuss the problem with nutrition staff if someone is available, otherwise they call the dietitian at the local hospital, who unfortunately has little expertise in nutrition for children with special needs.

A recent quality assurance review of the EI program revealed an unacceptable rate of nutrition assessment and follow-up, and identified three children with significant unmet nutrition needs—one overweight spina bifida child and two children on complex tube feeding (one because of cleft lip and palette reconstruction and the other because of a metabolic problem).

Breast-feeding Task Force

Sue sits on the local Breast-feeding Task Force, which is developing plans to initiate a major breast-feeding community awareness campaign. The task force is leaning toward a media campaign, but a decision has not been made.

Also represented on the task force are both local hospitals, a lactation consultant, mothers' groups, business leaders, physicians, and the River Valley Nutrition Coalition.

Both hospitals report breast-feeding rates at discharge at 45 percent. Sue knows this is very low compared to state and national objectives. Based on information from the WIC program, Sue is also aware that among low-income women, less than half of the women who start breast-feeding continue to six months.

Health Promotion Disease Prevention

As part of the cancer prevention grant, the health department wants to use the WIC clinics to reach women for education about breast self-exam and cervical cancer screening. The WIC staff say there is too much going on in WIC now with an immunization program, the Family Nutrition Program operated by Cooperative Extension, and the required cross referrals to the Food Stamp Program.

The Snack Smart project was launched nine months ago. It is a small project funded by the Cancer Society with an objective of changing the snacking behaviors of workers. The intervention involves replacement of some traditional vending food items with fresh fruits and vegetables and juices and low-fat versions of some chips and cookies. Vending changes have been implemented in all county government buildings.

So far the focus has been on getting vending machines properly stocked. Little attention has been paid to evaluation. The Cancer Society is expecting a report of outcomes by the end of the year. In addition, the nutrition staff need to determine if the passive intervention (just making the new choices available) is effective or if a nutrition education message should be added. The vending company has been providing Sue weekly sales reports of all food and beverage items sold in the vending machines of each government building.

TODAY'S EVENTS

- In a hallway conversation this morning, the health director (the administrator of the health department) asked Sue if she thought it would be more cost effective for nutrition staff to do the assessments and follow-up of the children in the Early Intervention program themselves or if nurses and other staff should be trained to do it. With the latter approach, nutritionists would serve as consultants to the EI team members rather than spend large amounts of time providing direct service. Approximately fifteen children a month would need nutrition assessment and intervention. The health director emphasized that the problem of nutrition services in the EI program should receive priority attention.

- The health department is beginning preparation of its annual report. The first draft is due Friday. This report demonstrates the accountability of the health department to the County Board of Commissioners, the local citizens, the state public health agency, funders, and other interested stakeholders. It also serves as a status report and helps inform decisions about program directions and priorities for future years. For the annual report Sue must summarize nutrition program activities and outcomes for the past year.

- One of the nutrition staff members is part of the agency's CQI committee. He tells Sue that the committee successfully completed its project with the environmental health unit and is now available to begin a new performance improvement project. Sue knows the health director has a strong commitment to quality and she expects all health department employees to be attuned to opportunities to be responsive to the needs of the community, but to save dollars. Fortunately, performance improvement efforts have good support throughout the organization.

- Sue is expecting the monthly budget reports for the nutrition unit on Thursday. However, based on a call from the financial officer this morning, Sue already knows she exceeded her personnel budget last month. She plans to review the past month's scheduling to see where the discrepancy is. She wonders if the use of two part-time staff to cover one nutritionist's maternity leave could be a problem. Since this is the ninth month of the fiscal year, she can take corrective action to get things back in line before the end of the year; or she may have to reallocate resources, but this would require careful justification.

- At noon, Sue has lunch with a local leader of the Laotian community. According to Mr. Lo, the community is concerned about increasing rates of diabetes, obesity, and hypertension. These problems are evident in elders who came from Laos over fifteen years ago. They are less assimilated than the younger generation and they experience many barriers to using the medical system. Mr. Lo says the younger generation is very interested in knowing about ways to prevent these problems and ways to help their parents and grandparents deal with these health problems, which they don't understand because the diseases were not common in Laos.

- There is a WIC staff meeting this afternoon. The agenda has to do with nutrition education activities. WIC staff have been trying group classes rather than less efficient individual contacts. There is a question about the appropriateness of classes for high-risk clients. When clients have serious nutrition problems it is all the more important that WIC services have a positive impact on the identified problem area. How can the staff determine what education strategies are really effective?

Sue would like to address the question of what strategies are most effective for high-risk as well as regular WIC participants, because it has major implications for staffing and budgeting for next year. The WIC Nutrition Education plan is due in three months. Nutrition education strategies and procedures for the coming year will be outlined in that plan.

QUESTIONS

1. What evaluation issues do the community nutrition professionals at the River Valley Health Department face?
2. What evaluation challenges must Sue Feldby address today? this week? this month? in the future?
3. At what stage in the life span of programs are the various nutrition programs? What does that mean for the focus of evaluation efforts?
4. What evaluation systems are in place? Where are better systems of data collection and documentation needed?
5. How could Sue address the health director's question about the cost effectiveness of nutrition services for the EI program?
6. How should she address the financial officer's concern about the personnel budget?
7. What advice should Sue give the WIC staff who are trying to enhance the acceptance and effectiveness of nutrition education efforts?
8. What other program issues could be informed and aided by solid information from an evaluation?
9. Select one of the issues raised by the case and plan an evaluation. State the purpose of the evaluation. Identify the types of data needed. What performance standards would you use as criteria for success? How and when would you get information? Who would you involve in planning and conducting the evaluation? What kind of report(s) would you plan to generate from the evaluation? To whom would the report(s) be directed?

CHAPTER SIXTEEN

MANAGING MONEY
BUDGETING AND GRANT WRITING

*Vision is important; but it takes resources
to make the dream reality.*
—PATRICIA L. SPLETT

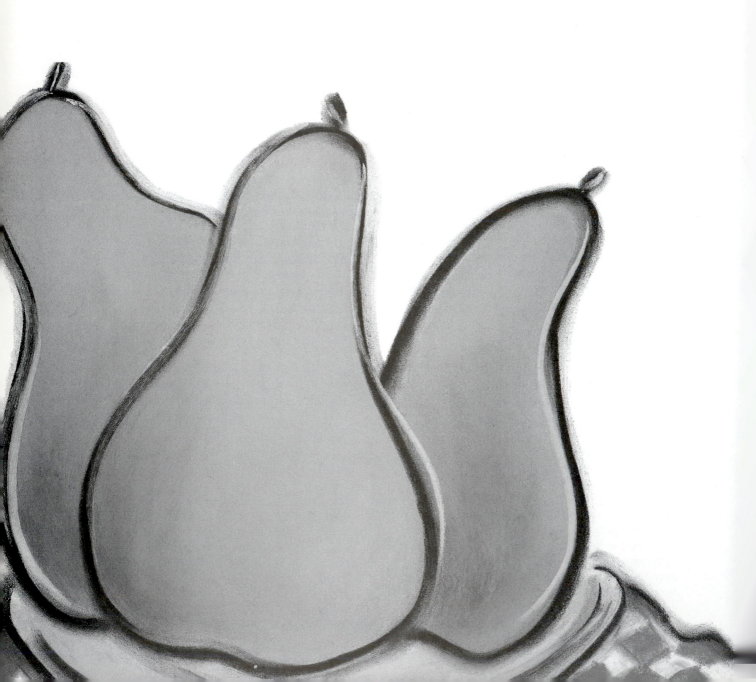

Core Concepts

The community nutrition professional must be skilled in securing and managing resources to operate nutrition programs and services. Budgeting is used to predict future operating expenditures and revenue needs. Financial management involves ongoing monitoring of resource allocation and utilization against plans and accomplishments and guides adjustments to assure efficient and responsible use of resources. Proposal writing and grantsmanship are important skills for securing the financial resources necessary to develop, operate, and evaluate nutrition programs and initiatives. The community nutrition professional must be an entrepreneur actively seeking funds from a variety of sources to assure essential nutrition services are available in the community.

Objectives

When you finish chapter sixteen, you should be able to:

~ Discuss the roles of community nutrition professionals in budgeting, financial management, and proposal writing.

~ Describe the budgeting process and the three parts of a budget document.

~ Calculate the total and unit cost for a nutrition program or activity.

~ Outline the overall process of proposal writing.

~ Identify several sources of funding for community nutrition programs.

~ Prepare a proposal for a nutrition project including all the component parts of a proposal.

Key Words

Word	Page Mentioned
Budgeting	483
Budgeting process	483
Revenue	483
Expenditures	483
Operating budget	483
Personnel budgets	483
Capital budgets	483
Conventional budgeting	484
Zero-based budgeting	484
Budget statement	485
Narrative	485
Line item expense categories	485
Statistics	485
Cost analysis	488
Flexible budgeting	490
Budget	491
Grants	493
Contracts	493
Formula grants	494
Block grants	495
Grantsmanship	496
Grantors	496
Grantees	496
Proposal	496
RFP	497
RFA	497

Money is not an evil; it is a necessary commodity used to purchase materials and supplies and compensate people who work to produce the products and services other people need and want. Nutrition goals and objectives become a reality only when sufficient resources are allocated to programs and when those resources are responsibly managed.

The first challenge is getting sufficient resources. That means community nutrition professionals must understand the grant or proposal writing process. But even be-

fore that, the community nutrition professional must be able to accurately estimate resource requirements. Costing and budgeting are used to make these estimates. Once the money or other resources are in hand, the community nutrition professional monitors and manages the resources to assure they are used efficiently. These are the processes of financial management.

This chapter follows the chapters on planning, implementation, and evaluation as a keystone that makes effective programs possible (see figure 16.1). Knowledge and

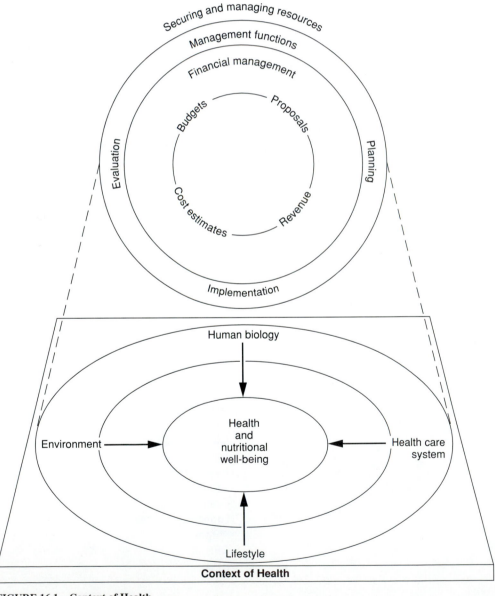

FIGURE 16.1   Context of Health
Managing money through budgets and grants.

skills related to budgeting, financial management, and proposal writing are closely linked with planning, establishing, and operating quality programs that make a difference in the lives of people. Community nutrition professionals who can estimate needs and talk money can go far in building the nutrition programs that are integral to assuring health and well-being of all community members.

BUDGETING AND FINANCIAL MANAGEMENT OF NUTRITION PROGRAMS

Budgeting

Budgeting is the process through which resource needs are identified and allocation decisions are made. The **budgeting process** is used to plan an organization's or program's finances in terms of predictions of where the money will come from (**revenue**) and how the money will be spent (**expenditures**) to accomplish specific purposes. The budgeting process takes into account minimum versus ideal levels of planned expenditures balanced against estimated revenues. Budgeting goes hand in hand with program planning, implementation, and evaluation and is an important tool of management.[10]

The Budgeting Process

The budgeting process begins with accurate projections of resource needs (for personnel, supplies and equipment, facilities, travel, contractual services, and administrative overhead costs) and potential revenue sources to accomplish program objectives. This formulation stage usually begins several months prior to the actual fiscal year for the budget. It leads to the preparation of a formal budget document (described later), which is submitted for administrator or funder review. Discussion, negotiation, and compromise follow; and ultimately, the budget is approved.[16] The community nutrition professional needs to anticipate challenges and be prepared to defend the budget and participate in negotiation. See the suggestions in box 16.1 for approaches to be successful with budget negotiations. Following budget approval, this document is used to guide implementation and control of ongoing nutrition programs and services. For example, regular financial reports enable assessment of program activities against expenditure and revenue projections. In this way, the budget becomes a management tool for monitoring and evaluating program performance. Occasionally, due to changing circumstances, the budget may be revised during the fiscal year. To do so may require further negotiation and approval.

WINNING AT BUDGET NEGOTIATIONS

1. *Be prepared to defend the budget.* Have accurate cost figures and a detailed plan including justification of need, program and service objectives, cost of additional resources, and potential sources of funding.
2. *Secure support.* Communicate developing plans and secure the support of interested parties before budgets are submitted. Adjust plans to incorporate valuable suggestions of others. Sell committee members and decision makers on program ideas and resource needs before hand.
3. *Anticipate challenges.* Consider opposition to the plan and its costs. Be prepared to defend personnel positions, salary levels, new equipment, and other cost items.
4. *Link budget to organization mission.* Be persuasive in showing others how the programs will further the mission and goals of the organization. Bring documentation of previous productivity and accomplishments.
5. *Work for win-win.* Know ahead of time the minimum level of resources at which you can conduct a quality, effective program. Identify where resource sharing, adjustments, or cuts could be made to achieve mutual benefits with partners. Negotiate to retain your essential base while supporting goals of the organization and collaborators.

Types of Budgets

The most common budget is the **operating budget.** It includes personnel and supplies and equipment (nonpersonnel). An operating budget defines resource requirements for activities to be conducted in a specific time period, usually a year or a contractual period. Personnel budgets may be separate or part of the operating budget. **Personnel budgets** itemize staffing needs by position, full-time equivalents (FTEs), wage or salary rate, fringe benefits, coverage for vacation and sick leaves, and anticipated overtime.[16] Because personnel costs commonly consume the largest percentage of nutrition program funds, personnel budgets merit special care and detail. Supplies and equipment needs are also estimated for the coming budget period.

Capital budgets estimate expenditures for improvements in fixed assets (e.g., buildings) and sources of funds to finance them. Capital budgets outline planned capital expenditures for the long term (i.e., more than one budget year). Nutrition program budgeting is infrequently involved in capital budgeting. However, creative programming to achieve education and behavior change goals may require new or remodeled facilities that are specifically designed to meet special needs of nutrition programs (e.g., major remodeling or securing facilities for cooking demonstrations that meet state codes for public food preparation and service). Capital expenditures for new clinic locations may be required to achieve a goal of reaching isolated target audiences.

Conventional and Zero-Based Budgeting

There are two ways to approach budgeting for future years: make incremental adjustments to the previous year's budget (historical or conventional approach) or start with a clear slate (zero-based budgeting).[10]

The tendency to let historical patterns drive the budgeting process favors existing programs. In **conventional budgeting** the manager focuses on justifying additional funding. However, a historical approach where activities are supported at about the same level as the previous year's (with adjustments for inflation and salary raises) does not lead to efficient use of resources or to achievement of program goals and objectives unless direct attention is given to shifting needs and measures of productivity or effectiveness. With reliance on historical trends, it may be difficult to secure dollars for development and pilot testing of innovations in service delivery, and it may be even more difficult to get dollars for implementation of a completely new program.

Figure 16.2 demonstrates how funding levels change over the life span of a program or project. Initially, funds are needed for market research, development, and pilot testing of new program ideas. Following successful development, additional resources must usually be invested to gear up for full implementation, which could include

staff recruitment or training, specialized equipment such as computers, opening new sites, and securing supply inventories. Once the program is implemented, funding needs stabilize until such a time as the program becomes obsolete or low priority. Then the program should be dismantled with resources reallocated to other programs.

In **zero-based budgeting,** which is also called the planning-programming-budgeting system (PPBS), there is no assumption that future needs match those of the past.[4] Budgets are projected across the life of the project and the entire budget, not just increases, must be justified. Nutrition unit activities are broken down into program decision packages consisting of a set of activities for which specific costs and outcomes (benefits) can be outlined and the consequences considered if the decision package is not approved. The decision packages are then ranked in order of importance using cost and outcome (benefit) projections. Finally, available funds are allocated to decision packages based on relative rank. Lower-ranking decision packages may be dropped or only partially funded. Zero-based budgeting is closely aligned with cost-benefit analysis. The advantage of zero-based budgeting is that it stimulates regular assessment and questioning of existing programs along with consideration of the development of new ideas in light of priorities and emerging needs in the environment. The disadvantage is that it is time consuming and requires a lot of paperwork.

Budget Statement or Proposal

A budget is the formal statement of proposed expenditures and anticipated resources (revenues) for a specified future time period. The budget is the backbone of a comprehensive plan of operation for an organization and its programs and services. It expresses plans in quantitative terms. The budget communicates organizational and program goals and objectives for a forthcoming period

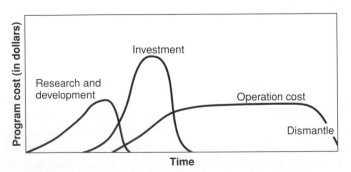

FIGURE 16.2   Costs Over the Life Span of a Program

and the allocation of resources to achieve those goals and objectives.[15]

Responsible budgeting implies the submission of a budget that accurately reflects resource requirements for accomplishing specific goals and objectives through nutrition programs and services. A carefully prepared formal **budget statement** or proposal helps reviewers understand resource requirements and thereby approve the allocation of adequate resources for development and ongoing operation of nutrition programs and services. The budget document not only projects dollars needed but it also must give an adequate description of what the program does, since some reviewers who approve budgets may not know.

Parts of a Budget

A budget consists of three parts: (1) a narrative section describing the program, its purpose (mission, goals, and objectives) and the services it provides, (2) the dollars needed to carry out the program, and (3) the statistics that will measure the outputs and outcomes of the program or services. A budget can describe resource needs for a single, small project, or it can present a package of services and programs that make up a complex nutrition department or unit. Box 16.2 illustrates a budget proposal for a small-scale nutrition project. Look for the three parts of a budget proposal on the budget example.

Budget proposals begin with a concise **narrative** that generally includes:

- The mission of the organization or sponsoring program
- Major program directions or strategies; target population expected to be served, including eligibility criteria and mandated and potential client numbers
- Goals and objectives for the budget period (including goals for downsizing, expansion, or reaching new target groups)
- Workload (personnel) expectations

In large nutrition units the narrative will identify the range of programs, projects, and services offered. The narrative establishes a clear rationale for the allocation of resources and communicates the plan for effective resource utilization. The budget narrative provides assurance that worthwhile activities will be delivered in a well-managed, responsible fashion.

The dollars section includes a line item summary of proposed expenditures by standard cost categories. Major cost categories (**line item expense categories**) and common subcategories with sample accounting codes are shown in Box 16.3. For ongoing programs, the estimated budget level and actual expenditures for the previous year, along with the current year's expenditures to date, are shown for comparison with next year's estimated amounts. The dollar section also shows how the line item amounts were estimated and alternatives were considered (e.g., cost of rental versus purchase), and gives an explanation of administrative overhead costs. This is called the cost "justification." Finally, the dollar section includes a complete listing of revenue sources and amounts anticipated.

The **statistics** section of a budget proposal defines the significant data that will be collected to manage and evaluate the program. These statistics (also called outputs, outcomes, or performance indicators) should be related to the objectives of the program or service and have a relationship to organizational and program goals. Examples include number of clients served, units of service delivered, and outcome indicators such as before and after rates of anemia or low-birthweight rates. This section should define realistic targets for output and outcomes since it becomes an important benchmark for assessing performance of the project or program.

How to Estimate Budget Needs

Resource needs to operate the program or project are estimated based on planned activities. Considerations, action steps, and timeline, described in chapter 14, provide the bases for estimating budget needs. The following steps, adapted from Swansburg,[16] are recommended as a way to develop sound estimates of resources needs. Steps 1 through 6 lead to estimates of personnel costs, step 7 addresses nonpersonnel expenses, and step 8 considers the possibility of capital expenses in future years. Accurate cost estimates and good planning develop a commonsense, defensible budget.

1. Determine performance levels based on activities to be completed and number of people to be served. (This should be the same as the statistics section of the budget proposal.) Performance levels are expressed in numeric terms. For example, certify 3,200 women, infants, and children for WIC; hold six one-day Healthy Mother-Healthy Baby events at separate locations in the community.

2. Forecast personnel needs to conduct activities using expected time per unit of service or activity. For example, 20 minutes per WIC certification × 3,200 × 2 times each year = 2,133 contact hours; add 20 hours

BOX 16.2

AGED TO PERFECTION: A COMMUNITY-BASED HEALTH PROMOTION PROGRAM FOR SENIORS
Budget Proposal

The mission of the Aged to Perfection program is to foster healthy aging among seniors in Vision City. The goal is to prevent physical decline and increase the years of healthful life of seniors (aged sixty-five and older) by collaborating with existing seniors' groups to offer services that encourage regular physical activity and positive food choices.

OUTCOME OBJECTIVES

Program participants will engage in moderate physical activity at least five days per week.

Program participants will reduce dietary fat intake to an average of 30 percent of calories.

Program participants will increase fruit and vegetable consumption to five servings per day.

In this pilot project, seniors' groups in one neighborhood of the community will be contacted and a core of eight seniors will be trained as peer leaders. In collaboration with peer leaders and seniors' groups, physical activity and nutrition activities will be organized in the neighborhood. A total of 180 seniors will be reached by the program in the first year.

SERVICES AND OUTPUTS

- By the third month, collaborating seniors groups and eight or more potential peer leaders will be identified in a neighborhood with a high concentration of elderly. Using a community development approach, the nutritionist will involve them in a planning process to identify and organize exercise and nutrition activities that use resources available in the community and are of interest to senior community members.
- By the end of six months, eight peer leaders will complete training.
- During the second six months, nutrition activities will be offered on a biweekly basis in the neighborhood, and one or more programs to foster physical activity will be operational in each neighborhood. Peer leaders will work jointly with project staff to arrange and offer the activities.

- Activity sign-in sheets will indicate an average participation rate of fifty per month.
- Community members over age sixty-five will be offered voluntary nutrition and fitness screening. We expect over 180 will take advantage of this service. Screening data will serve as a baseline for assessing impact of the pilot project on participants.
- An evaluation will be conducted to determine the level of satisfaction with the program, actual participation in scheduled activities, and self-initiated physical activity and food practice changes.

PROPOSED BUDGET AND JUSTIFICATION FOR TWELVE-MONTH PILOT OF AGED TO PERFECTION

Personnel

Nutritionist 0.25 FTE (responsible for community development, peer leader training, and community–based activities)	8,000
Secretary 0.10 FTE (responsible for scheduling activities, reserving meeting space, preparing education materials)	2,400
Fringe benefits at 25%	2,600
Education Materials	
nutrition/exercise booklets 240 at $6	1,440
screening questionnaires 180 at $1.25	225
exercise equipment	800
Travel	
Staff use of personal auto 30 miles per week at $0.29/mile	452
Total Direct Costs	**15,917**
Indirect Costs at 14% of direct costs	2,228
Budget Total	**$18,145**

---

of planning, add 1/2 day set up, and 1 day of supervision for each community event.

3. Add on staff time for other work related activities. For example, documentation and reporting (one hour per clinic day), planning time (four hours per month), staff meetings (two one-hour meetings per month), confer-

ences (one day per year per employee), in-service training (one and a half days per year per employee).

4. Add in supervisory and management activities.

5. Add in nonproductive hours for vacation, holidays, illness, and education leave for staff members. For example, two weeks vacation, eleven holidays, five

BOX 16.3

TYPICAL LINE ITEM EXPENSE CATEGORIES

PERSONNEL
110	Professional salaries
120	Technical salaries and wages
130	Hourly employees
	Personnel total

Fringe Benefits
171	Life insurance
172	Disability
173	Health insurance
180	Retirement
	Fringe benefits total

Personnel total

NONPERSONNEL
Office Supplies
210	Consumable supplies
220	Computer supplies
	Office supplies total

General Supplies and Services
311	Purchased education material
320	Printing services
331	Telephone—local service
332	Telephone—long distance
341	Postage
342	Shipping
	General supplies and services total

Equipment
410	Laboratory equipment
420	Computer hardware
	Equipment total

Travel
510	Local auto expense
520	Out-of-state transportation
530	Lodging
	Travel total

Contractual services
610	Professional services
620	Graphic design
	Contractual services total

Nonpersonnel total

INDIRECT COST
Administrative Overhead
710	Space rental
720	Insurance
730	Administrative services (e.g., planning, accounting, statistics)

Administrative overhead (indirect) total

Expense Total (personnel + nonpersonnel + indirect)

sick days for each full-time employee, and five weeks of education leave for one staff member.

6. Lay out preliminary staffing schedules to verify coverage of all activities and service areas. Based on calculations and schedule, identify the number and job classification of all full-time and part-time personnel needed. Use salary levels and fringe benefit rate to estimate personnel costs.[1] For an example see the personnel calculations in the budget of box 16.2.

7. Estimate cost of supplies and equipment to be purchased in the budget year. For example, office supplies and services at $120 per staff member, education materials at $15 per client served, one computer and monitor at $1,600, software update for six workstations at $200 each = $1,200.

8. Anticipate capital expenses for coming and future years. For example, construction of nutrition education center at $135,000.

Cost Accounting and Financial Management

Accounting is concerned with measuring financial resources and obligations and their changing levels. It follows set procedures that are standardized within an organization and are based on accepted accounting conventions.[15] Community nutrition professionals must be familiar with the following concepts to participate in financial matters in a responsible manner.

Cost Centers A cost center (sometimes called a responsibility center) is a defined area of accountability.[15,16] Costs and/or revenues are accounted and reported separately for each cost center. For example, at a state health department, the WIC accounts are maintained separate from the health promotion program, which is separate from the special demonstration grant for diabetes. Each cost center has a designated manager who is responsible for overseeing the operation as well as the expenditures and revenues of the center. Costs within the cost center are broken down into major cost categories and subcodes, which are standardized across the organization's cost accounting system. There are two types of cost centers—those that generate income by charging for services rendered and those that provide a function that is not tied directly to revenue.

Cost Categories The major cost categories, also called line items, that are common to most accounting systems are listed in box 16.3 with examples of subcodes under each cost category. The names and code numbers for cost categories are standardized within an organization.

Fixed, Variable, and Semivariable Costs   Some costs are constant regardless of the volume of activity, others increase as the number served or the intensity of service increases. Fixed costs such as facility, insurance, equipment, and the salary of the director are stable. Variable costs such as education materials and supplies are used in greater amounts as the size of the program or number of participants increases. Semivariable costs (also called step-variable costs by some authors) are constant up to a point, then another unit is needed.[3] For example, one nutritionist may be adequate for a case load of 200 to 300 people, but at the threshold of 300, another part-time or full-time nutritionist would be required. In this case, nutrition staffing is a step-variable cost.

Direct and Indirect Costs   Direct costs are those resources that are used at the front line of program operation, such as personnel, supplies, education materials, and equipment. Indirect costs are behind-the-scenes expenses necessary to maintain and administer a facility and its programs; sometimes these are referred to as administrative overhead. Examples of indirect costs are accounting services, computer assistance, insurance, rent, cleaning, maintenance, and security. A cost center tracks and controls direct costs as resources are expended. A rate for indirect overhead is usually calculated by administration and allocated to each cost center based on a formula (e.g., 20 percent of each cost center's direct costs).

Units of Service   Most programs and projects have a set way of counting the outputs or activity produced by the cost center. It might be number of individual encounters or visits, number enrolled, contacts with other organizations, classes held, and so forth. Service units are a measure of productivity, which is usually defined in program objectives. A performance budget closely monitors service units with expenditures. An average cost per unit of service (unit cost) can be calculated to determine the efficiency of the program or project over time.

Chart of Accounts   The director of a nutrition unit receives the chart of accounts monthly. This includes a table of expenses and revenues (budget report) for each

cost center, plus a summary report for the whole unit.[15] Monthly budget reports are important tools for managing performance and controlling expenditures.

Performance Reporting   Cost center managers track performance by examining the level of activity compared to objectives, actual line items and total costs compared to budgeted levels, and cost per unit of service on a regular (monthly or quarterly) basis.[16] Discrepancies signal the need for adjustments in program operations. Community nutrition professionals are accountable when they conscientiously monitor performance and identify discrepancies and make timely adjustments.

Costing Nutrition Services

Cost analysis is a procedure used to determine the total and unit costs of nutrition services.[14] Accurate cost information is necessary to plan and negotiate budgets, determine rates for fees and contracts, and to generate cost data for cost-effectiveness and cost-benefit analyses. Cost information is also used to relate resource consumption to outputs and outcomes for accountability purposes such as performance measurement. Cost analysis involves seven steps:

1. Specify the service to be costed and the reason for doing cost analysis.
2. Identify the number of units of service.
3. Define the activities involved in delivering the service.
4. Determine direct costs for personnel.
5. Determine other direct costs (nonpersonnel).
6. Determine indirect administrative overhead costs.
7. Total costs (personnel + nonpersonnel + indirect) and calculate unit cost.[14]

The steps of cost analysis are illustrated with an example in box 16.4. Cost analysis provides accurate estimates of the cost to conduct programs, projects, or services. Costing can be done prospectively to estimate future costs; and it can be done retrospectively to calculate the value of resources expended to provide specific activities in the past. Total and unit cost information is used to make decisions about future budget commitments and resource allocation, and to assess past performance. Note from the discussion at the end of box 16.4, how cost data is used to guide proposals and negotiations. Cost analysis provides solid estimates of costs, which informs planning and deliberations such as those faced by Acme Corporation and the health department in box 16.4.

BOX 16.4

COSTING A WORKSITE NUTRITION CONSULTATION SERVICE

Step 1. The Acme Corporation wishes to contract with the health department to conduct an employee weight management and strength training program called Healthy Weighs. Trained staff from the health department (a nutritionist with experience in weight management programs and a health educator with expertise in physical activity and weight training) will lead a series of twelve weekly group sessions plus provide at least one individualized nutrition consult to each participant. The core program to be used in the session is based on a commercially available program. The purpose of cost analysis is to determine the full cost of conducting the program so a contract can be negotiated with Acme.

Step 2. Based on a survey of employee interest, the health promotion director at Acme estimates that forty employees will enroll in the class. Because of the large number interested and different employee work schedules, the class will be offered in two groups—one meeting in the early morning on Wednesdays and the other meeting on Fridays at noon.

Step 3. The following activities are involved in delivering the program over a six-month period:
- Advertising and recruitment
- Setting up and equipping a weight lifting room
- Preparation for and conducting twenty-four separate class sessions
- Scheduling individual consultation sessions
- Staffing individual consultation session
- Printing education materials
- Printing and distributing evaluation forms
- Analyzing evaluation data and writing a report

Step 4. Personnel needs and costs were estimated:

Nutritionist 124 hours at $23/hour =	$2,852
20 hours review of curriculum and class preparation	
2 hours per session x 24	
3/4 hour per consult x 40	
1/2 hour per follow up consult x 20	
2 days data analysis and report writing	
Health educator 78 hours at $22/hour =	$1,716
6 hours to plan and prepare weight room	
20 hours review of curriculum and class preparation	
2 hours per session x 24	
4 hours data analysis and reporting	
Secretary 26 hours at $15/hour =	$ 390
6 hours word processing	
2 hours photo copying and collating	
8 hours data entry from evaluation forms	
10 hours appointment scheduling	
Personnel salary	$4,958
Fringe benefit rate (27 percent of salary)	$1,339

Total personnel costs	**$6,297**

Step 5. Other direct costs (nonpersonnel) include:

Purchase of curriculum		
1 at $350	=	$350
Printing of advertising brochures		
1,200 at $.05	=	$60
Nutrition and exercise posters for weight room		
6 at $8.00	=	$48
Education packet for Healthy Weighs participants		
40 x $7.00	=	$280
Total other direct costs		**$738**

Step 6. Determine indirect administrative overhead costs. Administrative overhead is calculated using the organizations indirect cost rate of 23 percent of direct costs

$$(\$6297 + \$738) \times 0.23 = \$1,618$$

Total indirect costs	**$1,618**

Step 7. Calculate the total program cost and cost per participant

Total program cost	= **$8,653**

Unit cost or cost per participant

$$\frac{\$6,269}{40} = \$216.33$$

Based on this cost analysis the health department has information to use in determining what to propose to Acme. They could charge exactly $8,653 and break even. They could also choose to charge by the participant at a rate of $216 per person who signs up. There is a risk in this approach because most of the costs are fixed cost and will be incurred whether twenty-five or forty-four employees enroll. They could also propose a charge of $10,000 and retain a small excess of revenue over expenses to use for planning other programs.

If Acme wants the program but is willing to pay only $6,000, the health department has several options. It can withdraw from negotiations, do the program but subsidize it with resources from other internal sources, or seek external funding for the $2,653 gap. The health department and Acme could also agree to revise the program plan to make it less costly by reducing the number of sessions or cutting the individual consultation. The potential danger of this is that the effectiveness of the program could be undermined if essential components are cut.

Monitoring the Budget

Box 16.5 illustrates a year-to-date summary of expenditures. This type of report is produced monthly by the accounting department and is made available to cost center managers. They, or a member of their staff, examine the monthly report to verify the accuracy of postings for the recent month and review year-to-date levels to identify cost categories where expenditures exceed or are under projected levels. Reasons for overspending and underspending are investigated. This is called variance analysis.[10] Cost categories that exceed projected levels must be brought into control or additional funds must be identified to cover a possible deficit. When a pattern of underspending is expected, plans should be made to reallocate these funds to overspent cost categories, to some other purpose, or to save them for a future opportunity.

Organizations that use a performance reporting system routinely link budget performance with output statistics. This compares the dollars and statistics projec-

tions from the approved budget with actual performance during the fiscal year. The report illustrated in box 16.5 is a performance report.

Flexibility in managing the budget is advocated by Osborne and Gaebler in *Reinventing Government.*[12] When managers have the leeway to control expenditures and retain saved resources for other worthwhile opportunities, they tend to manage resources more efficiently and be more entrepreneurial in the way they approach their work.

In traditional government systems, all budgeted dollars must be spent by the end of the fiscal year or the money is lost. In addition, if all the budgeted dollars are not spent, the budget is cut the following year. This "spend it or lose it" approach does not reward creative use of resources and efficiency. It leads to spending sprees at the end of the fiscal year. **Flexible budgeting,** called an *expenditure control budget* or *operational budgeting,*[12] gives the program manager the responsibility to manage resources to accomplish goals and objectives while taking into account changing circumstances and new opportunities.

BOX 16.5

MONTHLY EXPENDITURE AND ACTIVITY REPORT

Cost Center: Nutrition Program   Reporting Period: March 1–31, (year) (month 3 of fiscal year)

	Actual		Budget	Performance	
	Current Month	Year to Date	Fiscal year total	Percentage of total, current month	Percentage of total, year to date
Expense Category					
Personnel					
Salaries (2.7 FTEs)	7,900	23,700	90,800	8.7	26.1
Fringe	2,054	6,162	23,608	8.7	26.1
Supplies					
Telephone	47	141	720	6.5	19.6
Equipment rental	150	450	2,400	6.3	18.8
Printing	228	228	500	45.6	45.6
Travel	0	0	1,200	0	0
Direct total	10,379	30,681	149,228	7.0	20.6
Indirect cost	1,868	5,523	26,861	7.0	20.6
Total	12,247	36,204	176,089	7.0	20.6

	Actual		Planned	Performance	
	Current month	Year to date	Fiscal year, total	Percentage of total, current month	Percentage of total, year to date
Service Statistics					
Client contacts	840	2379	10,000	8.4	23.8
Community events	4	11	44	9.0	25.0

Within a nutrition unit, some sources of funds may require close control and budgets are zeroed out at the end of the fiscal year. Other funding sources may allow carry over of unspent funds to met project-related expenses in future years. The community nutrition professional must be alert to the responsibility and accountability associated with monitoring the various reports and managing budgets.

The Budget as a Tool for Nutrition Program Management

An accurate budget is an essential ingredient in successful management. The **budget** is a primary tool for matching resources with identified program priorities. It provides a financial guide to program operations. Participation in the budgeting process leads to greater understanding of the political nature of resource allocation and the necessity of soundly justified program priorities and accurate estimates of resource needs. With involvement, nutrition program managers gain skill in accurately estimating and convincingly communicating resource needs. As an informed participant in the organization's budgeting process, the community nutrition professional has a better chance of securing sufficient support for the nutrition services necessary to meet priority needs. However, planning the budgeting isn't enough. Community nutrition professionals should expect to monitor cost center budgets and make adjustments to maximize the use of resources to accomplish important projects. Use box 16.6 to check your level of involvement in budgeting and financial matters.

Reallocation and Reengineering and Downsizing

The realities of shrinking government and health and welfare reform seriously constrain the funds available for public programs. In times of tight resources, the budgeting process frequently involves identifying programmatic areas that can be cut. A more optimistic approach is to view the process as a way to identify funds that can be reallocated for performance improvement or for new initiatives that more effectively and efficiently achieve overall goals and objectives. Although the immediate and long-term goal may be to reduce costs, quality must not be sacrificed. Assurance must be given that changes will not compromise the quality of care, as is currently defined by professional practice and is perceived by clients; also, effectiveness in terms of achieving program outcomes must not be compromised. Sometime this is called "rightsizing."

When new initiatives or ideas for change are proposed, sources for additional resource requirements must be identified. Very often resources must be freed up from within the existing nutrition unit budget to fund new initiatives. Funds could also be from internal reallocation from other programs or departments; increased funding from state and federal contracts and grants; or new outside funding from government agencies, foundations, or corporations. Raising money through external sources of funding is addressed in the grantsmanship section of this chapter.

Funds for new projects or initiatives must be justified in terms of the necessity and benefits of instituting the proposed changes. A proposal should include descriptions of current performance based on evaluation criteria, specific plans for change along with the costs and benefits of the change, and methods to be used to document and assess the results of the change that are specific, quantifiable, and valid.

Major initiatives for change, whether performance or quality improvement projects, program expansion, or the more difficult change of program reduction, require well-thought-out and soundly justified plans. The criteria outlined in box 16.7 should be applied in all situations of major change. When these criteria are met, the community nutrition professional is prepared for the planning, proposing, advocating, negotiating, and compromising that will undoubtedly follow.

These criteria are also guidelines for cutting programs in times of budget cuts and reallocation, organizational reengineering or restructuring, and labor force reductions. Prioritization and decision making, as discussed in chapter 13, are especially relevant to making difficult decisions about what to cut and how. Data from performance indicators and evaluation studies help the nutrition program manager identify the most productive and effective programmatic areas and the highest-performing employees.

Responsible financial management means concentrating resources available where the greatest potential for results exists. The nutrition program manager must be prepared to tackle some difficult challenges in allocating scarce resources to nutrition programs and activities that meet the needs of the community.

Budgeting as a Political Process

Budgeting is not merely estimating, allocating, accounting, and reallocating; it is also a political process. Budgets can be viewed as an instrument of policy in that allocation of resources is the ultimate expression of

BOX 16.6

RATE YOUR FINANCIAL CONTROL

Instructions: Rate your financial control by circling the way your current organization is structured.

	Lowest level of control			Highest level of control
Budget preparation	Administration informs programs as to allocation for future year.	Administration requests from your supervisor expected future expenditures for coming year.	Administration requests your presentation of report to define what money is needed for the coming year.	Administration requests budget proposal with various levels of budgets, contingent costs, and various objectives and levels of service. Justification for each budget level is required according to community need.
Decision of budget allocation	Administration has complete control of funds.	Administration considers your boss's request for needed funds.	Administration considers your request for needed funds and may discuss your justification.	Administration evaluates demonstrated community need and your budget proposal, negotiates your level of budget with you.
Monitoring	Administration notifies program when it is overspending.	Administration provides fiscal reports twice or quarterly to program manager.	Administration provides monthly reports of revenue and expenditure for each cost center.	Administration requires program manager to monitor fiscal reports on a monthly basis and compare them to projected levels. Program manager can shift services to meet fiscal constraints.
Level of reporting	No program-specific data provided.	Program-specific data provided on a yearly or six month basis.	Program-specific data is hand monitored to assure meeting budget levels.	Program-specific data is inputted into a program-specific MIS on a monthly basis and compared to projected levels.
Flexibility	Shifting of resources and changing service delivery is not allowed. Development of new programs and risk-taking is not encouraged.	Shifting of resources is allowed as long as total costs to organization do not increase. Development of new programs are encouraged as long as new costs are not incurred.	Shifting of resources and development of new programs are encouraged. However, organization has some difficulty dealing with fiscal changes necessary for implementation.	Shifting of resources and development of new programs is encouraged as long as new resources are identified along with community need. Fiscal procedures are varied to accommodate new revenue and expenditures.

Source: Adapted from Bouchard C: *Financial management II,* University of Minnesota, 1991, ISP Executive Study Programs.

priorities. Program and service activities and outcomes, and accomplishment of goals and objectives should follow the allocation of resources. Political pressures influence the determination of priorities, resource allocation, and the budget approval process. Clearly, sound documentation of nutrition needs, along with good communication of needs and their potential solutions, is necessary to build political support for the allocation of dollars to nutrition programs and services. Building political support is particularly challenging for new initiatives and innovative program ideas that may compete for support,

not only with existing nutrition programs that are mandated or expected by various constituencies, but also with other nonnutrition priorities and emerging community and societal problems, such as violence.

Results from evaluations can be used to leverage political support. In times of scarce resources, which remains the case throughout the public as well as private sectors, cost-benefit and cost-effectiveness analyses can be used as tools to aid resource allocation decisions. Results of cost-benefit and cost-effectiveness studies carry a lot of weight in political decisions. (Refer to chapter 15 for details on evaluation including economic analysis.)

BOX 16.7

CRITERIA FOR REALLOCATION AND RESTRUCTURING

1. All initiatives must be central to the mission and goals of the organization and program. In community health and human service programs, this means that the possible impact of the change on the health and nutritional well-being of the community must be considered.
2. Essential programs and services must continue to be appropriate, acceptable, and accessible to the target population.
3. The needs of employees for job security, personal and professional development, reassignment, and retraining if necessary, must be included in the plan.
4. Costs and benefits of the plan in the immediate and future budget years must be estimated as carefully as possible. Financial implications of staff or service reductions (or expansions) must be calculated. Freed (or required) monetary or personnel resources must be clearly identified. In expansion projects, be sure all internal resources are used at maximum efficiency. Show internal reallocation of resources to indicate serious commitment to balance efficiency aims with program expansion.
5. Develop a flexible plan with actual or projected data as supportive evidence for the change. Identify evaluation procedures to be used to assess the implementation of the plan.
6. Good communication is essential throughout the process. Administration should be involved early in the process of formulating changes. Regular informational and problem-solving sessions must be held with staff, as well as collaborators and affected clients and constituents.

SOURCES OF FUNDS FOR NUTRITION PROGRAMS AND SERVICES: REVENUE

After an understanding of budgeting and program planning, the next phase is to identify sources of funds. Financing nutrition programs and services involves creatively obtaining and using public, private, and nonprofit funding sources. This includes **grants, contracts,** payment for services and products, and third-party reimbursement. Box 16.8 defines these types of revenue.

Community nutrition professionals can build a solid foundation for nutrition programs by marshaling financial support from several sources. A range of funding sources provides assurance of ongoing existence in spite of shifting political winds, changing funding priorities, and the unpredictable changes of the economy.

BOX 16.8

Grant: any form of sponsorship that usually includes a sum of money that is given to an individual or organization that has originated an idea.

Contract: any form of sponsorship that usually includes a sum of money *and* contains the work requirements specified by the funding agency.

Third-party reimbursement: Anyone paying for care who is not the patient (the first party) or the caregiver (the second party). It includes public and private insurance providers such as Medicaid, Medicare, and most commercial health insurance companies. Generally, the patient (or employer) pays a premium to the third-party payer, and the third-party payer then pays the bills—or a percentage of the bills—incurred by the patient.

Payment for services or products: Direct expenses paid by an individual or organization.

Box 16.9 gives examples of sources used by community nutrition professionals to seek funding for various types of programs.

The types and sources of funding for a program depend on financial management and project goals. Single-source funding ties the program to a defined set of regulations and a narrow target audience. On the other hand, multiple funding sources enable development of programs for a broader range of the population and allow for greater flexibility in responding to needs as they emerge. A drawback of multiple-source funding is the increased demands for proposal writing, record keeping to account for funds, and reporting to funding sources. This, however, is offset by the enhanced capacity to offer innovative and effective programming. Box 16.10 illustrates the funding sources used by a health department nutrition unit serving a metropolitan city.

Government Funds

Governmental agencies provide the largest percent of support for research, education, health, and social welfare programs. Within the United States government, there are three types of grants: categorical, block, and general revenue sharing.[11] Categorical grants are distributed for specific purposes or a specific project topic that the government is concerned about; and the amount of money distributed can be based on a specific formula. Project grants provide funding for fixed or known

periods and are for specific projects or the delivery of specific services or products (e.g., training grants and demonstration projects).

Formula grants refers to funds that are allocated according to a set of criteria (i.e., formula) prescribed by law or administrative regulation and for activities of a continuing nature not confined to a specific project. Formula grants allow some flexibility in use of the

---

BOX 16.9

SOURCES USED BY COMMUNITY NUTRITION PROFESSIONALS

- Federal government
- Private foundations
- Professional organizations
- Drug companies and private industry
- Food companies
- Local civic organizations
- Voluntary health agencies
- Combined nonprofit organizations (e.g., the United Way)
- Voluntary nonprofit religious organizations
- Sale of a product or service
- Third-party payor (i.e., insurance, Medicaid)

BOX 16.10

MULTIPLE SOURCES OF FUNDING SUPPORT THE ACTIVITIES OF A NUTRITION UNIT IN A METROPOLITAN HEALTH DEPARTMENT

GOVERNMENT FUNDS

USDA annual contract for WIC program

MCH Block Grant to county for breast-feeding support program

Community Services Block Grant for project with families in transitional housing

County funds for 0.5 FTE nutritionist for home health

Local school district payment for nutrition classes in community education program

FOUNDATIONS

McKnight Foundation three-year grant for homeless project

American Heart Association grant for primary prevention program with school children

American Cancer Institute grant for media campaign related to fruit and vegetables

BUSINESS AND CORPORATIONS

Corporate loan of an executive for assistance with market research

Local business prints monthly newsletters

Food company donation of food supplies for cooking classes in housing project

CHARGES AND FEE FOR SERVICES

Sales of nutrition education materials

Charges for individual nutrition consults

IN-KIND CONTRIBUTIONS

University-coordinated program with six dietetics students per year

funds as long as they are applied to the overall purposes for which they were appropriated. Major federal categorical health programs have been "blocked" into five health **block grants:** Maternal and Child Health, Primary Care, Social Services, Community Services, and Preventive Health and Health Services. Dollars are awarded to states based on a formula.

The most frequently used sources for funding state and local nutrition programs are WIC, the federal block grants to states, state revenues, and internally allocated funds. Increasingly, local public health agencies are seeking reimbursement of personal health services through Medicaid, private insurers, and managed care organizations. Some health departments are preferred providers within managed care systems.

The Maternal and Child Health (MCH) Block Grant pays for some state and local nutritionist positions including several nutritionists who work in programs serving children with special health care needs. The Primary Care Block Grant provides full or partial funding for some nutritionist positions in community health and migrant health centers. The Preventive Health and Health Services Block Grant funds nutritionist positions as part of health promotion programs. Many states have programs that focus on cardiovascular risk reduction, diabetes control, or cancer prevention; community nutrition professionals are employed in these programs. Federal discretionary grants, particularly from agencies of the U.S. Departments of Health and Human Services (DHHS), Agriculture (USDA), and Education (DOE) can be used for nutrition programs.

Other funding opportunities exist for community nutritionist professionals involved in programs supported by the Community Services Block Grant, which funds community food and nutrition programs directed to emergency feeding and commodity distribution programs. Often these programs are operated at the local level through community action agencies rather than health departments.

WIC is the major funder of nutritionist positions in state and local health departments. In fact, WIC funds make up the largest revenue source for most state health departments. The largest portion of funds, however, goes directly to pay for WIC foods.

Several positions in state departments of education are funded by the USDA Child Nutrition Program to oversee and operate the National School Lunch, School Breakfast, Child and Adult Care Food, Special Milk, and Summer Food Service Programs. Opportunities exist for state and local nutritionists to collaborate with personnel in these programs as they attempt to reach the Healthy People 2000 Objectives of bringing these food programs in alignment with the Dietary Guidelines.

Another major funder of nutrition programs by the federal government is the Administration on Aging's Nutrition Program for Older Americans. Congregate dining and home-delivered meals programs are important access sites for reaching the elderly population.

Nutrition counseling of low-income women in childbearing years can be provided through the Title X Family Planning Program. Nutrition counseling of the elderly is reimbursable through Medicare Part B if provided under the supervision of the physician. Nutrition services can also be funded within home health agencies as a part of the agencies' administrative costs.

The recent emphasis on early identification of children with special needs increases opportunities for funding dietitian or nutritionist positions or reimbursement of services provided. Contractual services (payment for a defined scope of work) may be secured through the Early Intervention Program (zero to three years) of DOE or the Head Start Program of DHHS. Reimbursement for nutrition screening, assessment, and counseling of low-income children up to age 21 is available through Medicaid, especially within the Early and Periodic Screening, Diagnosis, and Treatment (EPSDT) program.

General revenue-sharing grants are federal programs that provide federal assistance to states and localities for broad purposes and the grantee has great discretion in the use of funds. General tax revenues in many states and local communities fund nutrition programs or nutritionist positions. The state of New York, for example, has funded a large program to reduce hunger, and Montana has passed legislation enabling support for nutrition initiatives. Other state and local health agencies make internal decisions to allocate a portion of their state or local funding to dietitian or nutritionist positions or activities.

Foundation Funding

Innovative programs designed to meet important needs in the community or needs experienced by a special segment of the population could be proposed to private foundations. A foundation is a nonprofit, nongovernmental organization with a principal fund or endowment of its own that aids charitable, educational, religious, or other activities serving the public good.[5] Foundations represent a flexible source of funding. The essential requirement is a good idea and a well-written proposal. Similar to all funding sources, the competition is stiff. Credibility in the community and a good track record with previous nutrition programs increase the chances of securing foundation grants.

Health and Civic Organization Funding

Another source of small grants for special projects or special equipment needs are voluntary health organizations such as state affiliates of the American Heart Association or the March of Dimes Birth Defects Foundation and civic organizations and clubs. Local civic organizations routinely support activities that benefit the community. They may be pleased to be asked to support or become involved in nutrition-related activities.

Funding from Corporations

Corporations can provide donations up to 5 percent of pretax earnings toward projects at their discretion. This type of giving provides valuable public services—usually in communities where the corporation operates. It helps maintain a positive public image, and often supports special projects related to the corporations interests. Corporations may claim a tax deduction for the value of materials and equipment donated to tax-exempt 501(c)(3) organizations. Examples of items that are donated include chairs; desks; tables; computer hardware, software, and paper; office supplies; typewriters; bookshelves; and file cabinets. Corporations and businesses also donate *in-kind* gifts including services such as photography and graphic keylining, or donated products such as McDonald's providing free food or beverages.

Another avenue is to sponsor special activities through a corporation's operating budget. To do this community nutrition professionals must outline program or project benefits as they relate to the short- or long-range goals of the corporation or its executives.

Many large corporations give grants from their company-sponsored foundation to nonprofit organizations (which can include other foundations).

A community nutrition professional can seek financial support for a complete project or a single aspect of a project. For example, a drug company might be willing to cover the cost of printing a newsletter, and an-

other company who is upgrading their computer technology may be willing to donate their used computers to the nutrition project.

Contractual services paid to community nutrition professionals by individuals, businesses, or corporations offer the greatest opportunity for creative planning and negotiation for support of nutrition programs. Packaged programs may be offered to businesses and corporations as part of workplace health promotion activities. They often include employee screening, counseling, and education, as well as cafeteria programs designed to alter the type of food available to employees.

Other programs such as weight-control programs or heart-healthy cooking classes may be offered to members of the community for a fee.

GRANTSMANSHIP

The essential ingredients for securing any source of financial support are a good plan for nutrition programs and services, knowledge about what works, and a commitment to serve the client with high-quality services designed to meet their needs. Most potential grantors (whether in government agencies or the private sector) and individual contributors can recognize these ingredients. They have a review and approval process in place to assure that their limited funds go to organizations and programs where the resources will have the greatest payoff in terms of a positive impact on important community health problems.

Grantsmanship is the art and skill of being able to organize information (your organization's capabilities, experience, and capacity to implement a nutrition project offering benefits to the community), use knowledge and experience to locate potential resources, and communicate well with others to obtain a grant. "It involves lots of hard work, a 'state of readiness,' and sometimes trial and error prior to a successful outcome."[7] If done well, **grantors** (agency providing grant funds, such as government, foundations, businesses, corporations, or nonprofit organizations) award money to **grantees** (an individual or organization). This collaboration assures successful outcomes to all—the community, the grantor, *and* the grantee.

The primary tool used to communicate a funding request is a written **proposal.** Proposal writing requires a sound idea, organizational skills, and time to be clear, concise, and convincing. A written proposal may only take a half day and be a two-page letter to a civic group asking for participation in a health fair. Alternatively, it may be a forty-page proposal to the National Institutes for Health for a large community intervention project and take a year to write. Whatever the time allotment, writing proposals to submit to a government agency or organization offers a dynamic opportunity to collaborate and promote health in a community.

Grant and contract opportunities are announced as either request for proposals (**RFP**) or request for applications (**RFA**). They include the funding purpose; time schedule for submission of proposal, special provisions to be included, criteria used to evaluate proposals, who is eligible, special forms or procedures to be followed; and the address where the proposal should be sent. An RFA has broader goals and gives the applicant greater latitude in defining the project; whereas an RFP is very specific.

SEVEN PROCESS COMPONENTS TO DEVELOP AND IMPLEMENT GRANT PROPOSAL WRITING

Getting down to actually writing a proposal occurs within the context of a process that builds relationships, communicates ideas, and improves the program or project. This process must be organized in such a manner that it can manage a multitude of information and be accessible to direct your grant-seeking work—within your organization and with potential funders. This process has the seven components listed in box 16.11.

BOX 16.11

SEVEN STEPS TO THE PROCESS OF GRANTSMANSHIP

Step 1: Possess a creative idea and begin to inspire others.

Step 2: Communicate your great idea within your organization.

Step 3: Search for the match and initiate communication with funders.

Step 4: Develop, write, and "sell" the proposal.

Step 5: Get others to review the proposal.

Step 6: Submit the proposal on time and follow all the rules.

Step 7: Follow up with potential funders.

Step 1: Possess a Creative Idea and Begin to Inspire Others

A good proposal succeeds because there is a creative idea that addresses a community problem and potentially offers a cost-effective or cost-beneficial solution. Many funders also look for an able, committed, persevering and effective person behind the proposal.[13] Gitlin and Lyons offer seven major sources from which to formulate a great idea[7] (See box 16.12). Once an imaginative idea is developed around a nutritional problem area, the process moves on to the next step.

Step 2: Communicate Great Idea Within Your Organization

Communication of a great idea operates according to an internal set of organizational rules and an individual's own experience. For success, a community nutrition professional must begin by gaining support within his or her own organization. Communicating the importance and excitement of an idea that solves a nutritional problem involves many forms, including written reports, body gestures, speeches, personal contacts, and letters. Interaction with others develops the idea, builds the commitment of the organization, and helps create a viable plan for implemention.

Bauer refers to this internal assessment step as "capitalizing on your capabilities."[2] It is a process of taking inventory of what your needs are and what makes your organization *good* at what you do. One approach is to answer the following statement: "Our organization is uniquely suited to implement this project because _____." A more comprehensive approach is to review your organization's mission

BOX 16.12

MAJOR SOURCES OF PROPOSAL IDEAS

- Professional experience
- Interaction with others
- Societal trends
- Legislative initiatives
- Public documents
- Agency goals and priorities

statement and related structures to ensure that the proposed program supports this mission and can be managed effectively. This strengthens your understanding and capabilities and prepares you to match your project to the internal capabilities. The key is to know yourself and the interests and capabilities of your organization so that as you begin to share the idea outwardly it will be accurately represented to those outside of your organization. As a result of this step, persons within the organization will know their role and contributions toward the project. Trust and mutual understanding are developed when you are communicating well within your organization, and they are best developed when you know yourself and your organization. You will be able to identify the persons and procedures necessary to contact future funders.

Step 3: Search for the Match and Initiate Communication with Funders

To succeed with funding, you need to research potential funders and look for a "best fit." This part of the process should establish a clear match between what your project has to offer (i.e., goals, objectives, features, and outcomes) and what the potential funders are interested in supporting (i.e., their priorities and fields of interest and what the benefits are to them). This step is time-consuming but is critical to the success of being funded. Each potential grantor must be researched to identify their mission, past funding areas, and current interest areas. A match between your idea and a potential funder is found when the funder has a record of giving monies to or a recent interest in your type of activity. Geographic locations and submission dates must also be taken into consideration.

Several national collections or reference centers index and summarize foundation information. For example, the Foundation Center collects information on large foundations and makes it available at no or minimal cost. They publish *The Foundation Directory* and *Supplements.* Table 16.1 identifies written resources for locating government, foundation, and corporate grants. Table 16.2 identifies computer and electronic access to search for available grants. Many of these resources are available through the Foundation Center Library Services, which disseminate current information on foundation and corporate giving through approximately 210 cooperating libraries in all fifty states.

You will also want to determine if your organization holds a tax-exempt status so that donors can receive tax deductions for their contributions. Many organizations contribute only to 501(c)(3) organizations. To qualify, the organization or individual must meet the stipulations under section 501(c)(3) of the Internal Revenue Code of 1954.

Be prepared before making the first contact. Information to compare *before* initiating a contact is shown in figure 16.3. The burden of understanding your organization's capabilities and being able to discuss these intelligently with potential funding sources is the grantee's responsibility and is an important step in building partnerships and credibility.

The first contact may take the form of a letter of intent, a telephone call, or a visit. This first contact should include identifying your organization and a discussion on your organization's predetermined concern for a problem, summary of the project for how you plan to solve the problem and credentials (institutional and individual) of who will be accountable. Your initiative and preparedness builds a strong foundation in this step of the grantsmanship process.

If you have been given the opportunity to discuss your project in person or with a telephone call, then listen closely to the important concerns of the funding source. This will help you identify ways to adapt the project to fit the grantor's values and concerns so there will be an increased potential for a "perfect match." Grantors and grantees will need to view one another as partners in solving problems and satisfying needs.

Complete the telephone call or personal visit with the project officer or trustee by verifying with the potential funder that they support a program in this topic area and clarify the application deadline. Request an application packet, if necessary.

There is also the possibility that the changes a potential funder expects will reshape the project so that it will not meet your organization's purpose or that your organization does not qualify. *Do not apply to this funder.* It is better to stop the proposal-writing process for a particular project with a particular funder when you have determined your organization cannot qualify with regards to eligibility or adaptability. You should ask if the agency anticipates future funding in your project area and make a note of this on your screening worksheet (figure 16.3). Keep a separate worksheet on each potential funder and their defined priorities. In this way, you will organize important information for later reference, if needed.

TABLE 16.1

Resources for Locating Government, Foundation, and Corporate Grants

Name	Source	Location
Catalog of Federal Domestic Assistance (CFDA); 202–783–3238	A listing and description of federal programs and activities that provide assistance or benefits to the American public; gives information on grants, loans, scholarships, insurance and other financial assistance	Superintendent of Documents U.S. Government Printing Washington, DC 20402 or Government depository libraries
Annual Register of Grant Support Marquis Who's Who 4300 West 62nd, Suite 2, Indianapolis, IN 46206	Annually revised directory of grant support programs of government, foundations, corporations and other organizations	The Foundation Center cooperating library nearest you
Foundation Center Directory [Part 1] Directory Part 2, Supplement The Foundation Center 79 Fifth Avenue New York, NY 10003–3076 800–424–9836 Fax: 212–807–3677 http:. .fdncenter.org	The Foundation Center lists resources about the country's major and midsize foundations; entries are arranged by state and include financial data, program policies, names of donors, trustees, and administrators *The Directory, Part 2* provides information on foundations with annual grants totaling between $25,000 and $100,00 The *Supplement* provides updates	The Foundation Center cooperating library nearest you
Grant Guide Series Grants for Public Health and Diseases The Foundation Center 79 Fifth Avenue New York, NY 10003–3076	Covers grants $10,000 or more for specific medical descriptions, multipurpose health associations, and related health organizations to promote the prevention or treatment of specific disorders	The Foundation Center cooperating library nearest you
America's New Foundations The Taft Group 12300 Twinbrook Parkway, Suite 520 Rockville, MD 20852	Gives information on newly created philanthropies having $100,000 in grants paid; information provided includes foundation philosophy, financial summaries, and recent grants	The Foundation Center cooperating library nearest you
The Directory of Corporate and Foundation Givers The Taft Group 835 Penobscot Building Detroit, MI 48226 800–877–8283	Information on corporate and foundation funding sources. There are nine indexes by which to search; includes grant types, nonmonetary support types, grant recipients by state	The Foundation Center cooperating library nearest you
Corporate Giving Directory The Taft Group 835 Penobscot Building Detroit, MI 48226 800–877–8283	The Directory provides profiles of 1,000 largest company, foundation, and corporate direct giving program and includes gifts, cash, corporate sponsorships and volunteer programs; also described are the application process, and evaluation criteria	The Foundation Center cooperating library nearest you
State and Local Foundation Directories	Information on state and local foundations; includes smaller foundations	The Foundation Center cooperating library State government libraries

Source: The Foundation Center: *The Foundation grants index*, ed. 25, NY, 1997, The Foundation Center. Used with permission of The Foundation Center, 79 Fifth Avenue, New York, NY 10003–4230.

Step 4: Develop, Write, and "Sell" the Proposal

A written proposal is a systematic working plan that describes the importance of the project, what it will accomplish, and the funds needed. This plan should present state-of-the-art knowledge and indicate that you have the expertise and capability to implement the project.

Resources are available to guide organizations and individuals on how to write grant proposals in a manner that concisely describes a program or project and

TABLE 16.2

Electronic and Computer Resources for Locating Government and Foundation Grants

Name	Source	Location
The Sponsored Programs Information Network (SPIN) InfoEd 453 New Karner Road Albany, NY 12205 800–727–6427	A database of federal and private funding sources	University libraries Federal government depository libraries
GrantSearch CFDA Capital Publications 1101 King Street, Suite 444 Alexandria, VA 22314 800–847–7772	An electronic edition of the Catalog of Federal Domestic Assistance (CFDA)	The Foundation Center cooperating library nearest you
Federal Assistance Program Retrieval System (FAPRS) Domestic Assistance Catalog Staff General Services Administration 300 6th Street, SW Washington, DC 202–708–5126	A computerized guide to federal grants that includes all the information on federal programs found in CFDA; you can use your computer modem to link directly to the database	University libraries State and county offices Cooperative extension offices
Foundation Center Search, 1996 Version 2 The Foundation Center 79 Fifth Avenue New York, NY 10003–3076 800–478–4661 fcsearch.@fdncenter.org	Most comprehensive data files on grantmakers and awarded grants; grants awarded equal $10,000 or more; searches can be done using twenty-one key selection criteria and text searching; Combines all the Foundation Center's resources on a CD-ROM	The Foundation Center cooperating library nearest you
Federal Information Exchange *Federal Register* *GrantsNet* *NIH Contracts & Grants* *CRISP* (U.S. Public Health Service) (Information about grants awarded)	http://web.fie.com http://www.lib.purdue.edu/gpo http://www.os.dhhs.gov:80/progorg/grantsnet/index.html http://www.nih.gov/grants http://www.nsf.gov	

Source: The Foundation Center: *The Foundation grants index,* ed. 25, NY, 1997, The Foundation Center. Used with permission of The Foundation Center, 79 Fifth Avenue, New York, NY 10003–4230.

convinces a potential funding agency of your competency and uniqueness.[6,8,9,13,17] All proposals should have the following components outlined in Table 16.3. A more detailed discussion of how to write each component of the proposal is discussed later. Every proposal will be different and some parts of the proposal can be combined into one section. Overall, the proposal reflects your organization's ability to accomplish a plan of action for an important project.

A *"master"* proposal is drafted and then is modified to fit each potential funders criteria. Writing one proposal and sending it to many funders is *not* recom-

mended. Rather, each proposal must be written to address specific concerns or interests of the funder. For example, perhaps one organization can fund a specific component of the project, such as providing nutrition software for a nutrition screening project at a seniors' center. The budget section of the proposal would need to reflect this. It would also be important to ensure a clear, concise description about the computerized nutrition assessment in the methodology section. For another potential funder, this proposal may need to be changed due to the funder not providing monies for staff training (i.e., training of nutrition personnel regarding use of the

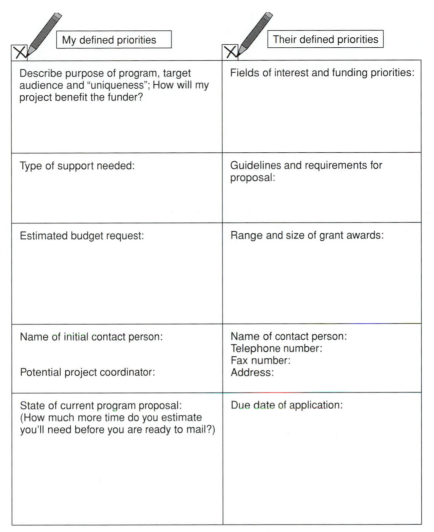

My defined priorities	Their defined priorities
Describe purpose of program, target audience and "uniqueness"; How will my project benefit the funder?	Fields of interest and funding priorities:
Type of support needed:	Guidelines and requirements for proposal:
Estimated budget request:	Range and size of grant awards:
Name of initial contact person: Potential project coordinator:	Name of contact person: Telephone number: Fax number: Address:
State of current program proposal: (How much more time do you estimate you'll need before you are ready to mail?)	Due date of application:

FIGURE 16.3   Worksheet for Screening Potential Funding Sources

nutrition software). It is always important to know the types of support and limitations of financial giving. Always "tailor-fit" the written proposal for each organization so that the grantor "feels" as if he or she is walking through the door of the potential project and can visualize and participate in the success.

Throughout the writing and drafting process of grantsmanship, improvements to your great idea and all aspects of communication should be optimized. Generous hours of presenting, writing, and networking are needed to build commitment toward the proposal. It is important to continue to network within your organization so that the best combination of ideas and resources are offered toward the project. Individuals working for

the applicant organization need to be cohesive and demonstrate enthusiastic support. Networking outside the organization and within the community also builds partnerships with potential consumers of the program and evaluates the best approaches for implementation. Finally, continuing to build support through editing, revising, and completion of the written proposal increases your potential for successful funding from the grantor. Marketing this proposal is based on building effective partnerships, communicating clear and concise ideas, and demonstrating creditability. Potential funding organizations notice enthusiasm toward the project and support the benefits of working within a community to promote positive outcomes.

TABLE 16.3
Components of a Grant Proposal

Component	Description	Length(depends on type of proposal)
Title	A name that captures interest and communicates the topic of the proposal	Not many words
Executive summary/abstract	A brief summary of the entire proposal	One paragraph to one page
Introduction	Establishes organization's credibility and record of accomplishment related to project area	One paragraph to two pages
Statement of need	Why this project is necessary and that the project can address the problem	One to four pages
Goal and objectives	The overall purpose and expected results in specific, measurable terms	One half to one page
Project description/methodology	The nuts and bolts of how the project will be implemented and managed	One to ten pages
Evaluation	Plans for process and outcome evaluation	One half to two pages
Budget and budget justification	Resource requirements to conduct the project; and budget justification, as necessary	One to three pages
Attachments	Information that can include references, credentials of project and primary staff, verification of 501(c)(3) status, and/or letters of support for the project	One to ten pages

Source: Adapted from Geever, JC, McNeils, P: *The Foundation Center's guide to proposal writing,* New York, 1993, The Foundation Center; Gitlan, L, Lyons, KJ: *Successful grantwriting: strategies for health and human service professionals,* New York, 1996, Springer Publishing; Kiritz, NH: *Program planning & proposal writing,* Los Angeles, 1980, The Grantsmanship Center.

Step 5: Get Others to Review the Proposal

Seek review of the proposal and feedback from others before you submit it to the potential funding organization. Use this feedback to clarify and refine the proposal. Bauer has provided excellent information regarding how to improve your proposal and increase chances of funding by implementing a "grants quality circle."[2] This type of confidential, peer review can improve the quality and succinctness of your written proposal. It is important to remember that the "mock" reviewers should be given only the amount of time that the time the actual proposal reviewers would spend.

Step 6: Submit the Proposal on Time and Follow All the Rules

It is important to follow the specific application procedures and deadlines that foundations and other potential grantor agencies provide. Final application procedures and deadlines for each government program are printed in the *Federal Register*. One criteria for moving your application from the "maybe" funded category to the "likely" funded category could just be that you completed the application process following all the directions. After submission, wait patiently for an answer. Figure 16.4 provides an ex-ample of how to track the funding status of various resources using hypothetical cases from Vision City and Aged to Perfection. This form can provide a summary of all the various sources used to fund a particular project.

Step 7: Follow Up with Potential Funders

Always follow up any type of funding notification with a thank you. If your idea is approved, make every effort to send a thank you and expect to communicate with the funder about payment procedures and any reporting requirements. Place the grantor's name(s) on any organizational newsletters or mailing lists. Finally, recognize the grantor's contributions in all publications and presentations.

If your proposal is not funded, also send a thank-you letter. State your appreciation for the time and effort that the staff spent on reviewing your proposal. Ask for suggestions on improving your proposal and reviewers comments, if available.

Government proposals are given the following responses: approved, deferred, or not recommended for further consideration. Those that are rated the latter should still consider reapplying in the future. For additional information about understanding the government review process, please see Gitlin and Lyons.[7]

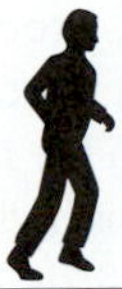

Proposed project title: Aged to perfection: A community-based health promotion program for seniors

Project goal: Prevent physical decline and increase the years of healthful life of seniors using collaborations with existing seniors groups.

Name of organization	Date appli-cation due	Budget item requested	Amount	Date of response	Yes	No	Budget item funded	Contact person Comments
Vision City Hospital	4/25	.1 FTE RD	$3060					Jan Smith, Director of Dietary; She has to meet w/hospital administrator on 5/1.
ABC Foundation	2/18	.5 FTE Project coordinator	$30,000	4/28		X		John Dean, Exec. Director; Unable to support grants to local campaigns to eliminate or control specific disease.
Vision City State Bank	3/29	Meeting place to provide the peer training	"in-kind" donation	4/15	X		O.K. as long as they do not interfere with board meetings the first Thursday of every month	Tucker Jackson, President
XYZ Foundation	3/1	Peer leader salaries	$8000					Exec. Director *On vacation

FIGURE 16.4   Example of How to Track Prospects and Success

PARTS OF A GRANT PROPOSAL

The components of a grant proposal are identified in table 16.3. All proposals should contain these components as this format provides for describing the project and assures a potential funder that your organization has thoroughly examined the project components and will be accountable for how their money will be spent. The length of the proposal is variable, but an overall concern is to use simple, informal, concise words that avoid jargon. For some foundations, a letter may *be* the proposal.[9]

The title needs to capture interest and identify the topic of the proposal. The executive summary/abstract is succinct, clear, and interesting and presents the essential points necessary to give the reviewers within a funding agency an overview of what is being proposed. This section, although placed first on the application, is always written last. Kiritz recommends that the summary should:[9]

- Identify the applicant and describe the applicant's credibility.
- State the reason for the grant request such as an issue, problem, or need to be met.
- Outline the objectives to be achieved through this funding.
- Briefly report the activities that will be conducted to accomplish the objectives.
- State the total cost of the project, funds already committed, and the amount asked for in the proposal.

The introduction section of your grant proposal will introduce your organization to the funding agency. This section should describe what is unique about your organization and how long you have been established, and should provide evidence that you have effectively intervened in an area similar to the proposed project. You will also want to list some of your sources of funding received in the past. If available, provide quotes from satisfied clients, colleagues, and experts to support your credibility.

The statement of need connects a solution (idea, method, or program) with a problem that exists and needs attention. This section develops the rationale or philosophy behind a proposed activity or program. Chapter 13 describes the process of conducting a needs assessment. This information is condensed even further to integrate how your organization's mission statement and goals clearly commit to resolving a problem or need within a geographic community. The information

presented must be "well thought out, procedures explained thoroughly, the necessary data precisely presented but through it all the message to the reader must be: 'This is a good idea; it will yield worthwhile results; it is in good hands.' "[17] The "need" or "problem" should always be stated in terms of the client or program recipient, not the organization. If the problem is of national scope, the section within the needs statement needs to be applied to your community. Again, Kiritz has developed a checklist for a problem statement or needs assessment.[9] Does the problem statement or needs assessment

- Relate to the mission and goals of the organization?
- Present an idea, program, or project with reasonable expectations?
- Have support from authorities? Have support of statistical evidence?
- State benefits in terms of clients or program recipients?
- Use professional jargon, only when necessary, and is defined?
- Present a concise and interesting description?

Developing a program goal and objectives is the next section of writing the grant proposal. A written goal is a positive statement of what would exist if the problem were no longer there. For example, a goal might be "to reduce the number of overweight adults related to decreased physical activity levels and high-fat dietary intakes." Goals are future-oriented, simple, easily understood, and broad.

"Program objectives are 'outcomes' of your activities. . . . They are measurable and become the criteria by which you judge the effectiveness [of your intervention]."[9] Objectives (discussed in chapter 13) should be specific and measurable.

The project description/methodology section states the plan in a step-by-step sequence and outlines the amount of time estimated to complete the project. In this grant component, you will need to "sell" the reader on the many aspects of the project. The reader will need to join your concern and motivation about the importance of the project, believe you can do it, and understand how the project works. Any uniqueness or unusual ways to solve a problem will need careful, concise descriptions. The methods section lays out a general plan of work that guides the reader through how the project will be implemented. Many times a Gantt chart (see chapter 14) is used to outline the project and describe the sequence of important activities as a way to outline your management plan. In addition, the methodology section should implicate what resources are needed so the budget section (found later) will be clear. Any facilities and equipment, special techniques, or provisions needed have to be identified. This includes how you will select and train staff, and how persons participating in the project or program will be selected. Finally, all of the activities planned should be "do able" in the time suggested and within the resource capability of the applicant. Overall, methods identify what will be done, who will do it, how long it will take, and the materials and equipment needed. Adapted from Bauer[2] and Kiritz,[9] the following checklist is helpful to review your methods section:

- Describe your program activities and demonstrate how they fulfill your objectives.
- Describe the sequence, flow, and interrelationship of the activities.
- Describe the planned staffing for your program and designate who is responsible for which activities; include the names and credentials of persons responsible for overall management of the project.
- Describe your client population and method for outreach and determining client selection.
- State a specific time frame for the project.

Evaluations should address both process and outcome components. Success is measured from an intervention management perspective. Were the activities conducted on schedule and at a sufficient quality? (process evaluation). The outcome evaluation focuses on the client: Is there concrete evidence that clients achieved desired outcomes? (outcome evaluation). Using the community-based health promotion program for seniors example cited in box 16.2, a process evaluation objective is: "Project staff will have trained eight or more peer leaders by the end of six months." As part of monitoring outcomes, a follow-up survey of elderly program participants could measure how many participants continue with moderate physical activity at least five days per week. Outcome evaluations compare results of the program at a defined period; with the specific, measurable outcome objectives established earlier. Chapter 15 discusses outcome and process evaluations in more detail. Of note is that one challenge of outcome evaluation for the community nutrition profession is tracking clients after their involvement with nutrition programs so that the outcomes indicators can be measured.

The budget part of the proposal contains projections of resources needs (for personnel, supplies and equipment, facilities, travel, contractual services, and administrative overhead costs) and revenue sources. Costs are usually divided into two categories: personnel and non-personnel costs. In addition, costs are also divided into two columns: the amount of money requested from the funding organization and the amount of money donated by either the organization or other collaborators. Box 16.3 shows a sample of the line item expense categories necessary to a complete budget.

Finally, don't forget to obtain and include attachments. These may be a financial statement, verification of 501(c)(3) status, letters of support, and certifications attesting to the compliance with protection of human subjects or any pertinent regulations which are applicable. You may also want to include position descriptions for the project's primary staff as well as references for any statistical data presented.

An important motto to keep in mind after completion of all the components is, "You won't get it right the first time." Therefore, it is important to review each section thoroughly and examine how each section is organized and fits into the entire grant proposal. Is the proposal tailored to your specific audience? Does it match with a potential funder's goals? Did you use informal language and avoid jargons? Does your executive summary/abstract summarize your project in a concise and accurate manner? Does your proposal generate a perception of value in the minds of reviewers?

Once the proposal is completed, it is necessary to write a cover letter to the executive director, project officer, or to whomever you were instructed to direct the proposal. If you are submitting a proposal to the government, the cover page is a transmittal letter. If you are writing to a foundation or corporation, the cover letter accomplishes more. In this case, your cover letter should reflect the innovative proposal and offer a unique, distinctive, effective, and financially accountable project. Good luck!

As more organizations use proposals to obtain revenue, competition and the challenge to improve grant-writing skills also increases. Clear, concise writing and effective organization throughout the process are successful strategies. In addition, it is important to understand your organization's unique capabilities to achieve the goals outlined in any proposal. Finally, good communication skills through out the process are also necessary for success.

IMPLICATIONS FOR COMMUNITY NUTRITION PROFESSIONALS

There is a big gap between being a passive recipient of budget allocation and being a proactive player by preparing proposals, seeking resources from a range of sources, and participating in financial management and resource allocation decisions. Go back to box 16.6. Where are you on the continuum of involvement in the financial control of your nutrition programs? Where would you like to be on this continuum?

Learning and practicing now will prepare you for expanded responsibility in financial management later. Community nutrition professionals who have skills and are confident in the areas of budgeting, managing resources, and proposal writing will be better able to assure essential nutrition programs and services are available in their communities. This is an essential area of competence for community nutrition professionals today.

COMMUNITY NUTRITION PROFESSIONALS IN ACTION

- Interview community nutrition professionals in government, nonprofit, and private organizations about the funding base for their program(s) and their roles in budgeting, financial management, and grantsmanship. Compare and contrast sources of funds for program operations and the level of involvement the community nutrition professionals have in financial matters.
- Develop a budget proposal for a small-scale nutrition program that would meet a nutrition-related need in your community or Vision City (as described in the chapter 13 case study).
- In conjunction with a local community nutrition professional, complete a cost analysis for a program or service.
- As a result of welfare reform, the number of families experiencing food insecurity has greatly increased. What can you do to secure resources to address this problem?
- You have identified a foundation that is interested in supporting a new nutrition intervention program to help frail elderly remain in their homes. The foundation staff director says they can only award the grant to a 501(c)(3) agency. How can you find out if your organization is a 501(c)(3)?
- Identify a local Foundation Center depository library that has the computerized grant search capabilities

available. Identify four potential funding agencies for the Aged to Perfection program identified in box 16.2.
- Review the sample form of how to track funding prospects for the Aged to Perfection program (figure 16.4). If you were a community nutrition professional in Vision City, where would you look for additional sources of financial support?

GOING ONE STEP FURTHER

- Request the budget reports for the nutrition project where you work or volunteer. What cost category is the largest? How do expenses to date compare with the year's budget. What adjustments, if any, should be made to prevent shortfalls or overspending within line item categories?
- Identify a need for a new project or the expansion of an existing nutrition project in your community. Use resources listed in the chapter to identify at least three potential sources of funding for the project. Prepare a complete proposal for submission to one funding source. Make sure the proposal includes all the essential parts of a proposal and is tailored to the guidelines or requirements of the targeted funding source.

REFERENCES

1. Association of State and Territorial Public Health Nutrition Directors: *The 1994 biennial salary profile of public health nutritionists,* Washington, DC, 1994, ASTPHND.
2. Bauer, DG: *The "how to" grants manual. Successful techniques for obtaining public and private grants,* ed 3, Phoenix, AZ, 1995, The Oryx Press.
3. Cleverley WO: *Essentials of health care finance,* Rockville, MD, 1986, Aspen.
4. Finkler, SA: *Issues in cost accounting for healthcare organizations,* Gaithersburg, MD, 1994, Aspen.
5. The Foundation Center: *The foundation index,* ed 25, New York, 1997, The Foundation Center.
6. Geever JC, McNeils P: *The Foundation Centers guide to proposal-writing,* New York, 1993, The Foundation Center.
7. Gitlin L, Lyons KJ: *Successful grantwriting. Strategies for health and human service professionals,* New York, 1996, Springer Publishing.
8. Hall M: *Getting funded: a complete guide to proposal writing,* Portland, OR, 1988, Continuing Education Publications.
9. Kiritz NJ: *Program planning and proposal writing,* Los Angeles, 1980, The Grantsmanship Center.

10. Liebler JG, Levine RE, Rothman J: *Management principles for health professionals,* Gaithersburg, MD, 1992, Aspen.

11. Nassau County Department of Senior Citizens Affairs and The Foundation Center: *National guide to funding in aging,* New York, 1987, The Foundation Center.

12. Osborne D, Gaebler T: *Reinventing government,* Reading, MA, 1992, Addison-Wesley.

13. Sladeck FE, Stein EL: *Grants, budgeting and finance. Getting the most of your grant,* New York, 1981, Plenum.

14. Splett PL, Caldwell M: *Costing nutrition services: a workbook,* reprint ed., Chicago, 1993, Region V, U.S. Department of Human Services.

15. Suver JD, Neumann BR: *Management accounting for healthcare organizations,* Chicago, 1985, Pluribus Press.

16. Swansburg RC: *Budgeting and financial management for nurse managers,* Sudbury, MA, 1997, Jones and Bartlett.

17. White VP: *Grant proposals that succeed,* New York, 1983, Plenum.

CASE STUDY

POPNM FOUNDATION

DESCRIPTION

This case study gives students the opportunity to practice writing a grant proposal for a foundation. Fictitious names and organizations were created. Students are encouraged to refer to Vision City statistics presented in chapter 13 to develop a project idea. Figures 16.3 and table 16.3 provide tools to build student skills and appreciation for the proposal writing process without becoming too overwhelmed. Box 16.2 in this chapter also helps provide an example of developing a project-specific budget. If time allows, students can be assigned to review proposals from the grantor's perspective.

TEACHING OBJECTIVES

After completion of the assignment, students will be able to:

• Identify the components of a grant proposal.
• Plan a nutrition service project and develop a grant proposal to secure funding.
• Review and evaluate a grant proposal according to the the application guidelines presented in the POPNM case study.

THE CASE

Imagine that you are a community nutrition professional working for a nonprofit organization. You completed a computerized Foundation Center Search and felt that the POPNM Foundation was a potential match for one of your organization's newly proposed nutrition intervention projects. You followed preapplication information and contacted Jane Smith who mailed you the application materials shown in the boxes. The next Board of Directors meeting is in one month. You are the designated nutrition unit director to manage the development and submission of the proposal.

RELATED QUESTIONS

1. Based on a review of the application materials received from the POPNM Foundation, what key components do you feel the Board of Directors are looking for in a nutrition service project?

2. What were some of the challenges faced when writing this grant proposal?

3. When you wrote your proposal, were you able to include the major components of a grant proposal discussed in table 16.3? Why or Why not?

BOX 16.13

POPNM FOUNDATION

Dear Prospective Grantee,

Thank you for your interest in The POPNM Foundation. At POPNM, we believe in collaborative, community-based services to promote healthier outcomes. The POPNM Foundation awards grants to many nonprofit organizations and institutions.

The POPNM Foundation Board of Directors meets six times per year and reviews grant applications. Board Members are looking for a broad range of innovative efforts that are based on collaborations within the community. We are interested in funding projects that enhance the nutritional well-being of people and build on current, cost-effective nutrition services. They must also demonstrate a commitment to empowering communities.

If you are interested in applying, please submit the POPNM Grant application to:

> POPNM Foundation
> P.O. 1000
> Healthy Pyramid, MO 77777
>
> Contact Person: Jane Smith

Thank you for your interest in the POPNM Foundation. We wish you success in efforts to serve your community.

Sincerely,

Jane Smith

Jane Smith
Executive Director,
POPNM Foundation

BOX 16.14

THE POPNM GRANT APPLICATION

TITLE OF PROJECT:

Name of Applicant
Organization: _____

Primary Contact Person: _____

Address: _____

_____

Telephone Number: _____

Fax Number: _____

E-mail Address: _____

> GIVE A BRIEF SUMMARY OF YOUR PROPOSAL (include the kinds of activities planned, target population served, the total cost of the project, and the amount asked for in this proposal).

IDENTIFY THE ISSUE IN YOUR COMMUNITY AND THE UNMET NEED. Be sure to include your approaches used to involve community members in helping define the issue and developing proposed interventions.

OUTLINE THE GOAL AND OBJECTIVES OF THE PROJECT.
Goal:
Objectives:
- _____
  _____
- _____
  _____

continued.

BOX 16.14 (CONTINUED)

(The following sections may be submitted on plain paper, not to exceed a total of six pages.)

DESCRIBE THE PROJECT

HOW WILL YOUR PROJECT BE IMPLEMENTED (Include collaborators), WHO IS GOING TO MANAGE THE PROJECT AND HOW WILL IT BE MANAGED? (Write clearly and concisely).

HOW WILL YOU RECORD AND TRACK YOUR PROGRESS TO LEARN WHAT WORKS, DOESN'T WORK, OR COULD BE DONE DIFFERENTLY? HOW WILL YOU KNOW IF YOU HAVE MET YOUR OBJECTIVES?

BUDGET REQUEST AND JUSTIFICATION
(Identify all budget line items required to conduct the project. Also specify the amounts requested from POPNM and provide a budget justification.)

LIST THE RESOURCES YOU HAVE SOLICITED FROM WITHIN YOUR OWN ORGANIZATION AND OTHER SOURCES?

ATTACHMENTS: (Include a letter of support from a collaborator, a position description of the project director, and verification from your organization of 501(c)(3) status.)

Signature

_____   _____
Applicant   Date

PART FOUR

ACHIEVING EFFECTIVE COMMUNITY NUTRITION PROGRAMS

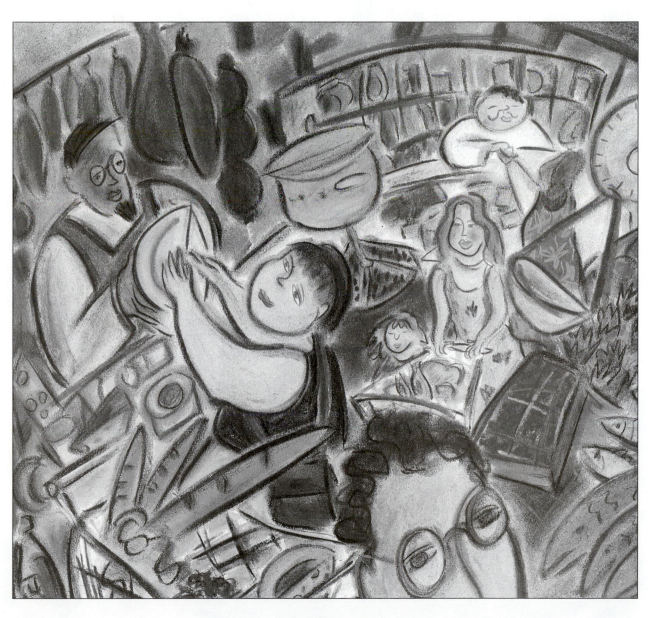

CHAPTER SEVENTEEN

COMMUNICATIONS

*It is time for the media to recognize the difference
between zeal and science. Freedom of press is not
only a basic right, it is also a privilege which must
be earned by a dispassionate pursuit of the truth.*
—WILLIAM WEISS, MD

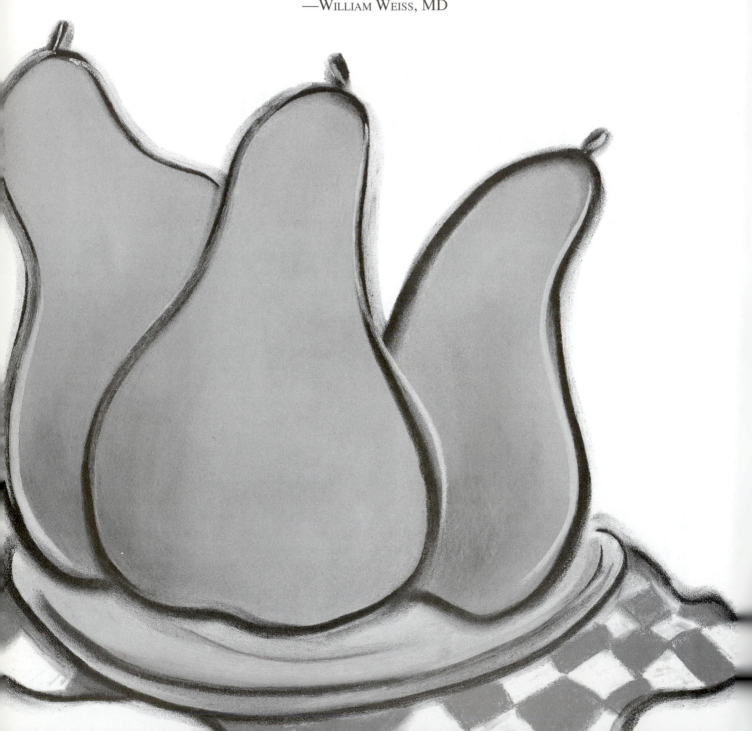

Core Concepts

Effective communication is an integral part of the community nutrition professionals' role of shaping food choices and having an impact on the nutritional status of the public. Nutrition intervention efforts cannot be effective without good communication. Understanding the communication process and the barriers that exist is the first step in effective communication. Communicating effectively can make a major difference in achieving health promotion and disease prevention outcomes. To be viable, nutrition and health communications programs must be based on an understanding of the needs and perceptions of the target audience. The six steps in health communications described include assessment of target audience needs, selecting appropriate channels, program and message development, implementation, assessing effectiveness and feedback, and refining the program.

Effective community nutrition and health programs are based on sound science. However, many nutrition and health messages that reach the public are not based on scientific fact. As a result, nutrition and health misinformation is prevalent.

Objectives

When you finish chapter seventeen, you should be able to:

~ Define the communication process and identify the barriers to effective communication.

~ Describe the role of communication in disease prevention and health promotion.

~ Examine the six stages in health communications and determine how they can be applied to programs in the community.

~ Describe the characteristics of mass media channels and identify the types of mass media outlets.

~ Discuss critically the factors affecting public acceptance of health messages.

~ Identify the special considerations that are necessary to develop messages and materials for ethnic minorities.

~ List the types of organizations and activities to consider when working with intermediaries (other groups).

~ Describe the factors contributing to nutrition misinformation and quackery.

~ Cite the skills needed to be an effective oral and written communicator, including mass media communications.

Key Words

Word	Page Mentioned
Communication process	514
Technical barriers	514
Language barriers	516
Psychological barriers	516
Listening	516
Health communication process	518
Qualitative research	519
Quantitative research	519
Messages	520
Mass media channels	521
Pretesting materials	524
Focus group	525
Intermediaries	525
Evaluation	527
Nutrition misinformation	528
Nutrition facts	529
Food faddism	529
Alternative medicine	531
Oral communication	531
Media presentation	532
Written communication	533

Effective communication skills are critical for the community nutrition professional. Understanding the **communication process** and applying it will determine your success as a practitioner. Communicating effectively about health is not an easy task. Health information is often complex and technical. In addition, the information may be inconclusive, controversial, contradictory, and subject to change as new research findings are released. New health information may conflict with long-held personal beliefs. The media and some scientists may add to the way health risks are inflated or distorted in medical and nutrition news. As a result, the potential exists for misdirecting or alienating the public.

THE COMMUNICATION PROCESS

Communication is defined as the transfer of information, ideas, and understanding or feelings among people.[21] A working definition of communication calls attention to three essential points:

- That communication involves people and that understanding communication therefore involves trying to understand how people relate to each other
- That communication involves shared meaning
- That communication involves symbols—gestures, sounds, letters, numbers, and words can only represent or approximate the idea they are meant to communicate

The basic elements of the communication process are shown in figure 17.1. This process is significant as we address the context of health. Each step in the sequence is critical to successful communication. The source (or sender) is the person who has an idea or message to communicate to another person or persons. As the first step in the communication process, the sender must encode (convert) the message or idea—put it into a set of symbols that the receiver will understand. Words on this page, for example, are symbols to the reader. The sound of a car's horn on a busy freeway may be a symbol of danger or of an impending accident.

When communication is attempted, messages are transmitted through various means such as speaking, writing, acting, and drawing. A number of communication channels may be used to transmit any message. Communication channels are the means by which information is transmitted to people. Words can be communicated orally, through such methods as face-to-face communication, telephone communication, radio, and television. Books, letters, and articles can serve as writ-

ten channels. The senses of touch, smell, and taste are nonverbal channels. Much meaningful communication takes place without a word being spoken.

Communication must also have a recipient. Shouting for help on a deserted island is not communication. Similarly, if a community nutrition professional is presenting information on the dietary guidelines and no one listens or understands, there is no communication. The receiver must decode (convert) the message—convert the symbols into meaning. The receiver may then act in response to the communication—this action can be to ignore the message, to perform some task, to store the information for future use, or something else. The receiver also usually provides feedback so the sender will know if the message was accurately received and the proper action was taken. In general, the more the receiver's decoding matches the sender's intended message, the more effective the communication has been.

BARRIERS TO COMMUNICATION

For communication to be effective, the receiver must correctly interpret the sender's message. Often, however, communication is ineffective because of breakdowns that can occur at any stage in the communication process. Barriers to communications are classified as technical, language, and psychological.[21]

Technical Barriers

Environmental barriers to communications are referred to as **technical barriers.** Timing, information overload, and cultural differences are three such barriers.

Timing   Timing involves the determination of when a message should be communicated. For many years, the clinical dietitian was called to give diet counseling to patients as they were about to leave the hospital. This obviously was an inappropriate time to present information.

Information Overload   This condition exists when an individual is presented with too much information in a period of time. With the many channels and media that are presenting nutrition and health information, some with conflicting messages, it is little wonder that information overload occurs. Another example is a presentation that has too many facts, figures, and statistics. A person can absorb only so many facts and figures at one

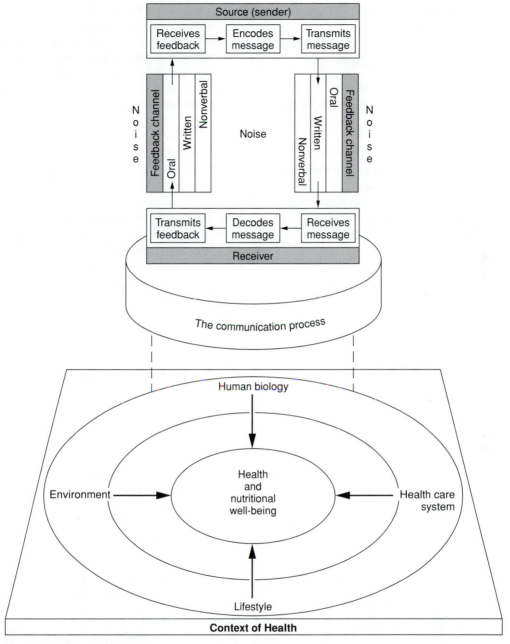

Figure 17.1   Context of Health
The communication process. (*Source:* Top of model from Mondy R, Premeaux SR: *Management: concepts, practices and skills,* ed 7 © 1995. Reprinted by permission of Prentice-Hall, Inc., Upper Saddle River, NJ.)

time. When excessive information is provided, a major breakdown in communication can occur.

Cultural Differences   Such differences can lead to a breakdown in communications. In the United States, time is a valuable commodity and a deadline suggests urgency. But in the Middle East, giving another person a deadline is considered rude, and the deadline is likely to be ignored. The community nutrition professional works with cultural diversity on a daily basis. Chapter

18 provides an extensive coverage of working in cross-cultural and multicultural settings.

Language Impediments

Language barriers can result from the vocabulary used and from different messages applied to the same word (semantics).

Vocabulary   The community nutrition professional must understand the type of audience being addressed. Physicians, teenagers, and a Hispanic immigrant likely have quite different vocabulary sets. Breakdowns in communication often occur when the sender does not tailor the message to match the knowledge base of intended receivers.

Semantics   When a sender transmits words to which a receiver attaches meanings different from those intended, a semantic (relating to meaning of words) communication breakdown will likely occur.

Jargon   This is a special language that group members use in their daily interaction. Virtually all health care providers use a jargon daily. The target population, too, has its own jargon. Understanding and using the jargon correctly can strengthen communications.

Psychological Barriers

Technical factors and language differences cause many breakdowns in communications, but **psychological barriers** tend to be the major cause for miscommunication. These barriers include various forms of distortion and problems involving interpersonal relationships.

Information Filtering   This is the process by which a message is altered through the elimination or modification of certain data as the communication moves from person to person. Most of us are familiar with the game of "telephone" in which one person whispers a message into the ear of another and so on around the circle. Inevitably, when the last person says the message out loud, it is quite different from what was first whispered.

Lacking Trust   A successful communication relationship must be based on trust. A receiver's trust or distrust of a message is, to a large extent, a function of the credibility of the sender in the mind of the receiver. Hopefully, consumers will place their trust in a professional health association such as the American Heart Association, the American Cancer Society, or The American Dietetic Association for health and nutrition information. In communities there are several sources of credible information that should be utilized. In the Case Study at the end of this chapter, the mothers were the most important sources of credible information for the women in the program described.

Preoccupation   Some people are so preoccupied with themselves that they do not hear or receive the message they are **listening** to or reading. Preoccupation may cause people to respond in inappropriate ways.

Hearing What We Expect to Hear   Most of us are conditioned to hear whatever we expect to hear, not what is actually said. Sometimes, because of past experiences, we hear what we want to hear.

Perception Set Differences   A perception set is a fixed tendency to interpret information in a certain way. Differences in past experiences, educational background, emotions, values, beliefs, and many other factors affect each person's perception of a message or of words. Perception set differences affect the meanings of tangible words such as chair, pencil, and hat—but the impact is much greater for such intangible words such as liberal and conservative.

Noise   Anything that interferes with accurate transmission or reception of messages is noise. It is the principal source of error in communications and it can occur at several or all points in the communication process. Although it cannot be completely eliminated from the communication process, its negative impacts can be lessened.

HOW TO BECOME BETTER COMMUNICATORS

When a breakdown in communication occurs, the result is often negative. Learning how to communicate effectively will help avoid a communication breakdown and can lead to successful nutrition intervention efforts in a community. Communication skills can be learned. Empathy, listening, reading skills, observation, word choice, and body language are all involved in effective communication.

Empathy

Empathy is the ability to identify with the feelings and thoughts of another person. It does not mean that you necessarily agree with the other person, but that you understand why that person speaks and acts in a certain way.

Listening

One of the most effective tools to facilitate communication is the ability to listen. Listening skills help community nutrition professionals identify problems and determine solutions. It has been observed that the average speaking speed is about 120 words per minute. The speed at which most people are able to comprehend words is more than four times the speed at which the words are spoken. The question therefore arises: What does the listener do with the "free time" that results from the difference in speeds?

As table 17.1 shows, at least three types of listening habits have been identified; marginal, evaluative, and projective.[21] The slower speed of the speaker provides the listener with an opportunity for *marginal* listening— letting the mind stray while someone is talking. This can lead to misunderstanding and even insult. Most of us have experienced a conversation in which we realize that the other person's mind is "a million miles away." The person may have heard a few words, but most of the message was not understood. *Evaluative* listening occurs when any free time is devoted to evaluating the speaker's remarks. As soon as the sender says something that is not accepted, communication ceases, and the receiver begins to develop a response. Instead of one idea being transmitted and held by two people, two ideas develop, neither of which is really communicated. If the listener allocates too much time to disproving or approving of what is heard, there may not be time to understand it fully. This is particularly true when the remarks are loaded with emotion or threats to the security or status of the receiver. *Projective* listening holds the greatest potential for effective communication. It is the communicator's role to set the stage for effective listening. Listeners attempt to project themselves into the position of the speaker and to understand what is being said from the speaker's standpoint. This requires the ability to listen for feelings as well as for words. After listening to and understanding what has been said, individuals are better able to evaluate the communicated message.

Reading Skills

The reading level of the consumer must be determined. Health and nutrition information materials such as pamphlets, flyers, posters, and magazine articles are usually designed for distinct target audiences. A readability test will indicate if a printed piece is written at a level most of the audience can understand.

Observation

Carefully observing important elements in the environment (such as eating, clothing, housekeeping, and furnishing patterns) can provide the community nutrition professional with much information and can lead to an increased understanding of target audience characteristics.

Word Choice

Community nutrition professionals who want to communicate effectively must choose their words carefully. The words transmitted by the sender should be in the vocabulary set of the receiver and appropriate for the intended audience.

Body Language

Research has shown that 90 percent of our first impressions are based on nonverbal communication (sometimes called body language) and only 10 percent on verbal communication.[20] An effective communicator strives to make a positive impression by using appropriate body language in the delivery of their message. The

TABLE 17.1
Types of Listening

Marginal	Evaluative	Projective
Majority of the message isn't heard or understood	Careful listening until hearing something that isn't accepted; listening ceases as a response is developed to the incomplete message	Listening without evaluation of the full message or attempting to understand speaker's viewpoint

Source: Adapted from Mondy RW, Premeaux SR: *Management: concepts, practices and skills,* ed 7, Upper Saddle River, NJ, 1995, Prentice Hall.

BOX 17.1

DEALING WITH COMMUNICATIONS

- *Have a plan.* Think of why you want to communicate a particular idea. Then consider the best way to get the message across.
- *Get organized.* Merely having a general idea of what you want to communicate is not sufficient, a logical thought process should be followed.
- *Develop the message from the receiver's viewpoint.* Do not try to impress the receiver with big words and long phrases. Remember, if the message is not understood, effective communication has not taken place.
- *Select the best way to communicate the message.* At times, a verbal exchange is best. At other times, a written memorandum will prove superior.
- *Look for feedback.* Communication is not complete until you know that your message is clearly understood. A

mere nod may be satisfactory. However, it is best to ask, "What do you think I mean?" rather than merely, "Do you understand?"
- *Follow up.* Even if the message is accurately received, the desired action may not occur. Your priority may not correspond to that of the receiver. You may need to check to see if what you wanted done has actually taken place.
- *Do not assume too much.* Sometimes, matters that seem obvious to you are not so obvious to your listeners.
- *Be a good listener.* Listening is more than just hearing.
- *Use a language that others can understand.* It is not what you say that counts; it is what the receiver hears.
- *Observe nonverbal cues.* This form of communication may be a more accurate indication of their response than spoken words.

body language of the audience may also be monitored to help determine communication effectiveness.

Guidelines for Dealing with Communications

A list of ten tips for dealing with communications is presented in box 17.1.

ROLE OF COMMUNICATION IN DISEASE PREVENTION AND HEALTH PROMOTION

Communication plays an essential role in disease prevention and health promotion. Programs designed to promote changes in health behavior and to encourage early detection and prompt treatment of illness have demonstrated that mass media and other communication strategies can be effective in reducing the risk of serious illnesses.[23] Health communication programs can be designed to inform, influence, and motivate institutional and public audiences (box 17.2).

THE HEALTH COMMUNICATION PROCESS

To be viable, the **health communication process** must be based on an understanding of the needs and perceptions of their target audiences. Figure 17.2 illustrates an approach to health communications incorporating assessments of target audiences, needs and perceptions at critical points in the program, development, implemen-

BOX 17.2

Communication can
- Increase awareness of a health issue, problem or solution.
- Affect attitudes to create support for individual or collective action.
- Demonstrate or illustrate skills.
- Increase demand for health services.
- Remind or reinforce knowledge, attitude or behavior.

Health communication programs cannot
- Compensate for a lack of health care services.
- Produce behavior change without supportive program components.
- Be equally effective in addressing all issue or relaying all messages.

tation, and evaluation. The six stages constitute a circular process (figure 17.2) in which the last stage feeds back to the first in a continuous process of planning and implementation.[23] The steps outlined constitute an ideal process. All of the steps may not be feasible or essential. In general, professional judgment must be used to decide which steps are appropriate for a particular program. The planning process is described in detail in chapters 13, 14, and 15. This same process is applied to communications planning.

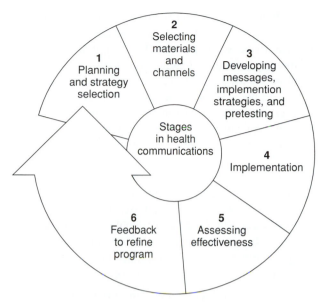

Figure 17.2   Stages in Health Communications
(*Source:* Adapted from National Cancer Institute, USDHHS: *Making health communications programs work: a planner's guide,* NIH Publication no. 89–1493, Washington, DC, 1992, Office of Cancer Communications.)

Stage 1: Planning and Strategy Selection

The planning stage of a program provides the foundation for the entire health communication process. Faulty decision making at this point can lead to the development of a program that is "off the mark." To begin the development of a communications program, the following questions should be asked:

- What is the nutrition/health problem to be addressed?
- Who is affected by it and how?
- Are they aware that the problem could affect them?
- Who is interested in the problem?
- What programs or activities have been addressing the problem?
- Are the media and other organizations doing anything about the problem?
- What do we want to accomplish?
- What resources do we have available?

The answers to these questions are necessary to design a communications program plan.

Review Available Data   Looking at existing data is called secondary research. Nutrition professionals should review all potential sources of information, noting gaps in what has been done. The purpose of this data collec-

tion is to describe the health problem or issue; who is affected; and what they know, believe, and do about it.

Identify Existing Activities   If another organization is already addressing the problem, it is important to contact this group to determine what they have learned, what information or advice they may have to help you plan and where additional needs may exist. Telephone networking can be an excellent, productive way to get a focus on the problem and resources. It also helps to build support. These discussions may provide an opportunity for cooperative efforts.

Address Gaps and Gather New Data   There may not be enough existing data regarding a particular health problem, its resolution or those who are affected to fully develop a communications strategy. At this point, new data needs to be collected. This is called primary research. Two types of primary research may be used, **qualitative research** and **quantitative research.**

Qualitative market research is designed to provide five important Ws

- Who
- What
- Where
- When
- Why

For example,

- Who in the population is most interested in reducing saturated fat intake?
- What does a particular population know about cholesterol?
- Where in the United States is dietary fat consumption the highest?
- When do individuals get serious about following a low-fat diet?
- Why do individuals lose interest in low-fat diets?

The methods that are most often used in qualitative research have been described in chapter 7. Although qualitative research can help identify and explore issues, because of the small number of participants and the lack of strength sampling, the findings cannot be projected to the population as a whole.

Quantitative research seeks to measure and confirm the type of information that has been obtained through qualitative research. The methods used in quantitative research are discussed in chapter 7. Information from quantitative research can provide numbers or percentages relative to a given study population and aid in understanding the magnitude of a health related issue.

Identify Target Audiences   Specifically describing the audience(s) for the program—who should be reached and influenced with the message—will provide a basis for relevant **messages** and materials and identify the channels most likely to reach them. Few messages are appropriate for everyone in the general public given the diverse interests, needs, concerns, and priorities among different segments of the public. Trying to reach everyone with one message or strategy may dilute your message so that it appeals to few rather than many people. In describing the target audience, it is necessary to think about all of the characteristics of the people you are trying to reach. These characteristics include

- *Physical*—sex, age, type and degree of exposure to health risks, medical conditions, disorders and illnesses, health history of family
- *Behavioral*—media exposure, membership in organizations, health-related activities or actions, and other lifestyle characteristics
- *Demographic*—attitudes, opinions, beliefs, values, cultural traditions, self-appraisal, and other personality traits

Primary target audiences are those you want to affect in some way; you may have several primary target audiences. If so, priorities must be set among the audiences to help order the planning and allocate resources. Secondary target audiences are those with influences on the primary audiences or those who must do something to help cause the change in the primary target audience. The process of identifying and defining audiences should lead to setting audience priorities.

Assess Resources   The following questions should be asked when determining availability and use of resources:

- Which activities will contribute the most to the desired change?
- What resources are available including staff and other people, budgeted funds, and time?
- What community activities and organizations or other contributing factors exist?
- What barriers are there?
- Which activities will best utilize the resources you have identified and best fit within the identified constraints?

Establish Goals and Objectives   Goals and objectives shape the communication program and determine what is to be accomplished. The program goal(s) describes the overall change such as a specific improvement in one aspect of the health of a certain population. Reaching the goal may encompass service delivery, financial and societal support, and other situational changes that can only be partially addressed by communication strategies. An example of a communication strategy goal may be to reach 75 percent of the audience with a communication message.

Objectives describe the intermediate steps that must be reached to accomplish the broader goals. These objectives should be specific, attainable, prioritized to direct the allocation of resources, measurable to assess progress toward the goal, and time-specific. An objective to meet the goal described above may be:

> Within one week of message implementation, conduct a phone survey with audience members to determine message receipt and level of understanding.

If objectives are not clear and actionable, the program will be unfocussed and ineffective. Refer to chapter 14 for additional information on writing goals and objectives.

Draft Communication Strategies   Now that what needs to be done is defined (goals and objectives) with whom (target audience), it is time to design the communication strategies most likely to get desired results. As the program develops and more is learned about the audience, refinement of the strategy(ies) may need to occur. In fact, constant reevaluation of strategy(ies) and appropriate redirection when necessary is a very important component of successful interventions.

Stage 2: Selecting Materials and Channels

After completing the program plan, communication tools must be developed. Care must be taken when developing new materials as this can be a time-consuming and costly process. It should be determined if creating new materials is really necessary. Materials may already be available that meet the needs of the communication program. State and local health departments, universities, voluntary organizations, health professional organizations, and community-based health promotion coalitions may have materials already prepared on the desired topic or may have materials that can be tailored to fit current needs. If it appears that materials from another agency or organization suit your needs, then it is important to test these promising materials for appropriateness with the target audience.

Discussions about what materials format (e.g., print or audiovisual) will best suit the program will be determined by

- The message—its complexity, sensitivity, style, and purpose
- The audience—will they want to read about the subject or would they rather watch a video
- The channels—whether you will be most likely to reach the audience through a school, library, physicians, the media, or a combination of these
- The budget and other available resources[23]

Selecting Channels   The decision regarding which channels your program will use is interdependent with the decision about materials format. Message delivery channels include

- Face-to-face (e.g., health care professional to patient, peers, family members)
- Group delivery (e.g., worksite or classroom)
- Organizational (e.g., constituents of a professional or voluntary association)
- Mass media (e.g., radio, television, magazines, direct mail, billboards, newspapers)
- Community (e.g., libraries, employers, schools, malls, health fairs, local government agencies)

Each channel offers different benefits and may require different message design (although not necessarily different messages) to fit the channel in length and format. Selecting and using multiple, complimentary channels usually improves message effectiveness. Those channels that allow for interpersonal contact provide a format for information discussion and clarification, motivation, behavioral influence, and message reinforcement.

Mass media channels, the larger channels, can transmit news quickly to a broad audience. Keep in mind, however, that the purpose of the mass media is to inform and entertain, not educate. Therefore, messages must be interesting as well as accurate, and fit within the media's agenda. Choice of mass media format(s) will depend on both the message and the intended audience. Table 17.2 shows characteristics of mass media channels.

Types of Media Outlets   "The media," often thought of as one great entity, is actually made up of numerous subcategories. The three basic media categories—print, broadcast, and wire services—include the subcategories in box 17.3, many of which can be further categorized into national, regional and local outlets.

The type of story that is being prepared influences the media list (reporters and editors to whom you will direct the news). It is important to know exactly who should receive the information. If sent to the wrong person, even the most compelling release can wind up in the trash can. To reach local audiences, call the publications and stations in your area to get the names of reporters or producers who cover the appropriate subject area. For national media, check the library for broadcasting and editors and publishers.

Understanding and Working with the Media on Food Safety and Nutrition Issues   American consumers rely on the news media for most of their information about nutrition and food safety. Given the central role media play in shaping the public's dietary outlook, the International Food Information Council (IFIC) Foundation completed a content analysis of food and nutrition reporting in the media nationally over a three-month period in 1995.[5] The media research showed many positive developments in food and nutrition reporting, but also highlighted many ways in which the communication process could be improved. The study's major findings are shown in the box 17.4.

Allen completed a content analysis to evaluate the coverage of the food labels in the print media.[1] Quotes in the articles indicated that less than 8 percent of the total quotes were from dietitians. These findings illustrate the need for community nutrition professionals to increase their exposure with the media and help the media translate complex nutrition labeling information to the public.[5]

Making Decisions about Channels   Using several different channels will increase the repetition of the information, increasing the chance that the audience will be exposed to the information a sufficient number of times to absorb and remember it. Channel selection should be determined prior to materials production since message format will be different for various channels. Consider these questions as you make decisions about channels:

- What channels are most appropriate for the health problem/issue and message?
- Which channels are most likely to be credible to and accessible by the target audience?
- Which channels fit the program purpose (e.g., inform influence, attitudes, change behavior)?
- Which and how many channels are feasible, considering your time schedule and budget?

TABLE 17.2
Characteristics of Mass Media Channels

Television	Radio	Magazines	Newspapers
Potentially largest/wide range of audiences, but not always at times when PSAs are most likely to be broadcast	Various formats offer potential for more audience targeting than television (e.g., teenagers via rock stations); may reach fewer people than TV	Can more specifically target to segments of public (young women, people with an interest in health)	Can reach broad audiences rapidly
Deregulation ended government oversight of station broadcast of PSAs, public affairs programming	Deregulation ended government oversight of stations' broadcast of PSAs, public affairs programming	No requirement for PSA use; PSAs more difficult to place	PSAs virtually nonexistent
Opportunity to include health messages via news broadcasts, public affairs/interview shows, dramatic programming	Opportunity for direct audience involvement via call-in shows	Can explain more complex health issues, behaviors	Can convey health news/breakthroughs more thoroughly than TV or radio and faster than magazines; feature placement possible
Visual as well as audio make emotional appeals possible; easier to demonstrate a behavior	Audio alone may make messages less intrusive	Print may lend itself to more factual, detailed, rational message delivery	
Can reach low-income and other audiences not as likely to turn to health sources for help	Can reach audiences who do not use the health care system	Audience has chance to clip, reread, contemplate material	Easy audience access to in-depth issue coverage is possible
Passive consumption by viewer; viewers must be present when message is aired; less than full attention likely; message may be obscured by commercial "clutter"	Generally passive consumption; exchange with audience possible, but target audience must be there when aired	Permits active consultation; may pass on; read at reader's convenience	Short life of newspaper limits rereading, sharing with others
PSAs can be expensive to produce and distribute; feature placement requires contacts and may be time consuming	Live copy very flexible and inexpensive; PSAs must fit station format Feature placement requires contacts and may be time consuming	Public service ads are inexpensive to produce; ad or article placement may be time consuming	Small papers may take public service ads; coverage demands a newsworthy item

Note: PSAs public service announcements.
Source: From National Cancer Institute, USDHHS: *Making health communications programs work: a planner's guide,* NIH Publication No. 89–1493, Washington, DC, 1992, Office of Cancer Communications.

Stage 3: Developing Messages and Pretesting

Developing Messages   The information gathered about the target audience(s) in stage 1 form the basis for developing message concepts. One of the first activities in message development is to determine how the public perceives health messages. This perception will help direct message development. There are several factors affecting public acceptance of health messages (see box 17.5).

Factors that help develop public acceptance of a presented message include clarity and consistency.[22,23] Clear messages contain as few technical, scientific, or bureaucratic terms as possible and eliminate unnecessary detail that the audience doesn't need to make informed decisions. Readability tests can help determine the reading level required to understand drafted materials and help writers to be conscientious about carefully selecting words and phrases. Consistency refers to con-

BOX 17.3

MEDIA CATEGORIES

- Daily and weekly newspapers
- News and business magazines
- Specialized consumer publications (i.e., women's health, fitness, and parenting magazines)
- Local business journals
- Trade journals (often highly specialized for a business audience)
- Broadcast media
  Network television
  Network radio
  Local television
  Local radio
  Syndicated/cable television and radio programs
- Wire and news services
  National wire services (AP, UPI, Reuters)
  News services (Scripps-Howard, Knight Ridder, Gannett)
  State and local wire services (PR newswire, Business wire)
  Syndicates (*Washington Post, New York Times, Los Angeles Times*)

BOX 17.4

MEDIA REPORTING ON FOOD SAFETY AND NUTRITION[5]

- Media seldom provide the context needed to understand overall nutrition recommendation in news reports about individual foods.
- Media reports on scientific research often lack details that would allow consumers to judge a study's relevance to their own diets.
- The need to reduce dietary fat is the top story in food news, getting twice the coverage of any other nutrition topic and relegating other dietary recommendations to virtual obscurity.
- Local newspapers and news broadcasts deliver substantially more food safety and nutrition reports than national news outlets, but are less likely to accent positive messages.

sensus among government, industry, health institutions, and public interest groups on the meanings of new health findings. Consistency among these groups' messages may sometimes be difficult due to the varied foci.

Considerations for Message Construction   Both the channel and the purpose of community health information influence message design. Information may be designed to convey new facts, alter attitudes, change behavior, or encourage participation in decision making. Some of these purposes overlap, often they are progressive. That is, for persuasion to work, the public must first receive information, then understand it, believe it, agree with it, and then act on it. Audience needs will also influence message construction. The Dietary Guidelines Alliance project "It's All About You," is a good example of message construction based on target audience needs. Research was conducted to determine what consumers preferred when it came to health and nutrition information.[9] Research findings were then used to guide message development. It was found that consumers wanted health and nutrition information that was relevant to their lives, succinct, easily understood, fun, and beneficial to themselves. From these findings, five key messages were developed[9] (see box 17.6).

Developing Materials

Audiovisual Materials   If the decision has been made to develop audiovisual materials, there are several options to consider:

- *Demonstration*—The audiovisual format is ideal for demonstrating the desired health behavior, especially if skills must be taught.
- *Testimonials*—A credible presenter (e.g., the Surgeon General) can give credibility to the message. (Make sure the credibility of the presenter is verified.)
- *Slice of life*—A dramatization within an "everyday" or familiar setting may help the audience associate with the message. This style may be more memorable but it may also be "corny."
- *Animation*—this may be "eye-catching" for adults. It can be used to demonstrate desired actions on sensitive subjects such as AIDS, or several disparate target audiences (e.g., different ethnic groups) at once.
- *Humor*—Humor can be memorable, heart-warming, and effective. However, it is difficult to do well.
- *Emotion*—Emotion can make a message real and personal. It can also "turn off" the viewer. As with

BOX 17.5

FACTORS AFFECTING PUBLIC ACCEPTANCE OF HEALTH MESSAGES

- *"Health risk" is an intangible concept*—Many people do not understand the concept of relative risk, and so personal decisions may be based on faulty reasoning. For example, the public tends to overestimate their risk of car and airplane accidents, homicides, and other events that frequently make the news and underestimate their risk of less newsworthy, but more common health problems such as strokes and diabetes.
- *The public responds to easy solutions*—The public is more likely to respond to a call for action if the action is relatively simple (e.g., get a blood test to check for cholesterol) and less likely to act if the "price" of that action is higher, or the action is complicated (e.g., quitting smoking to reduce cancer risk). Therefore, when addressing a complex issue, there may be an intermediate action to recommend (calling for information, preparing to quit).
- *People want absolute answers*—Some people don't understand probabilities; they want concrete information on which they can make certain decisions. In the absence of firm answers from a scientist, the media will sometimes draw an inappropriate conclusion, providing the public with faulty but conclusive-sounding information that the public finds easy to accept and deal with. Therefore, you must carefully and clearly present your information to both the public and the media.

- *The public has other priorities*—New health information may not be integrated as one of an individual's priorities. For many people, intangible health information cannot compete with more tangible daily problems.
- *Individuals do not feel personally susceptible*—The public has a strong tendency to underestimate personal risk. An NCI survey found that 54 percent of respondents believed that a serious illness "couldn't happen to them" and considered their risk as less than that of the general public, regardless of their actual risk.[23]
- *The public holds contradictory beliefs*—Even though an individual may believe that "it can't happen to me," he or she can still believe that "everything causes cancer," and, therefore, there is no way to avoid cancer "when your time comes," and no need to alter personal behavior.
- *The public does not understand science*—Technical and medical terminology, the variables involved in calculating risk, and the fact that science is not static but evolves and changes over time are all poorly understood by the public. Therefore, individuals may hesitate to believe a scientist's prediction, especially if it seems to contradict a previous scientific finding. (Understanding science and what it means for consumers is discussed in Appendix G.

humor, the emotional approach may be a "high-risk" production choice and should be pretested and produced with care.

- *Music*—Use of music can enhance a message; it can also compete with the message.

Print Materials   Writing about health often requires the use of some technical language. However, the way the message is presented (vocabulary, typography, layout graphics, and color) can favorably affect whether it is read and understood. Table 17.3 describes how to make print materials more effective and easier to read.

There are several guidelines to be followed when producing print materials. These include:

- Ensure all messages reinforce each other and follow the communication strategy.
- Use the same approach or style in all campaign elements. Use the same or comparable colors, types of illustrations, and typeface throughout the campaign.

If you have a logo, use it throughout. Designing and using a good logo can produce a coordinated effect.
- Use graphics to gain attention and to aid understanding and recall. Use captions, headlines, and summary statements for additional reinforcement.

Pretesting Materials   **Pretesting materials** is a type of evaluation used to help ensure that communication materials will be understandable, relevant, credible, and acceptable to the target audience. Because materials production is one of the most costly steps in program development, it makes sense to test draft materials before a large investment is made in final materials. Draft materials should resemble the final product as closely as possible but without expensive production. For example, radio announcements may be produced in a nonstudio setting with nonprofessional voices for testing. A television announcement may be tested with a story board or with an animation (videotaped sketches with voice-over). Posters, print ads, and flyers can be produced in rough form for testing. Pretest

BOX 17.6

IT'S ALL ABOUT YOU[9]

Make Healthy Choices That Fit Your Lifestyle So You Can Do the Things You Want to Do

Be Realistic
Make small changes over time in what you eat and the level of activity you do. After all, small steps work better than giant leaps.

Be Adventurous
Expand your tastes to enjoy a variety of foods.

Be Flexible
Go ahead and balance what you eat and the physical activity you do over several days. No need to worry about just one meal or one day.

Be Sensible
Enjoy all foods, just don't overdo it.

Be Active
Walk the dog, don't just watch the dog walk.

TABLE 17.3
Make Print Materials Easier to Read

Text should be
- Introduced, stating the purpose, and summarized at the end to review major points
- Presented in short sentences, short paragraphs
- "Broken up" with visuals placed to emphasize key points, text as "bullets," underlined, boldfaced, or boxed and titles or subtitles to reinforce important points
- Written in the active, not passive, voice
- Underlined, boldfaced or "boxed" for reinforcement
- Clarified with use of examples
- Tested for readability
- Tested with the audience
- Explained, if necessary, in a glossary (with key words defined within the sentence)

Try to avoid
- Jargon, technical terms or phrases, abbreviations and acronyms
- Small type (less than 10 point)
- Lines of type that are too long or too short

Just as necessary as clear writing is text that is easy to read and graphics that help the reader understand and remember the text.

Graphics should be
- Immediately identifiable
- Relevant to the subject matter and reader
- Simple, uncluttered
- Used to reinforce, not compete with text
- Professional quality

Source: From National Cancer Institute, USDHHS: *Making health communications programs work: a planner's guide,* NIH Publication No. 89–1493, Washington, DC, 1992, Office of Cancer Communications.

every detail—even choice of colors can contribute to the success of materials and may be culture-specific.

Most pretesting involves presenting draft materials to a few persons chosen as representative of the intended target audience but not as a statistically valid sample (in number or selection). Thus, pretesting is generally considered qualitative research, which can be interpreted somewhat loosely to provide clues about audience acceptance and direction regarding materials production and use.

A variety of procedures can be used to test messages and materials. Methodology should be selected and shaped to fit each pretesting required, considering the objectives and resources available for each project.

Methods of Pretesting Health Concepts, Messages, and Materials

It may be wise to use several methods of pretesting in combinations that will help overcome the limitations of individual procedures. These include:

- *Focus group interviews* can be used to identify issues and concerns related to a particular audience, followed by individual interviews to discuss identified concerns in great detail.
- *Readability testing* should be used as a first step in pretesting draft manuscripts, followed by individual

questionnaires or interviews regarding materials with target audience respondents.[23]

- *Critical location interviews* or theater testing of messages for television or radio permit contact with a large number of target audience respondents.
- *Self-administered questionnaires* enable planners to elicit detailed information from respondents who may not be accessible for personal interviews (e.g., physicians, teachers, or residents of rural areas).
- *Gatekeeper review* is important because public and patient education materials are routed to these intended audiences through health professionals or other **intermediaries** who can communicate for you to their members.

Some Limitations of Pretesting Given the qualitative nature of most pretesting research, it is important to recognize its limitations. Pretesting cannot absolutely predict or guarantee learning persuasion, behavior change, or other measures of communication effectiveness. It is not a substitute for expert judgment; rather, it can provide additional information from which sound decisions can be made. Perhaps the most common error is to overgeneralize pretesting results. Despite its limitations, pretesting is a vital and necessary step in the communication process.

Developing Materials for Special Audiences

As the link between diet and health has become clearer, the challenges for health professionals, educators, and the food industry is getting the message to minority communities that suffer higher rates of chronic illnesses most often related to diet.

Messages must be culturally sensitive to be effective. For minority communities, cultural identities may be closely linked to traditional customs, including foods, and the reluctance to change eating habits may be great. For many minorities, the source of the information is a large element in evaluating its relevance and worth.[13] For groups where language presents barriers, including many Hispanics and Asians, simply reaching these audiences with information is a challenge. Food cost and preparation time are issues with some minorities, and they need food choices that make it affordable and convenient to eat more healthfully. Grant indicates that a mixture of commitment, cultural sensitivity, community involvement, and cooperative efforts can lead to success in minority nutrition and health education, especially when something "creative and unique is thrown in for good measure."[23] The Sisters Together Calendar Case Study at the end of this chapter illustrates an effective community program for minorities that is culturally sensitive and geared toward the target audience's health problems.

Producing Materials for Ethnic Minorities

Although every target audience needs separate consideration to some extent, ethnic minorities may require special messages and materials. These audiences may benefit from the following considerations:[13,23]

- Interaction with the target audiences and intermediaries (community members and leaders) familiar with them is especially important in working with ethnic minorities.
- Do not assume that "conventional wisdom," published research studies, or "common knowledge" will hold true for ethnic minority audiences. The degree of assimilation and "mainstreaming" is ever-changing, so current information will be needed to choose the best channels and message strategies.
- Use of language and graphics may vary for different cultural groups (e.g., a word or illustration may have a different meaning to different groups).

- Using bilingual materials will ensure that intermediaries and family members who are most comfortable with English can help the reader understand the message content.
- Print materials should never be simply translated from the English; concepts and appeals may differ by culture just as the words do.
- Difference in target groups extend beyond language to include diverse values and customs, needs, and beliefs.

Stage 4: Implementing the Program

As preparations are being completed to introduce a program, a number of actions occur simultaneously. These actions should address the following concerns:

- Do you have a list of all the relevant media outlets to be contacted?
- Does every organization that should be involved know about your program?
- Have you prepared the staff and others to respond to inquiries?
- Do you have sufficient materials to start the program and to respond (i.e, press kits, leaflets for the public)?
- Are the materials in place (i.e., in television stations, physicians' offices, schools or supermarkets)?
- Are health/nutrition professionals in the community aware of the new program and prepared to respond if asked?
- Do you have mechanisms in place to track progress (i.e., number and nature of inquiries) and identify potential problems (e.g., insufficient supply of materials)?

When all issues have been addressed and a complete implementation schedule developed, the program "kickoff" may begin. The program kickoff can accomplish more than just the message introduction. In the Sisters Together case study, the kickoff was used creatively for multiple purposes such as qualitative research on the calendar, obtaining mailing lists, pretesting materials in progress, and looking for partnerships to make the program successful.

Establishing Process Evaluation Measures   To help avoid overall program dysfunction because specific tactics aren't working, program checks should be put in place. Checks may be placed to verify work performed, time schedules, and functioning and quality of response systems (such as distribution and inquiries from consumers). Other strategies that may be helpful in program implementation include conducting weekly materials inventory review and using 'bounceback' cards or follow-up phone calls to identify problems and monitor interest.

Working with Intermediaries (other Groups) To reach a target audience, working with organizations and individuals outside of the agency where you are employed is usually necessary. These organizations (e.g., television stations, hospitals, or PTA) or individuals (e.g., public health nutritionist, extension service, or family physician) are intermediary channels to reach target audiences. It is also important to consider cooperative ventures with the business sector (industry) that will benefit both your program and the company. Private sector companies with an interest in health information include supermarkets; insurance companies; hospitals; managed care groups; and producers of pharmaceuticals, foods, and other health-related products. Table 17.4 describes the types of intermediary organizations and activities to consider in health communication programs.

Review and Revise Program Components Whether or not other media outlets or organizations are involved in the program, it is important to periodically assess whether activities are "on track" and on time, if the target audience is being reached, what aspects of the program need alteration or elimination, and if time schedules and budgets are being met.

Stage 5: Assessing Effectiveness

The process measures discussed in stage 4 were designed to monitor the program by tracking the number of materials distributed, meeting attendance, and so forth. These measures will not provide information on the program effects (whether the target audience learned, acted, or made a change as a result of the program). Therefore, it is important to evaluate the results of your program—its effects on outcomes.

Outcome **evaluation** methodologies casually consist of a comparison between the target audience awareness, attitudes, and behavior before and after the program. Going a step beyond process measures, outcomes evaluation should provide more information about value than quantity of activity. The discussion on evaluation and what types of evaluation should be completed should take place in the initial stages of the program. Chapter 15 "Evaluating Nutrition Services" presents extensive coverage of the evaluation process.

Determining What Evaluations to Do

Every program planner faces constraints to undertaking evaluation tasks. These constraints may include limited funds, staff time, and capabilities; lack of management support for well-designed evaluation activities; and difficulties in separating the effects of program influences from other influences on the target audience in "real-world" situations.

Some of the questions that should be considered before deciding what kind of evaluation will be used to test the program include these in box 17.7.

Stage 6: Feedback to Refine Program

If the program is continuing or if similar programs are planned, take the time to apply what has been learned.

- Reassess goals and objectives.
  - Has anything changed (e.g., with the target audience, the community or your agency's mission) to require revisions to the original goals and objectives?
  - Is there new information about the health issue that should be incorporated into program messages or design?
- Identify effective activities or strategies.
  - Which objectives have been met as a result of successful activities?
  - Can they be expanded to apply to other audiences or situations?
- Determine areas where additional effort is needed.
  - Are there objectives that are not being met? Why?
  - Are there strategies or activities that did not succeed? Are more resources required? Do you need to review why they didn't work and what can be done to correct any problems?
- Compare costs and results of different activities.
  - What were the relative costs (including staff time) and results of different aspects of your program?
  - Are there some activities that appear to work as well but cost less than others?
- Reaffirm support for the program.
  - Have you shared the results of your activities with the leadership of your agency?
  - Did you remember to share this information with the individuals and organizations outside your agency who contributed?
  - Do you have evidence of program effectiveness and continued need to convince your agency to continue the program?
  - Do you have new or continuing activities that suggest the involvement of additional organizations?
- Determine to end a program that did not work.

TABLE 17.4

Types of Organizations and Activities to Consider in Health Communication Programs

Voluntary health associations—such as the American Cancer Society, the American Heart Association, the American Lung Association, the March of Dimes

Professional associations—local medical societies and chapters of the American Academy of Family Physicians and the American Academy of Pediatrics

Public health professionals—local health officers/department, school nurses, health teachers, university teachers, and departments of public health

Health-related institutions—hospitals, HMOs, insurance companies, YMCAs and YWCAs, other fitness centers

Nonhealth industries—television and radio stations, newspapers, employee assistance programs or personnel department of major employers, and labor unions

Nonhealth organizations—PTAs, 4H clubs, boys clubs, church groups, and other organizations concerned with youth and/or parents; fraternal organizations or other social/cultural groups related to the target audience; and public libraries

Suggested Activities

Planning

- Join program development committee
- Collect data to help target the program
- Assess community health and other resources
- Identify health and other organizations and media outlets in the community
- Identify available, appropriate health communication materials
- Help pretest materials

Resource Development

- "Recruit" volunteers, organizations, and media to participate in the program and/or provide "in-kind" contributions (e.g., printing, collating, mailing services, public service space, or time in media)
- Help raise funds
- Contribute staff or volunteer time

Program Implementation/Publicity and Promotion

- Provide conference rooms/space for program meetings and activities
- Join program development committee
- Organize or participate in attention-getting events (e.g., health fairs and press conferences)
- Prepare press releases
- Prepare exhibits for public places (e.g., shopping malls, building lobbies, schools, and public libraries)
- Distribute materials
- Write letters
- Publish articles in newsletters
- Sponsor presentations
- Offer individual counseling
- Provide recognized, credible spokesperson
- Provide media interview

Tracking and Follow-up

- Provide computer or manual services for program tracking
- Identify and train other organizations interesting in becoming involved
- Follow-up by telephone with participants to assure continued involvement
- Serve on "thank you" committee

Source: From National Cancer Institute, USDHHS: *Making health communications programs work: a planner's guide,* NIH Publication No. 89–1493, Washington, DC, 1992, Office of Cancer Communications.

Share What Has Been Learned   It is important to share what has been learned from implementing a communications program. Consider sharing information about what you have learned with the intermediaries who have worked with you. Develop a short paper for appropriate nutrition, public health, medical, and health education journals. Present results to state and local nutrition and public health associations. Letting others know about the program may prompt them to describe similar experiences, lessons, new ideas, or potential resources for further programs.

Food, Nutrition, and Health Misinformation   There are an overwhelming number of food, nutrition, and health messages that reach the public daily. Some of these messages are inaccurate, deceptive, controversial and often based on emotion or marketing, not on science. In a position paper on food and **nutrition misinformation,** the American Dietetic Association stated "Nutrition misinformation, misbeliefs, frauds and quackery prevent the public from attaining optimal nutritional health."[27]

Food has long been endowed with metaphysical, moral, and theological meaning. The folklore and tradi-

BOX 17.7

CONSIDERATIONS TO DECIDE TYPE OF EVALUATION

- How long will the program last? Will the implementation phase be long enough to permit measurement of significant effects and periodic adjustment?
- Will the program be repeated or continued?
- Are the objectives measurable in the foreseeable future?
- What program components are most important?
- Is there management support or public demand for program accountability?
- What aspects of the program fit best with your agency's priorities?
- Will an evaluation report help communication efforts compete with other agency priorities for future funding?

BOX 17.8

TERMS ASSOCIATED WITH MISINFORMATION

Nutrition facts are those that have been established using the scientific method.

Nutrition misinformation consists of erroneous statements or misinterpretation of nutrition science.

Food faddism is a dietary practice based on an exaggerated belief in the effects of nutrition on health and disease. These are beliefs that special attributes of a particular food may cure disease, that certain foods should be eliminated from the diet because they are harmful, and that certain foods confer unique health benefits.[27]

Food quackery is the promotion for profit of special foods, products, processes, or appliances with false or misleading health or therapeutic claims. Food quackery is exploitive and entrepreneurial.[34]

Health fraud shares many of the characteristics of food faddism and food quackery, yet it is always deliberate and done for financial gain. In cases of health fraud, a person or group knowingly disseminate erroneous nutrition information or make false claims of nutrition benefits.[34]

tions of cultures throughout history have attributed healing and harmful properties to certain foods. Food folklore continues today despite enormous advances that have been made with the sciences of food and nutrition. Contemporary food fads often make claims that are not substantiated by available scientific evidence.[34]

Angell has indicated that Americans follow news of medical research as closely as sports and the stock market.[2] Consumers are particularly avid for new findings about the health effects of diet and lifestyle because Americans have come to believe that good health is a matter of doing the right thing with the corollary that illness is a failure of some sort.

Therefore, effective communications must be based on sound scientific principles and findings to counter the effects of inaccurate messages, and need to present medical research findings in a clear and appropriate manner.

The terms in box 17.8 are associated with food, nutrition, and health misinformation.

Factors Contributing to Nutrition Quackery and Health Fraud At least four problems promote the growth of quackery.[30] These include the first amendment (right of free speech), loose use of the term "nutritionist," misrepresentation of scientific studies, and the vague definition of a dietary supplement.

Freedom of Speech Two forms of misinformation are protected by the First Amendment, which guarantees

the right to free speech. First, nutrition books published for the public can be grossly inaccurate. Second, nutrition misinformation is often disseminated as promotional material with dietary supplements, herbal remedies, or special preparations for weight control, constituting a form of hidden advertising.[19]

Inappropriate Use of Term "Nutritionist" The title "nutritionist" is not regulated in many states and, as a result, anyone may call themselves a nutritionist. Nutrition advisors with dubious credentials represent themselves as being legitimate nutritionists.

Misrepresentation of Scientific Studies Some research scientists go public with their findings before their study can be duplicated and the results confirmed. One research study or one epidemiological survey does not prove a scientific theory. The public does not know what to believe because, unfortunately, much of the public does not understand the scientific method and does not know how to interpret scientific data (if and when it is provided).[30]

Goldberg and Shuman completed a paper entitled "Is Anything Safe to Eat? Making Sense of the Research,"[12] for FANSA on how to interpret scientific evidence. (The Food and Nutrition Science Alliance [FANSA] is comprised of four professional societies: the American Dietetic Association [ADA], the American Society for Clinical Nutrition [ASCN], the American Society for Nutritional Science [ASNS], and the Institute of Food Technologists [IFT]. The purpose of FANSA is to provide consumers with consistent, accurate nutrition information.) The paper appears in Appendix G and can be used for the lay public in helping consumers to understand the science. In addition, chapter 3 "Community Assessment: Clinical and Epidemiological Approaches" describes sound scientific methods.

FANSA, concerned about the proliferation of reports that exaggerate and distort science, issued a list of ten red flags to help consumers spot "junk" science[11] (see box 17.9). The group indicated that any combination of these red flags should raise suspicion about the accuracy of the information.

Dietary Supplements   There is no legal definition of a dietary supplement at the present time. In addition, legislation now pending in Congress on health claims for supplements would be less strict than those required by the Nutrition Labeling and Education Act (NLEA). A significant problem with the proposed bills in Congress is that the burden of proof of safety would be the overburdened FDA, not the manufacturers.[10,14,26] All of

---

BOX 17.9

RED FLAGS FOR SPOTTING "JUNK" SCIENCE[11]

- Recommendations that promise a quick fix.
- Dire warnings of danger from a single product or regimen.
- Claims that sound too good to be true.
- Simplistic conclusions drawn from a complex study.
- Recommendations based on a single study.
- Dramatic statements that are refuted by reputable scientific organizations.
- Lists of "good" or "bad" foods.
- Recommendations made to help sell a product.
- Recommendations based on studies published without peer review.
- Recommendations from studies that ignore differences among individuals or groups.

---

these issues lead to confusion about and lack of control over supplement use.

Food supplements in the form of food adjuncts have a long history in the practice of medicine. In contrast, the use of dietary supplements, primarily vitamins and minerals, is a phenomenon that has evolved during the last half century. This phenomenon reflects the advances in our knowledge of nutrition science; our knowledge and understanding of vitamins and minerals; the growing recognition of the role that some nutrients play in energy metabolism, immune function, and psychological effects; and the growing trend for people to take responsibility for their own health. As a result, there has been a major growth in the sales of supplements in recent decades. In 1993, some 60 million Americans spent $4 billion on dietary supplement products available in virtually all groceries and pharmacies, by mail order, door-to-door sales, and in health food stores.[26]

For certain segments of the population who are identified at high nutritional risk, dietary supplements may be part of therapy. For example, folate is beneficial for women of childbearing age and iron is recommended for older infants and toddlers.[26] However, many consumers self-prescribe supplements for various reasons including concern about the adequacy of their diet, a desire to prevent or treat illness, or a desire to be more healthy. Herbal remedies represent one of the many ways that consumers medicate themselves. At present, many herbal remedies are not sold in standardized doses in the United States. Consumers may be unaware of possible side effects that could result from taking these products. They may be toxic to the liver and affect response to other medications.[26]

Indiscriminate use of dietary supplements raises safety and economic questions. Since there is no cap on potency of dietary supplements, many high-potency (up to several hundred times the RDA) are promoted for a variety of reasons, many of which are not related to possible health benefits. History is replete with overzealous use of nutritional supplements resulting in adverse rather than beneficial effects. There is a need for emphasis on public education that stresses the scientific basis for any dietary supplement to ensure nutritional safety for individuals using dietary supplements.

Harmful Effects of Health Fraud   Health fraud, including food faddism and quackery, has become big business in the United States. Twenty-five years ago, quackery was said to cost $1 to $2 billion a year. Today, it probably totals at least $10 billion.[17] A substantial portion of the health fraud is nutrition related. Louis Harris and Associates studied American adults use of questionable health products for fifteen different conditions and found that nutrition products were by far the most commonly misused.[17]

Health consequences of quackery may result from failure to seek legitimate medical care or continue essential treatment, effects of nutritional toxicities or potentially toxic components of products, undesirable nutritional-drug interaction, nutrient deficiencies, and interference with scientifically based nutrition education and assistance. Economic harm occurs when purported remedies and cures do not work and when products are purchased needlessly. Another potential harm results when public opinion based on conflicting information affects public policies including resource allocation, legislation, and law enforcement. Lawmakers have to sort through a mass of facts and misinformation to shape legislation.

Alternative (or "Complementary") Medicine   Complementary medicine has been flourishing in the United States for several decades. The term complementary medicine covers a broad range of healing philosophies and approaches. Some approaches are consistent with physiological principles of Western medicine, while others constitute independent healing systems. Examples of complementary or **alternative medicine** include macrobiotics, biofeedback, yoga, meditation, acupuncture, aromatherapy, chelation therapy, and homeopathic and naturopathic medicine.

To address the growing interest in alternative forms of medical care, the Office of Alternative Medicine (OAM) was initiated through congressional mandate under the FY1992 National Institutes of Health (NIH) appropriations bill. The congressional mandate establishing the OAM stated that the office's purpose is to "facilitate the evaluation of alternative medical treatment modalities" for the purpose of determining their effectiveness and to help integrate effective treatments into mainstream medical practice.

The Role of Community Nutrition Professionals
Community nutrition professionals need to take an active role in helping consumers recognize misinformation. Qualified processionals in partnership with other members of the health care team, educators, and representatives of the food industry can be a forceful voice against food and nutrition misinformation. Consumers need to be aware of credible sources of nutrition information. This can be done by directing the media and consumers to these sources.

BUILDING COMMUNICATION SKILLS

To become effective communicators, community nutrition professional must develop skills that enable them to be heard above all of the competing, and often conflicting, nutrition messages that consumers receive on a daily basis.[28]

The ADA has developed several documents that can assist the practitioner with skill building. *Communicating as Professionals* provides comprehensive discussions on how to communicate in various settings; its a primer for community nutrition professionals who want to develop these skills effectively.[6] *The Competitive Edge: Advanced Marketing for Dietetic Professionals*[14] and the chapter by Simko and Gilbride on "Bringing Research into Practice"[31] are invaluable resources for the community nutrition professional.

Oral Communication

Deborah Tannen, a professor at Georgetown University in Washington, D.C., has indicated that **oral communication** isn't as simple as saying what you mean. How you say what you mean is critical, and differs from one person to the next, because using language is learned social behavior.[32] Sarnoff suggests that there are four positive "vibes" that a commanding speaker gives out[29] (see box 17.10).

BOX 17.10

FOUR POSITIVE VIBES FROM COMMANDING SPEAKERS

- *Joy and Ease*. If a speaker isn't comfortable, you feel uncomfortable listening to them. When the speaker is at ease and seems to enjoy presenting to you, you feel at ease.
- *Sincerity, Credibility, and Concern*. These create instant trust.
- *Enthusiasm*. Enthusiasm, energy, intensity, and belief in yourself infect the listener. The expression "fire in the belly" describes the enthusiasm that is considered the greatest business asset in the world.
- *Authority*. Authority communicates the message. It says to the listener that "I know that I know."

Becoming an Effective Speaker   Effective speech delivery blends the verbal message with appropriate, complimentary nonverbal communication. In fact, more than half of all communication takes place on the nonverbal level. Mannerisms and physical behavior make messages more meaningful and memorable, and provide visual stimuli that capture your audience's attention.[18] It is important that your posture, gestures, facial expressions, and eye contact be natural, varied, and help convey the essence of your message.

Presentation to Professional Audience   Professional audience formats include lectures, workshops, and roundtable skill workshops, among others. Regardless of format, keep in mind that the audience is the most important factor, so you must know your audience and tailor messages to them. Visual support almost always enhances an oral presentation for professional audiences and should be used to add depth to the presentation.[6]

Presentation to the General Public   Planning a speech for a general audience begins with a clear focus on the central idea you want to convey. Analyzing your audience is critical to successful presentation planning and delivery. Two common errors made in presentations to the general public include speaking in "nutrition jargon" and audience overload.

Nutrition Jargon   As community nutrition professionals, we often use terms that may not be understood by the audience. For example, in a presentation on nutrition and cardiovascular disease, we may lapse into the LDL *versus* HDL cholesterol discussion. What is more meaningful for a lay audience is to discuss the "good" cholesterol and the "bad" cholesterol.

Audience Overload   Conveying too much material in a short time is a real problem for an audience. Select a few major points and reinforce them.

Developing the Presentation

The success of a presentation is judged by one criterion: whether the audience believes it got the information it came for. A speech has three main parts: an opening or introduction, a body or middle, and a summary or conclusion. Clear organization and logical flow of information that follow the format are essential to a good presentation. The following simple speech format works every time.[4]

- Tell them what your are going to tell them.
- Tell them.
- Tell them what you told them.

Delivering quality oral presentations requires adequate preparation and practice. To reiterate, the six steps for successful presentations include:

- Know your audience.
- Know your topic.
- Organize your presentation to include an introduction, middle, and summary or conclusion.
- Choose and use appropriate visual aids.
- Practice your presentation.
- Deliver your presentation with enthusiasm.

Media Presentations

In **media presentations** one of the keys to success is communicating in "sound bites," which are concise statements that effectively capture your primary message. For example, the message

> Children like sweet breakfast cereals but parents should encourage their children to eat cereals that are less sweet and higher in fiber.

can be reduced to

> Look for cereals that are low in sugar and high in fiber.

Mastering this skill can help community nutrition professionals improve their skills in any setting. The ability to distill and communicate the essence of a complicated issue in consumer-friendly terms in thirty seconds is a skill of benefit to any presentation in any work setting.[8]

Carolyn O'Neil, a registered dietitian and Executive Producer and Correspondent, at Cable News Network (CNN), indicates that the communicator has to think how the message can be summarized in twenty-five words or less. This helps identify the "take home message," the bottom line that message receivers will remember.[24]

The better one knows his or her message, the easier it will be to communicate it to the media. Start by identifying a SOCO (single overriding communication objective). For example, in an interview on heart disease, the SOCO might be for the audience to know which foods tend to be high in fat. Next, develop three key message points that support the SOCO and form the backbone of the interview. Review the message points before the interview, putting them in consumer-friendly language and rehearsing them so that they will flow easily during the interview.[15] Table 17.5 presents additional examples.

TABLE 17.5
Examples of SOCOs Development for Media Interviews

Topic	SOCO	Message points
Heart disease	"Know your numbers"	• Cholesterol testing is as close as the local doctor's office.
		• Diet can make a difference in lowering your number.
Picnics	"Make your picnic safer and healthier"	• Dietetics professionals are your best resource.
		• Keep hot foods hot and cold foods cold.
		• Look for lower fat burger and hot dog options.
		• Plan plenty of physical activity for children of all ages.

Source: © 1994, The American Dietetic Association. *Communicating as professionals.* Used by permission.

Ask the following questions as you develop message points:

- Who will be listening to or watching the interview?
- What are they interested in? What are they interested in knowing?
- What is the news or human interest angle of the story?
- Which visuals would help make a point?

Broadcast Interviews

On television, appearances can be more powerful than facts. How you say something and how you look saying it can have more impact on the perceptions of the audience than what you say.

On radio, the quality of your voice greatly affects how listeners "see" you. Your vocal tone, inflection, volume, and conversational style should communicate your concern, confidence, honesty, and authority (see box 17.11).

Cultivating Media Relations

Opportunities to work with the media come in many different ways. The key is to be responsive and make yourself available. Sometimes, the media will call on you to answer a question. Other times, they may want you to appear personally. People in the media like to receive mail. It alerts them to stories that have made an impression on their audiences. A topic that generates many letters from their audience is sure to be covered again and again.

As a community nutrition professional, you have the responsibility to know the broadcast media in your community and to work with them as often as possible. When you receive a call from the news media, follow established guidelines and contact the communications department for further assistance. Table 17.6 provides information needed to work with the media effectively.

BOX 17.11

TALKING FOR BROADCASTING

- *Be Positive*—Be candid and confident. Show your conviction.
- *Be Specific*—Use facts, examples, easily understood statistics, analogies or anecdotes to illustrate your point.
- *Be Right*—Your credibility is at stake. Don't lie, exaggerate, or mislead.
- *Be Human*—Be open, likable, and concerned. Find common ground with the audience.
- *Be Quotable*—Tell stories. Don't lecture. Keep it conversational. Use first-person, active tense ("I believe . . . We try").
- *Be Calm*—Ghandi is credited with saying: "When you're in the right, you can afford to keep your temper. When you're in the wrong, you can't afford to lose it."

Written Communications

Good writing comes from training and practice. Every community nutrition professional must be capable of producing clear **written communications.** The best way to approach a writing project is to clarify why you are writing (your objective), who the audience is, what the format and content should be, and how you'll write (attitude and diction).[3]

Why? Your Purpose The first thing that should be done is to write a clear statement of purpose or what you hope to accomplish. Its only to keep you on track, not a part of the finished product. For example, it may be your goal to have clients know about the Step One Diet for cardiovascular disease risk or to motivate clients to use Step One as part of their lifestyle pattern.

TABLE 17.6
Media Reference Card

ASK QUESTIONS AND TAKE NOTES
Be sure you understand:
- *Who* is calling and her or his telephone number
- *What* publication or broadcast station the caller represents
- *Why* the reporter wants to interview you
- *What information* is being requested (statistics, background, personal opinion, organizational policy, reaction to an event or disclosure)
- *What* is the reason for doing the story
- *Who else* is being contacted for information (associates, competitors)
- *When and where* will the interview be held
- *How long* the interview would take
- The *deadline*
- The probable *time* or *date* of publication or broadcast

DO NOT ANSWER IMMEDIATELY IF YOU ARE NOT WELL-PREPARED
A timely answer is important but you do not have to answer on the spot. Tell the caller you are busy at the moment but you will call back by a certain time. Or you may want to schedule a person-to-person interview.

ESTABLISH ANY GROUND RULES IN ADVANCE such as length of interview, whether you will be filmed or photographed, topics you cannot discuss. Assume everything you say will be on the record.
ANTICIPATE DIFFICULT QUESTIONS What are your answers to them?
PREPARE ONE TO THREE KEY MESSAGES Make them as positive as possible.
REHEARSE IF TIME PERMITS Have someone ask you sample questions.
ANSWER TRUTHFULLY Do not mislead with an answer. Be accurate.
ANSWER CLEARLY AND CONCISELY State the important facts first. Have statistics, examples, comparisons, or other backup information available for follow-up questions.
IF YOU DO NOT KNOW THE ANSWER TO A QUESTION, ADMIT IT If appropriate, say you will check on it and call back.
At the end, **ENCOURAGE THE REPORTER TO CALL BACK** if any clarification is needed.

Source: Adapted from Shandwick: *Management communication training*. Minneapolis, MN.

Who? Your Readers   Understanding your target audience is critical. You'll need to know the demographics, gender, age, ethnic background, subject knowledge, and the like about your audience. Another point to consider is where and when they will most likely be reading your message and if there are other materials on the same subject that are competing for their attention.

What? Appropriate Form and Content   Identifying "why" and "who" will go a long way toward helping you select the "what."[3] Ask yourself what information your readers need to achieve the desired results. A detailed outline is an important goal at this stage. The outline should take into consideration whether some information would be best presented graphically. Plan to write the introduction and the title last.

How? Diction and Attitude   Before you begin writing a specific piece, determine the vocabulary that is appropriate to you readership and to the format in which the writing will be presented. For example, a column on osteoporosis written for a booklet sent to persons who have osteoporosis could assume that the audience is familiar with the disease and the recommended diet. To create a sense of intimacy, use first and second person primarily. "You will benefit from consuming a diet high in calcium." If you need to distance yourself, use a pas-

sive voice. "The reduction in funds for the program was made because of a smaller tax base." This doesn't let the reader know who specifically made the decision to reduce funding. Be aware that the use of passive voice may sometimes lead to weak and unclear writing.[3,7]

Writing for the Lay Press

With food, nutrition, and health issues constantly in the news today, there are many opportunities for community nutrition professionals to get their "foot in the door." Having a fresh idea and being able to deliver it in words that readers understand is key to getting something published.[33] To come up with a novel idea or a new angle on an old or existing problem begins with listening to the consumers you see on a daily basis. In addition to listening to the consumer, keeping abreast of trends, scientific literature, and current events is a must. Ideas generated from reading and listening can be refined in the following ways:[33]

- Build on new research by finding a way to make it relevant and understandable to the average consumer.
- Localize a national story for a regional publication.
- Take a seasonal angle on topics. For example, topics on eating healthfully could highlight available fruits and vegetables.

Writing for Newpapers and Magazines

Deadlines Daily newspapers have a much shorter turnaround time than do monthly magazines. A feature story in the newspaper may be published the week after completion, whereas a completed story for a national magazine will not be published for three to six months.

Editing differences Newspapers, with their quick deadlines, will often undergo just one editing. If you are working with the food editor of a small paper, he or she may be the only staff person. Magazine pieces often undergo several layers of editing. If any questions or problems are spotted, the article goes back to the writer for revision.

Service Service articles provide information that readers can incorporate into their lives. Newspapers do more reporting of facts, events, and studies geared toward a general audience; magazines tend to provide how-to service articles that are geared to specific readers.[25,33]

Guidelines for Writing for Newspaper/Magazine Columns

- *Outline*—Organizing your thoughts and developing an outline is the best way to begin.
- *Sources*—Build credibility into an article by quoting references, such as research papers found in nutrition and medical journals. You may want to contact the researcher who did the work for a quote.
- *Writing*—Write copy that flows and use a good lead or an exciting opening to draw the reader (or editor) into the story. Leads include amazing statements, anecdotes, questions, wordplay, paradox, and late breaking news.
- *Highlight*—Articles made up solely of text can become tedious and difficult to read. Highlighting copy by underlining words, using bullets, sidebars, and simple graphs or charts can add interest and retain the reader's attention.
- *Revisions*—Rewrites and revisions are a way of life in writing for scientific journals and magazines.[33] These processes help refine and tailor communication messages.

Writing News or Press Releases

The news release is the main form of communication between the community nutrition professional and the media. It is used to announce the results of data gather-

TABLE 17.7
Guidelines for Writing a News or Press Release

- Print on regular sized paper ($8^1/_2''$ by $11''$).
- Write about 300 words for news story and 700 words for a feature story.
- Type your organization, name and title, address, and your telephone and fax numbers and e-mail address in the top right corner.
- Skip four lines, then on the left side of the page, type the date the news release is sent to the media and, in capital letters, the date the news can be released to the public (e.g., FOR IMMEDIATE RELEASE or FOR RELEASE FRIDAY 18 SEPTEMBER 1997).
- Continuing on the left side of the page, skip two lines and type a catchy title in capital letters.
- Then follow the guidelines for writing a news story, using a "hook." Writing should be simple and descriptive for quick reading. Use quotes from individuals to emphasize main points. Write in the third person.
- If release is longer than one page, type "—more—" at the bottom of the first page, and "—end—" at the end of the release. Ideally, a news release shouldn't be more than two pages long.
- Proofread carefully for spelling, grammatical, and typing errors, and double check all facts and figures.
- When writing a news release, include the name of your organization as frequently as possible. You want to publicize not only the primary message but the good work coming out of your organization.

ing, the outcome of a community meeting, or an upcoming event. If the data are to be published in a refereed journal, the professional community should receive the information prior to press notification. A well-written release can generate huge publicity at relatively little cost. Because the news media is bombarded with releases from all over the country, use of an established format is vital to ensure that the release is read.[16] Table 17.7 presents guidelines for writing news or press releases.

IMPLICATIONS FOR COMMUNITY NUTRITION PROFESSIONALS

Communicating effectively about nutrition and health is a major function of the community nutrition professional. Understanding the communication process, including the barriers, is necessary to be successful in communicating. Empathy, listening, observation, word choice, body language, and action are all involved in improving communication.

Health communication programs designed to promote changes in health behavior and to encourage early detection and prompt treatment of illness have demonstrated that communication strategies can be effective in reducing the risk of serious illness. Health communication programs can be designed to inform, influence, and motivate public audiences. A six-stage process is described to effectively plan and implement communication programs. The process is based on an understanding of the needs and perceptions of the target audience. The stages in health communication development include planning and strategy selection, determining channels and materials, developing and pretesting materials, implementing the program, assessing effectiveness, and providing feedback to refine the program.

To determine the best format for a program, consideration must be given to the message, its complexity, its purpose, the audience, the channels, and the available resources

Nutrition misinformation, which consists of erroneous statements or misinterpretation of nutrition science, is a major problem in developing healthy lifestyles in communities. Alternative or complimentary medicine has been flourishing in the United States. Some therapies are far outside the realm of accepted medical theory and practice and may pose some health hazards to individuals.

The community nutrition professional must communicate scientific information in both oral and written forms at levels appropriate for different audiences including the general public. Knowledge of media strategies using various communication channels, such as print, radio, television, and videotape will enhance the nutrition professional's ability to communicate effectively and to achieve health and nutrition outcomes.

COMMUNITY NUTRITION PROFESSIONALS IN ACTION

- Develop a scenario with a group of your classmates (three to four) and present to the class a demonstration of how the barriers to communication (behavioral, language, and psychological) can make communications ineffective.
- Using the scenario from the previous action, show how the barriers can be overcome by utilizing the skills (such as empathy, listening, body language, etc.) necessary to improve communications.
- Compare and contrast what health communications can and cannot do in disease prevention and health promotion.

- Describe the six stages in health communications. Determine the important elements in each stage that are necessary to design a program that will work.
- Compare and contrast the characteristics of mass media channels including radio, television, magazines, and newspapers.
- Describe the factors affecting public acceptance of health messages.
- Develop two health messages for cardiovascular disease in adults giving consideration to the desired outcome you want to achieve. Also, consider the factors of clarity and consistency in developing these messages.
- Identify the strategies needed to develop successful educational messages and materials for minority communities.
- Review the factors contributing to nutrition misinformation and quackery. Monitor the 6 P.M. television news for one week and identify a story or commentary that may have contributed to nutrition misinformation.
- Monitor your local daily newspaper for one week and identify any stories or advertisements that could be classified as alternative or complimentary medicine.
- Develop three sound bites on nutrition that may be used in broadcast media for a TV show on teen pregnancy.
- Identify the four positive messages ("vibes") that a speaker should project when presenting information to an audience.
- Develop a press release for a program in which you have been involved. Highlight the results of your activities and who benefited from the program. Determine where the press release should be sent based on the population that was served by the program.

GOING ONE STEP FURTHER

- Using the six stages in the health communication process, design a communication program for a community that has a high prevalence of cardiovascular disease risk. Its a group of adults who do not exercise, eat whatever tastes good, and dismiss all the health advice they have heard because it is confusing. Consider reviewing the existing data on the group and identify gaps in data before completing your plan. Review the factors affecting public acceptance of health messages and construct your message(s) with clarity and consistency. Select a channel or channels of communication that will best suit the audience based on the data that you have gathered. Present your program to the class and have them give feedback on each of the six stages.

- Develop a series of health messages (five to eight) for a minority population in your community. Select the message types based on the health problems that affect the community. Identify the needs, values, and beliefs among the group before you complete your planning. Identify a person or persons in the minority community who will be willing to work with you on this project. Pretest your ideas with the person you have selected to assist you. Review the information in chapter 18, "Working Effectively in Cross-Cultural and Multicultural Settings," before you embark on the program.
- Select a media channel (radio, TV, magazine, or newspaper) where you feel misinformation has been given on a nutrition issue. Write a letter to the channel indicating why you object to the reporting, citing appropriate scientific information to bolster your objections. Present your draft letter to the instructor and class for input before you proceed with the letter so that you can make a strong case in support of science.

ADDITIONAL INFORMATION

Several professional organizations have trained members to work on communicating sound health, nutrition, and food safety information to the media.

The American Dietetic Association (ADA)

The ADA spokespeople provide accurate food and nutrition information to the media in the United States using a region approach. In addition, state media representatives deal with the state and local media.

The ADA develops position papers and timely statements for its members and the public. The following position papers relate to communications:

1. Nutrition education for the public, *J Am Diet Assoc* 96:1183, 1996.
2. Food and nutrition misinformation, *J Am Diet Assoc* 95:705, 1995.

The American Society for Clinical Nutrition (ASCN) and the American Society for Nutritional Science (ASNS)

The ASCN and the ASNS have a joint Public Information Committee that has published a *Guide to Experts* (2nd edition), which identifies nutrition professionals with specialized knowledge in nutrition science and clinical nutrition. This guide is available to all members of the mass media.

Institute of Food Technologists (IFT)

The IFT has a national network of eighty scientists trained to deliver credible and timely messages to the news media and lawmakers. The IFT develops Scientific Status Summaries for its members. The following Scientific Status Summary relates to communication:

1. Assessing, managing and communicating chemical food risk, *Food Technology* 51:85–92, 1997.

REFERENCES

1. Allen AM: The new nutrition facts label in the print media: a content analysis, *J Am Diet Assoc* 95:348–51, 1995.
2. Angell M: Overdosing on health risks, *New York Times Magazine,* May 4, 1997, p. 45.
3. Beuoy C: *Keys to good writing.* In Chernoff R, editor: *Communicating as professionals,* ed 2, Chicago, 1994, The American Dietetic Association, pp. 44–55.
4. Brown MB: *Presentation to the general public.* In Cherenoff R, editor: *Communicating as professionals,* ed 2, Chicago, 1994, The American Dietetic Association, pp. 12–34.
5. *Changing channels: how the media report on food safety and nutrition,* Washington, DC, 1996, Food Insights, International Food Information Council (IFIC).
6. Chernoff RC, editor: *Communicating as professionals,* ed 2, Chicago, 1994, The American Dietetic Association.
7. *Chicago Manual of Style,* ed 14, Chicago, 1993, University of Chicago Press.
8. Derelian D: President's page: demonstrating leadership by working with the media, *J Am Diet Assoc* 95:597, 1995.
9. The Dietary Guideline Alliance: *A handbook for nutrition and food communicators: reaching consumers with meaningful health messages, Chicago, 1996, The American Dietetic Association.*
10. Dietary supplement regulations 59(002), *Federal Register.* 350–437, 1994.
11. Food and Nutrition Science Alliance (FANSA): *Junk science: scientists issue 10 red flags for consumers,* Chicago, 1995, FANSA.
12. Goldberg JP, Shuman JM: *Is anything safe to eat: understanding the research,* Washington, DC, 1997, Food and Nutrition Science Alliance.
13. Grant A: *In a different voice: reaching minority audiences,* Washington, DC, 1996, Food Insight, International Food Information Council Foundation.
14. Helm KK: *The competitive edge: advanced marketing for dietetics processionals,* ed 2, Chicago, 1995, The American Dietetic Association.
15. Hermann M, Levy GA: *Media presentations.* In Chernoff R, editor: *Communicating as professionals,* ed 2, Chicago, 1994, The American Dietetic Association, pp. 35.

16. Hudnall M: *News releases, advertising copy and brochures.* In Chernoff R, editor: *Communicating as professionals,* ed 2, Chicago, 1994, The American Dietetic Association, pp. 111–119.

17. Louis Harris and Associates: *Health information and use of questionable treatments: a study of the American public,* Washington, DC, 1987, USDHHS.

18. McNeal T: *Effective public speaking. Dietitians in business and communications,* Chicago, 1996, DBC Dimension.

19. Milner J: Devious claims—the anatomy of marketing schemes, *Nutrition Forum* 23:8–17, 1988.

20. Mizock M: What you aren't saying may be everything, *Data Management* 24:33, 1986.

21. Mondy RW, Premeaux SR: *Management: concepts, practice and skills,* ed 7, Englewood Cliffs, NJ, 1995, Prentice-Hall, Simon & Schuster.

22. Morreale SJ, Schwartz NE: *Helping America eat right: developing practical and actionable public education messages based on ADA Survey of American dietary habits,* Chicago, 1996, The American Dietetic Association.

23. National Cancer Institute, USDHHS: *Making health communication programs work: a planners guide,* NIH Publication no. 89–1493, Washington, DC, 1992, Office of Cancer Communications.

24. O'Neil C: Nutrition in broadcast journalism, *Top Clin Nutr* 10:55–59, 1995.

25. Petersen D: How to write the how to articles, *Writer's Digest* 83:110, 1992.

26. Position of the American Dietetic Association. Enrichment and fortification of food and dietary supplements, *J Am Diet Assoc* 94:661–663, 1994.

27. Position of the American Dietetic Association. Food and nutrition misinformation, *J Am Diet Assoc* 95:705–707, 1995.

28. Position of the American Dietetic Association. Nutrition education for the public, *J Am Diet Assoc* 96:1183–1187, 1996.

29. Sarnoff D: *Never be nervous again,* New York, 1987, Crown.

30. Short SH: Health quackery: our role as professionals, *J Am Diet Assoc* 94:607, 1994.

31. Simko MD, Gilbride JA: *Bridging research into practice.* In Monsen ER, editor: *Research successful approaches,* Chicago, 1991, The American Dietetic Association, pp. 421–431.

32. Tannen D: The power of talk: who gets ahead and why, *Harvard Business Review* Sept–Oct: 138–148, 1995.

33. Tribole E, Hermann M: *Writing for the lay press.* In Chernoff R, editor: *Communicating as professionals,* ed 2, Chicago, 1994, The American Dietetic Association, pp. 105–108.

34. *U.S. Surgeon General's report on nutrition and health,* DHHS Publication no. 88–50210, Washington, DC, 1988, USDHHS.

CASE STUDY

SISTERS TOGETHER CALENDAR

JEANNE P. GOLDBERG, PHD, RD AND
J. HELLWIG, MS, RD

TITLE: SISTERS TOGETHER: MOVE MORE, EAT BETTER

"Sisters Together" is a community-based health communication intervention to prevent obesity in Boston-area African-American women aged eighteen to thirty-five years.

DESCRIPTION

This case illustrates the creation of a twelve-month wall calendar as a tool to communicate the central messages of a community-based health campaign. The challenge in this case was to design a communications tool that was culturally sensitive, economical, and usable for the target audience, with the objective that the calendar would teach basic skills and, ultimately, facilitate behavior change in the target population.

OBJECTIVES

- To illustrate the role formative research plays in designing a health behavior intervention
- To identify the different communication outlets available for use in a community-based intervention and how to utilize them
- To define how to best utilize available resources, while operating within a limited budget
- To interpret the role culture and ethnicity plays in designing health behavior interventions for specific target populations
- To learn how to adapt a general nutrition teaching tool, such as the USDA Food Guide Pyramid, to a specific target population

THE CASE

Background

The Weight-Control Information Network (WIN), a service of the National Institute of Diabetes and Digestive and Kidney Diseases (NIDDK), and Matthews Media Group, Inc., under a contract with the National Institutes of Health (NIH), set out to design and execute a pilot communications campaign aimed at preventing obesity among African-American women in the Boston area. The pilot program was titled "Sisters Together: Move More, Eat Better." Funding for the project was provided by the NIDDK, under a subcontract from the NIH, to Matthews Media Group, Inc.

An advisory group comprised of experts from New England Medical Center, Tufts University School of Nutrition, Science and Policy, and Harvard School of Public Health was assembled and referred to as the WIN-Boston advisory group.

Collecting Information and Defining a Population

One of the first tasks of the WIN-Boston advisory group was to analyze existing data on the topic of prevention and treatment of obesity. This analysis consisted of three parts: analysis of existing survey data, a literature review, and interviews with experts in health and communication. Results revealed that African-American women have better body images and lower rates of eating disorders than their White counterparts, but have higher rates of obesity and obesity-related chronic diseases than White women, irrespective of education level.

Analysis of existing information, including demographic data from the Massachusetts Department of Public Health and interviews with nutritionists working in local community health centers and representatives from the Massachusetts League of Community Health Centers led to the selection and specification of the target population. The primary target audience was African-American women between the ages of eighteen and thirty-five years, because this is the age range when weight gain typically begins, and this population is generally not targeted for health information. A secondary target audience was defined as children and mothers of the primary target audience.

The Target Community

Three Boston neighborhoods, Dorchester, Mattapan, and Roxbury, comprised the target community. The combined population of the neighborhoods is approximately 180,000, ranging from 50 to 90 percent African-American. Average per capita income is approximately $12,000 per year. Close to 20 percent of the population is below 100 percent of the poverty line; almost 50 percent of children under the age of eighteen years live in poverty.

The three target neighborhoods are served by eight neighborhood health centers, six of which are also WIC centers. There was general agreement among nutritionists at these centers that young African-American women represented an appropriate focus for the project, particularly if messages were prevention-based.

The Goal and Objectives for the Sisters Together Program

The goal of "Sisters Together" was to develop media-based intervention strategies aimed at the prevention of obesity among young African-American women, which were replicable for populations in other communities. The two main objectives were (1) to heighten the awareness of the benefits of healthy eating and increased physical activity, and (2) to provide information that could lead to healthier eating and increased physical activity.

Results of Focus Group Research

Qualitative research in the form of focus groups was conducted to explore attitudes about healthy eating and physical activity among the target population. Key findings were

- There was some confusion among target audience members when attempting to define healthy eating. This was especially clear when groups were asked to define low-fat foods.
- The two most common means of preparing foods were frying and baking. For some, baking was perceived as the "lazy" way of cooking.
- Participants cited numerous benefits associated with healthy eating and physical activity including looking good, having more energy, living longer, feeling better about oneself, reducing stress, and maintaining current weight.

- The two major complaints about healthy foods were taste and cost. Fresh fruits and vegetables, along with other foods perceived as healthy (e.g., fish), were viewed as more costly.
- Barriers to physical activity included lack of reliable day care, soreness, pain, and lack of immediate results.

These findings guided the development of the calendar.

The Calendar

The WIN-Boston advisory group decided that a twelve-month wall calendar would be a useful communications tool, therefore a 1996 calendar was developed as the major nutrition teaching instrument of the "Sisters Together" campaign. The focus groups revealed that target audience members lacked information on healthy recipes that tasted good and the skills necessary for preparing healthy foods. Therefore, the calendar was to provide members of the target audience with recipes and tips on how to prepare healthful foods, information on how to use the USDA's Food Guide Pyramid to eat healthfully, and practical tips on how to increase physical activity. A calendar format was chosen because it provides one convenient package for timely and useful information. As well, each month would have a fresh look to engage the target audience.

A committee of three registered dietitians and members of the WIN-Boston advisory group wrote the calendar, while the rest of the advisory group was involved in editing. The calendar's authors worked closely with a professional graphic designer and illustrator, to ensure that the calendar was readable, usable, and visually engaging. Test calendars were prepared to aid in formative research on several aspects of design, including color, format, and content.

Each month, the calendar focused on one of the Food Guide Pyramid's food groups, with a corresponding recipe, complete with nutrient analysis, and a menu incorporating the recipe. As well, each month featured an "eat better" and a "move more" tip, along with an inspirational phrase.

Recipe Selection and Testing

The process of selecting the recipes for the calendar included several steps. First, the authors reviewed books and magazines for traditional African-American recipes. Other suggestions came from focus group results. From there, the authors developed several recipes, modified for calories and fat, and prepared and taste-tested the recipes.

The authors then pretested various written recipes with the target audience to determine acceptance. At the "Sister's Together" kickoff fair, target audience members could visit a booth where they were asked to read a variety of recipe cards, including entrees, side dishes, and desserts, and to comment on whether or not they would be willing to make the recipes. The participants were enthusiastic about providing feedback, and thus, the pretesting yielded considerable valuable information regarding what target audience members looked for in a recipe, including ease of use, necessary ingredients, and perceived taste. For example, one recipe for sweet potato pie, a traditional favorite among African-American women, included low-fat cottage cheese as an ingredient. Nearly all the women who read this recipe commented on how unfamiliar that was to them, and that they probably would not make the recipe because of it. As a result, a different, more acceptable, but still reduced-fat sweet potato pie recipe was included in the calendar. Other popular foods that were included in the calendar as a result of feedback at the kickoff fair included collard greens, macaroni and cheese, chicken, black-eyed peas with rice, and peach crisp (a low-fat version of peach cobbler). As a result, it was possible to narrow the choices and select the final twelve recipes after the calendar team prepared, taste-tested, and conducted nutrient analysis.

Distribution and Evaluation of the Calendar

The calendar was distributed to the "Sisters Together" target audience members free of charge. Participants at the kickoff fair placed their names on a mailing list to receive the calendar. As well, a local radio station advertised the "Sisters Together" toll-free phone number, which audience members could call to request a calendar. Calendars were also made available at neighborhood health centers, beauty parlors, and at community meetings where "Sisters Together" was represented.

To help evaluate the calendar, a preaddressed, stamped postcard requesting feedback was included in each calendar. The postcard questions were:

1. How many recipes have you tried?
2. Are you using the eat better tips?
3. Are you using the move more tips?
4. Do you have any other thoughts about this calendar?

SUMMARY OF EVALUATION FINDINGS

Returned postcards were received from fifty-three calendar recipients. Responses from the postcards were uniformly positive. Respondents used words such as "wonderful," "beautiful," "great," and "fun," to describe the calendar. Several respondents expressed interest in a 1997 calendar.

With regard to content, respondents commented primarily on the tips and recipes, describing them as "creative," "fun," and "excellent." Some suggested having photographs of recipes rather than illustrations. Gratitude for addressing issues of African-American women was also expressed within the responses.

With regard to style, many respondents described the calendar as "beautiful" and "eye-catching." Some would have liked larger squares depicting the days of the week.

QUESTIONS

1. What skills did the nutrition professionals employ to create a calendar that would correlate to the campaign's goals and objectives?
2. What are some other ways to illustrate the guidelines of the Food Guide Pyramid in a community-based health campaign?
3. Which factors are important to remember when creating recipes geared to a specific population?
4. Discuss some other methods of distributing the calendar to the target population.
5. How might you extend the reach of this calendar?

CHAPTER EIGHTEEN

WORKING EFFECTIVELY IN CROSS-CULTURAL AND MULTICULTURAL SETTINGS

Reflecting a cultural system in which individualization and independence are highly valued, American health care has traditionally acknowledged and emphasized individuals as the locus of problems and of intervention. The influence of patterned cultural and subcultural characteristics, the symbolism and meaning attached to those characteristics, and the impact of those and other population level factors have not been consistently incorporated into providers' knowledge bases.

—KAVANAGH AND KENNEDY[32]

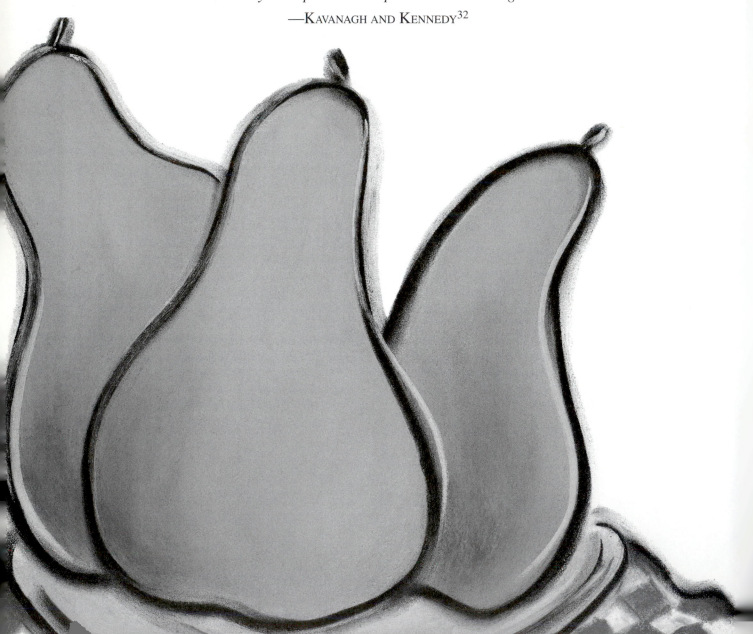

Core Concepts

Maintaining cultural sensitivity and implementing culturally relevant programs will be among the greatest challenges faced by nutrition professionals given the current economic and demographic trends toward globalization. The ability to work effectively with persons from different cultures and in settings where several cultures coexist is of critical importance for community nutrition professionals planning to work either within or outside the United States. In the United States, the cultural issues for community nutrition programming are defined primarily in conjunction with racial or ethnic minority groups and are influenced by the socioeconomic and health status of minority groups as well as the cultural and social climate regarding race relations.

Objectives

When you finish chapter eighteen, you should be able to:

~ Discuss the concepts and principles of cross-cultural relations.

~ Identify steps to take for increasing cross-cultural competence.

~ State the demographic profiles of U.S. racial and ethnic minority populations.

~ Compare and contrast the health profiles of U.S. racial and ethnic minority populations.

~ Use programming approaches that are culturally sensitive and client-centered.

Key Words

Word	Page Mentioned
Cross-cultural	544
Multicultural	544
Norms	544
Values	544
Worldview	544
Pluralistic	546
Assimilation	546
Political correctness	546
Cultural imposition	546
Ethnocentrism	546
Cultural competence	547
Codes	547
Stereotyping	548
Nonverbal communications	550
Excess deaths	555
Cultural sensitivity	559
Cultural specificity	559
Empowerment-oriented interventions	561

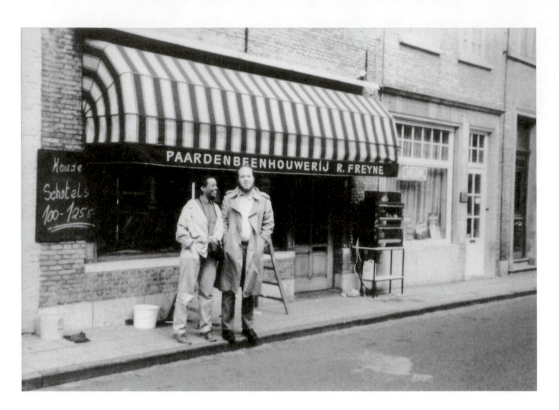

The authors of this chapter, pictured standing in front of a horse meat butcher in Belgium, have a cross-cultural marriage. Eating horse meat is entirely acceptable to Chris (right), who was born and raised in the Netherlands, but is unthinkable to Shiriki (left), who was born and raised in the United States. Whose attitude is "right"?

The principles of effective cross-cultural and multicultural programming apply to domestic as well as international settings, but the application of these principles can be very different in different contexts. This chapter focuses on cultural issues in community nutrition programming within the United States. In this chapter, the term **cross-cultural** refers to situations in which the provider or the provider institution is from the mainstream U.S. culture (generally White, middle-class, of European ancestry) and the client or client population is from a racial or ethnic minority group. The term **multicultural** is used to distinguish situations in which several cultural groups are represented in the client population; this is in contrast to a relatively homogenous cultural group. The issues and principles discussed can be applied generally to any setting in which different cultural frames of reference are operating.

Working effectively with another cultural group requires an awareness of and ability to work around one's own cultural biases, a knowledge of the other culture, and skill in cross-cultural interaction. *Cultural biases,* as used here, include social class biases, which are relevant because many community nutrition services are delivered in low-income communities. Everyone has cultural biases to some degree. Knowledge of another culture includes assessment of facts not only about the relevant **norms, values, worldview,** religions, and practicalities of the other's everyday life but also about how the services provided and the providers are viewed by those others. Skill in cross-cultural programming requires translation of *cultural self-awareness* and knowledge of the other culture into effective ways of communicating (asking questions and hearing what is said as well as what is not said). Effective cross-cultural programming also requires the ability to think about program design, content, and logistics from a client- or community-centered perspective.

In this chapter we begin by clarifying some key concepts in cross-cultural relations and then discuss practical steps that can be taken to improve competence in cross-cultural relations. We subsequently provide and discuss some selected demographic and health indicators for U.S. racial and ethnic minority groups. The chapter concludes with a discussion of community nutrition programming strategies from a perspective of achieving optimum effectiveness in cross-cultural and multicultural settings. Figure 18.1 illustrates how these

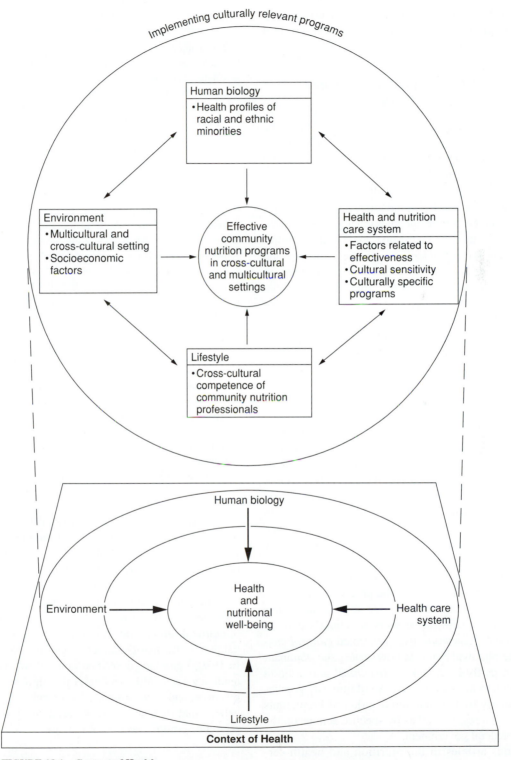

FIGURE 18.1   Context of Health
Concepts important to nutrition programming in cross-cultural and multicultural settings.

concepts work together to achieve effective community nutrition programs in cross-cultural and multicultural settings within the context of health.

CONCEPTS IN CROSS-CULTURAL RELATIONS

The original concept of American society incorporated the idea of a mixture of diverse cultural groups, that is, groups who had different customs, beliefs about how society and the people within it should function, and, in some cases, languages and *nonverbal communication* styles. The founding fathers primarily had religious and language diversity in mind. Over time, the traditional view of American society became one of a melting pot in which cultures mix and blend through intermarriage, the economy, and education to produce a new culture[45] and, further, in which the norms and values of the Anglo-Saxon population segment would be the point of reference. In contrast with this older view, demographic and cultural realities have led to a new, more culturally **pluralistic** view of American society. Pluralisms represented by the "salad bowl" (box 18.1) recognizes the value to individuals and to society when ethnic differences are preserved.

The changing view of diversity in American society has profound implications for the way education and health services are delivered. Under the view of American society as a melting pot, the professional's role, even responsibility, would be to foster cultural **assimilation** (adoption of mainstream attitudes and behaviors), which translates into a scenario where the burden is on the minority client to move toward the mainstream. In W. M. Parker's words, the result is that service providers have a hidden agenda, "a plan to fix minority clients so that they begin to think, feel, and behave as white people do."[54] With a view of America as culturally pluralistic, the burden is on the professional to work with the client or community so that services are delivered in a manner compatible with the client's cultural and situational framework, usually termed *cultural sensitivity*. The pluralistic view is now clearly the dominant one, driven partly by a lack of *structural assimilation* (integration into the social structure) of minority populations and partly by the continuous influx of immigrants from other cultures, as well as by specific actions on the part of the federal government.

Numerous articles in the nutrition and health services literature of the 1980s and 1990s advocate increased attention to and respect for cultural differ-

BOX 18.1

Replacing the metaphor of the melting pot with that of the "salad bowl" reflects a shift in paradigm that is more a change in values than a change in facts.[2] Underlying this paradigm shift is a fundamental change in the perception about the (global) struggle for human equity—a struggle that is a direct inheritance of the founding doctrine of the American nation. In this context, the shift toward a "serious pursuit of multiculturalism is rightly perceived as a threat to the status-quo" (reference 14, p. 563). It is, therefore, not surprising that the pluralist movement is under attack from the more conservative sectors of society. For example, proponents of multiculturalism have been described as "robotic arbiters of political correctness" (reference 14, p. 563, citing Susan Schweik), where **political correctness** refers to a forced standard of adherence to certain socially acceptable language and attitudes (e.g, what one is allowed to say publicly about minority groups or women). Tensions surrounding affirmative action policies, attempts to restrict services to immigrants, or passing legislation allowing English as the only language used in schools or in official transactions are other examples of conservative opposition to cultural pluralism. The social demand for loyalty to a particular group is also increasing[24,33] meaning that people who might previously been open to several points of view may feel obliged to take one side or the other.

Thus, while the melting pot concept may have lost its luster, the acceptance of the salad bowl of multiculturalism is variable. Multicultural awareness is essential in any organization or profession.[26,71]

ences.* Even if one is not motivated by a sense of equity, recognition of the powerful influence of culture on food- and health-related behaviors remains necessary on practical grounds. Programs that inadequately address cultural norms and values simply do not work.

Although harsh-sounding to Americans who pride themselves on being fair and unprejudiced, the concepts of **cultural imposition** and **ethnocentrism** are an essential part of the dialogue on cross-cultural programming.[42] In 1970, Leininger described cultural imposition—"the tendency for health personnel to impose their beliefs, practices, and values upon another culture because they believe that their ideas are superior to those of another person or group"—as one of the most serious continuing

---

*See references 4, 5, 19, 22, 35, 37, 42, 57, 58, and 67.

problems in the health field and one largely unrecognized by many health practitioners.[42] She refers to the deliberate cultural imposition associated with political domination (e.g., British or American colonization) and to the less clearly intentional cultural imposition that occurs when Western health practitioners attempt to introduce new ideas and services to people in developing countries without fully recognizing and accounting for indigenous, culturally embedded health care values and norms.

Ethnocentrism can be defined as "the universal tendency for any people to put its own culture and society in a central position of priority and worth"[33] or as the tendency for people "to see their own way of doing things as the only way of doing things."[3] Implicit in the concept of ethnocentrism is "the tendency to evaluate other cultures in terms of one's own and to conclude that the other cultures are inferior."[3] The current culturally pluralistic view of American society moves us away from the ethnocentric superiority implications of the Anglo-Saxon-oriented melting pot concept. Nevertheless, the context of community nutrition practice is very conducive to such ethnocentric attitudes and practices on the part of the professionals involved, that is, attitudes that what is offered by the health care system is superior to and preferred over existing practices of the client or the community. Clients, in general, are at the powerless end of the hierarchy in the traditional service delivery model. When, as in most federally funded nutrition programs, eligibility for services is limited to persons with low incomes, negative attitudes about poor persons may contribute to the perceived inferiority of the client, and such perceptions can be aggravated when the poor person is also a member of a stigmatized minority group. The high value attached to objective scientific evidence in mainstream American culture also means that advice or prescriptions made "from a sound scientific perspective" will be viewed as superior to client beliefs and practices. Thus, community nutrition professionals who want to work effectively in cross-cultural settings must be vigilant in evaluating their own ethnocentrism and take deliberate steps to work around it.[42]

PRINCIPLES OF CULTURALLY SENSITIVE PROGRAMMING

Cultural Competence

In all societies, being an adult means to be considered culturally competent by staying within certain bound-

aries and following certain rituals. A minimum level of **cultural competence** is usually taken for granted. For example, adults are expected to be fluent in speaking their "native" tongue and to have internalized cultural norms, attitudes, and values to such a degree that they even convey emotions in the accepted and recognized verbal and nonverbal expressions, including gestures and signs (termed **codes**) of their social group. Those who are most competent in the culture receive praise and prestige and honors are bestowed on them to identify them as cultural role models.

Cross-Cultural Competence

Cross-cultural competence is competence on a different scale. It refers to the ability to understand the behavior of other peoples or other groups, and grasp the meaning of their spoken language and codes. Persons who know only the language or a few rituals but nothing about the culture are "tourists" at best and, at the worst extreme, "fluent fools."[7] Knowing language and customs are important, but cross-cultural competence requires what the anthropologist Clifford Geertz calls a "thick reading," a willful exercise in absorbing the "text of the lives of the others."[24]

Skills in cross-cultural competence are generally developed through either of two pathways. One pathway, often dictated by situational factors, leads to the development of bicultural awareness[9,53] through immersion in or association with one other culture. Multicultural awareness could result from cultural awareness of several different cultures learned one at a time. The other pathway starts with an attitude of willingness to explore and try to understand the world from the perspective of those with whom one comes into contact in interpersonal and professional relationships.[36,55] It is this latter, generalized attitudinal change that is needed in the United States to guarantee what Sumida calls a "systematic multicultural education that will 'transform and not merely crowd' our visions of an egalitarian society" (reference 65, p. 565).

Cross-cultural competence in service delivery can be defined as "a set of congruent behaviors/practices, attitudes and policies that come together in a system or agency or among health professionals, enabling effective work to be done in cross-cultural situations."[12] Cross-cultural competence can be viewed along a continuum from incompetence to proficiency and in which extreme incompetence is associated with negative consequences (cultural destructiveness).[12]

STEPS TOWARD CROSS-CULTURAL COMPETENCE

Experts in cross-cultural training recognize that most people in helping professions and management positions, although not immune to the ethnocentrism that affects all human beings, can be helped to become more effective in cross-cultural interactions by progressing through various stages of development that include increasing awareness, knowledge, and skill.[27,30,54,56] Four steps toward cross-cultural competence are outlined in box 18.2.

BOX 18.2

STEPS TOWARD INCREASING CROSS-CULTURAL COMPETENCE

INCREASING PERSONAL READINESS
- Cultural self-awareness
- Comfort level in cross-cultural situations
- Awareness of stereotypes and of your own stereotypic beliefs
- Willingness to learn from others
- Learning to value differences

ACQUIRING CULTURAL KNOWLEDGE
- Learning about other cultures
- Assessing how people in other cultures view you and your culture
- Sharing experiences with persons from other cultural groups
- Finding common ground with persons from other cultures

DEVELOPING CROSS-CULTURAL INTERACTION SKILLS
- Verbal communication
- Nonverbal communication
- Flexibility
- Overcoming fears
- Obtaining feedback

MAINTAINING CROSS-CULTURAL ALERTNESS
- Regular evaluation of your own feelings and reactions
- Continued assessment of overall climate for race relations
- Setting incremental goals toward increased appreciation of cultural differences
- Building cultural bridges extending beyond professional boundaries and into your personal sphere
- Remaining well informed about the client populations

Source: Adapted from references 17, 22, 34, 35, and 44.

Increasing Personal Readiness

Cultural Self-Awareness   Although there are overt aspects of culture (e.g., traditional clothing and religious symbols or specific rituals), a great deal of culture is subconscious and invisible to members of the cultural group. Checklists such as the one in box 18.4 on page 550 can be helpful for learning to identify the more subtle aspects of one's own cultural framework. Recognizing that many attitudes are culturally driven is an important first step in increasing self-awareness of attitudes promoted by one's own culture and how they may differ from those of another. The temptation to consider one's own cultural attitudes to be the "correct" ones (e.g., placing a high value on punctuality or on being thrifty) should become obvious once one begins this process.[46]

Comfort Level in Cross-Cultural Situations   Another step in the process of increasing self-awareness is for a person to determine how bound he or she is within a culturally ingrained way of perceiving things as opposed to being relatively comfortable in situations that permit or are dominated by other cultural attitudes. Parker's "multicultural interaction index" for self-evaluation on a low, moderate, or high comfort level with ethnic differences includes items such as how comfortable a person would feel having an ethnically different person for a personal physician or a spouse or attending a religious service of a culturally different group.[55]

The ability to recover from mistakes in cross-cultural communications is essential to achieving a high level of comfort in cross-cultural situations.[32] Even when rapport has been established between a provider and client or in a group setting, circumstances in which something said or done will offend or create distance between people from different cultures will arise inevitably. Most mistakes in cross-cultural communication can be corrected. Some ways to deal effectively with such situations and reestablish rapport are shown in box 18.3. However, remember that the wide latitude that one usually has for making mistakes in cross-cultural situations will erode without signs that progress toward mutual understanding is being made. Repetition of even small mistakes can lead to breakdown of the communication.

Awareness of Stereotypes   **Stereotyping** can be defined as "the categorization of individuals in ways that ignore their uniqueness and limit their potential."[54] It may be easier to practice identifying stereotypes used in your family or work about any group of people, for ex-

BOX 18.3

THE INEVITABLE MISTAKE
What to Do When Cross-Cultural Communications Go Awry

1. Redirect attention from the topic that has caused tension in the interaction and back to the basic problem.

2. Apologize for your blunder or error. Don't overapologize. Neither you nor the client should expect perfect communication.

3. Recognizing that the client knows more than you about his or her culture and situation, orient the direction of the interaction to allow the client to be the primary source of information for generating appropriate solutions and alternatives; in some interactions, this may constitute a client-provider role reversal, at least temporarily.

4. Allow a period of silence to intervene (e.g., if you realize that you have said the wrong thing, count to ten before you say anything else). Better a reflective silence than a stream of words that makes the problem worse.

5. Involve another person or persons who can act as cultural mediators or "brokers" in a difficult situation.

Source: Based on Pedersen (reference 56) as adapted by Kavanagh and Kennedy (reference 32, p. 564).

ample, about old people or young people, Northerners or Southerners, people from certain neighborhoods, rich versus middle-class persons, or men or women before trying to assess your own tendency to stereotype persons of other races. Analyze stereotypes in terms of their content and how rigidly or aggressively they are promulgated. Keep in mind that overly positive stereotypes can be as damaging as negative ones (for example, expecting all Asian-American students to be very smart in math can be as problematic as expecting all African-American students to be academically weak in this area). Develop a plan, not to rid yourself of stereotypes (which may be unrealistic), but to bring them out into the open. Also, listen carefully to see whether other groups have stereotypes about you. Find the unfairness and illogic in these stereotypes, try to neutralize them, and assess your reactions.

Learning to Value Differences   Valuing differences can be somewhat problematic for some people because of the uncertainty it involves. To improve in this area one might practice seeing the positive side of diversity

about things such as clothes, music, cars, architecture, hair designs, and foods—areas that are not as politically charged as race relations—and then try to think of human diversity in the same light. Think of people as "of many colors" rather than as "nonwhite." Recognize the inherent ethnocentricity in a term such as nonwhite, which implies that being White is the primary ethnicity from which others deviate. See Yanov[70] for a specific discussion of the inequity problems hidden in the English vocabulary, especially on gender issues, but also regarding color.

Acquiring Cultural Knowledge

Learning about Other Cultures   Although one can never learn all there is to know about another culture, studying aspects of another culture's general outlook and principles of living can go a long way toward contradicting latent stereotypes and helping to anticipate issues that arise in cross-cultural interactions. It is here that Geertz's concept of "thick reading"—the process of studying another culture—becomes important. This process may involve reading, observations, talking or sharing experiences with persons from other cultures, and reflecting on what is similar or different about underlying attitudes.

Learn external expressions of cultural such as ethnic food and language. Then become more aware of specific cultural differences in attitudes in the areas shown in the checklist in box 18.4. Seek and catalog information about how certain attitudes may differ between your culture and another.

Assessing How Other Cultures View You   There is usually a history between groups that affects how members from one cultural group view and interact with those from another. In the United States, this history includes decades of open or latent conflicts between the Americans of European descent, the most powerful ethnic group, and less powerful native born or immigrant racial or ethnic "minority" populations and in which the less powerful are at a disadvantage. Think about how attitudes derived from acculturation within this context might influence the way a client views you? For example, are you seen as a do-gooder? In spite of any efforts on your part, are you viewed as an extension of an institution that has a bad reputation in the community, whether earned or not? Acknowledge the sociopolitical context that may shape how you are viewed by a client apart from how you present yourself, especially in the

BOX 18.4

A CHECKLIST FOR IDENTIFYING CULTURAL DIFFERENCES IN ATTITUDES

What are your attitudes toward . . . ?

Assess the attitudes of some of your relatives and colleagues. Take note of the difficulty you encounter.

Picture yourself in a meeting with representatives from the community. Do you have at least a rough idea of the types of attitudes you might encounter in relation to the issues listed below or as to whether these attitudes might be different from yours? How could you find this out? Is what you think you know based on knowledge or on stereotypes?

- Time
- Education
- Work
- Aggressive behavior
- Expression of emotion
- Competition
- Innovation
- Sexual behavior
- Self-reliance
- Self-sufficiency
- Individualism
- Industriousness
- Supernatural phenomena
- Status seeking
- Sobriety
- Thriftiness
- Authority
- Independence
- Intermarriage
- Children

Source: Adapted from Mithun JS:The role of the family in acculturation and assimilation in America: a psychocultural dimension. In McCready WC, editor: *Culture, ethnicity, and identity: current issues in research,* New York, 1983, Academic Press.

people in which elements of communication and behavior are evaluated as objectively as possible, suspending the value judgments that ordinarily take place in a cultural perspective, and freeing the practitioner to accept communications or behaviors at face value. For example, a person's interdependence with other family members might be viewed negatively as passivity or low self-esteem and rejected by a practitioner from a culture that places a high value on personal independence. However, when the professional and client meet in an access zone in which the professional is vigilant against the tendency to impose such value judgments, interdependence might be accepted without prejudice and recognized as an important factor in treatment.

Developing Cross-Cultural Interaction Skills

Verbal Communication   People born in the United States are generally monolingual, requiring that persons whose native language is not English speak English to communicate. Although the overall ethic of acculturation to an Anglo-Saxon orientation has softened, the view that persons living in the United States must ultimately learn to communicate in English is still firmly held. However, as a practical matter, being able to communicate with people in their native tongue is indispensable for effective community nutrition programming and does not necessarily deter people from learning English.

Cultural differences in language usage and connotations and in literacy level also affect communications among native English speakers. What is said may be misunderstood or not understood, even though the words used are familiar to both parties. Strategies to avoid communication problems include being informed about potential problems of this type, using the most widely understood terminology wherever possible, and using a communication style that builds in numerous opportunities to obtain direct feedback from the client as to what has been heard and understood.[16]

Nonverbal Communication   Nonverbal communications—messages communicated through silence, distance, eye contact, facial expressions, touching, or position of the body—can be as complicated and potentially helpful to effective cross-cultural relations as verbal communications.[67] Persons working in cross-cultural settings should be keenly aware of the nature of nonverbal communication and of the potential pitfalls of inter-

initial stages of an interaction. In other words, be aware of how you or your institution might be stereotyped. What are realistic ways that you can demonstrate that these stereotypes do not apply?

Finding Common Ground   Finding common ground does not mean finding aspects of other cultures that are like yours. We can create a false comfort level for ourselves by emphasizing to persons from other cultures how much they are "just like us," giving a message that the person can please us by suppressing differences. This closes off communication or throws it out of balance. Finding common ground means establishing in your professional approach an access region in which the people are able to meet you on mutual terms. In practice, this means developing ways of dealing with

preting nonverbal behaviors outside one's known cultural context. A person from one culture may expect some periods of silence during a conversation, whereas a person from another culture may find silence awkward and search for something to fill the void as quickly as possible. A close seating arrangement in an office or a room may be uncomfortable for a client from a culture that prefers a greater physical distance between people. With respect to eye contact, looking directly at someone from a culture that finds it inappropriate may seem intimidating or rude. Not looking directly at someone who expects it may be interpreted as trying to conceal something or being uninterested. Different patterns of preferred eye contact among Black, White, and Native Americans have been described. Informality such as addressing someone you have just met by their first name may be inappropriate in some cultures and therefore be interpreted as showing disrespect.

Being Flexible   Working with others requires sufficient flexibility to respond to them as things progress rather than only in ways that are predetermined from the outset. One way to promote flexibility is to have realistic expectations about what you can accomplish and to be able to modify those expectations when indicated. Also, it is necessary to respect people's rights to think and feel in unique ways in order to be willing to modify your approach in response to what is presented by the client. In addition, because people who are angry or upset tend to be rigid, it is important to ride out situations in which your emotions become aroused until things can be discussed in perspective. To anticipate such situations, reflect on things that upset you or your coworkers and evaluate them.

Overcoming Fears   Fears are among the primary factors predisposing to inflexibility. A person who is uncertain of his or her ability to be effective with another cultural group might be afraid to work with that group. A person who feels unable to overcome prejudice against members of a certain group may try to avoid working with this group for fear that this underlying prejudice will be revealed. These fears may affect the desire of people to work with clients of other ethnic backgrounds or the desire of middle-class professionals to work with persons from lower socioeconomic groups of the same or different ethnicity. Stereotypes or social conditions may cause a person to fear physical harm

from members of a minority group or when working in certain communities. Colleagues who openly express politically conservative or prejudiced views may raise fears of reprisal or disapproval among other colleagues. Professionals who are themselves members of minority groups may fear that they will lose status among their colleagues by working too closely with other minorities.

Practitioners should assess their apprehensions about working with clients from other cultures and should express these openly to elicit feedback and suggestions from coworkers about how they might be overcome. It will probably be possible to identify some aspect on which to focus as a first, manageable step. Self-acceptance of the natural tendency to be somewhat fearful in uncertain situations will help in taking things step by step and in avoiding the tendency to overreach by trying to conquer these apprehensions too quickly.

Obtaining Feedback   Always be open for feedback—before, during, and after cross-cultural encounters. This is especially important since the knowledge base about any culture changes over time and includes many subtleties. View feedback as a way to obtain information about how you are perceived by others, how well you get your message across, and how well you listen. Solicit and attend to as many forms of feedback as possible, from both verbal and nonverbal communication and from both clients and coworkers. Realize that in many cultures, open feedback may be considered rude, and critical feedback may reach you only after several contacts or through subtle messages.

Maintaining Cross-Cultural Alertness

Maintaining cross-cultural competence is an ongoing process.

Regular Evaluation of Your Own Feelings and Reactions   Reevaluation of feelings and reactions is necessary because cultural biases are deeply ingrained and continually resurface and because growth in cross-cultural interactions skills must be incremental. It is important to pause and reflect.

With exposure and involvement in cross-cultural situations, one may develop an overappreciation of one's own culture, especially if the cultural distance being bridged is wide, if there are historical political dimensions, or if numerous pitfalls emerge that damage rapport. Another possibility is that a person will fear "marginalization," that is, of losing the emotional and social anchors that tie him or her to their professional or social group. A third scenario is one in which the person develops an exaggerated attachment to the other culture.

Continued Assessment of Overall Climate for Cross-Cultural Relations   We are living in a dynamic situation in which cultures are continually interacting and changing and in which the environmental context for delivering programs is also continually changing. Thus, when involved in a community nutrition program in a multicultural setting, make a habit of reading newspapers and magazines and listening to reports in the mass media through the "lens" of your client group. Think about the issues presented not only with respect to your locality but in the context of political views and events at the national and international levels, which are interpreted and reported to Americans daily and which ultimately affect our day-to-day lives.

Setting Incremental Goals Toward Increased Appreciation of Cultural Differences   Just as you know that losing weight is an incremental process and that developing a regular exercise program has to be done in steps, so too must one approach multicultural contacts and work relations as an incremental process of attitudinal and behavioral change. Sincere efforts to bridge cultures are usually met with a fair amount of latitude for learning and making mistakes. Thus, one should feel comfortable in taking small sequential steps toward learning, allowing time to appreciate the personal growth that comes from mastering cross-cultural competencies. One's eagerness to immerse more in the "other side" of things will increase as cross-cultural understanding and skill increase. The incremental process of learning about a culture involves cycles of experiences, reading and reflecting—finding new meanings and more subtleties as you go along. Experiencing the growth of knowing about others and, thus, about yourself is the biggest intrinsic reward of becoming and staying cross-culturally competent.

Building Cultural Bridges That Extend Beyond Professional Boundaries and into Your Personal Sphere   While you may be motivated to enter into a cross-cultural experience solely for professional purposes, this endeavor will invariably have more far-reaching implications. The cross-cultural experience

needs to be supplemented by personal commitments that go beyond the work responsibilities. Separations of work and personal life can take place in time, place, and ritual, but not within the professional as a person. It is unnatural and highly stressful to keep trying to be two persons in one mind. It is more natural to gradually replace the original "ferry" between the two cultures with a permanent, two-way, toll-free bridge.

Remaining Well-Informed about the Client Populations   Staying well informed about your client population helps in being effective. Having good information about the community you work with facilitates the interaction and portrays your own competence in a positive manner. It is important to know about daily life and significant events in the client's community and to understand it from their perspective. For a constant refreshing of your perspective, keep your radio tuned to the stations that serve communities with which you are working. Much ethnic community-oriented information comes from local radio stations. Staying well informed also helps you to keep your goals on target and to understand the impact of your work on the lives of your clients. Be aware that the process of cross-cultural learning may be one-sided. The client population is not the active agent here and may not meet you halfway. There is no equivalent of the professional drive for cross-cultural sensitivity among clients. Sensitivity of clients is based on their vulnerability to actions and policies of individuals and institutions in the majority or dominant culture.

U.S. MINORITY POPULATIONS

Demographic Profiles

Racial and ethnic minorities in the United States include persons designated in the U.S. Census as Black or African American, Hispanic American, Asian-Pacific Islander American, and Native American or Alaskan Natives. Estimates place the aggregate number of persons in these minority groups at 64.3 million, approximately 25 percent of the U.S. population.[52] The major subgroups in the Hispanic-American and Asian-Pacific Islander categories are shown in figure 18.2 and box 18.5, and selected demographic data for the four major minority grous are in table 18.2. More than 500 American Indian groups are included in the category Native Americans as well as Eskimos, Aleuts, and Alaskan

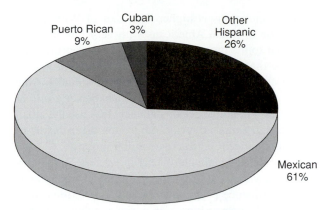

FIGURE 18.2 Breakdown of the Hispanic Population, 1990
(*Source:* From O'Hare, WP: America's minorities. The demographics of diversity, *Population Bulletin;* 47(4):1–47, 1992.)

ASIAN-PACIFIC ISLANDER SUBPOPULATIONS IN U.S. CENSUS—COUNTRY OF ORIGIN

China	India
Japan	Pakistan
Korea	Bangladesh
Philippines	Sri Lanka
Vietnam	Burma
Cambodia	Hawaii
Laos	Guam
Thailand	Samoa
Malaysia	Tonga
Singapore	Fiji
Indonesia	Micronesia

TABLE 18.1
Demographic Comparison of U.S. Racial/Ethnic Groups

Indicator	White	Black	Hispanic	Asian-Pacific Islander	American Indian
Percentage of U.S. population, 1992	74.8	11.9	9.5	3.1	0.7
Percentage population growth, 1980–1992*	5.5	16.4	65.3	123.5	30.7
Age distribution, 1992					
Percentage < eighteen years of age	24	32	35	29	35
Percentage ages eighteen to forty-four years	41	44	47	48	43
Percentage of population ages forty-five to sixty-four years	20	15	13	17	15
Percentage of population over sixty-five years of age	15	8	5	7	6
Percentage in poverty, 1991	9	33	29	14	32
Percentage in deep poverty, 1991†	3	16	10	7	14
Percentage of persons ages ≥ sixteen years who were working, 1992	62	54	59	61	53
Percentage of persons ages twenty-five to forty-four with < twelve years education	9	19	40	8	22
Percentage of persons ages twenty-five to forty-four with ≥ four years of college	28	14	10	47	11
Percentage of female-headed households, 1991	13	44	23	12	27
Number of births to mothers ages ten to fourteen years per 1,000 women, 1992	0.8	4.7	2.6	0.7	1.6
Number of births to mothers ages fifteen to nineteen years per 1,000 women, 1992	51.8	112.4	107.1	26.6	84.4
Total fertility rate, 1992‡	1.9	2.5	2.7	2.3	2.9

*Mexican, Puerto Rican, and Cuban data are from 1980–1990.
†Below 50% of the 1991 official poverty threshold.
‡Average number of children born per woman under current age-specific fertility rates.
Sources: From O'Hare, WP: America's minorities. The demographics of diversity, *Population Bulletin;* 47(4):1–47, 1992; National Center for Health Statistics: *Monthly vital statistics report;* 43(5), suppl, DHHS Publication (PHS) no. 95–12204–0677, Hyattsville, MD, 1994, Public Health Service.

Indians.[59,68] Native Hawaiians are not usually listed as a separate census category but are grouped with either Native Americans or Asian-Pacific Islanders. Table 18.1 also shows that Asian-Pacific Islanders and Hispanic Americans are the fastest-growing minority populations and have high proportions of immigrants. Definitions of minority populations may eventually change to keep pace with the growing diversity and changing sociopolitical climate of the U.S. population. Current classifications overlap (i.e., persons of Hispanic ethnicity may also fit into categories defined by race, such as Black or White) are not necessarily appropriate for people of mixed ancestry.[52]

Minority populations are generally younger than the majority White population. Therefore, comparisons within age categories or data that have been statistically adjusted to account for age differences are the most useful for comparing health indicators across groups. However, the absolute burden of a problem in a population is a function of the actual age distribution (e.g., a population with proportionately more women in their childbearing years needs more services for pregnant women and children).

The socioeconomic and health profiles of U.S. minorities are disadvantageous relative to those of the majority White population. Minority groups are therefore overrepresented in the service populations of programs targeted to low-income and high-risk groups. For example, although Black and Hispanic persons are, respectively, 12 and 9.5% of the overall U.S. population, Black and Hispanic persons comprised 51 percent (25 and 26 percent, respectively) of the population served by the Special Supplemental Food Program for Women, Infants and Children (WIC) in 1994.[20] The proportions of households headed by females, of teenage pregnancies, and of mothers with four or more children are generally higher among minority groups than among Whites. Educational attainment tends to be lower in minority groups as a whole, although there are wide variations (table 18.1).

Overall data for Asians and Pacific Islanders do not follow the pattern of socioeconomic disadvantage seen for the other minority groups. However, summary statistics for Asian-Pacific Islander Americans can be very misleading, because this category includes population subgroups with markedly different socioeconomic and health profiles. Some subgroups of Asian-Pacific Islanders are better off than the majority population, whereas others are notably disadvantaged. For example, although the median income of the Asian-Pacific Islander populations is higher than that of Whites, the proportion of Asian Americans with very low incomes is similar to the proportion seen in other minorities and is twice that in Whites.[52] This example of problems within certain subgroups being hidden in data for the larger group should be remembered as a general rule of interpreting minority health statistics, because the small numbers in some minority subgroups often result in "oversummarized" data across similar groups.

Regional and community-level differences in the proportion of various minority groups in the population can greatly influence program perspectives. National data show that the composition of minority populations differs in different regions of the country.[52] More than half of Black Americans live in the southern United States, fewer than 10 percent live in the West, and approximately 85 percent live in urban areas. These data mean that, although Black Americans are a minority of the U.S. population overall, they constitute the majority of the population in certain areas. For example, Black Americans constitute about 65 percent of the population of the District of Columbia and about 75 percent of the population of Detroit and can be approached as a majority population from a programmatic point of view. In other cities or localities throughout the country, other minority populations are in the majority or at least are a larger proportion of the population than in the national averages. In 1990, 48 percent of American Indians lived in the West. The four states with the largest American Indian populations were Oklahoma (0.25 million), California (0.20 million), Arizona (0.20 million), and New Mexico (0.13 million), and American Indians made up 6 to 15 percent of the populations of Arizona and New Mexico. In 1990, Asian-Pacific Islanders made up 62 percent of the population of Hawaii, 14 percent of the population of California, and 3 to 4 percent of the population of Washington, Nevada, and New York. The 1990 census figures indicate that Hispanic Americans made up 38 percent of the population of New Mexico; 37 percent of the California population; 26 percent of the population of Texas; 23 percent in Arizona; 12 to 13 percent in Colorado, New York, and Florida; and from 8 to 10 percent of the populations of Illinois and New Jersey.[52,69]

Health profiles

One perspective on minority health comes from comparing health indicators among minorities and Whites and noting whether minorities have higher or lower rates.

This approach was taken by the Secretary's Task Force on Black and Minority Health that resulted in the identification of several nutrition-related health problems—cardiovascular diseases, cancers, diabetes, and infant mortality—as four of the primary causes of **"excess deaths"*** among U.S. minority populations,[59] along with homicide, suicide, and cirrhosis of the liver, for which handgun activity or alcohol and drug use were viewed as the major modifiable risk factors.

In making such comparisons, one should keep in mind that the rates in Whites may be higher than is desirable in the an absolute sense and that bringing rates in minorities into line with those in Whites is only an interim objective on the way to bringing overall rates down to acceptable levels. One should also be aware that cross-sectional comparisons of rates may be misleading as to relative group status if disease or risk factor trends are changing over time.[40] For example, during certain periods Black Americans appeared to have had relatively lower rates of deaths from colon cancer than Whites, but after several years during which rates increased in Black and decreased in Whites, rates of colon cancer deaths in Blacks are higher. Because of problems of low data availability on some groups, inaccuracies in racial and ethnic identification in health statistics (data that contribute to the numerator of disease rates) and the different set of problems in determining how many people are in the population base for calculating certain rates (data that make up the denominator for disease rates), no single data source should be taken as absolute evidence about the status of a minority group. Further, no impression given about the overall status of a minority group in a national data should be applied directly as an indicator of the status of specific minority subgroups in a given locality. The importance of local needs assessment to support community-level programming cannot be overemphasized.[25]

With the increased attention to minority health issues as a critical subset of overall U.S. health care issues, national data are more frequently reported in a way that permits comparisons of minorities and Whites or across minority groups. Such data for several health indicators that have implications for nutrition programs (i.e., data relating to infant mortality, heart diseases, cancer, diabetes, end-stage renal disease, tuberculosis, self-rated health, and health insurance coverage) are shown in the tables on the following pages. Ratios in which rates in the minority population are divided by a comparable rate for Whites have been calculated to provide an impression of whether rates in minorities are in "excess," as defined previously, or are equivalent to or below those of Whites (either all Whites or specifically non-Hispanic Whites).

For example, among Black Americans, almost all health indicators are in the direction of higher risk or poorer health status than whites (table 18.2). Rates of infant mortality and related determinants are approximately twice those in Whites. Rates of death from stroke are three times higher in Black than in Whites. Rates of tuberculosis are six to eight times as high in Blacks as in White.[13,64] Black Americans are more likely to be uninsured than White Americans. More Black than White Americans report that they are in only fair or poor health; this disparity is higher among persons with a high school education or more[47] (not shown in the table). The excess occurrence of diabetes, identified in Blacks as well as in all other minority groups, is associated with marked excess incidence of end-stage renal disease in minority populations.[1,66] Teutsch and coworkers estimated that in 1983 to 1985, the rate of occurrence of new cases of end-stage renal disease was four times higher among Blacks than Whites and seven times higher among American Indians than Whites. Data from 1988–91 indicate that these disparities persist.

Data on Native Americans indicate excess risks in several areas, including infant mortality (postneonatal), diabetes, and tuberculosis (table 18.2). Diabetes and obesity are widespread problems among American Indians.[1,8,59] The issue of health insurance coverage is not applicable to Native Americans eligible for services through the Indian Health Service, however many who have low incomes have the same problems of noncoverage observed in other minority groups.

Some data for Hispanic Americans are available for separate subgroups such as Mexican Americans, Puerto Ricans, and Cuban Americans (table 18.3), but other indices are reported only for Hispanics overall (table 18.2). The consistent picture of a health status disadvantage seen for Black Americans is not observed in Hispanics. Heart disease and cancer death rates are lower among Hispanic than non-Hispanic Whites. However, tuberculosis is nearly six times as common among Hispanics than

---

*Excess deaths were defined by comparing death rates in minority populations with those in Whites within age and sex groups and calculating the actual number of deaths among minorities that would not have occurred if death rates were comparable to those in Whites.

TABLE 18.2

Selected Health Indicators for Racial and Ethnic Groups and Excess Ratio Compared to Whites

Annual indicator	Population subgroup	Rate in Whites	Rate in Blacks	Ratio	Rate in American Indians/ Alaskan Natives	Ratio	Rate in Hispanic Americans	Ratio	Rate in Asian Americans	Ratio
Infant mortality and determinants										
Beginning prenatal care after first trimester (%)	Pregnant females	19.2	36.1	1.9	37.9	2.0				
Beginning prenatal care during third trimester or no prenatal care (%)	Pregnant females	4.2	9.9	2.4	11.0	2.6				
Live births weighing <1,500 g (%)	Infants < 1 year old	1.0	3.0	3.0	1.0	1.0				
Live births weighing 1,500–2,499 g (%)	Infants < 1 year old	4.8	10.4	2.2	5.3	1.1				
Neonatal deaths per 1,000 live births	Infants < 28 days old	5.2	11.7	2.3	6.0	1.2				
Postneonatal deaths per 1,000 live births	Infants 28 days to 1 year old	3.0	6.2	2.1	7.3	2.4				
Chronic diseases and related risk factors										
Deaths per 100,000 due to heart disease	Adults 45–64 years old	219.4	403.9	1.8	188.0	0.9	143.0	0.7	89.9	0.4
Deaths per 100,000 due to cancer	Adults 45–64 years old	281.9	414.9	1.5	156.0	0.6	159.6	0.6	147.1	0.5
Deaths per 100,000 due to stroke	Adults 45–64 years old	26.3	82.2	3.1	25.2	1.0	29.2	1.1	30.3	1.2
Deaths per 100,000 due to diabetes	All ages	10.1*			25.8	2.6				
Undiagnosed diabetes (%)	Adults 45–74 years old	6.1	9.3	1.5						
Diagnosed diabetes (%)	Adults 45–74 years old	5.9	10.1	1.7						
Diabetes (%)	Males 45–74 years old	12							20	1.7
	Females 45–74 years old	14							16	1.1
Diabetic end-stage renal disease (new cases\1 million)	Males	49.7	158.3	3.2	240.8	4.8			68.4	1.4
	Females	42.0	185.5	4.4	295.2	7.0			63.9	1.5
Smokers (%)	Males ≥ 18 years of age	27.4	35.1	1.3	27.9	1.0	25.2	0.9	24.2	0.9
	Females ≥ 18 years of age	23.8	24.4	1.0	35.2	1.5	15.5	0.7	7.5	0.3
Other indicators										
No health insurance, 1993 (%)	Persons < 65 years of age	16.2	23.2	1.4					16.9	1.0
Poor or fair self-rated health (%)	Adults 45–64 years of age	15.3	32.0	2.1*						
	with < 12 years education	31.1			39.6	1.3			23.2	0.7
	with ≥ 12 years education	10.8			18.7	1.7			8.9	0.8
Tuberculosis case rate per 100,000	All ages	4.0	31.7	7.9	16.3	4.1	22.4	5.6	46.6	11.7

*Rate for all races.

Source: Compiled from National Center for Health Statistics: *Health United States, 1990,* DHHS publication (PHS) no. 91–1232, Hyattsville, MD, 1991, Public Health Service; National Center for Health Statistics: *Health United States, 1993,* DHHS publication (PHS) no. 94–1232, Hyattsville, MD, 1994, Public Health Service; Center for Health Statistics, *Health United States, 1994,* DHHS publication (PHS) no. 95:1232, Hyattsville, MD, 1995, Public Health Service; Federation of American Societies for Experimental Biology, Life Sciences Research Office: *Third report on nutrition monitoring in the United States,* Washington, DC, 1995, US Government Printing Office; American Diabetes Association: *Diabetes 1996. Vital statistics,* Alexandria, VA, 1996, American Diabetes Association; CDC: Cigarette smoking among adults—United States, 1991, *MMWR,* 42(12):230–233, 1993; Cantwell MF, et al.: Epidemiology of tuberculosis in the United States, 1985 through 1992, *Journal of the American Medical Association;* 272:535–539, 1994.

TABLE 18.3
Selected Health Indicators in Hispanic Subgroups and Excess Ratio Compared to Whites

Annual indicator	Population subgroup	Rate in Whites	Rate in Mexican Americans	Ratio	Rate in Puerto Ricans	Ratio	Rate in Cuban Americans	Ratio
Infant mortality and determinants								
Beginning prenatal care after first trimester (%)	Pregnant females	19.2	37.9	2.0	32.2	1.7	13.2	0.7
Beginning prenatal care during third trimester or no prenatal care (%)	Pregnant females	4.2	10.5	2.5	8.0	1.9	2.1	0.5
Live births weighing < 1,500 g (%)	Infants < 1 year old	1.0	0.9	0.9	1.7	1.7	1.2	1.2
Live births weighing, 1,500–2,499 g (%)	Infants < 1 year old	4.8	4.7	1.0	7.5	1.6	4.9	1.0
Neonatal deaths per 1,000 live births	Infants < 28 days old	5.2	5.0	1.0	7.2	1.4	5.3	1.0
Postneonatal deaths per 1,000 live births	Infants 28 days to 1 year old	3.0	2.9	1.0	3.9	1.3	2.0	0.7
Cardiovascular risk factors and diabetes								
Undiagnosed diabetes (%)	Adults 45–74 years old	6.1	9.6	1.6	11.8	1.9	9.9	1.6
Diagnosed diabetes (%)	Adults 45–74 years old	5.9	14.3	2.4	14.3	2.4	5.9	1.0
Overweight (%)	Males 20–74 years old	32.0	39.8	1.2	25.6	1.1	27.6	1.1
(BMI ≥ 27.3 kg/m² female; ≥ 27.8 kg/m² male)	Females 20–74 years old	32.2	48.1	1.5	40.2	1.7	31.6	1.3
Hypertension (%)	Males 20–74 years old	25.2	27.1	1.1	21.4	0.6	20.7	0.6
(Systolic pressure ≥ 140 or diastolic pressure at ≥ 90 mm Hg)	Females 20–74 years old	19.0	20.5	1.1	19.2	0.8	14.4	0.6
High blood cholesterol (%)	Males 20–74 years old	18.8	20.5	1.1	17.7	0.7	16.1	0.7
(serum cholesterol ≥ 240 m/dL)	Females 20–74 years old	20.1	19.0	0.9	22.7	0.8	16.9	0.6
Other indicators								
No health insurance (%)	Persons < years of age	16.2	39.5	2.4	21.0	1.3	23.3	1.9
Poor or fair self-rated health	Adults 45–64 years old with < 12 years education	31.1	31.0	1.0	41.4	1.3	23.1	0.7
	with ≥ 12 years education	10.8	14.4	1.3	17.3	1.6	13.1	1.2

Source: Adapted from the National Center for Health Statistics: *Health United States, 1993,* DHHS publication (PHS) no. 94–1232, Hyattsville, MD, 1994, Public Health Service; CDC: Cigarette smoking among adults—United States, 1991, *MMWR;* 42(12):230–233; Cantwell MF, et al.: Epidemiology of tuberculosis in the United States, 1985 through 1992, *Journal of the American Medical Association;* 272:535–539.

TABLE 18.4

Selected Perinatal Health Indicators in Japanese, Chinese, Filipino, and White Americans

Annual indicator	Population subgroup	Rate in Japanese Americans	Rate in Chinese Americans	Rate in Filipino Americans	Rate in Whites	Ratio*
		Infant mortality and determinants				
Beginning prenatal care after first trimester (%)	Pregnant females	11.8	16.2	21.3	19.2	0.6
Beginning prenatal care during third trimester or no prenatal care (%)	Pregnant females	2.4	2.9	4.3	4.2	0.6
Live births weighing < 1,500 g (%)	Infants < 1 year old	0.9	0.7	1.1	1.0	0.9
Live births weighing 1,500–2,499 g (%)	Infants < 1 year old	6.2	4.3	6.4	4.8	1.3
Neonatal deaths per 1,000 live births	Infants < 28 days old	4.4	3.3	4.5	5.2	0.8
Postneonatal deaths per 1,000 live births	Infants 28 days to 1 year old	2.5	2.5	2.4	3.0	0.8

*Japanese to White ratio; ratios for Chinese and Filipinos can be calculated from data presented.
Source: Adapted from National Center for Health Statistics: *Health United States, 1994,* DHHS publication (PHS) no. 95–1232, Hyattsville, MD, 1995, Public Health Service.

non-Hispanics, and being overweight and having diabetes are also notably more prevalent among Hispanic subgroups. Lower rates of health insurance coverage affect all three Hispanic subgroups.

As with Hispanics, some data for Asian-Pacific Islander Americans are subgroup specific (see for example, perinatal indicators in table 18.4), while other data are aggregated over the entire group (tables 18.1 and 18.2). Tuberculosis is a striking area of excess risk in this population,[13,64] whereas for other indicator shown, this minority group is on par with whites or has a relatively better health status. The aggregate data do not, however, reflect the high prevalence of diabetes in Asians and Pacific Islanders, the high prevalence of obesity in Pacific Islanders, the higher risks of hypertension in Filipinos as compared to some other Asian-Pacific Islander subgroups, or the high risks of cardiovascular diseases and cancer among Native Hawaiians.[15,18,28,38,43,59]

Nutrition priorities compete within the overall priorities in minority communities. Therefore, it is also useful to have a perspective on the relative importance of various health and social problems for minority groups versus the majority population. Ranking of causes of death (shown in table 18.5) is a crude indicator of differences across population subgroups for males and females. The causes of death listed are those ranked 1 to 10 in 1992 for each sex-racial\ethnic group, as published by the National Center for Health Statistics.[48] Diseases of the heart are the top-ranked cause of death for all populations except Asian\Pacific Islander females, for whom this cause ranks second. Stroke is among the top three causes of death for White and Asian males and for most females. Cancer is among the top two causes of death

for all populations except American Indian males, for whom cancer deaths are displaced by unintentional injuries (accidents) to third ranked. Diabetes deaths are among the top ten causes of death for all populations shown and rank higher among Black, American Indian, Hispanic, and Asian-Pacific Islander females than among White females. Other noteworthy differences include the relatively higher rank of deaths associated with chronic liver disease in American Indians and of suicide in American Indian males, and the importance of homicide and legal intervention and of HIV infection among Black males and females compared to the other populations. The relatively higher mortality from traumatic causes and HIV among minority populations may substantially influence their relative risks of dying from chronic diseases. Persons who would ultimately be at risk for heart disease, cancer, or stroke may die before these risks take effect.

Both the similarities and differences in the rankings should be noted. In regard to similarities, nutrition-related interventions for heart disease, cancer, stroke, and diabetes are of high priority for both men and women in all groups, even though the death rates in some groups are lower than in the White population. However, interventions that are not within the direct purview of nutrition programs, for example, interventions to lower rates of accidents, homicide, or HIV infection, are also of high priority for many minority communities and may be more immediate on a day-to-day basis. Being sensitive to the nonnutrition priorities that are addressed in a comprehensive context will improve the cultural relevance of nutrition programs. Being sensitive to potential differences in disease rates and rank-

TABLE 18.5

Ten Leading Causes of Death by Race and Ethnicity for Males and Females, U.S. Population, 1992

Cause of death	White	Black	Hispanic	American Indian/ Alaska Native	Asian-Pacific Islander
Females					
Heart disease	1	1	1	1	2
Cancer	2	2	2	2	1
Stroke	3	3	3	5	3
Chronic obstructive pulmonary disease	4	9	8	8	7
Pneumonia and influenza	5	6	6	7	5
Unintentional injuries	6	5	5	3	4
Diabetes mellitus	7	4	4	6	6
Atherosclerosis	8				
Nephritis, nephritis syndrom, nephrosis	9			9	10
Speticemia	10				
Certain conditions arising in the perinatal period		7	7		
Chronic liver disease and cirrhosis				6	
Suicide					8
Homicide and legal intervention		10			
HIV infection		8	10		
Congential anomalies			9	10	9
Males					
Heart disease	1	1	1	1	1
Cancer	2	2	2	3	2
Stroke	3	6	6	6	3
Unintentional injuries	4	5	3	2	4
Chronic obstructive pulmonary disease	5	8		10	6
Pneumonia and influenza	6	7	10	9	5
Suicide	7		8	5	8
Chronic liver disease and cirrhosis	10		7	4	
Diabetes mellitus	9	10	9	7	9
HIV infection	8	4	4		10
Homicide and legal intervention		3	5	8	7
Certain conditions arising in the perinatal period		9			

Note: Blanks indicate causes of death ranked higher than 10 for the racial/ethnic group in question.
Source: Adapted from National Center for Health Statistics: *Health United States, 1994,* DHHS publication (PHS) no. 95–1232, Hyattsville, MD, 1995, Public Health Service.

ings across racial and ethnic groups and across genders improves the cultural specificity of nutrition programs in multicultural communities. For example, priorities may be different between Black and Puerto Rican or between Mexican-American and Filipino-American communities within the same locale or between native-born Asian Americans versus recent immigrants.

ACHIEVING CULTURALLY SENSITIVE AND CULTURALLY SPECIFIC NUTRITION PROGRAMS

In her thoughtful book, *Within Our Reach,* Schorr elaborates the lessons that can be learned from successful pro-grams, after analyzing the high costs of poor outcomes of inadequate programs (see Chapter 10 in reference 62). Core elements of success are trusting and respectful relationships and what we characterize as **cultural sensitivity** and **cultural specificity.** Cultural sensitivity and specificity are two important but somewhat different dimensions of the effectiveness of community nutrition programs. Cultural sensitivity can be defined as a characteristic of the service provider: an awareness of cultural factors relevant to interventions in a given population and a willingness to incorporate these factors into program design and implementation. Cultural specificity can be defined as a characteristic of an intervention program that results from cultural sensitivity on the part of the provider: the extent to which the program design, content, and delivery strategies incorporate and reflect the specific norms, values, and situational context of the population served by the program. This distinction helps to clarify that the ultimate goal in cross-cultural programming is cultural specificity. Cultural sensitivity is a means to achieving this goal. A key principle to remember in thinking about culturally sensitive and specific programming is that everyone operates within a cultural framework. Approaches for improving the effectiveness of programs involving easily identifiable cultural subgroups are also useful for improving effectiveness with cultural contexts that are less visible. Insights into ways to increase effectiveness with minority groups can lead to general insights about improving community nutrition skills. In one sense, the comments that follow simply represent the application of sound community nutrition programming principles in situations where very different cultural frameworks are operating.

Needs Assessment

Culturally sensitive needs assessment requires knowing what to measure as well as being aware of cultural variables that influence the validity of assessments made. Consistent with approaches described elsewhere in this book, the entire spectrum of factors that potentially influence the effectiveness interventions should be assessed in relation to a proposed program (see the box 18.6). The environmental factors and provider and program variables would be assessed at the institutional or locality level and the client variables through surveys, reference to medical or program records, and specialized techniques such as focus group interviews or discussions with key informants like community leaders or client advocates.

Environmental and provider variables are intentionally listed before client variables in the box to counteract the tendency toward "victim blaming," in which client behaviors or circumstance are viewed as barriers that make clients seem hard to reach with the approaches that may be the most convenient for or familiar to service providers.[22]

The needs assessment variables in box 18.6 are highlighted here because they vary systematically by race or ethnicity and social class. Therefore, it cannot be assumed that these variables are homogeneous among racial or ethnic or socioeconomic status groups within the same locality or that, within the same racial or ethnic

---

BOX 18.6

FACTORS RELATED TO THE EFFECTIVENESS OF NUTRITION INTERVENTION IN MINORITY COMMUNITIES

ENVIRONMENTAL VARIABLES
- Health care system
- Other health and social problems
- Extant media campaigns
- Risk factors
- Cultural changes in general population

PROVIDER AND PROGRAM VARIABLES
- Nature of services offered
- Intervention approach
- Credibility, legitimacy in community
- Structural and cultural accessibility

CLIENT VARIABLES
- Family history
- Health problems
- Health insurance coverage
- Income, occupation, education
- Household composition
- Social orientation
- Generation
- Worldview
- Religious beliefs
- Literacy level
- Skill in cross-cultural communication
- Alienation from government
- Health care–seeking practices
- Food preferences and dietary practices
- Food ideology and folk beliefs
- Other health-related attitudes and practices
- Experience with prior programs

Source: Adapted from references 11, 31, and 51.

---

or socioeconomic status group, they are similar across localities. For example, Leininger has developed a rather practical health care assessment tool used in transcultural nursing.[42] However, as with many other tools, using this assessment tool without sufficient training and a firm, cosmopolitan understanding of the underlying concepts may reduce it to a mere checklist of superficial characteristics. Each item in the box is worthy of detailed consideration that is beyond the scope of this chapter.

Deciding on the Type of Intervention

The continuum of intervention possibilities extends from a totally provider-centered approach on one extreme to a totally client-centered approach at the other extreme. The most client-centered approaches are oriented toward empowerment. Kent defines empowerment "as the capacity to define, analyze and act on your own problems."[34] **Empowerment-oriented interventions** are not viewed as necessarily working within existing environmental constraints but rather as challenging these constraints and attempting to remove them. From a culturally sensitive perspective, programs that focus on empowerment are the ideal. Recently, Neighbors et al.,[50] putting an emphasis on empowerment with responsibility for self-empowerment, recommended that "health providers and health educators need to find ways of strongly encouraging black clients to take personal responsibility for their health actions . . . health messages phrased within the context of self-help, self-reliance, *community control* [emphasis added], empowerment, and self-pride should be firm and culturally sensitive" (reference 50, page 564).

The classical model for empowerment approaches is that of Paulo Freire.[23] A program in a Micronesian community is often cited as an empowerment approach applied in the community. In this program, community residents were helped to understand the system behind the promotion of a commercial soft drink. The resulting motivation to gain more control on this issue led to identification of locally produced coconut milk as a more profitable and nutritious alternative to soft drinks that could be promoted by community residents to the advantage of both merchants and consumers.[61]

Having institutional policies that are culturally sensitive and genuinely oriented toward the goal of improved nutritional status and that take a long-term rather than short-term view is critical to the ability to design and implement effective cross-cultural programs. Intervention programs that attempt to empower clients to develop their won analysis and problem-solving approaches generally require more effort, time, and resources as well as institutional tolerance for decentralized programming, lower cost-efficiency, client-centered attitudes among staff, and a possible apparent lack of results in the short term.[61] Urban gardening programs are another example of programs that attempt to improve dietary intake by helping people to take control of their food resources at the production level.[6]

A review of the literature on programs for "special populations," as minority groups are sometimes termed, provides many useful examples of the effective use of community-based programming strategies. Such strategies can help to achieve programs that, although less ambitious than some that would reach the empowerment ideal, do incorporate the concepts of forming partnerships with the community, seeking solutions from the community, planning *with,* rather than *for* the community, and permitting the pace and nature of efforts to achieve the goal to be shaped in the relevant cultural framework.* A clear advantage of such approaches is that they build in legitimacy and credibility and can lead to mechanisms for reaching those who are in the community but currently outside the usual health care delivery system (see Gonzalez et al.[25]).

Two other important characteristics of effective programs in minority communities are the use of multiple strategies—recognizing that there is not one best strategy for reaching everyone—and integrating or linking programs that address multiple outcome. Fragmentation of services that results from categorical programming approaches in which separate and often duplicate systems are established to meet different nutrition program objectives is legendary in the U.S. health and welfare system. Such approaches place a large burden on members of the client group to access all of the different service components they need. The health profiles of minority and low-income populations indicate a coexistence of multiple problems. Client-centered approaches that reduce artificial divisions and competition among an individual's health problems or among the needs of members of the same family can reduce the burden on the individual or family who needs to access those services.

IMPLICATIONS FOR COMMUNITY NUTRITION PROFESSIONALS

Cultural variables potentially apply to all program settings. Within the United States, cultural factors that influence the effectiveness of programs for racial or ethnic minority groups are of particular interest because the health and socioeconomic profiles of these groups are disadvantageous relative to the majority population.

---

*See references 10, 11, 21, 29, 31, 39, 41, 60, and 63.

The heightened *awareness* of the need to be effective with minority populations reflects the changing demographics of the United States, in which minority populations now constitute nearly one fourth of the population overall and the majority of the population in some areas. *Acceptance* of the need to be effective with minority populations reflects the changing image of American society and the realization that the melting pot concept in which ethnic groups acculturate toward an Anglo-Saxon reference culture will probably never take place but, more important, *should* never take place. There is recognition that the suppression of ethnic diversity, largely motivated by ethnocentric devaluing of other cultures, deprives both minority group members and the population as a whole of the richness of a multicultural environment.

The steps toward improving cross-cultural competence and cultural sensitivity are much easier to outline than to accomplish. A process including cultural consciousness-raising, self-evaluation, unlearning of stereotypes relaxation of professional style, and shift to client-centered programs is needed. Given the willingness to think carefully about and respect cultural differences, the requirements for achieving culturally specific programs include facilitative institutional policies, willingness to extend oneself—psychologically and physically—to the client population, and the willingness and ability to approach program design and implementation in a client-centered and goal-oriented manner.

Maintaining cultural sensitivity and implementing culturally relevant programs will be among the greatest challenges faced by community nutrition professionals in the next century. The sociopolitical context for race relations in America and in the world will determine how members of different cultural groups view each other. Competition for resources will determine how far an agency can extend itself by using approaches in which the practitioner's role is to empower members of the community to identify their problems and develop the solutions. Changing demographics may redefine which cultural groups are in the minority. Changing health patterns among economically advancing minority populations may result in even greater health disparities than are now seen.

COMMUNITY NUTRITION PROFESSIONALS IN ACTION

- An African American colleague finds a statement in a book on multicultural issues to be particularly prob-

lematic. In fact, she is outraged over the following statement and wants the book banned from further use in a course at your institution:

> A popular image of the African American woman is that of "Mammy," the affectionate nursemaid of both white and black children. This image has some basis because historically motherhood has been an important role for the black woman—even more meaningful than the role of wife (reference given).

Why do you think your colleague is so upset? What do you think the instructor should do? What kind of statement would make *you* want to have a book banned from further use?

- At the wrap-up of a training seminar for cardiologists on nutrition issues in diverse populations, one of the participants refers to "minorities and their *peculiar* foods." Would you be offended by such a statement? In any case, can you explain why this statement is problematic? Use this situation to explain to a colleague what it means to be ethnocentric. In what way could the cardiologist have made her point about others' unfamiliar food choices without seeming ethnocentric.

- Some treasured food choices in any culture can be deemed unhealthy. Think of one such "unfavorable" food habit among the people of your culture and describe a potential intervention program that could eventually curb this habit without "imposing" on the culture. Identify an unhealthy food habit from a culture *other than your own*. Describe a potential intervention program that could eventually curb this habit without "imposing" on the culture. What do you think or do differently in this case, compared to when considering a food habit from your own culture? Give some specific examples of aspects that make this second part of the exercise feel *cross*-cultural?

- You are a staff member of the U.S. Department of Agriculture headquarters in Washington, D.C. The California WIC program has requested an exemption to the regulations for content of the WIC food package to provide foods that meet the cultural preferences of the Asian-Pacific Islander clients. You are told that this is impossible and contrary to policy and are asked to draft the agency's official response? What clarifying questions might you need to ask you supervisor, and why? What do you think is your agency's rationale for this policy? What questions, if any, might you ask the California WIC director, before preparing your response, and why? What cultural issues do you need to address in your response? If you were the director of your agency and had the authority to change the policy, would you change it? If so, how and why? List the pros and cons of your decision.

GOING ONE STEP FURTHER

Your university has an exchange program with universities in several other countries. Next year ten graduate students (five from Venezuela and five from Indonesia) will arrive for an intensive training (ten weeks) in nutrition intervention and education programs, to be followed by a sixteen-week practical internships in several nutrition programs across your state. The ten students are free to absorb as much as possible of the techniques used in the programs. Cultural diversity in the service delivery has been a main focus of these programs. The goal of the internships is to assess the programs and to analyze the feasibility of using the programs or parts of them in Indonesia and Venezuela. Each group of five students will provide a report to advise the national Ministry of Health of their country.

You are asked to chair a planning and support team for the visiting students. The team is composed of faculty and graduate students. Your first task is to provide this team with a work plan that pays attention to arrangements for the visit, including aspects of housing, social, religious, and other needs. However, you have been told that one faculty member is of the opinion that the ten visiting students need only a lot of technical data and very detailed facts. Another faculty member has made it clear that in her opinion training in U.S. nutrition education for foreign application is unwise. You realize that the quality, scope, and direction of your first draft of the work plan will heavily influence the outcome of the deliberations of the support team. You decide to make an all out effort and be as specific as possible in your first draft.

Write a first draft based on what you perceive to be a successful visit. Make also a rough sketch on how you plan to guide the deliberations of the support team so that the goal of a successful learning experience will be accomplished. Use advise of experts and trusted people as you see fit.

REFERENCES

1. American Diabetes Association: *Diabetes 1996. Vital statistics,* Alexandria, VA, 1996, American Diabetes Association.
2. Airhihenbuwa Co: *Health and culture. Beyond the Western paradigm,* Newbury Park, CA, 1995, Sage.
3. Bassis MS, Gelles, RG, Levine A: *Sociology: an introduction,* ed 2, New York, 1984, Random House.
4. Berg J, Berg BL: Compliance, diet, and cultural factors among black Americans with end-stage renal disease, *J Natl Black Nurses Assoc* 3:16, 1989.
5. Bertorelli A: Nutrition counseling: meeting the needs of ethnic clients with diabetes, *Diabetes Educ* 16:285, 1990.
6. Blair D, Giesecke CC, Sherman S: A dietary, social and economic evaluation of the Philadelphia Urban Gardening Project, *J Nutr Educ* 23:161, 1991.
7. Brislin R, Yoshida T: *Intercultural communication training. An introduction,* Thousand oaks, CA, 1994, Sage.
8. Broussard BA et al: Prevalence of obesity in American Indians and Alaska Natives, *Am J Clin Nutr* 53:1535S, 1991.
9. Brown, RD: Affirmative action and workforce diversity, *Public Manager* 24(3): 43–45, 1995.
10. Bruerd B, Kinney MB, Bothwell E: Preventing baby bottle tooth decay in American Indian and Alaska Native communities: a model for planning, *Public Health Rep* 104:631, 1989.
11. Burrell-Roberson N: Outreach programs: community networking, in Proceedings of the Fourth National Conference on Cancer Nursing, Atlanta, 1983, American Cancer Society.
12. Campinha-Bacote J: The Process of Cultural Competence, Wyoming, OH, 1991, Transcultural C.A.R.E. Associates.
13. Cantwell MF, Snider DE, Cauthen GM, Onorato IM: Epidemiology of tuberculosis in the United States, 1985 to 1992, *JAMA* 272:535, 1994.
14. Coiner CB, Sumida SH: Is multiculturalism enough? *Women's Studies* 20:209, 1992.
15. Curb JD, Wilson RH, smith J, Leonard BB: Cardiovascular risk factor levels in ethnic Hawaiians, *Am J Public Health* 81:164, 1991.
16. Doak C, Doak LE, Root JH: *Teaching patients with low literacy skills,* Philadelphia, 1985, JB Lippincott Co.
17. Eliades DC, Suitor CW: *Celebrating diversity. Approaching families through their food,* Arlington, VA, 1994, National Center for Education in Maternal and Child Health.
18. Ernst ND, Harlan WR: Obesity and cardiovascular disease in minority populations: proceedings of conference held in Bethesda Md, August 28–30, 1990, *Am J Clin Nutr* 53(suppl):1507, 1991.
19. Fleming J: Meeting the challenge of culturally diverse populations, *Pediatr Nurs* 15:566, 648, 1989.
20. Food and Consumer Services, Office of analysis and Evaluation, United States Department of Agriculture: *WIC participant characteristics,* Alexandria, VA, 1994, USDA.
21. Foreyt JP, Ramirez AG, Cousins JH: Cuidando el Corazon: a weight reduction intervention for Mexican Americans, *Am J Clin Nutr* 53:1639S, 1991.
22. Freimuth VS, Mettger W: Is there a hard-to-reach audience? *Public Health Rep* 105:232, 1990.

23. Freire P: *Predagogy of the oppressed,* New York, 1970, Seabury.
24. Geertz, C: *The interpretations of cultures,* New York, 1973, Basic Books.
25. Gonzalez VM, Gonzalez JT, Freeman V, Howard-Pitney B: *Health promotion in diverse cultural communities,* Palo Alto, CA, 1991, Health Promotion Resource Center.
26. Gudykunst WB: *Bridging differences: effective intergroup communication,* Newbury Park, CA, 1991, Sage.
27. Harris PR, Moran RT: *Managing cultural differences,* ed 2, Houston, 1990, Gulf Publishing.
28. Havas S, Fujimoto W, Close N, McCarter R, Keller J, Sherwin R: The NHBLI Workshop in Hypertension in Hispanics, native Americans, and Asian\Pacific Islanders, *Public Health Reports* 111: 451, 1996.
29. Heath GW et al: Community-based exercise and weight control: diabetes risk reduction and glycemic control in Zuni Indians, *Am J Clin Nutr* 53:1642S, 1991.
30. Hofstede, G: *Culture's consequences: international differences in work-related values,* Newbury Park, CA, 1980, Sage.
31. Hutchins V, Walch C: Meeting minority health needs through special MCH projects, *Public Health Rep* 104:621, 1989.
32. Kavanagh KH, and Kennedy PH: *Promoting cultural diversity; strategies for health care professionals,* Newbury Park, CA, 1992, Sage.
33. Keesing FM: *Cultural anthropology: the science of custom,* New York, 1965, Holt, Reinhart, and Winston.
34. Kent G: Nutrition education as an instrument of empowerment, *J Nutr Educ* 20:193, 1988.
35. Kittler PG, Sucher KP: Diet counseling in a multicultural society, *Diabetes Educ* 16:127, 1990.
36. Krupat A: For multiculturalism, *Women's Studies* 20:242, 1992.
37. Kuhnlein HV: Culture and ecology in dietetics and nutrition, *J Am Diet Assoc* 89:1059, 1989.
38. Kumanyika S: Diet and chronic disease issues for minority populations, *J Nutr Educ* 22:89, 1990.
39. Kumanyika SK, Charleston JB: Lose weight and win: a church-based program for weight and high blood pressure control among black women, *Patient Educ Counseling* 19:19, 1992.
40. Kumanyika SK, Golden PM: Cross-sectional differences in health status in U.S. racial\ethnic minority groups: potential influence of temporal changes, diseases, and lifestyle transitions, *Ethnicity Dis* 1:50, 1991.
41. Lasco RA, Curry RH, Dickson VJ, Powers J, Menes S, Merritt RK: Participation rates, weight loss, and blood pressure changes among obese women in a nutrition-exercise program, *Public Health Rep* 104:640, 1989.
42. Leininger M: Becoming aware of types of health practitioners and cultural imposition, *J Transcult Nurs* 2:32, 1991.
43. Lin-fu JS: Population characteristics and health care needs of Asian Pacific Americans, *Public Health Rep* 103:18, 1988.
44. Locke DC: *Increasing multicultural understanding. A comprehensive model,* Newbury Park, CA, 1992, Sage.
45. Luhman R, Gilman S: *Race and ethnic relations: the social and political experience of minority groups,* Belmont, CA, 1980, Wadsworth.
45. Lysaught JP: Toward a comprehensive theory of communications. A review of selected contributions, *Educational Administration Quarterly* 20:101, 1984.
46. Mithun JS: *The role of the family in acculturation and assimilation in America: a psychocultural dimension.* In McCready WC, editor: *Culture, ethnicity, and identity: current issues in research,* New York, 1983, Academic Press.
47. National Center for Health Statistics: *Health United States, 1990,* DHHS publication (PHS) no. 91–1232, Hyattsville, MD, 1991, Public Health Service.
48. National Center for Health Statistics: *Health United States, 1994,* DHHS publication (PHS) no. 95–1232, Hyattsville, MD, 1995, Public Health Service.
49. National Diabetes Data Group: *Diabetes in America,* ed 2, NIH Publication no. 95-1468, Bethesda, MD, 1995, National Institutes of Diabetes, Digestive, and Kidney Diseases.
50. Neighbors HW, Braithwaite RL, Thompson E: Health promotion and African Americans. From personal empowerment to community action, *Am J Health Prom* 9:281, 1995.
51. Nickens HW: Health promotion and disease prevention among minorities, *Health Aff (Millwood)* 9:133, 1990.
52. O'Hare WP: America's minorities. The demographics of diversity, *Population Bulletin* 47(4):1–47, 1992.
53. Palmer TC: Changes in the neighborhood: integrating the academy and diversifying the curriculum, *Women's Studies* 20:217, 1992.
54. Parker WM: *Consciousness-raising: a primer for multicultural counseling,* Springfield, IL, 1988, Charles C Thomas.
55. Pearce WB: *Communication and the human condition,* Carbondale, 1989, Southern Illinois University Press.
56. Pedersen P: *A handbook for developing multicultural awareness,* Alexandria, VA, 1988, American Association for Counseling and Development.
57. Perkin J, McCann SF: *Food for ethnic Americans: is the government trying to turn the melting pot into a one-dish dinner?* In Brown LK, Mussel K, editors: *Ethnic and regional foodways in the U.S.: the performance of group identity,* Knoxville, 1984, University of Tennessee press.
58. Report of the Expert Panel on Populations Strategies for Blood Cholesterol Reduction: A statement from the Na-

tional Cholesterol Education program, National Heart, Lung, and Blood Institute, and National Institutes of Health, *Circulation* 83:2154, 1991.

59. *Report of the Secretary's task force on black and minority health, executive summary, vols 1 and 2, Crosscutting issues in minority health,* Washington, DC, 1985, U.S. Department of health and Human Services.

60. Robbins K: Heart, body, and soul: the gospel of good health, *Hopkins Med News,* Spring 1991.

61. Rody N: Empowerment as organizational policy in nutrition intervention program: a case study from the Pacific island, *J Nutr Educ* 20:133, 1988.

62. Schorr LB: *Within our reach. Breaking the cycle of disadvantage,* New York, 1989, Anchor Books.

63. Shintani TT, Hughes CK, Beckham S, O'Connor HK: Obesity and cardiovascular risk intervention through the ad libitum feeding of traditional Hawaiian diet, *Am J Clin Nutr* 53:1647S, 1991.

64. Snider DE, Salinas L, Kelly GD: Tuberculosis: an increasing problem among minorities in the United States, *Public Health Rep* 104:646, 1989.

65. Sumida SH: Have we had enough? *Women's Studies* 20:234, 1992.

66. Teutsch S, Newman H, Eggers P: The problem of diabetic renal failure in the United States, *Am J Kidney Dis* 13:11, 1989.

67. U.S. Department of Agriculture: *Cross-cultural counseling: a guide for nutrition and health counselors,* FNS-20, Washington, DC, 1986, USDA.

68. U.S. Department of Commerce, Bureau of the Census: We, the first Americans, SuDoc No C3.2:Am 3/9, Washington, DC, nd, U.S. Government Printing Office.

69. U.S. Department of Commerce, Bureau of the Census. 1990 U.S. Census Data, http://venus.census.gov/cdrom/lookup.

70. Yanov D: American ethnogenesis and public administration, *Administration and Society* 27:483, 1996.

71. Yutrzenka BA: Making a case for training in ethnic and cultural diversity in increasing treatment efficacy, *J Consult Clin Psychol* 63:197, 1995.

THE ROAD TO CRITICAL COSMOPOLITAN PROFESSIONALISM

CHRISTIAN B. MORSSINK MS, MPH

SOCIOLOGIST, AND HEALTH PLANNER

Who is to say what constitutes expertise in multicultural interaction? Sailors, pilots, journalists, and diplomats should be among the most expert if expertise were a simple count of contacts with "others." Sure, "globe-trotters" have many good stories to tell and their experiences are important in understanding other cultures. But this is not enough. Expertise also implies a certain attitude and "awakeness" in analyzing these experiences. This attitude, which we will term *the willingness to accept the existential equality of all human beings, combined with a reflective curiosity for the uniqueness of one's own place in the universe* is a core factor in defining multicultural expertise. Such willingness is a necessary condition for true multicultural effective interactions.

Domination "colors" many multicultural encounters. When Granman Aboikoni of the Saramacaner people in Suriname received the queen of Holland in his residence in Dejoemoe, a Dutch journalist suggested that he must be rather pleased that the queen came so far into the rainforest to meet with him. The Granman's answer was: "Why should I be? She came to the center of the universe, didn't she?" This was a perfect rebuke of the journalist's implicit arrogance and showed, at the same time, the Granman's sense of the relativity of ethnocentrism. We all have our perceptions of a center of the universe.

Most of humankind's multicultural encounters took place in terms of conquest, exploitation, genocide, and annihilation. Over the centuries the tendency of one group to want to dominate others has taken many forms, some more benign than others. Recent forms include such phenomena as the "ethnic cleansing" in Bosnia, the violent relocation of Indian tribes in Brazil, the underfunding of public schools in districts that happen to be mainly African-American or Hispanic, the denial of tribal rights that are documented in treaties, the refusal to let U.S. soldiers wear the blue United Nations helmets, or the removal of Princess Irene of the Netherlands from the line of succession when she became Catholic. The shift to an ecumenical approach to cultures and religions is rather young (witness the Kennedy candidacy for president and the willingness to learn about the Jewish faith and culture or about the Native-American history and philosophies) and is definitely not universal (witness the conflicts in Northern Ireland).

Ideas of universal human rights and global human equality are still not commonly accepted. Domination is still a key issue in most forms of cross-cultural encounters. We need to remain keenly aware of this history and the ensuing attitudes when developing a strategy of developing common ground and cooperation. Think about the explicit irony when a Palestinian girl on the West Bank reads the *Diary of Anne Frank*. Or, think about the rejection of cultural domination expressed in the remark about the Barbie Doll made by Majid Ghbaderi of Iran's Institute for the Intellectual Development of Children and Young Adults: "Barbie is like a Trojan horse. Inside, it carries its western cultural influences, such as makeup and indecent clothes. Once it enters our society, it dumps these influences on our children." Ghaderi created Sara, a new female doll, dressed in a traditional Iranian flowing gown (*Chicago Tribune*, October 25, 1996).

I lived for several years in Suriname, a country that definitely has its share of problems, but one that has been more successful than many in balancing many ethnic groups and language while at the same time defining a national identity. This balance has some good lessons for other parts of the world. For example, in the 1970s, the small Suriname Jewish community offered a building site for the newest and biggest mosque in South America, which now stands next to the oldest synagogue of South America. In Suriname there is no majority, there are only larger and smaller minorities. The question of dominance in the daily exchange between groups is absent or takes place in a political arena of debate, coalition building, and winning through voting and "pork-barrel" tactics. In the absence of a majority, cultural expressions are highlighted and there is frequent exposure of cultural differences between groups.

(For example, on national TV each national religious organization is allotted the same amount of air time.) National holidays embrace three major religions; professionals such as doctors, nurses, and dietitians have already learned in elementary school how to interact across the cultural divides. Predictions are that the United States will become a no-majority (in demographic terms) country around 2025. The United States can and needs to learn from countries such as Suriname in preparing for those times.

Besides the domination aspect, which is a constant yardstick for minorities and for societies at large in their dealings with majorities, the fear of loss of social anchors is a real problem for those individual who want to commit to a cosmopolitan attitude. When, several centuries ago, Rousseau walked out of the gates of the city-state of Geneva, he ventured on a road of scientific rebellion against the status quo and the established powers of church and state. Over time, he became a socially marginalized person, making him vulnerable to psychological stress and creating fears of paranoia in his mind. Starting on a road of critical cosmopolitan professionalism may bring such fears of marginality to the nutrition professional, especially as she or he works with the intensely cultural topics of food and health. We are all social animals and we need others to survive. It is rare that people roam freely beyond the confines of culture and structure. We use reference groups and individuals for bonding. Without them, we become adrift to the point of losing our humanity. The ease of committing to a cosmopolitan approach is then much influenced by the groups, families, and organizations that we interact with on a daily basis.

It is much more difficult to become cosmopolitan for persons from a strong ethnocentric culture, especially if that ethnocentricity is driven by a sense of hegemony. It may even be dangerous for one to exercise a deviant view in countries that don't condone freedom of expression. You may have to accept the relative powerlessness of the employee position in many professional situations and, thus, you have to be careful. However, commitment to a cosmopolitan approach does not mean to picking each and every fight; rather, it implies that you keep your eyes on the goals. Every voyage starts with a first step, and it may be necessary to go two steps forward and one step backward. Find solidarity among other "marginals" and choose the times and places where you want to be exemplary in your "global awareness."

Acknowledging that each group and culture has its own *equal* "right" to specific values and norms is termed *"cultural relativism."* However, this does not mean that our values and norms become relative for ourselves. *Au contraire.* By embracing a cosmopolitan view, we have to be intensely aware of our own values and norms. One cannot successfully enter a multicultural relationship—professional, familial, or geographical—without being aware of *all* the core values, habits, norms, and sanction mechanisms that play a role, including one's own. Learning about food and health habits of others should stimulate you to immediately also evaluate your own habits. Or, on a grander scale, tourism and immigration lead to an increased global awareness of the history and specificity of many ethnic and local cultures. Many old trades, habits, and architectures, for example, are consequently being revived. To use a nutrition-related metaphor: it is important that we understand the cultural *nourishment* that comes from such revival. Those who have been forcibly estranged from their cultures need the most nourishment. I think that the need for cultural and political nourishment of the African-American who visits Africa or the Jew who visits Israel must differ greatly from the needs I have when I return home to visit Holland.

Embracing the values of your own nest is not in itself inherently inconsistent with having a cosmopolitan attitude. Just try to define yourself by who you *are,* rather than by who you *are not.* You will be that much more sure of yourself in your cross-cultural interactions with others.

CHAPTER NINETEEN

ETHICS IN COMMUNITY NUTRITION

*In a world where wars may wreck any national or individual life,
where wealth and insecurity go hand in hand, where class still
divides, and religion no longer speaks with unquestioned
authority, the need of study and reflection [on ethics]
becomes increasingly evident.*
—J. DEWEY AND J. TUFTS

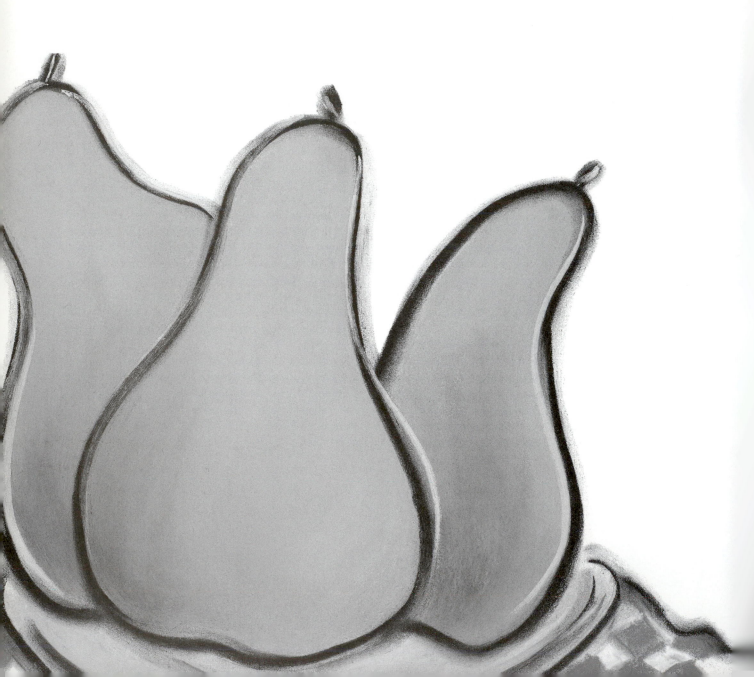

Core Concepts

In this environment of ongoing technological advancement, change in family and cultural systems, and pressure for health care and welfare reform, ethical leadership requires the ability to act on the strength of one's convictions, even when it may not be the most popular course of action. The study of ethics provides a base for decisions made between two conflicting choices and is guided by values and a motivation to support a principle viewed as worthwhile or desirable. This chapter presents a model for reflection on values and their application to specific cases through ethical principles and codes of conduct. Finally, tools for ethical decision-making are presented. Responsible, ethical decision making is a responsibility of all community nutrition professionals.

Objectives

When you finish chapter nineteen, you should be able to:

~ Define ethics and discuss its application in community nutrition.

~ Cite five ethical principles that apply to decision making in community nutrition.

~ Recognize an ethical dilemma as a situation where there is a conflict of values and a decision (action) is needed.

~ Apply deliberate steps of ethical decision making to resolve an ethical dilemma.

Key Words

Word	Page Mentioned
Ethics	570
Morality	570
Core values	571
Ethical principles	572
Autonomy	573
Paternalism	573
Beneficence	573
Justice	574
Rights	575
Duties	575
Burdens	576
Utility	576
Stewardship	576
Codes of conduct	577
Ethical dilemma	579
Ethical analysis or ethical decision making	579

The opening quotation, voiced over sixty years ago during the Depression, was written in a text designed to explore the meaning and consequences of conduct and social policies when adequate resources were limited. Today, limited resources are being faced but in a different context and in a changing environment. Downsizing and cross-training are changes in the business community. Competition and mergers of health care providers with the movement toward managed care are changes addressing health in communities. Health care costs and the expanding elderly population are exceeding our ability to pay for services. The value of life has become blurred with the use of technologically advanced treatment. Welfare reform and state waivers are forging redefinition of persons considered to be poor and how to define eligibility for assistance. There is no shortage of conflicts and there are no predetermined answers. The moral conflicts of decades ago continue to challenge today's decision makers. There is renewed importance in the study of ethics.

Community nutrition professionals in all kinds of positions face choices and decisions that involve ethical considerations. Definition of quality standards, provision of nutritional services, policy implementation, collegial or client relationships, and resource allocation all require an examination and identification of contributing values and ethical principles. Decisions must be based on a defensible ethical position and then implemented in a way to assure achievement of desired outcomes. The overall goal of this chapter is to enable community nutrition professionals to develop a defensible ethical stance.

Responsible, ethical decision making develops respected community nutrition professional leaders. This is because ethics advances critical thinking processes and helps community nutrition professionals determine how to weigh conflicting values and make decisions. Personal beliefs, work experiences, and authority interplay with ethical decision making, which deeply affects lives and relationships. These are important in facing the myriad of issues related to promoting and advancing the health and nutritional well-being of communities. Figure 19.1 illustrates how ethics encircles these components that contribute to health. To confront the moral conflicts shaping health, the community nutrition professional needs to make decisions considering how all of the ethical realms shape wellness.

ETHICS AND MORALITY

Ethics is a branch of philosophy that evaluates how moral decisions affect a specific behavior. It is a science that deals with judging as right or wrong, good or bad.[12] **Morality** is the conduct of living what is right. For example, a moral person is aware that his or her actions contain consequences that affect others. The moral person selects from the behavior choices using ethical guidelines to advocate positive consequences for others.

To study moral behaviors, one has to identify the nature of relationships among people, individual's rights and duties in society, and the moral rules that individuals apply in decision making.[25] Ethics guides conduct by systematically evaluating choices and behavior from the standpoint of how close it is to an "ideal" right or wrong, good or bad.

Hundreds of ethicists; philosophers; and contributors from the fields of philosophy, economics, law, and religion have outlined theories, hypotheses, and principles to describe the characteristics of ethics. As Tom Peters stated,

> Anyone who is not very confused all the time about ethical issues is out of touch with the frightful (and joyous) richness of the world. But at least being actively confused means that we are actively considering our ethical stance and that of the institutions we associate with. That's a good start.[20]

The best starting place is to characterize the components of ethical theory commonly used in ethical decision making. Adapted from Beauchamp,[5] Holmes,[16] and Sobal,[24] figure 19.2 schematically outlines the components leading to ethical behavior. The bottom level (the base) approaches ethics from an individual's worldview and values, advances through ethical principles and area rules, and then addresses specific cases (the top level). Information received at all other levels is integrated into a specific situational decision. The base presents the more abstract, all-encompassing, universal areas of human concern and activity.[16] From this foundation, relevant principles and rules are selected to make judgments and implement decisions in specific cases.

VALUES AND PERSONAL LIFE VIEWS

Values are beliefs that guide and motivate attitudes and actions. Your internal values interact within your world and shape behavior and obligations. An *individual* living in a *community,* which is part of the *world,* must approach ethics by understanding how his or her values shape behaviors in these relationships to persons in the community and society at large.

The base asks an individual to first reflect within the self and then "step outside" of the self and reflect on

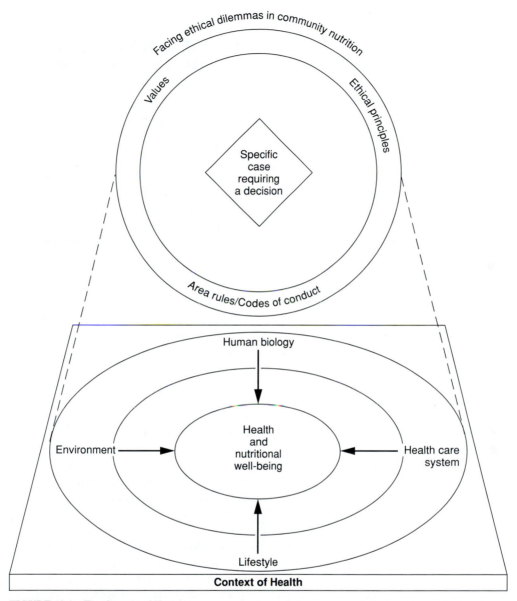

FIGURE 19.1   The Context of Health
Applying the components of ethical behavior within the context of community health and nutritional well-being.

what values are relevant for "good" and right behavior in the world. At this level, one brings any interpretations based on knowledge and experience (past and present) and evaluates his or her self-view as determined by personal values and the expectations of the external culture or society.

Core values that members of most societies accept as an ideal are shown in box 19.1. These virtues form the foundation of highest moral standards used to judge our actions and those of others. When found in a moral person, these values produce behaviors that are praised by others because they uphold high standards[22] Most cultures and societies respect these core values and believe individuals should possess these characteristics and use them in difficult situations.

There is an overlap where your internal values are shared with people in the society. Living a life according your values and values that your community also shares provides self-fulfillment. This gives a person a sense of "goodness" in life. The differences between

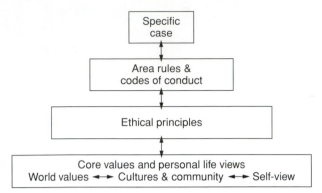

FIGURE 19.2   Applying the Components of Ethical Behavior
(*Source:* Adapted from Beauchamp TL, Childress JF: *Principles of biomedical ethics,* ed. 4, New York, 1994, Oxford University Press.)

BOX 19.1

EXAMPLES OF DEFINITIONS FOR VALUES ESTEEMED BY A GOOD SOCIETY

Respect for life—A value to assert that humans deserve respect as humans;[22] includes loving, caring, tolerance.

Responsibility—Something for which one has a duty, an obligation, or a burden;[2] includes concern for the "common good," fairness, civic duty, and citizenship.

Integrity—Soundness of and adherence to a moral principle; one who "maintains a consistent commitment to do what is best—especially under conditions of adversity";[14] includes honesty, trustworthiness, promise keeping, and loyalty.

Courage—The state or quality of mind or spirit that enables one to face danger or fear with self-possession, confidence, and resolution.

cultural values (business, geographic, racial, etc.) is how the values are perceived and applied within a group of people in the decision-making process.

STOP!! Take time to write your definitions of these core values in your own words. Then, give examples from your own experiences and professional work of how you apply that value to contribute positively toward society.

Try to imagine a perfect society where each person is free to make choices that do not harm the free choice of others. What is needed to make this community function together? Further your thoughts of what a "perfect world" would look like by answering the questions in box 19.2.

BOX 19.2

IDENTIFYING YOUR VIEW OF A "PERFECT WORLD"

1. When we can do anything we want, what should we choose to do? (How do you expect people to act in a perfect world?)
2. When we can do anything, but we can't do everything, what should we do? (How would you limit the action choices if given the constraint of scarce resources?)
3. When should society take action related to food distribution and accessibility? Health care? Housing needs? Job placement? The environment?
4. When should the decision be left solely to the individual?

Core values are routinely reflected in the behaviors of community nutrition professionals. An example of valuing fairness is when a community nutrition professional applies eligibility criteria equally. A firm advertising a food upholds honesty by accurately presenting product benefits after understanding the values of others. A working environment that promotes zero tolerance for sexual harassment or gender inequality is applying the value of respect.

Ask the following questions to identify the core values that define your view of the world. What values do you expect in your relationships with other people? What types of professional behaviors do you feel are morally right or wrong? Which value is the highest virtue? What types of values are morally good or bad for the harmonious functioning within your family, neighborhood, culture, workplace, country, and world?

Personal values and societal values relate to moral duties and obligations and direct our behaviors in relationship to others in the world. When applied, they are defined as **ethical principles.**

ETHICAL PRINCIPLES

Ethical principles give a person guidelines (i.e., tools) to use in evaluating "goodness" or "badness" of behaviors in a community ideal. In figure 19.2, the next component is labeled ethical principles and represents generalizations that guide a wide range of decisions and behaviors. At this level of application, the ethical prin-

BOX 19.3

PRINCIPLES OF ETHICS FOR COMMUNITY NUTRITION PROFESSIONALS

Principle of autonomy
Principle of beneficence
Principle of justice
Principle of utility
Principle of stewardship

ciples are a component in the final analysis of a specific case but do not give the community nutrition professional *the answer* on how to resolve a specific conflict. Ethical principles translate societal, professional, and personal values into impartial, equitable tools to apply toward judgment in a case (the top level in figure 19.2).

Early ethical thought focused on the understanding of universal principles or ideals that would remain consistent and unchangeable over time when analyzing and defining ethical behavior. Thus, ethical principles are the stable values by which society lives. They are generally accepted as fundamental; regardless of time, culture, or religion. Box 19.3 identifies five ethical principles particularly relevant to health and community nutrition. In reading about them, think how each one applies to your personal life and your professional practice.

The Principle of Autonomy

This principle refers to the rights of persons to make important decisions about their own lives even when viewed by others as the "wrong" decision. All individuals are entitled to self-choices about what is in their own best interests. The ethical principle of **autonomy** allows individuals to make their own choices as long as they do not harm or interfere with the autonomy of others. A libertarian defends personal autonomy as *the* highest value. Legal writings call for justification of any intervention that reduces the autonomy or right of the individual to determine his or her own actions. Laws guarantee autonomy for adults unless there is evidence of incapacity to do so.

The concept that an individual has the right to accept or refuse guidance once the benefits and burdens have been explained is an example of an autonomous deci-

sion. Note that autonomy implies being aware of the pros and cons so one can make an "informed choice." The dietary guidelines, which ask individuals to modify their behavior to reduce dietary fat intake to prevent chronic disease, can be viewed in terms of autonomy. The principle of autonomy is also reflected in the National School Lunch Program's policy of "offer versus serve." The food service staff must offer a nutritionally balanced meal to each child, but the child chooses what to take and eat. Intervention strategies to promote health behavior change described in chapter 6 are implemented with the principle of autonomy.

In contrast, some individuals are unable to make informed decisions. In these situations, other parties act on behalf of that person's well-being, using the principle of **paternalism.** A decision based on paternalism is a "purposeful, planned overriding of another's interest."[4] An example of paternalism is where the parents make decisions for young children or caretakers act on behalf of mentally incompetent adults. For example, in the case of an elderly person with dementia, a designated individual can make financial and health care decisions for that elderly person. Biomedical ethics has established that it is difficult to take away a person's right to make decisions about health treatments unless the harm prevented or the benefit provided justifies taking away the freedom of choice.

Examples of violating an individual's right to autonomy occur when interventions are manipulative or coercive. This can happen by (1) giving false, exaggerated, or incomplete information; (2) overwhelming individuals with excessive or complex information in an effort to cause confusion or reduce understanding; (3) provoking or taking advantage of fear, anxiety, or pain;[27] and (4) using powerful influence over less powerful, vulnerable persons. Strongly instructing persons using Food Stamps to purchase only nutritious foods rather than "junk" foods and implying their risk of losing benefits would be an example of manipulation.

The Principle of Beneficence

This **beneficence** principle refers to doing good for others. "A view of beneficence is that I ought to help my neighbor because everyone's life, including mine, will be better off if all of us (within reason) are helpful to each other" (reference 23, p. 53). Actively intervening to benefit individuals and communities is the essence of public health and health care interventions. For example, prenatal nutrition counseling offers education and support that can enhance the health and well-being of the mother and baby. If the supportive nutrition counseling gives the individual a sense of gaining control over her life and taking responsibility for the developing baby, improved self-esteem enhances motivations and benefits can extend beyond health. Examples of beneficence in health care include prevention of disease and disability, prolongation of life, relief from pain and suffering, and restoring a person to a useful function in life.

Today, most people believe that both the government and the business community have responsibility to act in the interest of society. "The sheer size of business and government, the two most powerful institutions in the country, obliges them to address problems of public concern and promote good."[25] However, because of limited resources, there is heightened awareness and questioning of how best to respond to human needs. For example, in managing health as a business, the philosophy of providing services (i.e., "good") without jeopardizing a business's profit mission (the limits of providing "good") is the area that managed care is defining.

The principle of beneficence also applies to giving aide to those who are in lower income classifications. Offering nutritional services to those who can work but perhaps are unable to earn enough to purchase adequate food and health services promotes a common "good" and contains the ethical component of beneficence. "The moral principle of beneficence recognizes that a person has an obligation to further the interests of others when those interests are both important and legitimate."[13] In community nutrition, discussions on the benefits of preventive nutrition services for persons in high-risk categories and where benefits are greater than the cost of input are important and legitimate. The resources (monetary and staff) used for these services are based on the sound ethical principle of beneficence. For example, if offering school breakfast promotes better learning and supports the nutritional well-being for children, then the benefits of having a motivated, learning child who will subsequently participate productively in society provides greater benefits to the community than the initial food and staff cost of preparing and serving the breakfast.

Related to the beneficence principle is *nonmaleficence*. This principle assures safety to members of society when they are under care or receive services from someone else. This principle requires interventions to not place harm on users and to reduce the risk of harm.

Since inaccurate information has the potential to harm others, the public health practitioner has the responsibility to maintain competence and attentiveness to the accuracy of information provided. For example, use of iron supplements must be clearly explained, since overdosing causes harm.

Another area of nutrition requiring ethical analysis on the basis of nonmaleficence is in policy making. What abundance of evidence is needed to make dietary recommendations for the public? To reduce the risk from diseases (i.e., harm), specific dietary interventions are recommended. However, many times, dietary recommendations are made before scientific evidence is conclusive. The community nutrition professional must carefully assess the weight of the evidence and the potential benefits and harm involved with establishing policy (or not establishing policy).[17] In addition, caution is advised to not promote dietary changes as more beneficial than what the limited knowledge has identified.[26] As science continues to provide new information about population-specific dietary guidelines, community nutrition professionals will need to be attentive to completing a periodic reassessment to modify policy recommendations, if necessary.[17]

The Principle of Justice

The principle of **justice** implies that equals should be treated equally and that those who are unequal should be treated differently according to their differences. Justice calls for fairness to all with considerations of what inequalities limit fairness. For example, Daniels suggests that "an individual's fair share of the normal range of opportunity for his society is impaired when disease or disability impair normal function".[10] Daniels argues that justice (in the sense of equal opportunity) begins if both are equal. A sick person's functioning level is unequal to a well person's functioning level. Thus, ill persons requiring more services to be restored to a "normal" functioning level is mandated because "equal opportunity" for health services is when both are offered an opportunity that protects and restores "normalcy."[10] "The fundamental issue is whether we are being fair to people by meeting the full range of their needs."[11] In the case of a child with disabilities, the principle of justice argues that more health care is needed to bring a disabled child's health to a normal functioning closer to fairness.[13] This leads to a discussion of the three elements within the principle of justice: rights, duties, and burdens.

Justice is a belief that people ought to get something based on what they have a *right* to. "If we have a right to something, it is morally wrong for anyone to take it away. . . . [For example,] when we talk about what is ours by right, we mean something we need not say 'thank you' for."[3] **Rights** are based on the view that each person has an intrinsic value and there are certain "freedoms" or guarantees because of this value. The principle of justice is the basis for a community nutrition profession to believe that all human beings are created equal and there is a minimum standard of nutrition services that all people deserve and need to contribute toward a "good" society.

According to one view of justice, people have rights because society grants them (reference 23, p. 35). Thus, justice is a fair distribution of rights among individuals or groups in society who have legitimate claims.[22] An example related to nutrition is the United Nations's Covenant of Rights (box 19.4). Do you agree with this statement of rights?

In applying the principle of justice, community nutrition professionals are continually faced with trying to distribute food and nutrition services equally based on rights. "There are times when persons have some special rights which differ from others. An aged person has different rights from those of a child. The rights of a disabled child are different from those of a healthy child. . . . One of the arts of managing a just community is recognizing when individual differences do create differences of rights" (reference 23, p. 35).

The 1996 accreditation manual of the Joint Commission on Accreditation of Healthcare Organizations (JCAHO) also include a new chapter entitled "Patient Rights and Organization Ethics."[7] The statement found in box 19.5 appears in the JCAHO manual. Notice how the JCAHO statement claims specific rights that include the principles of nonmaleficence and autonomy, discussed earlier. There is a right to "safeguard their dignity" (i.e., prevention of harm—a principle of nonmaleficence) and to respect their choices (the principle of autonomy). Overall, a "right" defines agreements, rules and practices within a community or organization to promote the moral values and conduct needed to make people better off.[15] They are developed through interrelationships and respect others' interest as equal in importance as their own.[15]

If one person has a right, then another person has a *duty* to honor it. If a client has a right to receive Food

---

BOX 19.4

AN EXAMPLE DEFINING INDIVIDUAL HEALTH "RIGHTS"

Everyone has the *right* to a standard of living adequate for the health and well-being of himself and his family, including medical care, and necessary social services and the right to security in the event of unemployment, sickness, disability, widowhood, old age or other lack of livelihood in circumstances beyond his control.

Source: The United Nations's Covenant of Rights. *United Nations International Covenant on Economic, Social and Cultural Rights,* Article 11.

BOX 19.5

AN EXAMPLE DEFINING PATIENTS' "RIGHTS"

Patients have a fundamental **right** to considerate care that safeguards their personal dignity and respects their cultural, psychosocial, and spiritual values. These values often influence patients' perception of care and illness. Understanding and respecting these values guide the provider in meeting the patients' care needs and preferences. The goal of the patient rights and organization ethics function is to help improve patient outcomes by respecting each patient's rights and conducting business relationships with patients and the public in an ethical manner.

Source: Joint Commission on Accreditation of Healthcare Organizations: *Comprehensive accreditation manual for hospitals,* Oakbrook Terrace, IL, 1996, pp. 76–78.

Stamps, then it is the duty of the caseworker to honor it. **Duties** are obligations toward individuals resulting from those persons having rights. In the case of the United Nations's Covenant of Rights, once adopted who "ought" to provide these and what "should" be provided?

STOP!! If food is considered as a "right," let's explore how identifying relationships and duties interact with offering food to the elderly. Chapter 11 described two meal distribution programs for seniors: Meals on Wheels and Congregate Dining Programs. If government funding was decreased and severely limited for these programs, who else could accept the duty of providing food for the frail elderly?

Equal treatment, or justice, also includes equal distribution of the **burdens.** Distributing the "costs" or the "undesirable" duties is part of the distribution of burdens. The principle of justice distributes difficult responsibilities as equally as rights. In community nutrition and health care, there are times when the limits of the resources become the burdens. The question becomes what basic, minimum of health (or nutritional) care is "adequate," given peoples' needs and the limitations of the resources?

Does "adequate health care" guarantee equitable access by all to quality health care? Members in a community include sick and well persons. An example of questions surrounding distribution of burdens in health services arise when persons with special health care needs require more services than those who are healthy. What criteria are used to determine an equitable distribution of services while not threatening the well-being of the one giving services? To many ethicists, evaluating if benefits are large enough to compensate for costs (i.e., benefit-cost analysis) *does not* meet the criteria of being ethically defensible.

There are times in community nutrition when clients cannot defend their own rights against the right of others. A community nutrition professional uses ethical decision making and intervenes to distribute resources based on the principle of justice. The interpretation of justice in practice considers whether service implementation includes equal treatment of all persons and provides equal access to community nutrition services. Alternatively, services are often based on entitlement, ability to pay, or on a first come first served basis?[19] In summary, a community nutrition professional's duty is to advocate for and respect the rights of others when applying the principle of justice, especially the rights of any vulnerable population groups. Overall, applying justice to populations is complex and requires understanding the process used to distribute resources and burdens.

Principle of Utility

The dilemma of distributing resources is a source of many ethical dilemmas in public policy, management, and social welfare. Managed care has begun to address concerns of what individuals and society want and what they are willing to pay for. Whether in health care in general or in community nutrition programs, a community nutrition professional must choose which services will yield the greatest benefit (beneficience), distribute the burdens of limited resources (justice) and pose the least risk for harming others (nonmaleficence). Apply-

ing all of these principles to distribute resources can lead to conflict between two principles.

The **utility** principle defends a position where there is "greatest good for the greatest number of people and no one is left worse off." It seeks to distinguish right from wrong on the basis of consequences and to prioritize benefits and resources. The moral individual must evaluate which course of action promotes the best outcome with the least amount of burdens shared by those unable to receive the action. This type of analysis is the essence of cost-effectiveness and cost-benefits analysis discussed in chapter 15.

> **STOP!!** Let's look at an example to review the principle of utility for a community nutrition professional in working in a clinic serving the homeless population. Suppose a grant of $10,000 was awarded to promote the nutritional status of the homeless population being served. Would you establish criteria to use all of the money to distribute the food to a certain number with the highest need (i.e., the most malnourished)? Or would you divide the total number of dollars received by the number of people served and give an equal share? Or would you use a portion of the money to develop counseling and education programs to educate homeless persons on how to better manage food dollars, find job employment, and access health care services? Would homeless *families* be given higher priority than single *individuals* due to the potential for a larger number of nutritional status improvements per contact? Would children be given greater attention due to the potential of reaching adulthood well nourished and being able to contribute toward a "good" society? Define the risks (i.e., harm) that would come to those persons to whom no food, counseling, or education would be given? Would there be an ethical difference if a person with a mental condition that impaired decision making refused to accept the nutritional services versus refusal by persons without mental conditions? Identify what other community relationships would accept the burdens and duties to provide food or nutrition services for the homeless?

Principle of Stewardship

The responsibilities of community nutrition professionals include managing services, finances, or the nutritional status of others within a context to enable others to fulfill their rights. To perform these roles, the principles of **stewardship** is important.

> Stewardship asks us to be deeply accountable for the outcomes . . . without acting to define purpose for others, control others, or take care of others. . . . Because it exercises accountability but centers on service rather than control,

stewardship is a means to impact the degree of ownership and responsibility each person feels for the success of our organizations, our society, and our lives.[6]

Stewardship includes a judgment of social responsibility and moral values and respect for property and puts resources to good and beneficial use. Spending your organization's time, money, and resources on programs and services is a commitment to meet a set of objectives within a determined level of cost.

Stewardship is usually discussed as financial accountability. A good steward is attentive to monitoring the implementation process and tracking how close the spending level is according to the allocations.

Finally, stewardship includes being answerable for outcomes. The community nutrition professional manages another person's trust and he or she implements changes to promote a more "good" society. The service component of stewardship includes active listening to cultural norms and distributing resources in a way that encourages vulnerable persons to also accept responsibility for their part in making changes to promote nutritional health and well-being.

Overall, when working in community nutrition, ethical principles provide tools for analyzing decision-making alternatives based on what society values. Reflection on the principles identified in box 19.6 is important to guide actions, as these principles remain unchangeable over time.

STOP!! Review the new terminology used in discussing ethical principles for community nutrition professionals (see box 19.6).

AREA RULES AND CODES OF CONDUCT

Your personal and professional values interacting with organizational values determine approaches to applying the principles of ethics. In the schematic levels (figure 19.2), area rules apply to a narrower set of guidelines for conduct. Area rules are unequivocal norms that guide conduct. They are present in the form of **codes of conduct** and professional ethics. Generally these can be applied to a case without a great amount of interpretation. Area rules do not resolve ethical controversy; rather, they define required standards of performance.

A survey of 1,900 international firms revealed that 84 percent of the U.S. respondents had codes of ethics.[18] Codes of conduct or ethics delineate behaviors expected of all members of the organization or group. The American Dietetic Association has adopted a Code of Ethics

---

BOX 19.6

ETHICAL PRINCIPLES FOR COMMUNITY NUTRITION PROFESSIONALS

Autonomy: The condition or quality of respecting the decision-making capabilities of an individual to make self-choices.

Paternalism: A policy or practice of treating or governing people in a parental manner, especially by providing for their needs without giving them rights or responsibilities. It can be justified only if (1) the harm prevented or the benefit provided outweighs the loss of patient's independence or (2) when the person's condition seriously limits the ability to choose autonomously.

Beneficence: An inclination to perform kind, charitable acts; to do good or the best possible.

Nonmaleficence: To prevent harm to persons or groups; provide safety to members of society.

Justice: The quality of being just or fair; the principle of moral rightness; conforming to moral rightness in action or attitude; the upholding of what is just, especially fair treatment and due reward in accordance with honor, standards, or law.

Rights: Very stringent claims that entitle a person to take a particular action; a person's freedom (i.e., self-determination) from interference with life. It can include entitlement to food, shelter, and health care. Rights can conform with or to justice, law, or morality.

Duties: A course of action required by moral and ethical principles. Moral bonds regarding what one ought to do and to whom. Obligations to take specific steps. These obligations can be *burdens* if the duties place unfavorable responsibilities on an individual or groups of individuals.

Utility: A belief that action should be directed toward achieving the greatest good for the greatest number of people and no one is worse off.

Stewardship: The individual's responsibility to manage property, finances, or other affairs with proper regard to the rights of others and maintaining accountability for outcomes and financial expenditures.

---

for Dietetic Practitioners (table 19.1). This code of ethics is intended to "reflect the ethical principles guiding the dietetic profession and to outline commitments and obligations of the dietetic practitioner to self, client, society, and the profession."[1] A professional code of ethics is

TABLE 19.1

Code of Ethics for Dietetic Practitioners

1. The dietetic practitioner provides professional services with objectivity and with respect for the unique needs and values of individuals.
2. The dietetic practitioner avoids discrimination against other individuals on the basis of race, creed, religion, sex, age and national origin.
3. The dietetic practitioner fulfills professional commitments in good faith.
4. The dietetic practitioner conducts himself/herself with honesty, integrity, and fairness.
5. The dietetic practitioner remains free of conflict of interest while fulfilling the objectives and maintaining the integrity of the dietetic profession.
6. The dietetic practitioner maintains confidentiality of information.
7. The dietetic practitioner practices dietetics based on scientific principles and current information.
8. The dietetic practitioner assumes responsibility and accountability for personal competence in practice.
9. The dietetic practitioner recognizes and exercises professional judgment within the limits of his/her qualifications and seeks counsel or makes referrals as appropriate.
10. The dietetic practitioner provides sufficient information to enable clients to make their own informed decisions.
11. The dietetic practitioner who wishes to inform the public and colleagues of his/her services does so by using factual information. The dietetic practitioner does not advertise in a false or misleading manner.
12. The dietetic practitioner promotes or endorses products in a manner that is neither false nor misleading.
13. The dietetic practitioner permits use of his/her name for the purpose of certifying that dietetic services have been rendered only if he/she has provided or supervised the provision of those services.
14. The dietetic practitioner accurately presents professional qualifications and credentials.
15. The dietetic practitioner presents substantiated information and interprets controversial information without personal bias, recognizing that legitimate differences of opinion exist.
16. The dietetic practitioner makes all reasonable effort to avoid bias in any kind of professional evaluation.
17. The dietetic practitioner voluntarily withdraws from professional practice under the following circumstances;
    a. The dietetic practitioner has engaged in any substance abuse that could affect his/her practice;
    b. The dietetic practitioner has been adjudged by a court to be mentally incompetent;
    c. The dietetic practitioner has an emotional or mental disability that affects his/her practice in a manner that could harm the client.
18. The dietetic practitioner complies with all applicable laws and regulations concerning the profession.
19. The dietetic practitioner accepts the obligation to protect society and the profession by upholding the Code of Ethics for the Profession of Dietetics and by reporting alleged violations of the Code through the review process.

Source: Copyright The American Dietetic Association. Reprinted by permission from *JOURNAL OF THE AMERICAN DIETETIC ASSOCIATION,* Vol. 88(5): 1592–1593, 1988.

designed to be a guiding principle or norm for professional behavior, to ensure minimal standards of practice for all members, and to protect the consumer from fraud.

Another set of code of ethics guiding the government-employed community nutrition professional is the Congressional Code of Ethics for Government Service (see table 19.2). Notice how many of the ethical principles discussed earlier are translated into specific behaviors in both of these codes of ethics.

Another set of rules guiding professional practices is quality assurance criteria. These form an implied contract with the public such that clients can expect to receive service or care that is technically (scientifically) sound. Quality assurance standards become accepted as the norm for all health care organizations. They form an implied contract with the public such that clients can expect to receive service or care that respects their free-

dom of choice (autonomy), to not be harmed (non-maleficence), and to be informed of treatment options.

Ethical analyses are needed to *develop* these standards. According to JACHO standards, patients have the right to refuse treatment.[7] This acknowledges the principle of autonomy as being a higher (i.e., more valued) ethic than the principle of acceptable professional standards of care to promote good (beneficence). For example, a person needing dietary intervention and counseling can refuse treatment even though the dietary modifications prescribed promote a "good."

When two ethical principles collide and one course of action must be chosen over another, there is an ethical dilemma. However, once written as a code of conduct and/or quality assurance standard for an organization, there is no uncertainty as to expected behavior. Area rules are important and guide behavior in specific cases.

TABLE 19.2

Congressional Code of Ethics for Government Service

Any person in government service should:

1. Put loyalty to the highest moral principles and to country above loyalty to persons, party, or government department.
2. Uphold the Constitution, laws, and legal regulations of the United States and of all governments therein and never be a party to their evasion.
3. Give a full day's labor for a full day's pay; giving to the performance of duties earnest effort and best thought.
4. Seek to find and employ more efficient and economical ways of getting tasks accomplished.
5. Never discriminate unfairly by the dispensing of special favors or privileges to anyone, whether for remuneration or not, and never accept, for self or family, favors or benefits under circumstances which might be construed by reasonable persons as influencing the performance of governmental duties.
6. Make no private promises of any kind binding upon the duties of office, since a government employee has no private word which can be binding on public duty.
7. Engage in no business with the government, either directly or indirectly, which is inconsistent with the conscientious performance of governmental duties.
8. Never use any information coming to employee confidentially in the performance of governmental duties as a means for making private profit.
9. Expose corruption wherever discovered.
10. Uphold these principles, ever conscious that public office is a public trust.

Source: From *United States Postal Service Employee Labor Relations Manual,* Issue 12, May 1, 1989.

SPECIFIC CASES *ARE* ETHICAL DILEMMAS

Ethical dilemmas arise when there is a conflict between two choices and each choice can be justified with an ethical principle. Decisions easily guided by rules or choices that become clear following appropriate data gathering are not ethical dilemmas. For example, an administrator is reviewing job applications for a community nutrition professional position and realizes that two persons who have applied are not qualified. The administrator does not interview these individuals because they lack minimum qualifications. If he is later notified that one of the individuals was from an ethnic group similar to the population with which the person in the community nutrition professional position would be working, there still is no ethical dilemma if the job requirements were valid for the position.

Ethical dilemmas occur when you must choose between opposing choices that each have merit depending on which or whose values you consider. At the top level of figure 19.2, the specific case is where ethical dilemmas are often confronted. Dilemmas involve the goodness of actions (means) and/or the goodness of outcomes or consequences (ends). Making a "good" ethical decision requires analyzing and ranking values and interests and then taking actions that distribute the "goodness" and lessens harm (or burdens) among community members.

ETHICAL ANALYSIS AND THE COMMUNITY NUTRITION PROFESSIONAL

Ethical analysis or ethical decision making is the process used to arrive at an ethically defensible decision. The challenge (and responsibility) of all ethical persons is to recognize potential ethical dilemmas, and then use appropriate questioning, analysis, and reasoning to understand and resolve the dilemma. Table 19.3 represents the steps to ethical decision making applied to community nutrition. This process reviews how the ethical dilemma impacts others at the societal level, the organizational level, individuals within a community, and your personal beliefs. Ethical conflicts occur in the context of professional, social, and economic pressures and obscure the moral issues discussed early. Careful study and judgment are necessary.

When considering eithics, it is important to remember that many times events outside of our control contribute to the outcome. Thus, even in the most analytical approach, the ethical dilemma takes on characteristics specific to each case. However, the community nutrition professional who has taken time to reflect and identify the ethical principles in conflict can be proactive in making the best choices given the circumstances. These factors underscore the attention needed for each step in the process of ethical decision making.

> **STOP!!** Let's look at an ethical code of conduct related to the value of respect: confidentiality. Any information related to any case (babies, pregnant teens, persons screened for the HIV virus, elderly, etc.) can be communicated in confidence to other care providers. However, many times discussion of diet concerns and interventions occur in areas where other clients can hear. What solutions are available to you, as a community nutritional professional to resolve this dilemma? Use the process outlined in table 19.3.

There are times when your ethical stance may not agree with the stance of your colleagues. Or, you may agree on the course of action and desired outcome, but dis-

TABLE 19.3
Ethical Decision Making in Community Nutrition

Values analysis
   What are my personal values and beliefs that will impact
   my decision making?

Examine the situation
   What are the facts?
   Who is responsible to act? (Duties Analysis)
   What are the consequences of action? (Benefit/Harm
     Analysis)
   What and whose rights are involved? (Rights/Principles
     Analysis)
   What is fair treatment in this case? (Justice Analysis)

Specify the problem or options
   Explore the options for action. What creative choices can
     be planned to resolve the problem(s)?
   Have I considered all of the creative solutions that might
     permit me to reduce harm, maximize benefits, respect
     more rights, or be fair to more parties?

Identify the stakeholders? Who or what is involved in the
   conflict?
   What people, information, services, systems, cultural
     beliefs, financial obligations, and other resources will
     contribute to discourage my decision?
   Is the client informed, competent, and able to state wishes?
     Have I listened to those wishes?
   Have I listened and identified the community's value
     systems?

Formulate the options and identify the consequences of each
   option
   What are the potential consequences of my solutions to
     each of the stakeholders?
   Which of the options considered does the most to maximize
     benefits, reduce harm, respect rights, and increase
     fairness?
   Are all parties treated fairly in any proposed decision?
   Does my organization usually provide this type of nutrition
     collaboration, intervention, or resources?
   Does my profession provide guidelines for this problem?

Identify and eliminate unethical options

Select the best alternative
   Assess the benefits, risks, and outcomes of each option on
     the individual, family, community, and societal levels.
   Evaluate the alternatives based on the values, principles,
     and area rules to defend the best alternative.

Implement the decision
   Who should be consulted and informed?
   What actions will assure that my decision achieves its
     intended outcome?

Evaluate and follow-up
   Was the decision implemented correctly?
   Did the decision maximize benefits, reduce harm, respect
     rights and treat all parties fairly?

Source: Adapted from Murphy, P: Implementing business ethics, *Journal of Business Ethics;* 7:907–915, 1988; Sims, R: The challenge of ethical behavior in organizations, *Journal of Business Ethics;* 505–513, July 1992.

agree on who is the proper authority to implement the action. In examining an ethical conflict, it is important to recognize potential causes for disagreement. Are there differences in amount or type of professional experiences? Are there traditional, cultural family system differences that your personal values are opposing? Does your organization have an institutional decision-making policy that is a barrier for recommending actions of an ethical nature? A community nutrition professional identifies important decision makers within the organization who will help discuss, evaluate, and recommend proper action.

With the change in health care delivery, more emphasis is on working together to produce healthier individuals and healthier communities. Consensus regarding *specific* behaviors is difficult to achieve. It is easier to agree on the ideals rather than the specific application of the ideals. Nonetheless, discussion unmasks the obscured values and increases sensitivity in the decision making. The process of ethical inquiry helps profes-

sionals critically reflect and actively participate in a decision-making process that contains controversial issues while respecting other people.

STOP!! Suppose you are working in a community where a managed care organization has collaborated with a health department to provide nutrition counseling and education to pregnant teenagers. In developing the program, this team has used research to identify appropriate intervention strategies and diet recommendation to meet the needs of pregnant teens. All agree on providing the best prenatal care for a mother to produce a healthy baby. Topics potentially addressed in the counseling sessions would include healthy weight gain during pregnancy, eating a well-balanced diet for two, breast-feeding versus formula feeding, drug use, and contraception following the birth of the baby. What might be some sensitive or controversial issues in applying the program?

Collaboration between these organizations offers an opportunity to expand services and provide a successful continuum of care. It is important to identify the ethical dilemmas caused by the internal policy making within each organization. Negotiating and respecting ethical differences of opinion clearly mark a nutrition leader. In the example above, your role would be to integrate interventions traditionally seen in public health with a market-based health care provider. It may also include collaborations with schools, migrant health centers, women's health clinics, and parent groups. The ability to identify and communicate any sensitive or potential areas of disagreement profits the client, the community nutrition professional, and the collaborating organizations.

ETHICAL ANALYSIS, THE COMMUNITY NUTRITION PROFESSIONAL, AND THE ORGANIZATION

How are values, ethics, and expectations for conduct communicated within your organization? Values and expectations can be written or unwritten. Answer the questions in table 19.4 to analyze your organization's commitment to ethical principles. Identify the role of written policies and consider if and how they are applied to daily activities. This is a review of your interpretation of how ethics is applied in your work life. Business experts report that in order to make and maintain visible ethical standards within an organization, an ongoing process for reviewing and establishing ethical behavior is needed.[18]

It is difficult to pioneer ethical sensitivity if workers (and more specifically, higher level managers) within the organization behave unethically. Business experts recommend yearly review of ethical standards through training and in yearly performance evaluations to imbue the importance and use of the code of ethics. Those organizations committed to ethical principles and yearly review inspire the importance of ethics at all service levels. An organization grounded in ethics is more apt to be financially successful as well as to achieve long-term stability because customers respect moral values. There are four business ethics principles that achieve this success[18] (see box 19.7).

Creating and maintaining high ethical standards within an organization, whether it is a for-profit business, a government public health agency, or a nonprofit community group requires regular "communication, encouragement, oversight, review, and revision."[18]

Community nutrition professionals face an important ethical "test" when developing nutrition policies on be-

TABLE 19.4
Evaluation of Organization's Ethical Culture

1. Does the organization have a vision statement, statement of purpose, ethical code, and/or statement of ethical policy? What do they say about the organization's ethics and values? Are these statements simply public relations ploys, or are they actually used in the organization?
2. Do the executives and managers ever talk about ethical matters? If so, in what way?
3. Is any ethical instruction provided for employees?
4. What is the role of ethical concerns in the decision-making process in the organization?
5. Are employees treated with justice and love; that is, are they treated with fairness and a concern for their personal development?
6. How are women and minorities treated in the organization?
7. Does the organization have a sexual harassment policy?
8. Does the organization have a policy on affirmative action or equal opportunity?
9. Does the organization view itself as having a social responsibility? If so, how does it carry it out?
10. In summary, what is the role of ethics in the organization? Is there a difference between the stated policies and actual practices within the organization?

Source: From Anderson, S: *Applying ethics in organizations,* St. Paul, 1997, Center for Continuing Studies, Bethel College, p. 17.

BOX 19.7

BUSINESS ETHICS PRINCIPLES

Principle 1: High-ethics firms are at ease interacting with diverse internal and external stakeholder groups.

Principle 2: High-ethics firms are obsessed with fairness.

Principle 3: High-ethics firms' responsibility is individual rather than collective; individuals assume personal responsibility for actions of the firm.

Principle 4: High-ethics firms see their activities in terms of a purpose.

half of their organization. Nutrition policy should reflect the food and nutrition needs of the public based on (1) results of formal scientific studies, (2) other assessments and market research, (3) consensus recommendations of health and nutrition researchers and practitioners, and (4) published national nutrition objectives and model standards for nutrition services.

To assess your readiness for a policy recommendation, complete the policymaking assessment in table 19.5. The

TABLE 19.5

Policymaking Assessment

Instructions: Read the statement, and answer based on the current status of your policymaking.

Yes	No	Statement
☐	☐	1. Have you stated the problem's impact on the numbers of people affected and the severity for the individual?
☐	☐	2. Have you gathered the scientific evidence indicating action?
☐	☐	3. Have you identified the uncertainty and imprecision in the scientific evidence?
☐	☐	4. Is there a need to act immediately?
☐	☐	5. Can you state the effectiveness (i.e., the ability to impact change and promote health) of the nutrition intervention policy?
☐	☐	6. Have you identified any secondary benefits of the policy?
☐	☐	7. Have you identified any barriers to the policy outcomes?
☐	☐	8. Have you compared the anticipated risks or other undesirable effects against the expected benefits?
☐	☐	9. Have you evaluated all of the costs of the beneficial public health policy?
☐	☐	10. Have you recognized or entertained any alternative proposals?
☐	☐	11. Have you addressed the social and political pressures certain population groups or political groups will place on the policymaking?
☐	☐	12. Can you defend whether the rights of the individual or rights of the community take precedence? That is, the degree the individual's rights are honored should bear an inverse relationship to the potential for community harm.
☐	☐	13. Have you developed a way to communicate the policy to consumers, the legal system, and other public health professionals?

If any of your responses to the self-assessment test were in the "no" column, then you will want to evaluate the urgency for making a policy guideline. To initiate or change a policy you must know (1) its importance to the policy maker(s), (2) who benefits, and (3) why it was initiated and adopted. Scientific evidence should provide a foundation for nutrition and health policies and should balance scientific evidence with the values, priorities, needs, and concerns of groups for which the policy tends to provide benefits.

Source: From Public health policy-making in the presence of incomplete evidence, *American Journal of Public Health;* 80(6):746–750,1990. © *American Journal of Public Health.* Used with permission.

professional assessment activity was designed (using the American Public Health Association's technical report) to diminish the risk of making policy too hastily and relinquishing ethical standards due to forceful demands. There are many internal and external stakeholder groups that can exert intense pressure. As the business ethics principles outline, a community nutrition professional needs to be confident and assume personal responsibility for the nutrition recommendations he or she is making. Overall, the APHA report gives support for implementing policy when the three criteria in box 19.8 can be met.

An example of policy setting in the presence of incomplete evidence is the setting of the Recommended Dietary Allowances. The subcommittee responsible for establishing the Recommended Dietary Allowances for the elderly did not have enough scientific evidence to support dividing healthy older people into two groups. Thus, the current RDAs for older adults are from ages fifty-one years and older. A more detailed discussion of applying scientific knowledge toward improving the public's health is discussed in Coughlin and Beauchamp.[8]

ETHICAL ISSUES THAT WILL CONFRONT COMMUNITY NUTRITION PRACTITIONERS

Issues with ethical implications are present in all areas of community nutrition practice. However, as we move into the next century, six challenges will confront community nutrition practice. Ethics will be at the heart of your responses to these challenges (see box 19.9).

Public health interventions have experienced acknowledging cultural diversity in the customer. The principle of beneficence encourages socially responsible community health interventions to examine outcomes and be sensitive to ethnic variations of what success is and what services (counseling, food accessibility, and health care) produce healthier communities. Allocating nutrition resources amid program mergers and collaborations will need ethics champions to address the customers served (or not served). Continuing to use the utility principle of promoting the greatest good for the greatest number of people will be a continuing ethical component.

BOX 19.8

CRITERIA FOR IMPLEMENTING POLICY

A. THE NEED IS GREAT.

The need for actions should be measured by the problem's impact, defined as the product of the numbers of people affected and the severity for the individual. Important also is whether subgroups in the population are particularly affected.

B. THE INTERVENTION IS ECONOMICALLY FEASIBLE.

Usually the costs of a beneficial public health measure are far less than those of the disorder or problem that is prevented and economic implications are usually a selling point. However, if the cost is exorbitant and the benefit small, intervention may not be deemed worthwhile. Further, given budgetary limitations, the costs of a new program may compromise other efforts, and therefore the expected benefits may be outweighed by harm done by cutting back other programs.

C. THERE ARE NO VIABLE, MORE SCIENTIFICALLY CERTAIN ALTERNATIVES.

It is important to evaluate the anticipated benefits and untoward effects of action. This evaluation includes secondary benefits and potential compliance with the dietary recommendations. The anticipated risks or other undesirable effects of the projected measure must be estimated and weighed against the expected benefits.

Source: From Public health policy-making in the presence of incomplete evidence, *American Journal of Public Health;* 80(6):746–750, 1990. © *American Journal of Public Health.* Used with permission.

BOX 19.9

CHALLENGES TO COMMUNITY NUTRITION PRACTICE

- Maintaining cultural diversity
- Developing collaborations and partnerships that prioritize health needs and are concerned with the health of communities
- Shifting to managed care accompanied with increased expectations for quality and access to advanced technology
- Expanding communication technologies and access to information
- Heightening personal responsibility amidst welfare reform
- Adjusting to budget cuts and government downsizing

When challenged by medical and social conditions that impact nutritional status, attention needs to be given to the rapid change in the health care system. The concept of managed care is to control health care expenses by ensuring that members receive only such treatment that is deemed appropriate and effective. In this environment, technologically advanced treatment of an individual competes against low-cost preventive interventions for many. Treatment of chronic diseases in an aging population will be more expensive and the outcome less substantial than health promotions for younger members. The new diversity of services will acknowledge the expanding socioeconomic classes where people who are underinsured or lack insurance need health care and may not be able to afford it. All of these demands renew the importance of ethics and proper ethical decision making.

Community nutrition professionals also need an ethical basis to form partnerships across public and private agencies. Nutrition interventions occur at primary, secondary, and tertiary levels. The nutrition programs historically implemented through public health may require change to respond to the new ways in which preventive, therapeutic, and rehabilitative services are provided. Community nutrition professionals seeking creative solutions to ethical nutrition intervention dilemmas in health care must take the lead in these changes.

Ethics is also involved in the world of technology. Electronic communication via cable and satellite provides quick access to information. There is an urgency to implement programs and information received via technology resources, but the same need exists for ethical consideration before deciding to take action. Even though technology broadens access and expedites receiving information, the demand to provide efficient services should not force a laxity in ethical reflection and decision making on the overall value of the information or services the technology introduces. Misuse or misrepresentation of nutrition information is not ethical behavior.

Respect of confidentiality measures to protect the public will also continue to be a high priority. For example, screening is a valuable tool for prevention and care, but it may also lead to discrimination and breaches of confidentiality. Ethical standards must be applied when planning procedures related to documentation and data access.

Our country has moved from small, isolated communities to one big company town. . . . We are united by our media and by what we consume. [Moreover,] accountability is different in the electronic community. Time and data has been blurred by nonstop information.[21]

It is our relationships with the customers that make our role compassionate and accountable. The principle of stewardship reflects a commitment from both the community nutrition professional and the community members to be accountable for change and to work toward a common good. With limited resources, there will be an increased emphasis on what additional burdens the community members can take on. The community nutrition professional will need to continue to identify the level of advocacy needed to respond to the needs with limited resources.

"Downsizing doesn't have to be ruthless."[9] Similarly, making program cuts doesn't have to be ruthless. Following the steps outlined in table 19.3 maintains a critical analytic view of the entire process and helps balance the benefits and burdens. In addition, proactive planning and intervention provides support for your ethical stance.

IMPLICATIONS FOR COMMUNITY NUTRITION PROFESSIONALS

The principles of ethics will continue to shape community nutrition practice in the year 2000 and beyond. One of the greatest challenges to community nutrition professionals is to participate in decision making so as to provide equitable access to nutrition information and necessary nutrition programs and services for all members of society. Decisions regarding the allocation of resources should value cost-effective nutrition interventions and maintain the clients' confidence in the benefits of nutrition and health. Community nutrition professionals must make decisions that balance priorities, standards of practice, and effective interventions in an interrelational contract with community members. Each component of ethical behavior requires a moral person to understand what questions are being asked, what comprises the relationship, and what ethical principles are relevant. This will be expected in a dynamic environment where integration of health promotion as well as treatment of acute and chronic illnesses occurs in ethnically diverse populations. Visible signs must exist that ethics matters to organizations interested in the nutritional care of human beings.

COMMUNITY NUTRITION PROFESSIONALS IN ACTION

- Review the excerpt from the United Nations's Covenant of Rights that defines an individuals right to health and well-being (see box 19.4). As a community nutrition professional, what nutritional components would you deem necessary to contribute toward "a standard of living adequate for the health and well-being of an individual and his or her family"? In your practice of community nutrition, what are the "nutritional rights" of individuals and families?

- Contact one of the centers on ethics listed below to obtain information addressing an ethical issue or locate an article that describes an ethical dilemma. Use the levels of analysis in figure 19.2 to identify values and the ethical principles involved. Clearly define the ethical dilemma and evaluate possible outcomes.

Kennedy Institute of Ethics
Georgetown University
Washington, DC 20057

American Association of Bioethics
FHP Center for Health Care Studies
2127 Annex Building
Salt Lake City, UT 84112

Hastings Center
255 Elm road
Braircliff Manor, NY 10510–9920

The Center for Biomedical Ethics
Suite 110, 2221 University Ave. S.E.
Minneapolis, MN 55414–3074

- Read the scenario below and follow the steps outlined in table 19.3 to determine your ethical response. Consider: What personal values influence your decision making? Which ethical principles are in conflict? Can you clearly define your organization's or profession's guidelines or codes of conduct that are applicable to this situation?

Your community nutrition program has been notified that budget cuts are necessary. To do so requires assessment of program usage and may require redefinition of eligibility criteria. An additional financial challenge is the need to purchase computers and software that would promote more efficient data processing, follow-up of clients, and information management. The new software would also allow your program access to the Internet. This would provide many opportunities to locate creative, innovative programs and access to libraries and journal resources. A grant has been awarded to initially purchase the hardware and software programs. However, as the director you realize that there will be an ongoing maintenance fee and computer training workshops for the professionals who use them. Money will also be needed for a computer programmer to update and link programs within the organization. The short-term loss of providing nutrition services to clients seems to weigh against the long-term advantage of investment in computers and better information management and follow-up of services. The overriding policy within your organization is to maintain your image in the community for helping provide food and diet counseling to low-income populations.

GOING ONE STEP FURTHER

- The essential feature distinguishing a classroom discussion on ethics and a community nutrition professional in practice making ethical decisions is that, at some point, the reflection must come to an end and a position must be taken. Identify one of your experiences as a community nutrition professional where the action implemented revolved around an ethical dilemma. Use table 19.3 to explore the approaches used when examining your decision making. Following this logical, systematic exploration, would you make any changes to your previous decision?

- Review current research journals to identify unresolved nutrition issues where policy recommendations are in progress. The nutrition issues can be in health promotion, disease prevention recommendations for populations, or it may be made with regards to specific individuals with a specific medical problem. Then, review the policymaking assessment checklist (table 19.5) and gather the appropriate background information needed. Finally, develop a recommendation statement for your organization. Ideas for policy recommendations are: What should be the infant feeding recommendations to young teen mothers (ages twelve to fifteen years)? What should be the weight guidelines for the aging population? What should be the recommendations regarding the use of antioxidants in the prevention of heart disease?

REFERENCES

1. American Dietetic Association: Code of ethics for the profession of dietetics, *J Am Diet Assoc* (12):1592–1953, 1988.
2. *The American heritage dictionary of the English language,* ed 3, Boston, 1993, Houghton Mifflin. Electronic version lic'd from and portions © 1994. Info Soft Intl, Inc.
3. Anderson S: Making Ethical Decisions, Presentation given at Bethel College on December, 1995, St. Paul, MN.
4. Bartels D: Ethics, Presentation given on March 3, 1997, Center for Bioethics of the University of Minnesota, Minneapolis.
5. Beauchamp TL, Childress JF: *Principles of biomedical ethics,* ed 4, New York, 1994, Oxford University Press.
6. Block P: *Stewardship: choosing service over self-interest,* San Francisco; 1993, Berrett-Koehler, p. 18.
7. *Comprehensive accreditation manual for hospitals,* Oakbrook, IL, 1995, Joint Commission on Accreditation of Healthcare Organizations.
8. Coughlin SS, Beauchamp TL: *Ethics and epidemiology,* New York, 1996, Oxford Press.
9. Cox C: High explosives. *Business Ethics* 8(1):33–35, 1994.
10. Daniels N: The ideal advocate and limited resources, *Theor Med,* 8(1): 69–80, 1987.
11. Daniels N, Light DW, Caplan RL: *Benchmarks of fairness for health care reform,* New York, 1996, Oxford University Press, p. 43.
12. Dewey J, Tufts J: *Ethics,* rev. ed., New York, 1959, Henry Hold & Company, p. 3.
13. Diekema D: Children first. The need to reform financing of health care services for children, *Health Care Poor Underserved* 7(1):3–14, 1996.
14. Halfon MS: *Integrity: a philosophical inquiry,* Philadelphia; 1989, Temple University Press, p. 36.
15. Hartman E: *Organization ethics and the good life,* New York, 1996, Oxford University Press, p. 15–19.
16. Holmes AF: Ethics: *approaching moral decisions,* Downers Grove, IL, 1984, InterVarsity Press.
17. Mortimer EA, Koplan JP, Lachenbruch PA, et al: APHA technical report. Public health policy making in the presence of incomplete evidence, *Am J Public Health* 80(6):746–750, 1996.
18. Nixon J, West J: Principles for infusing ethics in your company, *Business Forum* 18(4):12–14, 1993.
19. Pellegrino E: The anatomy of clinical-ethical judgments in perinatology and neonatology: a substantive and procedural framework, *Semin Perinato* 11(3):202–209, 1987.
20. Peters T: *Thriving on chaos: handbook for a management revolution,* New York, 1987, Harper & Row.
21. Pipher M: *The shelter of each other. Rebuilding our families,* New York, 1996, Grossett-Putnam & Sons.
22. Purtilo R: *Ethical dimensions in the health professions,* ed 2, Philadelphia, 1993, W.B. Saunders.
23. Smedes L: *Mere morality,* Grand Rapids, Wm Eerdmans, Pub. Co., 1983, pp. 35, 53.
24. Sobal J: Application of nutritional ethics in nutrition education, *J Nutr Educ* 23(4):187–191, 1991.
25. Stoner JAF, Freman RE, Gilbert DA Jr.: *Management,* ed 6, Englewood Cliffs, 1995, Prentice-Hall, p. 107.
26. Susser M: Improving Americans' diet. Setting public policy with limited knowledge, *Am J Public Health* 85(12):1609–1611, 1995.
27. Terry RD: *Introductory community nutrition,* Dubuque, IA, 1993, Wm. C. Brown Communications, p. 67.

THE EXPERT SPEAKS

ETHICS

NANCY R. CONNER

JUDGE, COURT OF LIMITED JURISDICTION, RETIRED
MARICOPA COUNTY, ARIZONA;
MEMBER, ETHICS TRAINING TEAM
ARIZONA SUPREME COURT 1994–1995

"No one is truly literate who cannot read his own heart."[2] There is no level of human endeavor poised to enter the twenty-first century that can afford to overlook the vital role of ethical conduct as it may affect success. The multiple manifestations of cultural decline in the 1990s are thankfully beginning to respond to a chorus of criticism from all corners. Hillary Clinton and Dan Quayle both wrote books urging a revaluing of family life. Public schools, which have resisted including ethics (a synonym for morals) in the curricula on the grounds of separation of church and state, are exploring the benefit of teaching manners (not which fork to use) and respect for fellow human beings. Corporations, which lament economic losses from employee petty theft and other misconduct, are seeking forums for continuing education that emphasize ethical self-expression for everyone from top management to entry-level hirelings. The professions are "dusting off" their codes or canons of ethics by stressing the practical application of these historical guidelines in modern-day practice. A special field of philosophy, axiology—the theory and study of values—is gaining new interest.[4] These emerging trends arouse hope for a cultural rebirth in America.

The study of professional ethics brings one of many dilemmas into focus: "the extent to which professionals must operate within different moral frameworks."[1] "Different" does not refer merely to the unique interpersonal relations defined by professional practices, but more interestingly, to special norms and principles that are taken in professional contexts to subdue normally relevant moral rights of the individual.

It is instructive (despite Webster's definitions) to consider the difference between *professional* ethics and *individual* morals. This becomes clear if we define ethics as firm standards for all members of a particular profession and morals as rooted in customs or individual choice of correct or incorrect action. This difference was illustrated by America's Founding Fathers. They worked with unflagging honor to establish a country based on

rights and freedoms (an ethical stance), while individually owning slaves (an individual moral decision based on the mores of the time). This dilemma was not quickly resolved. It was the sixteenth president, Abraham Lincoln, who finally called the country to consider a new way of thinking. The Civil War was hailed as having solved the problem, yet few can argue that remnants of deeply held beliefs entwined around slavery continue to run underground in our modern society.

The Founding Fathers had a right to own slaves. But by any measure of ethical standards, so clear for us today, it was not right. Similar dilemmas of modern times may become clear as history reviews them. But for today, the professional in any field must develop an informed, reliable practice of identifying, deciding, and acting on pressing ethical issues while recognizing that individual moral consequences may be confronted. Well-established examples of this axiom are experienced by judges who, sworn to uphold the law, rule accordingly but are often personally torn by the harsh results. For example, the law mandates a certain sentence following proof of criminal activity, such as, committing a third drug offense. The result is a young adult serving a lengthy prison term for smoking one marijuana cigarette. Similar disturbing results are experienced by medical professionals faced with differences between patient choices and proper treatment. Teachers, journalist, lawyers, accountants, and other professionals encounter similar moral dilemmas. However, immoral men and women need not worry about moral dilemmas.[3] Those who aspire to the "high road" will be faced with hard decisions. This will require serious thought and the willingness to give up some ideas we cling to.

One essential tool among many others discussed in this chapter, is a code of ethical conduct specifically developed for a profession. But, like any other tool, it is of little use if left to rust (or dust) without use. All members of a profession should embrace, be interested in, and be conversant with their code, its application to resolving common dilemmas, and its value as a basis for settling unique issues. As one judicial educator illustrated: Personally treat your professional code of ethics like a mine sweeper and you work every day in a mine filed. It can mean the difference between ethical decision making and an "explosion."[3]

Other valuable tools are so ordinary, so filled with common sense, that failure to recognize them can result in an ethical "explosion," completely surprising a professional despite years of serving as a pillar of personal morals and professional ethics. Stress management is one of these essential tools. Budget cuts, increased workload, associates who routinely engage in marginal ethical activity, and isolation from other responsible professionals are but a few of modern-day realities that distract us from well-established decision-making practices. Dr. Isaiah M. Zimmerman, PhD, a clinical psychologist in private practice in Washington, D.C., is unequivocal in the importance of stress management to judges, which clearly applies to many other ethically minded experts. He describes the topic as "definitely not a frill. It is a core subject: self management under severe work conditions. Without it, it is difficult to retain and practice the rest of the excellent available judicial education curriculum."

Here is a summary of actions suggested by Dr. Zimmerman.[6]

System Level Actions to Improve Wellness Under Stress

- Appoint a program director on the basis of proven capacity to lead, manage, and develop members of a team.
- Try to include as many members of a team as possible in ethical seminars, even those not professionally trained.
- Establish a mentor program for new team members after the initial orientation phase. On an informal basis, encourage family members to participate.
- When team members are isolated, allow a regular day for sharing a working day with another team member on a voluntary basis, to learn from each other and to reduce isolation.

Personal Level Suggestions to Improve Wellness Under Stress

- Develop and continue a regular exercise and health program.

- Build a supportive relationship with several other like professionals. Make it a point to chat together and share solutions for ethical dilemmas.
- During the workday, take three short breaks. Stretch, move about, or exercise.
- Maintain a careful separation between work hours and personal hours. If you take work home, do it for a set period instead of allowing it to use all or a significant part of your personal time.
- Cultivate a hobby or sports activity.
- Devote a period each day to meditate or pray, and reflect.
- When possible, attend a stress and wellness management seminar.

Of course, self-help need not stop here. Are there time-consuming (stressful) procedures in place simply because "that's the way we've always done it"? If so, try a new approach. Test it on another team member. Are there unexplained delays in getting things done? Develop a way to streamline the process.

In conclusion, moral disagreement is inevitable in America.[5] We life in a pluralistic democracy that was designed to deal with all kinds of differences of opinions. There are good arguments on all sides. No one has *all the answers*. Eventually someone will clash with your strongly held values. The literary critic, Lionel Trilling, in a 1947 essay remarked that he had been forced to question "his conventional education" by recognizing the complexities of life. "It taught us the extent of human variety and the value of this variety."[5]

REFERENCES

1. Goldman AH: *The moral foundations of professional ethics,* Totowa, NJ, 1980, Rowman and Littlefield, p. 283.
2. Hoffer E: *The passionate state of mind and other aphorisms,* New York, 1954, Harper and Row, pp. 97, 102.
3. Josephson M, President: Josephson Institute of Ethics, 4640 Admiralty Way, Suite 1001, Marina del Rey, CA 90292–6610.
4. Runes DD: *Twentieth century philosophy—living schools of thought,* New York, 1947, Philosophical Library, p. 59.
5. Tivan E: *The moral imagination—confronting the ethical issues of our day,* New York, 1996, Simon & Schuster, p. 266.
6. Zimmerman I: *Judicial stress management: coping with stress from the bench. National Judicial College Alumni Magazine,* X(1):15, 1994.

CHAPTER TWENTY

THE GLOBAL VILLAGE
NUTRITION AROUND THE WORLD

*Longer life can be a penalty as well as a prize. A large part of
the price to be paid is in the currency of chronic disease.*
—THE WORLD HEALTH REPORT 1996

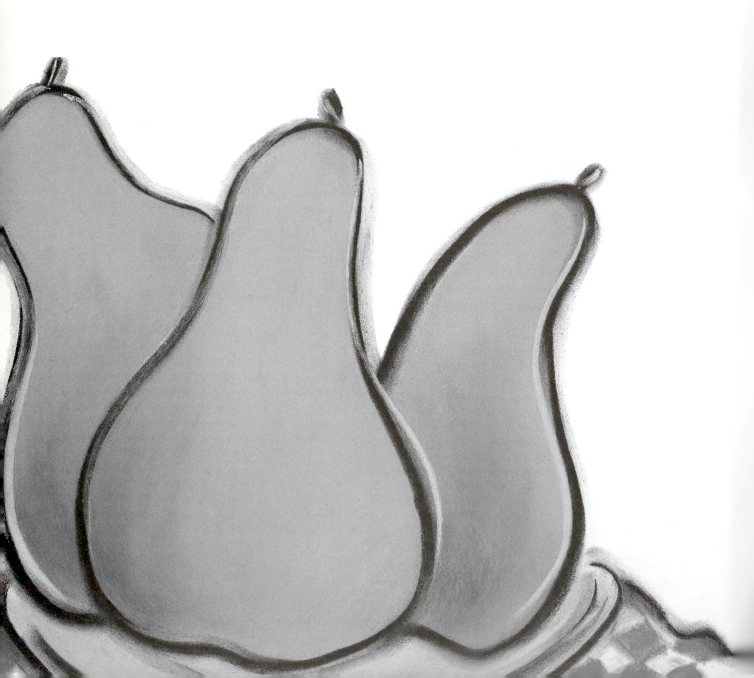

Core Concepts

Understanding nutrition in a global context will be a necessity in the twenty-first century as technology provides an opportunity to view the world as a global village. Major nutrition problems include starvation, chronic hunger, and deficiencies in micronutrients such as iodine, vitamin A, and iron. Undernutrition is prevalent among children, women, and the aged in developing countries. Inadequate sanitation, poor hygiene, and unsafe drinking water are environmental issues of major concern. To alleviate malnutrition, emphasis must be placed on community efforts that involve potential beneficiaries in planning and implementing interventions. The food supply and its quality, distribution, and nutritional balance are matters of global significance, not only in addressing the problems of hunger and malnutrition but also in addressing the interactions of diet, nutrition, health, and disease (see figure 20.1). Women's health status is affected by complex biological, cultural, and social factors that are interrelated. The biological determinants of women's health from birth through the postreproductive years are discussed. The nutrition-related problems of industrialized countries (coronary heart disease, stroke, obesity, hypertension, and diabetes mellitus) are increasing in developing countries, reflecting substantial changes in diet and physical activity.

Objectives

When you finish chapter twenty, you should be able to:

~ Describe the major demographic changes expected to occur in the world population in the next fifty years.

~ Describe the changing spectrum of nutrition-related diseases associated with economic development.

~ Discuss the major issues pertaining to production and distribution (availability) of nutritious food worldwide.

~ Identify where chronic hunger is most prevalent in the world.

~ Delineate the most important micronutrient deficiencies on a worldwide basis and discuss approaches to their alleviation.

~ Identify and discuss the biological and social factors that affect women's health throughout the life cycle.

~ Identify the critical areas of concern representing obstacles to women's advancement.

~ Discuss the interrelations of poverty, population growth, and environmental deterioration (PPE spiral) to child nutrition and health in developing countries.

~ Identify the most important aspects of behavior, policy, and community action in relation to alleviating malnutrition among young children.

~ Discuss the health and nutrition implications of economic development and the aging of the world's population.

Key Words

Word	Page Mentioned
World Declaration and Plan of Action for Nutrition	591
World Summit for Children	591
Micronutrient deficiencies	591
"Baby-friendly hospitals"	592
"Super rice"	593
Agricultural Biotechnology for Sustainable Productivity (ABSP)	593
Hidden malnutrition	595
Zero sum game for women	597
Discriminatory child care	597
Household behaviors	601
Community action	601
PPE spiral	601
International Committee of Dietetics Association (ICDA)	604

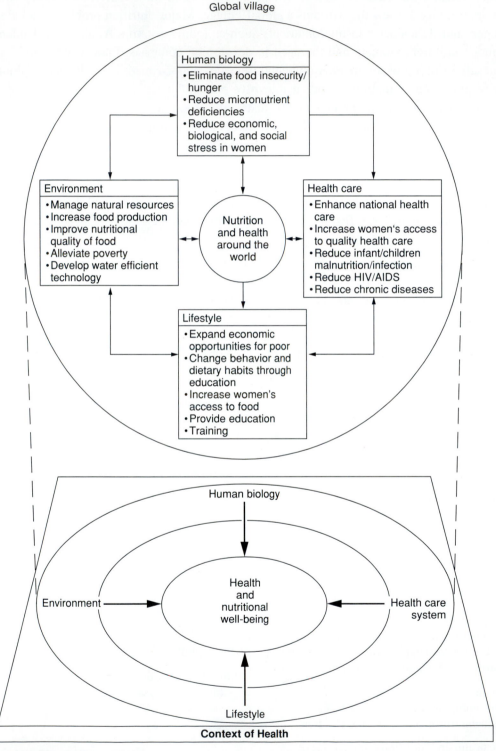

FIGURE 20.1   Context of Health
Applications to the global village.

GLOBAL NUTRITION PROBLEMS

In 1992, the **World Declaration and Plan of Action for Nutrition** was a product of the International Conference on Nutrition.[25] The conference involved some 1,300 delegates from 159 countries. The declaration is summarized in box 20.1. Signatories of the World Declaration and Plan of Action for Nutrition also reiterated commitment to the nutritional goals of the **World Summit for Children** (box 20.2).

What progress is being made in achieving the goals and objectives pertaining to mothers, infants and young children?

Starvation

Starvation and nutritional deficiency diseases continue to occur in communities affected by human-made disasters. Recent examples include Bosnia, Croatia, Cuba, North Korea, Somalia, and Zaire.

Under-Five Malnutrition

Under-five malnutrition is defined as having a weight-for-age that is more than two standard deviations (> -2 Z score) below the median weight-for-age using the international standard recognized by the World Health Organization (WHO). As shown in figure 20.2, there have been some downward trends in four regions (South Asia, East Asia/Pacific, Middle East/North Africa, and the Americas) between 1985 and 1995, but not much change has occurred since 1990. The rates in sub-Saharan Africa and Middle East/North Africa appeared to have gone up slightly since 1990.[20]

Low Birthweight

Low birthweight ($< 2,500$ g) is the best single predictor of growth of young children; children who are small at birth tend to remain relatively small. Approximately one third of all babies born in India have low birthweight (LBW) and nearly half of babies born in Bangladesh have LBW.[25] In contrast, only about 15 percent of infants born in sub-Saharan Africa have LBW, a proportion not much greater than that of Black

BOX 20.1

WORLD DECLARATION AND PLAN OF ACTION FOR NUTRITION

As a basis for the plan of action for nutrition and guidelines for the formulation of national plans of action, including the development of measurable goals and objectives within time frames, we pledge to make all efforts to eliminate before the end of this decade:

- Famine and famine-related deaths
- Starvation and nutritional deficiency diseases in communities affected by natural or human-made disasters
- Iodine and vitamin A deficiencies

We also pledge to reduce substantially within the decade:

- Starvation and widespread chronic hunger
- Undernutrition, especially among children, women, and the aged
- Other important **micronutrient deficiencies,** including iron
- Diet-related communicable and noncommunicable diseases
- Social and other impediments to optimal breast-feeding
- Inadequate sanitation and poor hygiene, including unsafe drinking water

BOX 20.2

NUTRITION GOALS FOR THE WORLD SUMMIT FOR CHILDREN
To Be Reached by the Year 2000

- Reduction in severe, as well as moderate, malnutrition among under-five children by half of 1990 levels
- Reduction of the rate of low birthweight ($< 2,500$ g) to less than 10 percent
- Reduction of iron deficiency anemia in women by one third of 1990 levels
- Virtual elimination of iodine-deficiency disorders
- Virtual elimination of vitamin A deficiency and its consequences, including blindness
- Empowerment of women to breast-feed their infants exclusively for four to six months and to continue breast-feeding, with complementary food, well into the second year
- Growth promotion and its regular monitoring to be institutionalized in all countries by the end of the 1990s
- Dissemination of knowledge and supporting services to increase food production to ensure household security

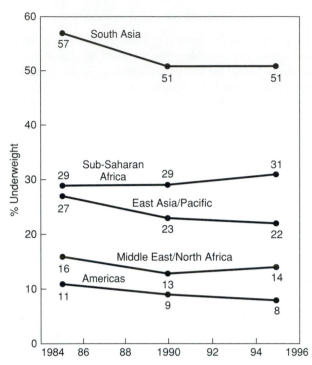

FIGURE 20.2   Underweight Children by Region
(*Source:* From *The progress of nations,* New York, 1996, United Nations Children's Fund, UNICEF House, pp. 10–21. Reprinted with permission.)

newborns in the United States.[9] As shown in table 20.1, the proportion of children under five years of age who are "underweight" (> 2 SD [standard deviation] below median weight-for age) and/or "stunted" (> 2 SD below median height-for-age) correlates rather well with the proportion of LBW infants,[10] just as their is an association between per capita gross national product (GNP) and growth retardation [26] (figure 20.3).

Vitamin A Deficiency

As of 1995, seventeen nations were moving rapidly toward the goal of adequate vitamin A for at least 80 percent of children under age two years. Large-scale programs are under way in 124 more countries. However, in thirty-five affected countries, the problem is not being acted on.[20]

Iodine Deficiency

An estimated 60 percent of the population in developing countries where iodine deficiency disorders were a

TABLE 20.1
Low Birthweight and Under-Five Malnutrition

Country	LBW (%)	Underweight (%)	Stunted (%)
Ethiopia	16	48	64
Burkina Faso	21	30	29
Tanzania	14	29	47
Zimbabwe	14	12	29
China	9	17	32
Indonesia	14	40	*
Vietnam	17	10	19

*Data not available.
Source: Adapted from Hautvast, JGAJ: Malnutrition in infancy around the world: state of the art at the end of the 20th century (Editorial), *Infant nutrition digest;* 3:4–7, 1997. Used with permission.

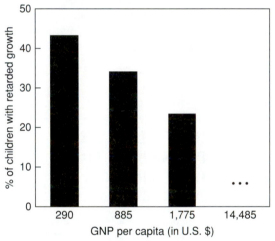

FIGURE 20.3   Growth Retardation in Terms of GNP
(*Source:* From Yunes J, Chelala C, Blaistein N: Children's health in the developing world: much remains to be done, *World Health Forum;* 15:73–76, 1994. Used with permission.)

problem are now consuming iodized salt. The goal of 90 percent salt iodination in all affected countries has been achieved by nineteen nations with eleven more passing the 70 percent mark.[20]

Breast-Feeding

Over 4,000 hospitals worldwide are following WHO/UNICEF guidelines on breast-feeding.[20] Specific information is not available to determine what effect **"baby-friendly hospitals"** have had on the rate of exclusive breast-feeding (no other fluids or foods) for the first four months of life.

FOOD AND THE ECONOMICS OF FOOD

Food production is an international activity. The food supply and its quality, distribution, and nutritional balance are matters of global significance not just where hunger and malnutrition exist but also in addressing the interaction of diets, nutrition, health, and disease.

The world population will have increased 50 percent (from 4 to 6 billion) between 1975 and 2000 and is expected to increase another 50 percent (from 6 to 8 billion) between 2000 and 2025. Nevertheless, the rate of population growth is slower than expected; for the period from 1990 to 1995, the worldwide growth rate was 1.48 percent per year, significantly lower than the 1.57 percent per year projected from the previous five-year period. This means there were 29 million fewer people in 1995 than expected. Only time will tell if the observed trend continues. Assuming that the production of food continues to increase, the slower rate of growth of the population has significant implications regarding food security issues.

As standards of living improve in developing countries, there is increasing consumption of meat and depletion of grain supplies (it takes 4 kg of grain to produce 1 kg of pork or beef).[4] At the same time, urbanization and industrialization in developing countries contribute to a loss of productive farm land. As a result of government farm policies and below average harvests for several years, grain supplies have been reduced in Europe and the United States to the lowest levels in thirty-five years. Experts estimate that the amount of global cropland used for growing grains can only increase about 3 percent. New technologies may offset the restrictions on available land for grain production in North America and other grain-exporting regions, but the application of current technologies to improve crop yields in developing countries is difficult because of concerns about intellectual property rights pertaining to biotechnology.[5] Of further concern in developing countries are problems related to production, storage, and distribution systems.

During the Green Revolution in the 1960s, intensive research efforts at International Agricultural Research Centers led to the development of high-yielding varieties of rice and corn. Work has continued at the Rice Research Institute in the Philippines to develop a "**super rice**" with increased crop yields of 20 to 25 percent. If efforts to make the super rice resistant to insects and disease are successful, the need for chemical pesticides will be reduced, which is good news for the envi-

ronment. The Consultative Group in International Agricultural Research believes the world has the resources needed to feed the world population well into the next century.[22] Along with super rice, strains of wheat and cassava are being developed that will substantially increase crop yields. Also, new varieties of fish are being developed that will double the production of small aquaculture farmers.

On the other hand, Lester Brown of the Worldwatch Institute doubts that technology will be able to match the increases of crop yields that occurred in the 1960s and 1970s.[3] He notes that in 1992, China had a net export of 8 million tons of grain, whereas in 1994, it had a net import of 16 million tons. He suggests that if China's rapid industrialization continues—with the associated loss of land and with water shortages—its import demands will overwhelm the export capacity of all grain-importing countries. He suggests that there will be no change in the world seafood catch, and predicts grain production will increase only modestly in the next thirty-five years (table 20.2). The grain output projection assumes slower growth in production almost everywhere and a decline in production in China, which in 1994 accounted for 20 percent of the world grain harvest.

During the period from 1950 to 1990, record economic growth was achieved because there were no natural constraints on the food supply. Brown suggests we may now be entering an era of scarcity with limits to the seafood catch, to water supplies, and to the production of grains (table 20.3). Future food security for China and the rest of the world may be accomplished with appropriate changes in a variety of strategies and policies (box 20.3).[3]

Because biotechnology is widely applicable to a variety of plants and animals, it is necessary to overcome issues concerning intellectual property rights and infrastructure inadequacies in order to apply the new techniques in developing countries. The U.S. Agency for International Development (USAID or simply AID) will continue to provide support to the International Agricultural Research Centers for their efforts to integrate the tools of biotechnology with their conventional research programs.[5]

In 1991, AID funded the **Agricultural Biotechnology for Sustainable Productivity (ABSP)** to "mutually enhance US and lesser developed countries institutional capacity for the use and management of biotechnology research to develop environmentally compatible, improved germplasm."[5] ABSP provides

TABLE 20.2
World Seafood and Grain Production

Commodity	1950	1990	2030	Projected change 1990–2030
Seafood catch	22	100	100	0
Grain output	631	1,780	2,149	+369

Note: All quantities are in millions of tons.
Source: Adapted from Brown LR: Who will feed China? *The Futurist,* January-February 1996.

TABLE 20.3
Food and Economic Indicators

Indicator	Era of surplus (1950–1990)	Era of scarcity (1990–2030)
Seafood catch per person	Up	Down
Grain production per person	Up	Down
Food prices	Down	Up
Grain market	Buyer's market	Seller's market
Politics of food	Dominated by surplus	Dominated by scarcity
Income per person	Up	May decline for much of world

Source: Adapted from Brown LR: Who will feed China? *The Futurist,* January–February 1996.

BOX 20.3

FOOD SECURITY FOR THE WORLD

- Reduce consumption of meat
- Convert to food production land now used for production of nonfood products, such as tobacco, cotton, and grain used to manufacture fuel
- Implement top-soil-saving agricultural techniques
- Reduce waste of water and encourage investment in water-efficient technologies
- Stabilize population growth

support for (1) postdoctoral research training in U.S. institutions; (2) constraint-oriented biotechnology research and development within public and private institutions; (3) activities in intellectual property rights; (4) increased host-country capacity in management of biotechnology through a commercially oriented industrial seminar series hosted by U.S. agricultural biotechnology firms; (5) net-working through regional and international conferences, newsletters, directories, database linkages, and the like; and (6) product devel-

opment via an incentive-based system for funding field-testing and commercialization activities for promising products of laboratory research in developing countries.

HUNGER

Hunger is a condition in which people lack the basic food intake to provide them with the energy and nutrients needed for active, productive lives. In recent years, the term "food security" has become part of the lexicology of hunger. Food security means access at all times by all people to adequate food for an active and healthful life. Hunger and food insecurity seem to be used almost interchangeably. If all people enjoyed food security, there would be no hunger.

We've all experienced brief or short periods of hunger with no harm. However, hunger can become life-threatening when it is allowed to continue over a long period of time. At some point, it becomes undernutrition, a chronic state of hunger. As defined by the Food and Agriculture Organization (FAO) of the United Nations (UN), "undernutrition is the state of having a dietary intake below the minimum energy requirement for a healthy body and a healthy, active life."[21]

The proportion of the world's population estimated to be chronically hungry decreased some 50 percent between 1970 and 1995, but with the 50 percent increase in the world population during the same period, it is likely there are nearly as many chronically hungry people in the world today as twenty-five years ago. Nearly three fourths of Asia's hungry or more than a third of the world total live in Bangladesh, India, Pakistan, and Sri Lanka (table 20.4). Two thirds of Africa's hungry live in seven countries—Ethiopia, Nigeria, Zaire, Tanzania, Kenya, Uganda, and Mozambique. More than 80 percent of the chronically hungry people in Asia and more than 60 percent in Latin America live in rural areas of their countries. Further, many of the urban hungry in developing countries have recently migrated there from the rural areas.

Except in cases of war or natural disasters, the cause of chronic hunger is not a lack of food. The fundamental reason is poverty.[21] At present, there is 20 percent

TABLE 20.4

Regional Distribution of Chronic Hunger

Region	World's people with chronic hunger (%)
Asia	57
Africa	27
Latin America	11
Middle-East	5

Source: From Raymond N, editor: *Fighting hunger: looking back, looking ahead,* Washington, DC, 1995, U.S. National Committee for World Food Day.

TABLE 20.5

Population Affected by Micronutrient Deficiencies by WHO Region

Region	Vitamin A	Iodine	Iron
Africa	13	39	206
America	0.1	30	94
Asia	10.0	100	616
Europe	—	14	27
Middle-East	1.0	12	149
China	1.4	30	1,058

Note: All figures are in millions.
Source: From *Micronutrient deficiency information system—iodine and vitamin A,* Geneva, 1992, Nutrition Unit, WHO.

more food per person in the world than there was twenty-five years ago. Of people in developing countries who are living on less than $1 a day, 75 percent live in rural areas. They depend on agriculture or agriculture-related business and services for that meager income. Some progress has been made in Latin America (Bolivia, Brazil, Columbia, and Mexico), in Southeast Asia (Indonesia, the Philippines, and Thailand), and in Egypt to improve life in the rural areas by improving the opportunities to achieve an adequate income, in some cases through land reform (redistribution), and in other cases through cooperative activity. In many cases, nonfarm rural employment is growing in food processing, light industry, rural services (health and education), and building roads and communications systems. This labor and employment strategy obviously requires a national policy with an emphasis on agriculture and rural development.

Sustainable development includes the reduction of poverty and hunger in environmentally sound ways. It also embraces the following broader objectives that are interrelated and mutually reinforcing:

- Expanding economic opportunities, especially for poor people, to increase their productivity, earning capacity, and chances to earn income in ways that are environmentally, economically, and socially viable over the long term
- Meeting basic human needs for food, clean water, shelter, health care, education, and fulfillment of the human spirit
- Protecting and enhancing the natural environment by managing natural resources in ways that take into account the needs of the present and future generations
- Promoting pluralism and democratic participation, especially by poor women and men, in economic and political decisions that affects their lives, with full respect for internationally recognized human rights.[17]

MICRONUTRIENT MALNUTRITION

The nutrition goals for the World Summit for Children (1990) and the World Declaration and Plan of Action for Nutrition (1992) both emphasized the need to eliminate micronutrient deficiencies, notably those resulting from insufficient intake of vitamin A, iodine, and iron. As shown in table 20.5, there are significant numbers of people affected with vitamin A, iodine, and iron deficiency. To grasp the cost of these deficiencies, consider a country of 50 million people with the level of micronutrient deficiencies that exist in South Asia. Such a country would suffer the following losses *each* year because of vitamin A, iodine, and iron deficiencies:

- 20,000 deaths
- 11,000 children born cretins (iodine deficiency) or blinded (vitamin A deficiency) as preschoolers
- 1.3 million person-years of work lost because of lethargy or fatigue (iron deficiency)
- 360,000 student-years wasted

The micronutrient content of foods is a hidden attribute, hence the term **hidden malnutrition** for specific micronutrient deficiencies. Hidden malnutrition is not necessarily due to a lack of food, but begins with reduced intake of a specific nutrient, which causes the body's stores or reserves to drop to a level insufficient to maintain normal functioning of tissues or organ systems linked to that nutrient. Biochemical tests or measures of physiological functions dependent on that nutrient may allow detection of deficiency long before there are overt clinical manifestations.

Alleviation of poverty, increasing food production, and enhancing national health care systems will not necessarily solve problems of micronutrient deficiencies. People do not spontaneously demand or select micronutrient-rich

TABLE 20.6
Serum Ferritin Levels in Guatemala Study on Iron Fortification of Sugar

Serum Ferritin (μg/L)	Community T		Community C	
	Basal	**Final**	**Basal**	**Final**
M & F (1–8 years)	16.5 (2.0)	26.0 (1.8)	15.4 (1.8)	15.8 (1.6)
M & F (9–17 years)	19.0 (1.8)	25.4 (1.9)	20.3 (2.0)	15.0 (2.3)
F (18–44 years)	15.3 (2.6)	25.3 (2.4)	19.9 (2.4)	19.1 (2.3)
F (> 44 years)	39.3 (1.9)	46.9 (2.2)	29.3 (2.1)	30.6 (2.3)
M (> 17 years)	30.0 (1.9)	46.9 (2.2)	21.8 (2.7)	24.4 (2.4)

Source: Adapted from Viteri FE, Alvarez E, Batres R, et al: Fortification of sugar with iron sodium ethylenediaminotetraacetae (FeNaEDTA) improves iron status in semi-rural Guatemalan populations, *Am J Clin Nutr;* 61:1153–63, 1995.

foods with increased income. People know when they are hungry and they know when they've had enough to eat. However, people have no natural appetite or craving for vitamin A, iodine, iron, or other micronutrients; those who are deficient in a micronutrient do not instinctively select foods that contain that nutrient.

Food and agriculture policies must be concerned not only with increasing the quantity of food but also with the nutritional quality through production, marketing, and consumption of micronutrient-rich foods. Policy makers must be informed of the economic and social costs of micronutrient malnutrition and they must learn about the political importance and cost-effectiveness of micronutrient programs.[7]

There are a number of ways to address the problem of micronutrient deficiencies:

- Agricultural policies with a nutritional focus
- Food fortification
- Direct delivery of supplements to target population
- Clinic-based programs to prevent and treat deficiencies during regularly scheduled visits
- School and worksite interventions
- Consumer education programs to modify diets to include micronutrient-rich foods.

One recently reported example of a fortification project in Guatemala concerned use of sugar as a vehicle for iron.[24] Sugar is consumed by all population groups at risk of iron deficiency and it does not impair iron absorption. In this project, iron sodium ethylenediaminotetraacetate (FeNaEDTA) was used as the source of iron for fortification. Iron in FeNaEDTA mixed with typical meals is better absorbed than other non-heme forms of iron. FeNaEDTA makes the total non-heme iron pool, including that contributed by food, as absorbable as that in FeNaEDTA, some 2.5 times greater than a similar amount of iron in ferrous sulfate.

Blood samples were obtained before the start of the study and again thirty-two months after iron-fortified sugar was made available. Results of serum ferritin determinations are shown in table 20.6 for participants in two communities in the Guatemala highlands, one of which "T" received iron-fortified sugar, and the other "C" served as the control community. The final values for all age and gender groups in community T were significantly greater than final values for community C.

Programs to educate, persuade, and change the behavior of consumers are essential to long-term elimination of micronutrient deficiencies. Social marketing of micronutrients and micronutrient-rich foods is necessary in virtually all developing countries, even where health service delivery is good and the food industry is well developed (see the Case Study at the end of this chapter). One aspect of sustainability is that once a behavior becomes a habit, it is more sustainable. These behaviors include industrial practices, medical routines, provider-client communications, and dietary habits. Integrated programs that generate good medical practices regarding micronutrients are more efficient than vertical programs, which require a single action isolated from specialized workers. Any behavior needs reinforcement to be perpetuated, and social reinforcement ultimately can replace public health messages.

WOMEN'S HEALTH AND NUTRITION

Women around the world play a major role in producing food, generating household income, childbearing and rearing, and overall household production. Throughout their life cycles, poor women experience stress because of conflicting time, energy, and economic demands made on them. Biological roles of pregnancy and lactation often compete for their time with child care, home production, and other social

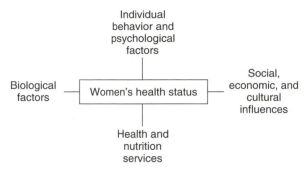

FIGURE 20.4 **Determinants of Women's Health Status**

roles. Women may also find conflicts between their biological needs and the ideal women defined by culture. Her nutrient needs may be belittled, her need for rest derided, and her desire for widely spaced children overridden. Because poor women lack resources, these conflicts engender a **zero sum game for women;** any extra effort devoted to one of her roles (economic, biological, or social) detracts from her fulfillment of other roles. Nowhere is this compromise more apparent than in nutrition—women grow food, women's income buys food, women prepare food and breast-feed, women's bodies nourish the fetus and suckling children, women use their physical energy for work, and women are responsible for prevention and treatment of most illnesses. To make a positive sum game in nutrition, women need to be able to increase their access to food, reduce the nutritional costs of their role conflicts, and enhance their control over nutrition-related resources.[13]

Biological Determinants of Women's Health

Women's health status is affected by complex biological, social, and cultural factors that are highly interrelated (figure 20.4). To reach women more effectively, health systems must take into account the biological factors that increase health risks for women and such sociocultural determinants of health as age, marriage, and attitude toward adolescent sexuality as well as psychological factors, such as depression arising from gender violence.[23]

Under optimal conditions for both men and women, a woman's life expectancy at birth is 1.03 times that of men. Many countries show a considerably greater advantage for women; in most industrialized countries, their life expectancy is more than 1.06 times that of men, and as great as 1.10 in Canada. In most developing countries,

however, the rate is much lower, even dropping below 1.00 in parts of Asia and to a low of 0.97 in Bhutan—a sign of socioeconomic conditions particularly inimical to women and girls.[12] Certain conditions can be exacerbated by pregnancy, including anemia, protein-energy malnutrition, hepatitis, malaria, tuberculosis, sickle-cell disease, diabetes, and heart disease.

Because of biological factors, women have a higher risk per exposure than men of becoming infected with sexually transmitted diseases including HIV. Cancer of the cervix accounts for more new cases of cancer each year in developing countries than any other type of cancer.

Women's Health and Nutrition Throughout Life

Biological and social factors affect women's health throughout their lives and have cumulative effects. That makes it important to consider the entire life cycle when examining the causes and consequences of women's poor health. Different health and nutrition problems affect females at different stages of the life cycle from infancy and childhood, to adolescence and the reproductive years, to the postreproductive period (see figure 20.5). For developing countries as a whole, 25 percent of females are less than ten years old, 21 percent are ten to nineteen years of age, 36 percent are between twenty and forty-five years of age, and 18 percent are over the age of forty-five years.[23]

Infancy and Childhood Discrimination in the care of girls can negate their innate biological advantage relative to boys. In many developing countries, girls are in poorer health than boys because of inadequate nutrition and health care. Such disparities are greatest in India and China, where more girls than boys die before their fifth birthday despite the girls' biological advantage. Key factors that adversely affect girls' health include:

- *Discriminatory child care:* In some societies girls receive less food and less nutritious food than boys, leading to malnutrition, impaired physical development, and laying the groundwork for future health problems.
- *Sex selection:* In countries where families have a strong preference for sons, there is evidence of selective abortion of female fetuses and female infanticide.[11]
- *Genital mutilation:* Each year an estimated 2 million young girls, mostly between four and eight years of age, are subjected to genital mutilation, also known as female circumcision. This invasive procedure can lead to death or to acute and chronic disability.[2]

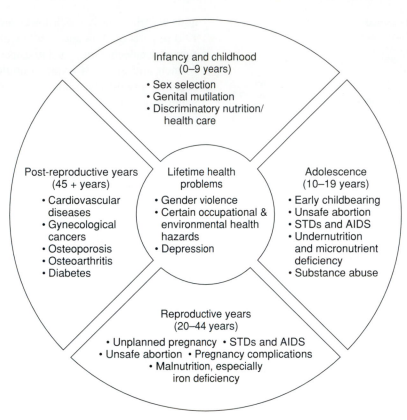

FIGURE 20.5   Health and Nutrition Problems Affecting Women Exclusively or Predominantly During Specific Stages of the Life Cycle
(*Source:* From Tinker A, Daly P, Green C et al: *Women's health and nutrition: making a difference,* World Bank Discussion Paper No. 256, Washington, DC, 1994, World Bank.)

Adolescence   Although women ten to nineteen years old are generally free of disease, their emerging sexuality and exposure to a variety of risks during the transition from childhood to adulthood can jeopardize their survival and well-being. Their status within the family and community is at its lowest in most countries during this part of the life cycle. To a large extent, adolescence sets the stage for health and nutritional status in the later years, yet health policies and programs are the least effective in addressing the needs of this age group.

• *Early childbearing:* The proportion of women giving birth during their teenage years ranges from 10 to 50 percent depending on the country. Although early childbearing is particularly common in traditional, often rural, settings, where early marriage is a norm, it is becoming increasingly prevalent among unmarried adolescents.

• *Unsafe abortions:* Because they often seek clandestine abortions and delay in obtaining the procedure and seeking medical attention for associated problems, adolescents have a higher rate of abortion complications.

• *Sexually transmitted disease:* Sexually transmitted diseases, including AIDS, are spreading rapidly among young women, mainly through prostitution and liaisons with older men. There is evidence that adolescent girls are biologically more vulnerable to contracting these diseases than are older women, and they are likely to have more difficulty negotiating safe sex practices with their partners. On average, women become infected five to ten years earlier than men.

• *Undernutrition and micronutrient deficiency:* Girls' nutritional needs increase in early adolescence because of the growth spurt associated with puberty and the onset of menstruation. Inadequate diets during this period can jeopardize their health and physical development, with lifelong consequences. A very common condition is iron-deficiency anemia.

- *Increased substance abuse:* Adolescents often experiment with harmful substances, including tobacco products, alcohol, and drugs. While diseases associated with lifestyle and behavior have been less of a problem for women than for men, this pattern is changing in some countries.

Reproductive Years   Women's risk of premature death and disability is greatest during their reproductive years. Many conditions that occur in these years affect the health of women long after their reproductive years are over. The health of their children is also affected.

- *Unplanned pregnancy and abortion:* In developing countries, one in five births is unwanted and one fourth of all pregnancies worldwide end in abortion.
- *Pregnancy-related complications:* More than 50 million women experience acute pregnancy complications and 15 million develop long-term disabilities.[1]

Strategies for Interventions in Women's Health

The United Nations Fourth World Conference on Women was held in Beijing, China, in 1995. The theme of the conference was "Action for Equality, Development, and Peace." In her address to the conference on September 9, 1995, U.S. First Lady Hillary Rodham Clinton stated that "families rely on mothers and wives for emotional support and care, families rely on women for labor in the home, and increasingly, families rely on women for income needed to raise healthy children and care for relatives. As long as discrimination and inequities remain so commonplace around the world—as long as girls and women are valued less, fed less, overworked, underpaid, not schooled and subjected to violence in and out of their homes—the potential of the human family to create a peaceful, prosperous world will not be realized."

Beijing Declaration and Platform for Action

Since the United Nations held the first world conference on women over twenty-two years ago (Mexico City, 1975), important progress has been made toward achieving equality between women and men. Women's access to education and proper health care has increased, their participation in the paid labor force has grown, and legislation that promises equal opportunities for women

BOX 20.4

TWELVE CRITICAL AREAS OF CONCERN REPRESENTING OBSTACLES TO WOMEN'S ADVANCEMENT

- Poverty
- Education and training
- Health
- Violence
- Armed conflict
- Economy
- Decision making
- Institutional mechanisms
- Human rights
- Media
- Environment
- Institutional and financial arrangements

---

and respect for their human rights has been adopted in more countries. As a result, important changes have occurred in the relationship between women and men.

Yet discrimination against women is still widespread. Violence against women remains a global phenomenon. Women's equal access to resources is still restricted, and their opportunities for higher education and training are concentrated in limited fields. A "glass ceiling" continues to bar women's advancement in business, government, and politics. Women are an overwhelming majority of the 1 billion people living in abject poverty and among illiterates. Decisions that affect women continue to be made largely by men. The Beijing Declaration and Platform for Action, adopted unanimously at the Fourth World Conference on Women by representatives from 189 countries, reflect a new international commitment to the goals of equality, development, and peace for all women everywhere.[14]

The platform identifies twelve "critical areas of concern" considered to represent the main obstacles to women's advancement. It defines strategic objectives and spells out actions to be taken over the next five years by governments, the international community, nongovernmental organizations, and the private sector for the removal of existing obstacles (box 20.4).

The platform defines reproductive health as a state of complete physical, mental, and social well-being and sexual health whose purpose is the enhancement of life and personal relations. Equal relationships between men and women in matters of sexual relations and reproduction require mutual respect, consent and shared responsibility. The platform recognizes that reproductive rights rest on the recognition of the basic human rights of all couples and individuals to decide freely and responsibly how many children they want to have, and when. They also have the right to obtain information and make decisions on reproduction free of discrimination, coercion, and violence.

The platform recommends actions to:

- Increase women's access throughout the life cycle to appropriate, affordable, and quality health care, information, and related services
- Reduce maternal mortality by at least 50 percent of the 1990 levels by the year 2000 and a further one half by the year 2015
- Encourage both women and men to take responsibility for their sexual and reproductive behavior
- Undertake gender-sensitive initiatives that address sexually transmitted diseases, HIV/AIDS, and sexual and reproductive health issues
- Increase resources and monitor follow-up for women's health

Gertrude Mongella, Secretary General of the Fourth World Conference on Women charged the participants to do the following: "Each government now must set priorities, specify the resources it will contribute, and declare what steps it will take to hold itself accountable to the world's women."[14]

CHILD HEALTH

It has been estimated that about 40 percent of the world's children under age five are chronically undernourished. The vast majority of these 141 million children live in the world's poorest communities. The principal threat to the poorest populations in developing countries comes from the mutually reinforcing problems of poverty, population growth, and environmental deterioration. The malnourished infant and young child is at great risk of death because of the combined effects of malnutrition and infection. Those children who survive the first four or five years of life may suffer long-term consequences of early malnutrition and infection, including stunted growth and decreased capacity to learn and to work.

Efforts to alleviate malnutrition have often failed to take into account the complexity of biological, social, and economic factors and relationships specific to a particular community. What might work in one community may not be applicable to other communities. Several issues and interventions need to be considered (box 20.5). From a review of various approaches to alleviation of malnutrition, Pinstrup-Andersen et al.[16] emphasize the need for understanding the community, no matter how small or how large, in which nutrition professionals are working.

Individual and Household Behavior

Taking into account their goals and preferences, relative power, and the constraints (resource, time, information and culture) within which they make decisions, most household members behave rationally. Accordingly,

BOX 20.5

ISSUES AND INTERVENTIONS NEEDED IN EFFORTS TO ALLEVIATE MALNUTRITION

- Household behaviors
    Demand for food
    Demand for health care
    Child care
    Breast-feeding
    Family planning
    Women's time allocation
- Interventions influencing behavior
    Nutrition education
    Growth monitoring
    Women's education and employment
- Interventions influencing health
    Child survival interventions
    Integrated health and nutrition programs
    Water and sanitation projects
    Family planning
- Interventions influencing access to food
    Food and income transfers
    Agricultural programs and policies
- Organization, information, and action
    Community participation
    Multisectoral nutrition planning
    Information
    Lessons for action

there are three entry points for nutrition intervention in households with malnourished members:

- Changing goals and preferences of the malnourished individual or his or her guardian
- Altering relative power of malnourished individuals
- Alleviating existing constraints

Nutrition education has generally aimed at changing goals and preferences. Prescriptive approaches, based on the medical model of compliance, have by and large not been very successful in nutrition education efforts. In contrast, the social marketing approach, which is more participatory, seems to be more successful. Social marketing takes into account past and current **household behaviors** and emphasizes transfer of pertinent information to the target audience (households).

Integrating efforts to alleviate household-level resource constraints—time and income—with efforts to reduce infectious diseases and increase nutrition knowledge will usually have positive nutrition effects in both the short and long term.

Policy-Level Interventions

Policies affecting cost of food, wages, employment, and health care affect nutrition without the need for **community action.** For example, promotion of breast-feeding in poor communities with an unsafe water supply and poor sanitation is an appropriate strategy to reduce infant mortality and malnutrition. Avoidance of use of foods other than human milk during the first six months of life may be desirable with respect to avoiding infection, but the intervention must take into account long-standing practices in the culture and the community. Availability of safe and appropriate weaning foods and education in their use are critical to the nutritional well-being of the older infant and young child.

Education of girls and young women has been shown to have a positive effect on child nutrition. This may result from delayed marriage, family planning with longer intervals between births, and alleviation of household constraints—time and material resources.

Health interventions such as oral rehydration therapy may reduce child mortality but not morbidity, and malnutrition may remain high. Access to primary health care services is of paramount importance in efforts to control infectious diseases and to alleviate malnutrition. However, health services alone may have negligible effects on nutrition. They must be accompanied by other interventions.

Policies and programs that reduce costs of production and distribution of food offer great potential for enhancing real income of low-income food consumers without adversely affecting low-income food producers. Keep in mind that in most low-income developing countries, the majority of the malnourished live in rural areas and many depend directly or indirectly on agriculture for their income and food security. Policies that impinge on costs and revenues in the agricultural sector will affect incomes of the poor, and policies that affect incomes of the poor and policies that affect food prices will affect the ability of poor consumers to meet energy and nutrient needs.

Community Action

The success of national policies and programs depends on implementation at the local level. Local communities can provide information to be considered in the design and implementation of feasible and cost-effective interventions. Realistically, local community participation in design of intervention programs is essential to their successful implementation. Growth monitoring of infants and young children provides information to the mother about health and nutrition problems and may be used to mobilize community action at the local level. It should be linked closely with household- and community-level assessments of the causes of growth failure and opportunities for alleviation through nutrition education, provision of food and health care services, or improvement in the water supply and sanitation in the community.

National and regional programs are needed to support local communities in developing and implementing appropriate intervention strategies. For example, the World Bank views community participation as an integral element in efforts to mitigate poverty and improve nutrition.[19]

In summary, appropriate investments in health, nutrition, education, and family planning are needed to solve the **PPE spiral** (figure 20.6). Community action with government participation, as opposed to government programs with or without community participation is likely to result in more sustainable improvements because actions will be problem-oriented and at least partly designed by the intended beneficiaries.

ADULT HEALTH

Of 52 million deaths worldwide in 1996, nearly 40 percent were caused by cardiovascular disease (including heart disease and stroke), 30 percent by infectious diseases (including AIDS, bronchitis, diarrhea, measles, pneumonia, and tuberculosis), and 10 percent by cancer (mainly lung, stomach, colon, liver, and breast).

In the twenty-first century, chronic conditions, largely affecting older adults, will be the world's greatest health problems (table 20.7). As shown in table 20.8,

the developing countries (Africa, Latin America, China, India, and other Asian countries) which comprised nearly 70 percent of the world's population in 1950, will account for 88 to 90 percent by the year 2050. The rate of increase in the population aged sixty-five and older in developing countries is substantially greater than that in

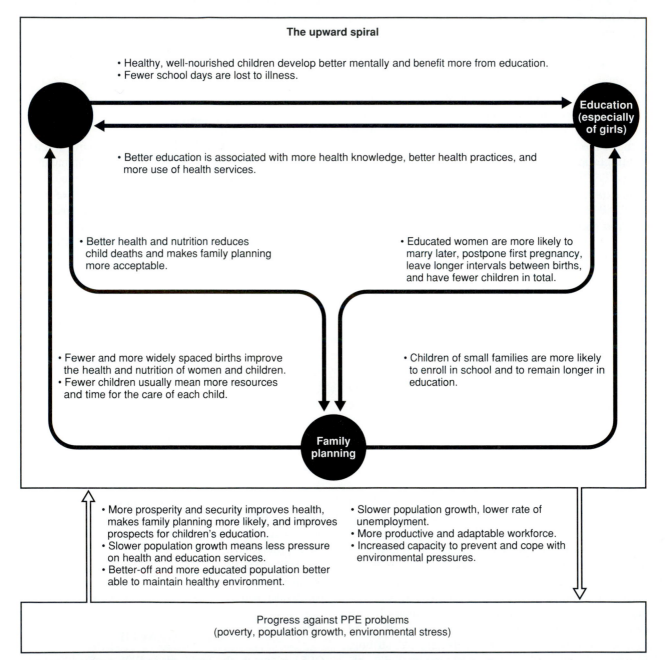

FIGURE 20.6   Investments in Health, Nutrition, Education, and Family Planning to Solve the PPE Spiral
(*Source:* From *The state of the world's children,* New York, 1994, UNICEF. Reprinted with permission.)

industrialized countries. It is estimated that during the first quarter of the twenty-first century there will be a two- to threefold increase in non-insulin-dependent diabetes mellitus (NIDDM) and cancer among adults in developing countries, reflecting three personal behaviors—diet, physical activity (exercise), and smoking. By 2020, tobacco-related disease will become the world's greatest killer, accounting for 10 percent of deaths.

As shown in figure 20.7, substantial changes in diet have occurred in Asia the past twenty years. As economies and GNPs grew between 1975 and 1994, the proportion of dietary calories from complex carbohydrates decreased and that from fat increased. The same trend was observed at all income levels.[6]

The relocation of people from rural to urban centers takes place with economic development and increasing industrialization. As may be appreciated, in the next twenty-five to thirty years, this change will be greatest among the lesser developed countries. With increasing urbanization and increasing income, the proportion of energy from animal fat and animal protein increases and that from carbohydrate decreases. These dietary changes and the decrease in physical activity (exercise) associated with relocation from rural to urban locations and increased income set the stage for increases in the prevalence of obesity, hypertension, NIDDM, coronary heart disease, stroke, and some types of cancer.

NUTRITION AND DIETETICS PROFESSIONALS IN THE INTERNATIONAL ARENA

With global expansion and new world trade agreements, nutrition and dietetics professionals are also actively involved in international activities. Dietetics is recognized by the International Labor Office in Geneva and classified among the paramedical professions; yet, there are no world standards for education and training within the dietetic profession.

T A B L E   2 0 . 7
Leading Causes of Disability

	World ranking	
	1990	**2020**
Heart disease	5	1
Major depression	4	2
Traffic accidents	9	3
Stroke	6	4
Chronic lung disease	12	5
Lower respiratory tract infections	1	6

Source: From *World health report,* 1996, World Health Organization.

T A B L E   2 0 . 8
Estimated and Projected Population of Major World Areas

Area	Year				
	1950	**1990**	**2000**	**2025**	**2050**
Developed					
Europe	393	498	510	515	486
North America	166	276	295	332	326
Oceania	13	26	30	38	41
USSR	180	289*	308*	352*	380*
Total	752	1,089	1,143	1,237	1,233
Developing					
Africa	222	642	867	1,597	2,265
Latin America	166	448	538	757	922
China	555	1,139	1,299	1,513	1,521
India	358	853	1,042	1,442	1,699
Other Asian countries	465	1,121	1,372	1,958	2,379
Total	1,766	4,203	5,118	7,267	8,786

Note: All figures are in millions.
*Countries comprising former USSR.
Source: Adapted from Wright W: *The universal almanac 1997,* Kansas City, 1996, Andrews & McNeal.

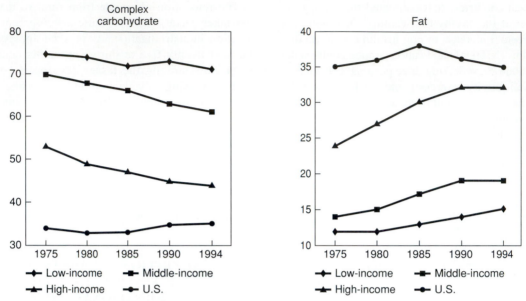

FIGURE 20.7   Relation among Availability of Carbohydrates and Fat to GNP in Asia
(*Source:* From Drewnowski A, Popkin BM: The nutrition transition: new trends in the global diet, *Nutr Rev;* 55:31–43, 1997. © International Life Sciences Institute. Used with permission.)

Nutrition and dietetic professionals must expand their interests beyond their national populations to the worldwide community. As education and technology cross defined boundaries, research and information are being shared among all cultures to improve the nutritional and health status of the world's populations. There are many good reasons for expanding our horizons. Box 20.6 describes some of the major opportunities for the nutrition and health community (community nutrition professional).[8]

The predecessor of what today is known as the **International Committee of Dietetics Association (ICDA)** pioneered the concept of collaboration across national borders. The American Dietetic Association became a founding member of this organization in 1952 and has been represented on the ICDA's executive committee ever since.[15]. The ICDA was begun by D. J. TenHoff of The Netherlands. The first international congress was held in 1952 in The Netherlands. Its mission conceptually asserts that the ICDA will support dietetic associations and their members through an integrated communication system, enhanced image, and improved awareness of ways to improve the standards of dietetic practice. The twenty-six member nations of ICDA pay biannual dues to help fund the congress. The permanent ICDA headquarters is located at the headquarters office

BOX 20.6

POTENTIAL BENEFITS OF INTERNATIONAL COLLABORATION FOR THE NUTRITION AND DIETETICS PROFESSIONS

- Broadened scope of cultural understanding
- Business and employment opportunities
- Commonality of education and practice standards
- Comparative research studies
- Cooperation among professionals in food, nutrition, dietetics, and agriculture
- Dialogues on creative solutions
- Expansion of job opportunities
- Increased electronic communications
- Joint problem solving
- Synergy and understanding of worldwide issues
- Technological advancements in databases

Source: Adapted from Gilbride JA, Leckowich K: International opportunities for the dietetics profession, *Top Clin Nutr;* 11:1–6, 1996.

of the Canadian Dietetic Association of Toronto. In February 1996, the Twelfth International Congress of Dietetics (ICD) was hosted by the Nutritionists-Dietitians Association of The Philippines in Manila. The next congress will be held July 23–27, 2000 in Scotland.

The American Dietetic Association's formal international partnership of longest standing is with Canada. Credential eligibility and membership reciprocity was established in 1984 and in 1992. The partnership expanded to include joint development and mutual adoption of position papers, the first of which was "Nutrition for Physical Fitness and Athletic Performance of Adults."[18]

One of the earlier efforts to foster international cooperation occurred in 1984 when the ADA granted representation to the American European Dietetic Associations (AEDA). The AEDA indirectly formed to provide networking and educational opportunities for ADA members living in Europe. It now includes outreach to dietetic associations of other countries, with over fifty countries being represented.

Another vehicle for international communication in nutrition and dietetics was established in 1993 with the development of the ICDA newsletter *Dietetics and Nutrition Around the World*. This newsletter focuses on nutrition news of international interest.[15]

Establishing and maintaining international alliances will be a necessity in the twenty-first century as technology brings the entire world within our reach. The community nutrition professional will have many opportunities for cultural exchange and personal growth as they work with, appreciate, and understand diverse cultures around the world.

IMPLICATIONS FOR COMMUNITY NUTRITION PROFESSIONALS

Community nutrition professionals must broaden their scope of cultural understanding to work with worldwide issues. Nutritional problems affecting people around the world include famine, starvation, and deficiencies of micronutrients (vitamin A, iodine, and iron). Widespread chronic hunger occurs with resultant undernutrition affecting primarily children, women, and the aged. Diet-related communicable and noncommunicable diseases are prevalent.

Food production and distribution are major concerns in many developing countries. Recommendations have been made to convert land now used for production of nonfood products (e.g., tobacco and cotton), to use for food production. In addition, reducing waste of water and investing in water-efficient technologies have been suggested. An important aspect of the concern about food is to stabilize population growth.

There are many impediments to achieving optimal nutrition for women. Women often face conflicts between their biological needs and the ideal woman defined by their culture. Because poor women lack resources, compromises on their health are made, and it is particularly apparent with respect to their own nutrition. The United Nations Fourth World Conference on Women held in Beijing in 1995 identified twelve critical areas of concern representing obstacles to women's advancement.

The malnourished infant and young child is at great risk of death because of the combined effects of malnutrition and infection. Efforts to alleviate malnutrition in infants and children have often failed to take into account the relationships specific to a particular community. The success of national policies and programs depend on understanding and solving problems at the local level.

Substantial changes in diet are occurring throughout the world. As the proportion of dietary energy from complex carbohydrates decreases and that from fat increases, chronic diseases (cardiovascular diseases, obesity, and diabetes mellitus) are becoming more prevalent throughout the world.

COMMUNITY NUTRITION PROFESSIONALS IN ACTION

- Utilizing figure 20.2, which describes underweight children by region, select one of the regions to study further. Determine the number of underweight children in the particular region and the potential causes, including undernutrition, poverty, social and cultural issues, and sanitation. Present this information to the class.

- Review figure 20.5, which identifies the health and nutrition problems affecting women around the world. Compare and contrast women's health problems around the world with those affecting women in the United States.

- Determine where the greatest amount of chronic hunger occurs in the world. Identify the economic, health, environmental, and nutritional variables that are causing this serious condition.

- Identify the micronutrient deficiencies that occur worldwide. Select one micronutrient to explore further in terms of root causes and possible interventions to alleviate the problem.

GOING ONE STEP FURTHER

- Prepare a paper to be presented to your local dietetic association or to a group on campus whose purpose it is to support women's issues. Consider developing a panel of student speakers (limit the number of students on the panel to four) with each taking a segment of the assignment and presenting the findings with you as the moderator. Based on the information from the United Nations Fourth World Congress on Women held in Beijing in 1995, provide information on the following:
  - Women's role in food production
  - Women's stress and conflict between biological needs and cultural issues
  - Biological determinants of women's health
  - Women's health throughout the life cycle from birth through the postreproductive years
- Contrast the twelve critical areas of concern representing obstacles to women's advancement from the Beijing Declaration and Platform of Action to the needs of women in the United States.
- Review the Case Study in this chapter on "Improving Nutrition in Nicaragua after War and Natural Disaster" by Dr. Ruth Dow. Identify additional strategies on nutrition, food, health, and economic and community development that you would employ to further assist the people of the Cerro Negro region. After identifying the strategies, meet with a faculty member from the international program on campus and determine if any, some, or all of the strategies you considered for implementation are appropriate to use in this community. This is an excellent learning situation in which to get some idea of what might be effective and what would in all likelihood be ineffective with this population.

ADDITIONAL INFORMATION

Professional societies develop statements, scientific status summaries, commentaries, and position papers to clarify an issue in which the particular society has expertise. The following societies have developed papers relevant to this chapter:

Institute of Food Technologists (IFT)

1. A backgrounder on: Genetically engineered foods, October 1996, IFT Science Communications Dept., 211 N. LaSalle Street, Chicago, IL 60601–1291.

The American Dietetic Association (ADA)

1. Position on: world hunger, *J Am Diet Assoc* 95:1160, 1995.

REFERENCES

1. *Approaches to adolescent health and development: a compendium of projects and programs,* Geneva, 1992, WHO.
2. Ascadi GTF, Johnson-Ascadi G: Socioeconomic, cultural and legal factors affecting girl's and women's health, World Bank Women's Health and Nutrition Work Program, Working Paper Series, Washington, DC, 1993, World Bank Population, Health and Nutrition Department.
3. Brown L: Who will feed China? *The Futurist* January-February 1996, pp. 14–18.
4. Burns G, Lindorff D, Carey J, Mandel J: The new economics of food, *Business Week* May 20, 1996, pp. 78–84.
5. Chambers JA: Creating new partners in global biotechnology, *Food Technology* 49:94–96, 1995.
6. Drewnowski A, Popkin BM: The nutrition transition: new trends in the global diet, *Nutr Rev* 55:31–43, 1997.
7. *Enriching lives: overcoming vitamin and mineral malnutrition in developing countries,* Washington, DC, 1994, The World Bank.
8. Gilbride JA, Leckowich K: International opportunities for the dietetics profession, *Top Clin Nutr* 11:1–6, 1996.
9. Guyer B, Strobino DM, Ventura SJ, et al: Annual summary of vital statistics—1995, *Pediatrics* 98:1007–1019, 1996.
10. Hautvast GJAJ: Malnutrition in infancy around the world: state of the art at the end of the 20th century (Editorial), *Infant Nutrition Digest* (3):4–7, 1997.
11. Heise L, Pitanguy J, Germain A: Violence Against Women; The Hidden Health Truth. World Bank Discussion Paper, Washington, DC, 1994, World Bank Health and Nutrition Department.
12. Keyfitz N, Flieger V: *World population growth and aging: demographic trends in the late twentieth century,* Chicago, 1990, University of Chicago Press.
13. McGuire JS, Popkin BM: Helping women improve nutrition in the developing world: Beating the zero sum game, The World Bank Technical Paper Number 114, Washington, DC, September 1992.
14. Mongella G: Fourth World Conference on Women: Action for Equality, Development and Peace, Beijing, China, 4–15 September 1995.
15. Parks SC, Bajus B: President's page: challenging the future—an evolving global perspective for the profession, *J Am Diet Assoc* 94:782–784, 1994.
16. Pinstrup-Andersen P, Pelletier D, Alderman H: *Enhancing child growth and nutrition: lessons for action.* In Pimstrup-Andersen P, Pelletier D, Alderman H, editors: *Child growth and nutrition in developing countries,* Ithaca, NY, 1995, Cornell Univ. Press.

17. Position of the American Dietetic Association, world hunger, *Am J Diet Assoc* 95:1160–1162, 1995.

18. Position of the American Dietetic Association and the Canadian Dietetic Association for physical fitness and athletic performance. *J Am Diet Assoc* 1993; 93:691–696.

19. *Poverty reduction handbook,* Washington, DC, 1992, World Bank.

20. *The progress of nations,* New York, 1996, United Nations Children's Fund, UNICEF House, pp. 10–21.

21. Raymond N, editor: *Fighting hunger: looking back; looking ahead,* Washington, DC, 1995, U.S. National Committee for World Food Day.

22. Scarcity or plenty? Food supply debated, *Arizona Republic* October 28, 1996, p. A5.

23. Tinker A, Daly P, Green C, et al: Women's health and nutrition making a difference. World Bank Discussion Paper No. 256, Washington, DC, 1994, World Bank.

24. Viteri FE, Alvarez E, Batres R, et al: Fortification of sugar with iron sodium ethylenediaminotetraacetate (FeNaEDTA) improves iron status in semirural Guatemalan populations, *Am J Clin Nutr* 61:1153–1163, 1995.

25. *World declaration and plan of action for nutrition,* Geneva, 1993, Office of Publications, World Health Organization.

26. Yunes J, Chelala C, Blaistein N: Children's health in the developing world: much remains to be done, *World Health Forum* 15:73–76, 1994.

CASE STUDY

IMPROVING NUTRITION IN NICARAGUA AFTER WAR AND NATURAL DISASTERS

RUTH M. DOW, PHD, RD, LD, FADA

GRADUATE COORDINATOR AND NUTRITION SCHOOL
OF FAMILY AND CONSUMER SCIENCES
EASTERN ILLINOIS UNIVERSITY, CHARLESTON, IL AND
PROGRAM DIRECTOR, ALFALIT INTERNATIONAL, INC., MIAMI, FL

DESCRIPTION

This case study illustrates the use of multifaceted approaches to improve food security and nutritional status of people in the Cerro Negro region near the city of Leon in Nicaragua. Following years of war and the natural disasters of drought, volcanic eruption, and a seaquake (offshore earthquake), the area was declared a disaster area. Homes, schools, food crops and animals, and the income-producing cotton crops were destroyed. Over 86 percent of the population lacked basic necessities, 42 percent of children under six suffered malnutrition, the infant mortality was 82/1,000 live births, and 42 percent of adults were illiterate. The most pressing nutrition-related problems were to provide adequate food and safe water, and to monitor the growth of infants and children. Longer range issues included enabling individuals and families to improve their own food availability and utilization.

The main questions raised in this case study relate to the chapter objectives:

1. To illustrate food and nutrition throughout the world and the challenges community nutrition professionals face

2. To compare and contrast the food and nutrition needs of developed versus underdeveloped countries

METHODOLOGY/TEACHING OBJECTIVES

The objectives are

1. To increase awareness of and cooperation with governmental and nongovernmental agencies, personnel and programs, organizations, foundations, universities, schools, churches, businesses, and other concerning national and community food-nutrition problems and means to alleviate those problems

2. To increase the availability of safe, nutritionally adequate food through food programs, gardens, small animal projects, and other means

3. To improve utilization of available and potentially available food through education in nutrition and food preparation.

Student review of this case study, followed by class discussion is recommended. Graduate students could submit a short report of proposed follow-ups to actions suggested by the class.

THE CASE

Problems related to nutrition and food security in Latin America are diverse and challenging. Malnutrition exists in every country, is primarily subclinical and hidden in some areas and ranges to a high incidence of second- and third-degree malnutrition in other areas.[1,2] Malnutrition often seriously impedes the human potential and productivity of nations as well as that of individuals.[2]

In Nicaragua, the largest Central American nation, cotton and bananas are the chief source of income. Of mixed Indian and Spanish ancestry, most Nicaraguans live in the fertile Pacific region where they work on large estates owned by wealthy landowners or the government. Rural houses often consist of pole walls and palm leaf roofs. Over ten years of war resulted in thousands of deaths and an economy marked by debt and unemployment.

In the Pacific region of Cerro Negro near the city of Leon, drought, volcanic eruptions, and a coastal earthquake further devastated the area. Homes, schools, crops and animals, and the income-producing cotton crops were destroyed. Over 86 percent of the population of 9,100 lacked basic necessities, 42 percent of the children under six suffered malnutrition, the infant mortality rate of 82/1,000 live births, and 42 percent of adults were illiterate. The rural communities lacked resources and distance and impassable roads complicated the situation.

Since 1962, Alfalit (Spanish for literacy and literature) has worked throughout Latin American to reduce illiteracy and to improve the lives and health of the most needy. The food-nutrition goal of Alfalit is to improve the nutritional status of the population, especially those at high risk, through improved food security and nutrition education. Alfalit has been active in Nicaragua for several years and has an agreement with the Nicaraguan Ministry of External Cooperation to supervise development work throughout the country, including programs in literacy, basic education, nutrition, and community development. Contracts and/or cooperation exist with churches, universities, medical facilities, ministries of education and public health, and other national and international foundations and nongovernmental organizations (see box 20.7). Examples of Alfalit programs used in Latin America include *La Buena Alimentacion para Todos*[3] (Good Nutrition for All), which includes basic nutrition, recipes, and effective, practical, "hands-on" nutrition education techniques.

"Wall libraries" made of plastic or fabric with pockets for pamphlets are popular and effective means to improve literacy skills and enhance personal, family, and community development. Participants usually make the attractive portable wall libraries, choose the booklets, and hang them

BOX 20.7

RESOURCES AND PROGRAMS

- Government ministries and agencies—education, public health, and the like
- National and international foundations
- Schools and universities
- International nongovernmental organizations (NGOs): UNICEF, UNESCO, FAO (Food and Agriculture Organization), the World Bank, and USAID
- Hospitals, clinics, and medical and public health personnel
- Churches and relief agencies, local, national, and international, for example, specific church denominations, the Red Cross, Catholic Charities, Church World Service, and CARE
- Radio, television, newspapers, and magazines
- Other print media, especially Alfalit booklets on food and nutrition; extensive literacy materials; and preschool materials for children, parents, and staff

---

on the walls of their homes, where they stimulate reading and use by household members and visitors who see the booklets. Literacy is only the first step, and many adults are motivated so they can read recipes, sewing and craft instructions, and in various ways increase family income.

Short segments of nutrition books have been read on the air by rural radio stations. Brief nutrition notes and "public service announcements" are broadcast to promote healthful eating and use of available foods. Audience call-in questions about food and nutrition on radio and TV programs also offer opportunities to address food safety and nutrition questions.

Local leaders are taught to teach others. Programs are based on local foods, needs, situations, materials, and interests, involving local leaders and participants in planning, implementation, and evaluation. In many rural areas nutritious foods such as eggs, and produce are sold for cash—to buy soft drinks and white bread. Fruits such as papayas and vegetables may be fed to the hogs. Wild greens could provide vitamins, minerals and fiber, but are usually ignored. Use of available but unused foods, especially complementary proteins, soybeans, and more fruits and vegetables is encouraged. Extensive preschool programs serve rural children with no access to schools, providing classes for the children's mothers or caregivers to practice safe, nutritious food preparation. When feasible, participants bring local foods to prepare. As adults and children enjoy the foods, they learn and are motivated to try them at home to share information with neighbors and others.

Children, youth and sometimes adults may lack the quantity and/or quality of foods for adequate nutrition. Funding for simple school meals is provided or facilitated through churches, foundations, UNESCO and others.

Home, school, and community gardens increase the use of fresh vegetables and fruits. Even in cities, small amounts of greens, tomatoes, carrots, peppers, and other vegetables can be grown in pots, window boxes, or patios. Small animal projects such as rabbits and guinea pigs improve dietary protein content and quality. Solar cooking has considerable potential, especially in tropical countries.

Under the circumstances described, Alfalit-Nicaragua's challenge was to find ways to address the immediate and long range problems related to food security and nutritional status in this area of Nicaragua.

In this case, Mireya Cano, the director of Alfalit-Nicaragua took the lead in dealing with the problems. She is not a nutrition professional. She made effective use of the nutrition booklets I wrote in Spanish and the nutrition training I had provided earlier in Nicaragua. She mobilized people, government, churches, NGOs, and others to provide food and nutrition education to help people help themselves and their families in the future. In some ways, what she did is more astounding than if a nutrition professional had done it. Although I was in the United States at the time, she used me as a resource. I provided her with anthropometric data, measurement procedures, kcalorie and nutrient standards for Central American children, and menu suggestions that she used and continues to use very effectively. There are many children alive today and learning in schools as a result of her work. I helped her make connections with USAID, but using the information I sent her, she did practically everything on her own. She is very talented in using resources and isn't afraid to knock on any door, no matter how high or low.

NUTRITION INTERVENTION

In addition to getting food from various sources, Mireya also had community programs where she combined teaching nutrition and using the limited foods available (using my books) with a community meal in which people took foods they had—some rice, a few carrots, and so on. It was a real-life version of "Stone Soup" in which everyone was able to eat better together than alone, and in which through "hands-on" activities they also learned applications to help themselves and their families in the future. Mireya was able to get dry milk, oil, and corn to feed the children at school, often the only food they had all day. She also acquired poles and tin roofing to make "schools" for the children. She has held hundreds of sessions for preschool children and their mothers, again teaching nutrition and parenting, and involving them in preparing simple nutritious foods- including some they bring home to improve the nutrition of families. All of these projects are continuing because they are still needed after hurricanes and ongoing economic and political problems. Funds and training were found to dig new wells and clean existing ones to provide safe water. Mireya said some Nicaraguans stood in line three days waiting to vote in a national election. Her story is truly inspiring and amazing.

RESULTS IN NICARAGUA

Nicaraguans in the case study shared their limited food items to make a "community soup" that was more nutritious and filling than their individual foods. They also learned about food and nutrition, an opportunity to nourish themselves in the present and in the future. Anthropometric measurements of preschool and school children in feeding programs have demonstrated significant improvement, although total daily nutrient intake often remains inadequate. Many of the other programs listed in box 20.7 were developed or utilized in Nicaragua. Increased use of fruits, vegetables, and wild plants, as well as complementary proteins has improved dietary intake. However, extreme poverty severely limits available food for many adults and children. More garden seeds, animals, and supplies are needed.

As the program director of Alfalit International, Inc., I have worked as a volunteer in nearly all Latin American countries about five to six weeks a year and learned Spanish to do this work. Staying with local people is very interesting, economical, and helps me be a part of the community. Initially, I worked with community groups and leaders, but in recent years I have also worked with nutrition, health, and education professionals, as well as utilizing radio and television to multiply the teaching and potential applications of food and nutrition information.

REFERENCES

1. Bread for the World Institute: *Hunger 1996: countries in crisis,* Silver Spring, MD, 1995, The Institute.
2. Bread for the World Institute: *Hunger 1995: causes of hunger,* Silver Spring, MD, 1994, The Institute.
3. Dow RM: *La buena alimentacion para todos,* ed 2, Miami, FL, 1992, Alfalit International, Inc.

CHAPTER TWENTY-ONE

ENTERING AN ERA OF DYNAMIC CHANGE IN HEALTH AND NUTRITION

I like the dreams of the future better than the history of the past.
—Patrick Henry

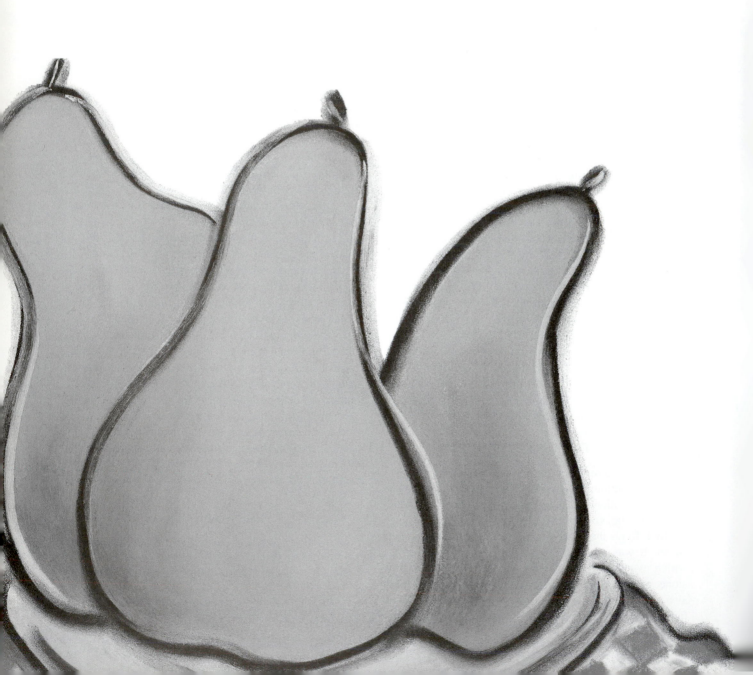

Core Concepts

As community nutrition professionals enter the twenty-first century, we must keep in mind there are many lessons to be learned from history. It is in times of wrenching change that some of the most significant advances have been made and the most enduring achievements are recorded. Keeping people healthy in the twenty-first century will require thoughtful planning on the part of health professionals because we will be expected to do more with less. Keeping people healthy not only requires the work of health professionals but it also requires an entire society to practice public health. In the twenty-first century, it will be necessary to keep up with and understand major developments in health and nutrition but equally important is knowledge of societal trends, each with their opportunities and challenges. Doing this will require a planned strategy to constantly look at the issues affecting society as a whole rather than just the field of health and nutrition. In the twenty-first century, we must be effective leaders to protect the public's health. With science and professional practice as our foundation, we must make our places of work innovative and effective instruments of health improvement. Leadership will be required to strengthen the effectiveness and efficiency of programs for the public. Collaboration with other sectors of society and the community will be critical to get the job done. We must work to assure conditions in which people can be healthy. Doing this will require advocacy to educate the public about their health.

Objectives

When you finish chapter twenty-one, you should be able to:

~ Identify the conditions in which people can be healthy.

~ Discuss critically the societal trends affecting public health.

~ Explain the impact that human genetics will have on nutrition in the future.

~ Describe the demographic changes that will occur in the twenty-first century, including the impact on children.

~ Identify how information technology will affect community nutrition professionals in their practice.

~ List the emerging areas of food and food technology.

~ State the leadership challenges that public health and community nutrition professionals face and identify the skills needed to address the challenges.

~ Identify the implementation strategies needed for education of the public in the twenty-first century.

Key Words

Word	First Mentioned
Human needs	612
Human rights	612
Equal access	612
Alternative and complementary health care	614
Human genetics	614
Point of service	614
Cultural Creatives	617
Information technology	618
Neutraceuticals	620
Thinking in the future tense	622
Pattern recognition	622
Cultural knowledge	622
Advocacy	624

We are about to be engulfed in future talk: new terms, new century, new millennium—what will it all be like? Futurists predictions for the twenty-first century offer prospects well worth celebrating. Science and medicine, surely the two great success stories of the past 100 years, are poised for fresh advances, exploring both the unimaginable frontiers of the universe and the microscopic secrets of the human body. The potential of computers to transform our work habits, our politics, and not the least, our shopping, is only the beginning to be anticipated. Our society will be older, wiser, and more ethnically diverse.

KEEPING PEOPLE HEALTHY
IN THE NEXT CENTURY

As we attempt to predict the future of the public's health, a good starting point is to review the definition in the Institute of Medicine report on *The Future of Public Health:* "Public health is what we as a society do collectively to assure the conditions in which people can be healthy."[11] Figure 21.1 describes the societal trends and challenges for the twenty-first century within the context of health. Public health professionals play profoundly important roles in our society, but it takes an entire society to practice public health. Levy addressed the question "What are the conditions in which people can be healthy?"[16] He lists twelve conditions that we as a society should be assuring. These conditions will be equally important as we move into the twenty-first century as they are now.

- *Basic **human needs:*** A sustainable system ensures that needs for food, clothing, and shelter are met.
- *Population-based health services:* Services and programs are adequately constituted and financially supported to meet community needs for promoting and protecting health and for preventing disease and injury.
- *Health care:* All people have access to affordable, quality health care for diagnosis, short-term and long-term treatment, and prevention of both physical and mental health problems.
- *Essential health information:* To take responsibility for protecting and promoting their own health and that of their families and communities, all people have access to understandable information and recommendations concerning health and health services.
- *Healthy and safe environments:* All individuals are able to live, work, and play in environments that promote health and present minimal or no risk of disease or injury, due to chemical, physical, biological, and psychological hazards.

- *Healthy sociocultural environments:* A framework of healthy sociocultural attitudes and behaviors supports individuals, families, and communities in being healthy.
- *Education, training, and employment opportunities:* All people have access to such opportunities to achieve their full potential and maintain their health and that of their families and communities.
- *Peace and security:* Conflicts at all levels—between individuals; within families, communities, and nations; and between nations—are resolved by nonviolent means. All people are secure from physical violence.
- *Development of new health-related knowledge:* Discovery, development, and dissemination of new knowledge and information concerning health and health services are supported.
- ***Human rights:*** Everyone, regardless of race, nationality, religion, gender, age, and political belief is entitled to "life integrity rights"—the right to live; the right to personal inviolability; the right to be free of arbitrary seizure, detention, and punishment; the right to free movement without discrimination; and the right to create and cohabit with family.
- ***Equal access:*** Access to health services, health-related information, and education and employment opportunities do not differ by gender, age, race, ethnic group, or socioeconomic status.
- *A framework for participation:* There is a sustainable framework for individuals and groups to participate in the decisions that shape their destiny and that of their communities. Disadvantaged and disenfranchised individuals and groups are empowered to participate. Individuals and groups are engaged in activities that assure the conditions in which they and their communities can be healthy.

How Will We Manage to Keep People Healthy?

Keeping up with major developments in public health and monitoring major societal trends will be even more critical in the twenty-first century. Knowing the issues will be the first step in being an effective public health professional.

The ten societal trends that have important implications for public health, each with their challenges and opportunities, are shown in box 21.1.[17] Each of these societal trends and their implications for change are discussed in this chapter.

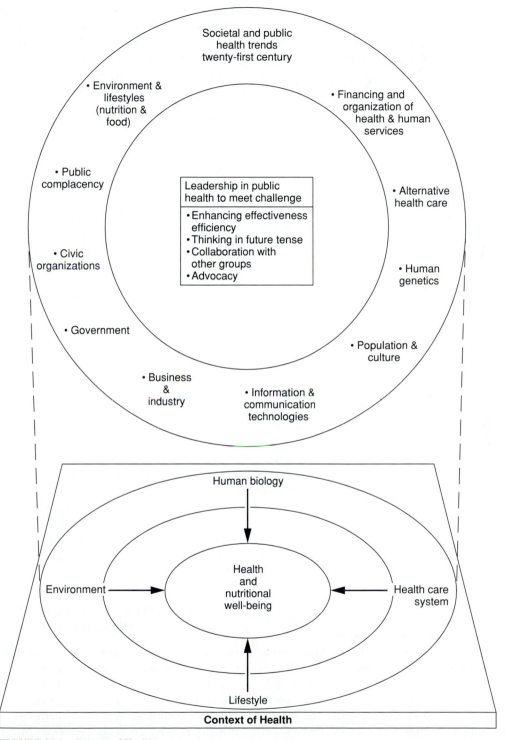

FIGURE 21.1   Context of Health
Health and nutrition in an era of dynamic change.

BOX 21.1

TEN SOCIETAL TRENDS AFFECTING THE PUBLIC'S HEALTH

- Financing and organization of health and human services
- **Alternative and complementary health care**
- **Human genetics**
- Population and emerging culture
- Information and communication technologies
- Business and industry
- Government
- Civic organizations
- Public complacency
- Environmental and lifestyle including nutrition and food

Source: Levy BS: Keeping up with societal trends and public health, President's column, *The Nation's Health,* May/June 1997, p. 2.

FINANCING AND ORGANIZATION OF HEALTH AND HUMAN SERVICES

Managed care poses challenges for public health. In the absence of legislated health care reform, the market has propelled the growth of managed care throughout the country. Even though managed care plans now cover nearly 60 million Americans, it is too early to draw firm conclusions about whether managed care will deliver more or less access and better or worse quality of care to patients.[2] While managed care offers possibilities to improve continuity of care, increase clinical prevention, and better monitor clinical outcomes, these possibilities remain largely unrealized.[17] Public health professionals, including those who support the concept of managed care, must be concerned by the findings of studies that managed care may adversely affect low-income and elderly patients with serious health problems.[32]

Consumers enrolled in managed care have sent a clear message. They do not want any more problems trying to get a timely appointment, a referral to a specialist, or approval for treatment. After years of mounting criticisms and a flood of proposed state and federal measures to limit their alleged excesses, HMOs and other managed care plans are trying to become less rigid and more consumer-friendly. The trend now is away from the restrictive type of managed care that has

dominated since the early 1980s. Plans are now offering enrollees new options and building integrated health care systems to provide seamless care ranging from preventative services to end of life needs.

The fastest growing form of managed care in the country, the so-called POS (**point of service**) plan is a prime example of the trend. Enrollees pay a 10 to 15 percent higher premium. In return, they can go to any physician, hospital, or health facility they want if they pay a portion of the bill, generally 30 percent. As of 1996, half of the nation's 630 HMOs now offer a POS option, up from 20 percent in 1990. Other changes include allowing enrollees to see specialists without having to get permission from primary care "gatekeepers."

The next level for managed care is in the pioneering stage. HMOs are creating teams of specialists to care for people with serious or chronic illnesses. For example, members with diabetes or heart disease will choose a team and have access to all of its specialists, which may include a dietitian, physical therapist, and a social worker, as well as a physician. Alternative medicine is also an option considered in some plans. Providers could include acupuncturists, naturopaths, chiropractors, and even yoga teachers. Managed care could be called a "work in progress." Where it will lead us in the next century is anyone's guess.

The number of uninsured people in this country continues to grow by 100,000 a month. The safety net for all human services is increasingly porous. For many, welfare reform passed in 1996 is welfare repeal. The nonpartisan Urban Institute estimates that the legislation will push 2.6 million more people, including 1.1 million children, below the poverty level.[23] It will reduce or deny essential benefits such as food stamps and financial support that sustain poor families, especially female-headed households.

ALTERNATIVE AND COMPLEMENTARY HEALTH CARE

One third of Americans purchase or use alternative health care products or services each year. These products and services should be assessed for efficacy and safety. Public health needs to build closer working relationships with practitioners of alternative and complementary health care.[17] The American Medical Association took a second look at alternative therapies in 1995. Responding to a culture in which a third of all patients were turning to some form of alternative treatment, often without telling their regular physicians, the AMA issued a formal statement advising its 300,000 members to "become better informed regarding the practices and techniques of alternative or unconventional medicine."[9] Until alternative medicine comes up with its own assessment standards, the future status of this treatment will remain unsettled. Without the proper proof, neither critics nor advocates will be able to demonstrate whether these approaches actually work. The alternative and complementary health care movement will no doubt be very much alive in the next century.

HUMAN GENETICS

Knowledge about the interaction between genetics and diet has been growing rapidly since the National Institutes of Health (NIH) started the Human Genome Project in the mid-1980s. The interaction of genetics and environment, nature and nurture is the foundation of all health and disease. Genetic factors determine susceptibility to disease and environmental factors determine which genetically susceptible individuals will be affected.[27] Figure 21.2 describes the makeup of genes, which include cells, chromosomes, nucleus, and DNA. It also shows how a flawed gene can lead to genetic disease. In a few situations, scientists and physicians have collaborated on ways to replace or to manipulate genes in the human body that have been flawed since birth or were damaged during fetal life. Many are touting gene therapy as the great medical savior that will bring treatment, even cures, within five to ten years.

Genetics and Nutrition

Major advances have occurred in the past fifteen years in both fields of genetics and nutrition.[28] Using the tools of molecular biology and genetics, research is defining the mechanisms by which genes influence nutrient

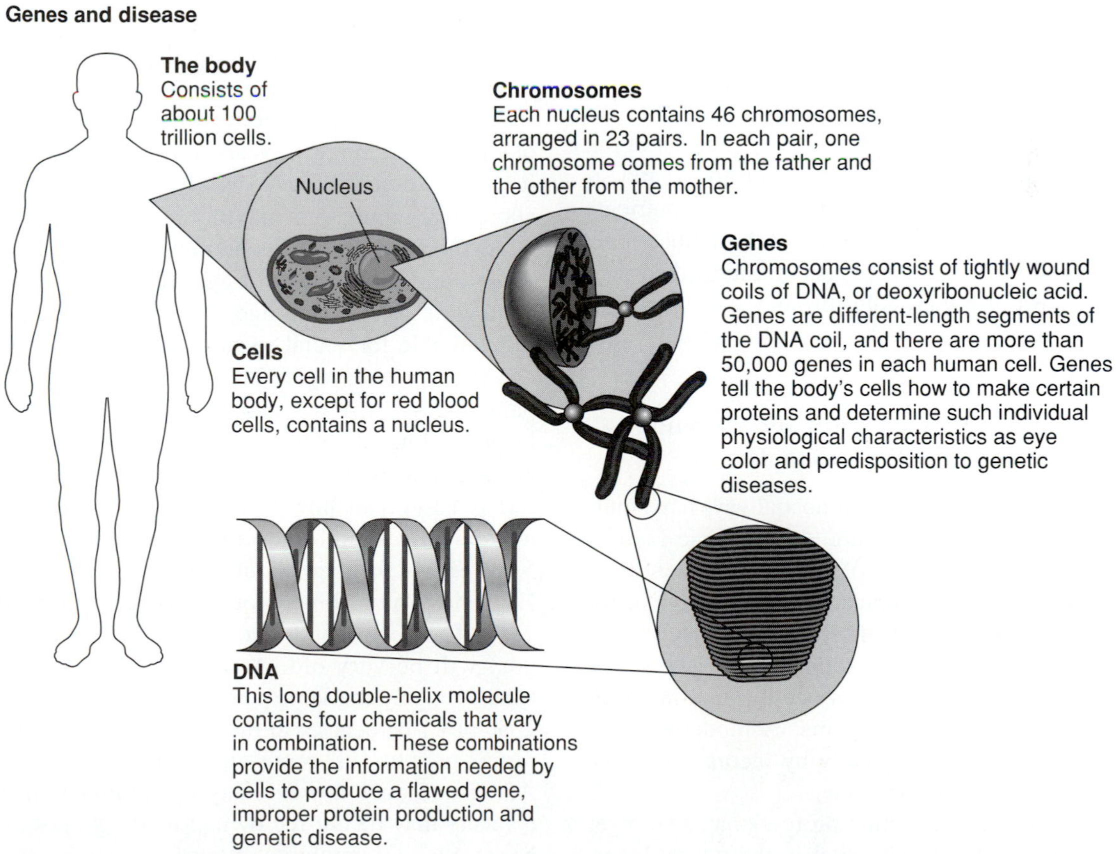

Genes and disease

The body
Consists of about 100 trillion cells.

Chromosomes
Each nucleus contains 46 chromosomes, arranged in 23 pairs. In each pair, one chromosome comes from the father and the other from the mother.

Nucleus

Cells
Every cell in the human body, except for red blood cells, contains a nucleus.

Genes
Chromosomes consist of tightly wound coils of DNA, or deoxyribonucleic acid. Genes are different-length segments of the DNA coil, and there are more than 50,000 genes in each human cell. Genes tell the body's cells how to make certain proteins and determine such individual physiological characteristics as eye color and predisposition to genetic diseases.

DNA
This long double-helix molecule contains four chemicals that vary in combination. These combinations provide the information needed by cells to produce a flawed gene, improper protein production and genetic disease.

FIGURE 21.2   Genes and Disease

Environmental	Genetic	Proteins
Supply Availability Consumption	Digestion Absorption Distribution Transformation Storage Excretion	Receptors Carriers Enzymes Hormones

FIGURE 21.3   Nutritional Health
(*Source:* Adapted from Simopolous AP: Genetic variation and nutrition. Part 1. Population differences due to polygenic defects, *Nutrition Today,* 30(4), 194–206, 1995.)

absorption, metabolism, and excretion, taste perception, and degree of satiation, as well as the mechanisms by which nutrients influence gene expression. Furthermore, advances in molecular and recombinant DNA technology have led to exquisite studies in the field of genetics and recognition in a much more specific way, through DNA sequencing, of how unique each one of us is and the extent to which genetic variation occurs in human beings.[29] Nutritional health is dependent on the interaction between the environmental aspects of diet in terms of supply, availability, and consumption and genetically controlled aspects of digestion, absorption, distribution, transformation, storage, and excretion by proteins in the form of receptors, carriers, enzymes, hormones, and so forth (figure 21.3). The interactions of certain nutrients with genetically determined biochemical and metabolic factors suggest different requirements for individuals, for example, familial hypercholesterolemia and familial combined hyperlipidemia.[28,29]

Implications for Public Health and Community Nutrition Professionals

The common chronic diseases almost always have multiple causes including interaction with genetic factors. For example, the prevalence of obesity and identification of subgroups in the population at specific risk for chronic diseases because of genetic predisposition should be a top priority for public health.[8] The scientific information about genetics needs to be incorporated into public health programs. A modern public health system will benefit greatly by incorporating the knowledge from genetic medicine.

For the community nutrition professional, a stronger emphasis on genetics will be vital in the future. Incor-

poration of genetics may be as broad as factoring in the potential of a family health history into counseling or as specific as teaming with other professionals to provide gene-tailored nutrition advice. In either case, it offers the potential of individualization, or personalization, of dietary guidance.[4]

POPULATION AND EMERGING CULTURE

Demography's crystal ball shows that twenty-first-century Americans will be older and more ethnically diverse. But children may face problems. These changes in the U.S. population will profoundly affect public health. The size and composition of the future population is determined by three factors:[24]

- Fertility (the average number of children born per woman)
- Mortality (the average life expectancy at birth)
- Migration

The Census Bureau projects higher fertility and faster improvement in mortality. As a consequence, the present U.S. population of 266 million will grow to 395 million by the year 2050.

Immigration is a subject that has caused a great deal of controversy in recent years. For the twenty-first century, one choice likely to be discussed is whether to allow more immigrants into this country.

As the population ages and taxes the social security system and medicare, old age may be redefined, by continuing to shift the age at which citizens become fully eligible for social security benefits up as high as age seventy-two years. This is likely to be the most palatable solution; it can be explained in terms of longer and healthier life spans and as a postponement, not an elimination of benefits.[24]

Discussions of how to support an aging population may acquire racial and ethnic overtones. By 2050, 53 percent of the total population is projected to be non-Hispanic White, down from 74 percent today (figure 21.4). The decline will occur after 2035 and this category will be very old. African-Americans will contribute roughly the same percentage of the population in 2050 (15.4 percent as in the 1990s (12.6 percent). The fastest growth will occur among Hispanic and Asian-Americans, fueled previously by immigration. Ethnic diversity may be blurred by intermarriage, just as it has been for earlier immigrant groups.

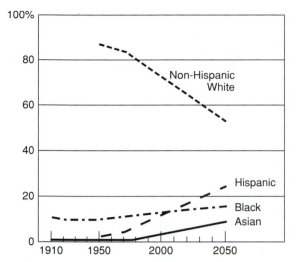

FIGURE 21.4 **U.S. Population by Race or Ethnicity**
(*Source:* From US Census Bureau, Washington, DC, September 1996.)

Children in the Next Century

Perhaps the most significant social change of the past fifty years has been the transformation of the American family. Most women are back in the workforce by a child's first birthday. More children are being born to unmarried women; 33 percent in 1994 compared with 5 percent in 1960. Overall, more than 60 percent of American children will spend some fraction of their childhood living with only one natural parent, typically the mother. Given these trends—the decline of two-parent family, an increasing proportion of children born into poverty (22 percent of American children lived in poverty in 1996), and a growing national focus on the problems of an aging population—one question stands out: will children in the future be sufficiently nurtured and equipped to keep the nation evolving in a healthy fashion? Support is likely to erode further as more children are born to minorities, with whom non-Hispanic Whites have difficulty identifying—they are "other people's children."[5,24]

American's will look back on 1997 as a turning point in the lives of poor children. The welfare reform bill, signed into law in fall 1996, eliminates major federal programs in exchange for block grants to states. America may be conducting an unprecedented social experiment with childhood, one with potentially profound effects on our nation's future. Community nutrition professionals must be constantly vigilant regarding the nutritional needs of children and must be innovative in their approaches to meet their needs.

The Emerging Culture in America

A major change that has been growing in American culture—a comprehensive shift in values, worldviews, and ways of life—applies to nearly one fourth of American adults or 44 million persons. People who follow the new path are on the leading edge of several kinds of cultural change. The emerging new group has been called "**Cultural Creatives**" and they tend to be affluent and well educated.

In numerous surveys, it has been shown that Americans live in three different worlds of meaning and value.[25] These include Traditionalism, Modernism and, more recently, Cultural Creatives. Traditionalism is the belief system for about 29 percent of Americans (56 million adults), who might also be called Heartlanders. They believe in a nostalgic image of small town and strong churches that define the "Good Old American Way." The second view is Modernism. It holds sway for about 47 percent of Americans (88 million adults). Modernists place high value on personal success, consumerism, materialism, and technological rationality.

The third and newest worldview is that of the Cultural Creatives. Their distinctive values separate them from the rest of American society. They tend to reject hedonism, materialism, and cynicism. For this reason, many are disdainful of modern media, consumer, and business culture. They may be disenchanted with the idea of "owning more stuff," but they have a strong emphasis on having new and unique experiences. The fact that six in ten Creatives are women is a major focus for understanding the subculture. Creatives are the core market for psychotherapy, alternative health care, and natural foods. What ties these together is the belief that body, mind, and spirit should be unified. Creatives may include a high proportion of people whom some physicians describe as "the worried well," those who monitor every twitch and pain in a minutely detailed attention to the body. As a result, they spend more on all forms of health care, even though most are fairly healthy. The appearance of the Cultural Creatives in America is a very hopeful thing for our society, for it offers a chance to create a more positive new culture. This group is on the leading edge of change. With their interest in preventive health measures, they may lead the way for a larger segment of the population to consider health promotion and disease prevention.

Women's Ideas of a Preferred Future

If women had their say, what would the future be like? Wagner addressed the issue of what is women's preferred future.[31] Based on a wide variety of submissions to *The Futurist* magazine on this topic, there were several elements of a preferred future that many of the scenarios share. However, it turns out that the preferred future for women must be one that benefits all humanity. The shared elements of a preferred future for women are described in box 21.2.

INFORMATION AND COMMUNICATION TECHNOLOGY

The pace of change is so fast that one year on the Internet is like seven years in any other medium. By this scheme, it has been nearly a century since the Internet was born. It has been more than a decade since the emergence of the World Wide Web as an electronic publishing vehicle. And by the year 2000, the Internet will have undergone another two decades worth of growth and development.[18]

The use of computers and communication technology to send and receive information is here to stay, and community nutrition professionals can capitalize on it to further demonstrate the value of comprehensive nutrition services including disease prevention and health promotion.[6] **Information technology** will affect community nutrition professionals in two important ways. Personal computers and expert systems will eliminate many of the routine functions we currently perform such as recording care plans.[21] The real benefit of this technology is that nutrition and dietetic professionals will spend less time on the business of the profession and more time on the purposes of the profession: helping people have healthy lives by promoting optimal nutritional health and well-being.[6] Further, information technology will be responsible for changing the basic

BOX 21.2

WOMEN'S PREFERRED FUTURE

- *No more glass ceiling:* In business, women become entrepreneurs, hiring and mentoring other women.
- *Equal representation of the sexes at all levels of government:* Some predict that a woman will be president or vice president of the United States by the year 2020 and that Congress and the Supreme Court will be made up of a proportional number of women.
- *Understanding and celebration of gender differences:* Gender differences become opportunities for learning and expansion and they are celebrated.
- *Understanding and celebration of diversity of all kinds:* Racism and homophobia will be relegated to the history books.
- *It's okay to be single:* More women are choosing to stay single and benefit humankind as leaders in government, religion, business, and humanitarian activities.
- *Control over childbirth:* All women should have knowledge about and free access to birth control that has no side effects. Methods of contraception have been so perfected by 2020 that not only is abortion outmoded but the majority of women worldwide will have fewer children.

- *Community- and business-based child care:* It does take a village to raise a child. Acceptance of broad responsibility for the care of children should be emphasized.
- *Human-scaled institutions:* Corporations and governments should be local and decentralized, down to the level of the neighborhood or even the home. Large corporate structures will diminish as women create smaller, home-based enterprises that blend their business and personal activities.
- *Equal education for women throughout the world:* This includes technological literacy.
- *A clean environment:* Based on principles of sustainability.
- *Less war, crime, and violence in general:* No more nuclear weapons. War should be abolished.
- *And men:* No one wants a "preferred" future that excludes men or in which men are subservient to women. The preferred future for women, however, must be one that benefits all of humanity—even men.

Source: Wagner CG: Women's preferred futures, *The Futurist,* May/June 1997, pp. 1–11.

definition of what we do. Many health professionals have already seen their work transformed by technology. Nutrition research has rapidly expanded assessment and intervention strategies for virtually every disease state. Technology will help us to remain current in the profession and to channel this knowledge into models that will ensure positive outcomes for many clients at once. The early twenty-first century will see us expand our abilities to work collaboratively with clients, practitioners, and scholars throughout the world. Practitioners will rethink old assumptions (e.g., does all counseling have to be face-to-face?), question old traditions (e.g., we can empower the client to do the major decision making), and abandon old processes (e.g., standards of practice, quality assurance, and outcome measures can be integrated into a single software package).[21]

Levy summarized the trends in information and communication technologies by indicating that opportunities include enhanced data analysis, improved communications among public health professionals, and more accessible education and training. He also states that the dangers include depersonalization of health services and the potential for violation of confidentiality.[17]

BUSINESS AND INDUSTRY

The very nature of work—what people do as members of organizations—is rapidly changing. Robert Reich, former U.S. Secretary of Labor, called this phenomenon the new work.[26] The new work involves less rote repetition and more problem solving. Value is added by customizing and continuously improving a product or service to meet customer needs. The new work is enhanced, not impoverished, by technology.[15,26]

Fortune magazine[15] painted the following picture of the workplace in the year 2000:

- The average company will become smaller, employing fewer people.
- The traditional hierarchical organization will give way to a variety of organizational forms, the network of specialists foremost among these.
- Technicians, ranging from computer repairman to radiation therapists, will replace manufacturing operators as the worker elite.
- The vertical division of labor will be replaced by horizontal division.

- The paradigm of doing business will shift from making a product to providing a service.
- Work itself will be redefined: constant learning, more high-order thinking, and less nine-to-five availability.

These changes in business and industry will have implications for the public's health and particularly for the way families work and live.

GOVERNMENT

Our elected officials want to downsize or "reinvent" government (this includes federal, state, and local public health agencies)—at least until an outbreak of disease is discovered. But a recent survey showed that most Americans want government to prevent disease and injury and ensure clean air, clean water, and control of toxic wastes.[17] Dangers from inadequate government services and protection are opportunities to translate latent public support into improved public health.

CIVIC ORGANIZATIONS

Participation continues to decline in civic groups where we can communicate public health information and discuss policy options. We need to participate in and strengthen these organizations. In May 1997, President Clinton convened a summit on the role of volunteer services to meet the nation's needs. The summit had strong bipartisan support. In a show of unity, every living former president (except Ronald Reagan, who was represented by his wife) met to salute mentors, tutors, and other involved citizens. There are many acknowledged benefits of volunteering. It helps build a sense of community, breaking down barriers between people, and often raises the quality of life. Volunteerism can be a two-edged sword. It is one thing to celebrate volunteers and their good work. The other side of the issue is to depend on volunteers to fill the gaps left by failures and cutbacks in welfare and other government programs.

PUBLIC COMPLACENCY

When public health is most effective, it is almost invisible. This breeds complacency. Public health professionals cannot work alone, for public health is what we, as a society, do collectively to assure the conditions in which people can be healthy. We need to put the public back in public health.

ENVIRONMENT AND LIFESTYLE (FOOD AND NUTRITION)

There is an inherent logic to health promotion and disease prevention. It has always seemed more sensible to prevent the occurrence of diseases, or to stop them early in their natural history, than to delay treatment until the process of pathogenesis has resulted in irreversible damage to the body. Prevention offers individuals and society a more rational strategy for dealing with disease and promoting health. This is true now and will be in the future. Society can practice health promotion and disease prevention through several channels:

- Controlling communicable diseases
- Protecting the environment
- Modifying personal behaviors that affect health
- Preventing or reducing the severity of noncommunicable and chronic diseases[33]

The main challenge in food and nutrition is how to inform and encourage the public to eat so as to improve their chances for a healthier life. The Institute of Medicine examined the needs and opportunities in nutrition and food sciences.[13] The report indicated the challenges in public health nutrition for the future, which include developing successful interventions and policies to reduce the risk of diet-related diseases and the incidence of hunger and food insecurity and monitoring the impact of these policies.

Previous nutritional interventions, which used either food fortification or vitamin and mineral supplementation approaches, were relatively simple to carry out and their results were easily observed. The nutritional challenges of today are much more complex, spanning dietary excesses and disease to inadequate food distribution and hunger. The targets of potential interventions range from the macro level of national agricultural and health policies to the micro level of household and individual food behaviors. Future interventions to deal with these complex problems will need to interpret findings from the basic behavioral science with agriculture, economics, political science, and the other social sciences. This process alone will provide many new exciting research opportunities for nutrition and food sciences.[13]

EMERGING AREAS OF FOOD AND FOOD TECHNOLOGY

The benefits of phytochemicals, functional foods, and **neutraceuticals** have been extensively publicized in the popular press, which has resulted in increased public awareness and interest in these foods as a method of enhancing health and well-being.

Confusion exists about how to describe this newly evolving area of food and food technology because numerous interchangeable and related terms have been suggested or published in the United States, Europe, and Japan. A "scheme" has been developed to describe the various terms being used that may have beneficial roles in prevention and treatment of disease[19] (see figure 21.5). Definitions for the three terms include:

- Phytochemicals are substances found in edible fruits and vegetables that may be ingested by humans daily that exhibit a potential for modulating tumor metabolism in a manner favorable to cancer patients.[22]
- Functional foods are any modified food ingredient that may provide a health benefit beyond the traditional nutrition it contains.[30]
- Nutraceutical is any substance that may be considered a food or part of a food and that provides medical or health benefits, including the prevention or treatment of disease.[30]

Common to all of these terms is the assumption that these foods, or components found within them, have a potential beneficial role in the prevention or treatment of disease. This area is an emerging field that holds great promise in the new millennium. The role of community nutrition professionals is clear.

How Will Americans Eat in the Next Century?

The best place to begin to look to the future is in the past. If we want to know what people will be eating ten years from now, let's look at today's list. Eight of the ten most popular foods today were on the list a decade ago. The form may be a little different, like turkey ham instead of real ham for instance, because people are eating healthier alternatives to some traditional foods. The top five items purchased in restaurants during 1995 were regular soft drinks, french fries, hamburgers or cheeseburgers, diet soft drinks, and heroes or sub sandwiches. Consumers like traditional foods—they are slow to change.[1] And when consumers change, it is usually to a version of the product that is perceived as having better value in terms of health, price, or convenience.

The aging population has fueled the extensive activity in the healthy foods area, which actually represents healthy alternatives across virtually all product cate-

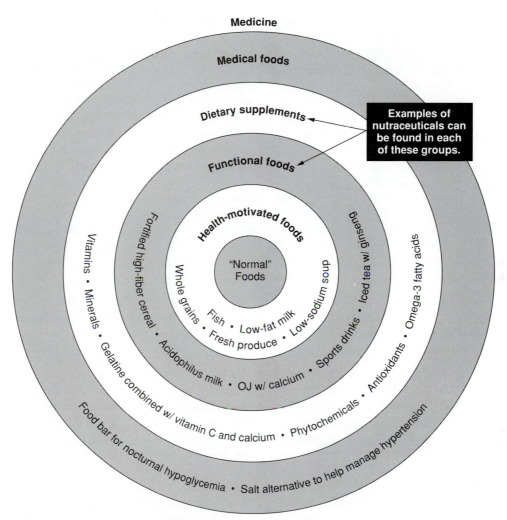

FIGURE 21.5 Nutraceuticals in Dietary Supplements and Functional Foods
(*Source:* From Beck C, Childs JM: Neutraceuticals: new aid for health promotion, *Nutrition Update,*
East Hanover, NJ, 1997, Nabisco Brands, Inc.)

gories.[10] Nearly one in three foods and beverage products consumed in the home is classified as "healthy." Fat-free and non-fat alternatives are sharing the most rapid growth. Consumption of ethnic foods is growing faster than any other main dish eaten at home. Mobility means convenience in packaging, product design, and distribution. To illustrate this point, as many as one in ten restaurant meals are eaten in cars.

Although it appears to many of us that the technology revolution in food is "old hat," it's really just beginning. The Internet, cellular phones, and high-powered and compact notebook computers are all new technologies in their infancy. Eventually, all information will be available via a single personal device.[10] This revolution is transforming the way consumers live, eat, work, and play. The truly mobile individual lifestyle is possible. The World Future Society predicts that supermarkets may become hydroponic greenhouses where shoppers pick up their own produce from the vine.[7] And for those who would not care for such a hands-on experience, groceries could be electronically ordered and automatically delivered into home refrigerators designed to open to the outside as well as inside the house.

How the meals of tomorrow might be prepared include the fanciful and the unbelievable. Cetron indicated that by the year 2006, people will have personal diagnostic and meal-preparation machines. If you eat too much, the diagnostic machine will tell you to exercise.[3] Many experts anticipate advances in biotechnology that could lead to cows that produce low-fat milk, and fat-free frying may be possible. Food companies are just now beginning to see how this transformation will shape eating patterns.

Consumers want more food but foods suited to their tastes, lifestyles, and pocketbooks. Americans want variety and healthy alternatives that translate into traditional foods without the fat or so many calories. The only thing that may be certain about food in the next millennium is that consumers will not compromise on taste. For community nutrition professionals the challenge is to recognize the complexity of our food supply and realize that food products are produced globally and will be developed to meet a global market with a demographically diverse population.

LEADERSHIP TO MEET THE CHALLENGE TO THE PUBLIC'S HEALTH

We have discussed how to keep people healthy in the next century and the societal trends that will affect public health. The societal trends and public policy challenges that we've discussed will require public health professionals (including community nutrition professionals) to reassert leadership over the changes that affect the public's health. Brown challenges the public health community to provide leadership in the next century. He indicates that "whether we are practitioners or scientists, whether we work in the university or service organizations, whether we are in public or private sector agencies or community-based organizations, we have the responsibility to be public health leaders."[2] Leadership is required to:

- Invigorate public health agencies with a commitment to effectiveness and innovation.
- Build collaboration with other sectors of the community.
- Advocate effectively for policies that meet public health needs.
- Build coalitions and make media our allies.
- Persuade policy makers to support health-promoting public policies.

Enhancing Effectiveness and Efficiency of Public Health Programs

The first task for leadership is to strengthen public health agencies. Public health programs and services must become more effective and efficient. Community

leaders and consumers are demanding more responsive service. Public- and private-sector policy makers are demanding increased accountability from public health. They are insisting on evidence that public health programs and services actually contribute to the health of communities and individuals, not just that they serve as many people as last year.[2] Public sector agencies must assure that services meet the needs of the larger community and must promote equity. If public health is to overcome bureaucratic constraints that impede innovation and improvements, managers and the public sectors must work together to increase an agency's flexibility and responsiveness. The present risk-averse behavior of agency heads stifles innovation and leadership, because leadership and innovation require risk-taking (see chapters 13, 14, and 15).

Leadership Skills for a New Age: Thinking in the Future Tense

American business, health care economics, and society are changing at the speed of light. At the dawn of the twenty-first century, the pressure is on and managers (including public health) need to learn faster, think smarter, and free themselves from conforming assumptions and old mind set. Many people view the future with fear and dread rather than excitement and anticipation. James indicates that to provide the missing framework, we must think "in the future tense."[14] **Thinking in the future tense** will help to identify the changes taking place around us, to interpret their meaning, and to benefit accordingly. Managers and public health professionals who do not learn the skills needed to separate old cultural beliefs from new realities will not survive.

We need to understand how the currents of technological change will affect our lives and our work in public health, how economic change will affect the global market, and how demographic and cultural changes will alter our perception of others and of society as a whole. In short, we need to know what the future will look like. James indicates that these are the skills we need:

- Perspective
- **Pattern recognition**
- **Cultural knowledge**
- Flexibility
- Vision
- Energy
- Intelligence
- Global values

These eight skills are the basic building blocks and are essential for everyone for understanding and adapting to change.

- *Perspective:* Perspective is the capacity to view things in their true relations or relative importance. A clear perspective is the linchpin in any process of change. Perspective is often the first casualty in rapid change. Tugged in opposite directions by a familiar present and an uncertain future, we can loose our balance and our ability to keep things in perspective. But it doesn't have to be this way—we can learn to recognize the many factors that may be distorting our perceptions. We can keep our eyes open and our minds open to the forces of change as they will affect our businesses and our lives.

- *Pattern Recognition (trends):* We need to train ourselves to determine when patterns or trends are changing, in our lives and in our work. The trick is to develop an eye for bits of information or clues that, when assembled, present us with a new visible pattern or trend. Levy's discussion on the importance of keeping up with societal trends and public health is the perfect example for this concept.[17] An example in nutrition is the trend that people are consuming lower fat foods. Twenty years ago, there was a recognition of chronic disease and the risks of high-fat diets. The trend began in the late 1970s when people were consuming 40 percent of their calories as fat. Food companies followed the low-fat trend. Now there are several thousand low-fat products in the marketplace and people are consuming 33 percent of their calories as fat.

- *Cultural Knowledge:* Know what is happening in society. In terms of change, knowing what old myths are losing power and what new myths are being created. Here are some myths that are being challenged by social analysts. Western civilization is the best civilization; secrecy is power; and, leaders must be strong and powerful. Watch for symbols; language is dense with symbols. When "techies" call managers "manglers" and bodybuilders call weaker men "wimps," these words symbolize what is being thought. The proliferation of politically correct terms such as "physically challenged" and "visually impaired" is another example of changing symbols.

- *Flexibility:* The key to handling change is, of course, your ability to be flexible. As a test of your flexibility, try to incorporate change into your daily routine. There are several tests and advice on how to change, but the one I like best is the vegetable test. Believe it or not, your attitude toward vegetables can tell you something about your level of flexibility. Most people are willing to add another vegetable to their edible list occasionally but we are cautious about it. The point is if you are not open to new tastes, you are probably resistant to change in general. Watch out for things that can keep you from being flexible: nostalgia for an imagined past, lack of awareness, workaholism, arrogance, the need to control, perfectionism, lack of confidence, need to be right, a closed mind, stress, waiting for someone else to change on your journey to the future—these are barriers that will trip you up and slow you down.

- *Vision:* Understand the past to know the future. Vision is unusual discernment and foresight. A person who thinks beyond the box. What is our view of the future? Where do we see public health moving in the future? That is what we need to address.

- *Energy:* The current trends in the expenditure of human energy is its increasing effectiveness. We can literally do more with less. It is rarely what we do or how much we do that tires us now. It is our mind-set in relation to what we do. It is our sense of security.

- *Intelligence:* The future will require a higher and more socialized process of reasoning and more sophisticated reactions. We need a new vision of intelligence, one that integrates the right brain of image and creativity with the left brain of words and calculations in the context of social environment. It has been called the "middle brain" because we need something in between to come with change.

- *Global values:* We need to make ourselves into global citizens, able to move easily among countries, currencies, language, and customs. We need to come to terms with diversity and enjoy the richness of other cultures.

"Thinking in the future tense" tells public health professionals how to adopt new management styles in time to help them manage more effectively and keep their jobs. This mind-set will make it possible to understand and apply the skills that will be crucial to success in the twenty-first century.

Collaboration with Other Groups

Public health groups cannot do the job by themselves, they must collaborate with other sectors of society and the community. Partnering with all sectors in the community involves those groups in solving public health problems, and it helps prevention practices take root in the community. Community organizations bring tremendous experience, expertise, and resources to deal with problems that affect them. These partnerships require leadership from public health, but control must be shared with community organizations. This textbook is replete with examples of successful partnerships that make a difference. The Arizona 5 a Day Program (Case Study in chapter 14) is an excellent example of cooperation between agriculture, public health, and the business community to meet a public health need.

Advocacy for Public Health

Even when we strengthen public health agencies and partner with community organizations, we still have to wage many policy battles for the public's health. We must work through agencies and professional organizations to make public health issues visible, build broad coalitions for public health and win support from elected officials at local, state, and national levels.[2]

Advocacy requires us to educate the public about public health. Most of the population, including elected officials, do not have a clue about public health. This invisibility isolates us from the support of potential allies, and makes us vulnerable when politicians decide to cut budgets or curtail public health agencies' regulatory powers. We must build support in our communities from virtually all sectors of the community: local business groups, labor councils, ministerial alliances, school organizations, medical societies, and neighborhood associations.

COMMUNITY NUTRITION PROFESSIONALS' ROLE IN IMPROVING NUTRITION AND HEALTH

The factors affecting food choices are numerous and complex. Some, such as inherent taste preferences and demographic trends, can be controlled little or not at all. Others more subject to modification include social norms, attitudes, skills, and availability of health-promoting foods. Over the past several decades, there have been important changes in food consumption patterns.[12] Some of these changes are consistent with dietary recommendations (e.g., an increase in fish and vegetable consumption) but others are not (e.g., an increase in the consumption of high-fat ice cream). Similarly, recent changes in consumer attitudes and beliefs provide cause for both optimism and concern. Although there is a general trend toward recognition of the role of diet in disease prevention, surveys indicate that people are sometimes confused about which food components are health promoting and which are not.

Nevertheless, a review of current theory and practice with respect to attitudes and behavior change suggests that modification of food preferences and eating patterns is possible but will require more than simply providing information to the public. People will need to be motivated to accept the information, see its personal relevance to them, integrate it into existing belief structures, acquire new skills and self-perceptions, and learn how to apply newly acquired attitudes to appropriate action and to prevent recidivism. Various studies conducted with schools, at worksites, and in communities have indicated that intervention programs based on the communication persuasion model and the social learning model can be effective in producing substantial reduction in risk factors for diet-related diseases, particularly when they involve several components that reinforce each other and include the mass media[12] (see chapters 7 and 17).

Six strategies and associated actions proposed for education of the public by the Institute of Medicine report are summarized below. These intervention strategies should be the guideposts as we enter a new decade for educating the public.[12]

Implementation strategies for education of the public in the twenty-first century are

- *Ensure that consistent educational messages about dietary recommendations reach the public:* This can occur if leaders of various national groups concerned with health develop a series of common educational objectives to implement the recommendations. Materials developed by these groups should be consistent and compatible with dietary recommendations.

- *Incorporate principles, concepts, and skills training that support dietary recommendations in all levels of schooling:* Mandating the inclusion of a food skills, nutrition, and health course in teacher preparation programs in each state would do a great deal to providing accurate nutrition information in the classroom. We should link classroom teaching about nutrition with the lunchroom and trained school food service personnel to prepare meals based on the lessons they have learned.

- *Ensure that children in child-care programs receive nutritious meals served in an environment that takes account of the importance of food to children's physical and emotional well-being:* National recommendations should be developed for legislation, regulation, and standards, as well as education and training guidelines for professionals and the public to ensure that these recommendations are achieved.

- *Enhance consumer's knowledge and skills needed to meet dietary recommendations through appropriate food selection and preparation:* Particular attention should be paid to cultural diversity in food selection and preparation.
- *Establish a system for designing, implementing, and maintaining community-based interventions to improve dietary patterns:* Relevant professional organizations should engage community leaders in the development of community-based programs that promote dietary recommendations.
- *Enlist the media to help decrease consumer confusion and increase the knowledge and skills that will motivate and equip customers to make health-promoting dietary choices:* This can be done through social marketing campaigns and by coordinating media activities to promote healthful diets (see chapters 7 and 17).

To take the lead in educating the public to improve and enhance their dietary patterns, community nutrition professionals will require a new vision of their roles and their work in the community. Most individuals will find that as work becomes more multidimensional, it will also become more substantive and rewarding.[20] Values will change from being protective or our disciplines to being productive problem solvers and decision makers (chapters 13 and 14). The reality that community nutrition professionals face is that the old ways of doing business simply will not work in the workplace of the future. Community nutrition professionals must take the lead in a new order of things and assume important leadership roles in moving the profession into the forefront. George Bernard Shaw, years ago, summarized the need to be proactive: "We are made wise not by the recollection of our past, but by the responsibilities of the future."

IMPLICATIONS FOR COMMUNITY NUTRITION PROFESSIONALS

The pace of change is more rapid than ever before. As we enter the twenty-first century, we are anxious to predict the future of the public's health, our life's work. A good starting point is to consider what the conditions are to keep people healthy. Conditions that fit this requirement include basic human needs, health care and services, safe physical and sociocultural environment,

human rights, a framework for participation in decision making, and peace and security.

Community nutrition professionals must keep abreast of major societal and public health trends. The trends that have implications for the health of the public in the next century include issues of organization and financing of health and human services. Alternative and complementary health care will grow; however, there will continue to be concerns about the efficacy and safety of some products and services. Human genetics will have a profound effect on health. Of all the recent advances contributing to our understanding of the role of nutrition in disease prevention and the variability in nutrient needs, the recognition of genetic variation as a contributing factor must be among the highest.

The population will be older and more ethnically diverse. There are some concerns about children in the next century. With the changes in the American family, the decline of two-parent households, a rising percentage of children living below the poverty level, and the national focus on the problems of the aging population begs the question—will children of the future be sufficiently nurtured and equipped to lead healthy lives?

Information technology will have an even greater effect on the community nutrition professional in the future. We will spend less time on the business of the profession (routine tasks) and more time on the purposes of the profession. Emerging areas of food and food technology including functional foods and nutraceuticals will be used to tailor diets to meet individuals health needs and to develop prevention strategies.

To meet the challenges of keeping people healthy, creative leadership will be critical. Leadership must be strengthened to enhance the effectiveness and efficiency of public health programs. This will be a new way of doing our jobs—it will require thinking in the future tense. In addition, collaboration with other groups will be necessary to extend public health programs and services. Community nutrition professionals will play an even greater role in keeping people healthy in the next century.

COMMUNITY NUTRITION PROFESSIONALS IN ACTION

- Search the Internet to find at least five sources that provide information on societal trends that affect the health of people.
- Develop a profile of the community in which you work or live using the twelve conditions needed for

people to be healthy. Rate each condition on a scale of 1 to 3 for programs and services with 1 offering the most services to meet a condition, 2 some services, and 3 limited or nonexistent services.
- Select one of the ten societal trends affecting public health to fully explore the implications of the trend on society. Write a report describing your research and present it to the class.
- Monitor the Internet for one week. Determine at least five products or services that could be considered alternative or complementary health care. Determine the positive and negative health consequences of using these products based on information in the scientific literature.
- Review the list of women's ideas of a preferred future. Determine if you agree or disagree with each of the issues. Based on your own interests (male or female) determine which of the issues you would see as having a high priority. Add to the list based on your experiences.

GOING ONE STEP FURTHER

- Information communication technology will help community nutrition professionals work more with the purpose of the profession and less with the business (routine tasks). Review your own work situation; determine the tasks that you now do that can be eliminated. With the additional time available, how would you better serve your clients and patients?
- Develop a paper for college or university students that describes the new foods and food technology including phytochemicals, nutraceuticals, and functional foods. Cite examples of each of these new areas of food technology. Determine how the future development of these substances will help reduce chronic disease in the United States.
- Review the information on *Thinking in the Future Tense* by Jennifer James (Simon and Schuster, 1996). Read the book and then develop your own personal and professional strategy to think in the future tense. Apply the eight skills that are basic building blocks for understanding and adapting to change to your own situation. Share this information with your professor and classmates.

REFERENCES

1. Balzer H: *Eating trends,* Park Ridge, IL, 1995, NPD Group.
2. Brown ER: Leadership to meet the challenges to public health, *Am J Public Health* 87:554–557, 1997.
3. Cetron GJ: *What's in store for the next century?* Arlington, VA, 1996, Forecasting International, Ltd.
4. Dodd JL: Incorporating genetics into dietary guidance, *Food Technology* 51:80–82, 1997.
5. Edmondson B: Children in 2001, *American Demographics* March: 15, 1997.
6. Evers WD: Communications technology and the profession, *J Am Diet Assoc* 96:756–757, 1996.
7. *Foods and dining in the next century,* Bethesda, MD, 1996, The World Future Society.
8. Foreyt JP, Poston WSC II: Diet, genetics and obesity, *Food Technology* 51:70–73, 1997.
9. Henig RM: Medicine, *Civilization* April/May: 43–49, 1997.
10. Hollingsworth P: Developing foods for the next millennium, *Food Technology* 50:110–118, 1996.
11. Institute of Medicine, National Academy of Sciences: *The future of public health,* Washington, DC, 1988, National Academy Press.
12. Institute of Medicine, National Academy of Sciences: *Improving America's diet and health: from recommendation to action,* Washington, DC, 1991, National Academy Press.
13. Institute of Medicine, National Academy of Sciences: *Improving America's Diet and Health from Recommendations to Action,* Washington, DC, 1991, National Academy Press.
14. James J: *Thinking in the future tense: leadership skills for a new age,* New York, 1996, Simon and Schuster.
15. Kiechel W III. How we will work in the year 2000, *Fortune* May 17, 1993.
16. Levy BS: Conditions in which people can be healthy, President's column, *The Nation's Health* April 1, 1997, p. 2.
17. Levy BS: Keeping up with societal trends and public health, President's column, *The Nation's Health* May/June 1997, p. 2.
18. McGrawth P: The Web: Infotopia or marketplace: America's new century 2000, *Newsweek* January 27, 1997, pp. 82–84.
19. *Nutraceuticals: new aids for health promotion,* Nutrition Update, East Hanover, NJ, 1997, Nabisco Brands, Inc.
20. Parke SC: Impact of the health care reform on career opportunities in the profession, *Top Clin Nutr* 10:1–7, 1995.
21. Parks S: Challenging the future impact of information technology on dietetics practice, education and research, *J Am Diet Assoc* 94:202–204, 1994.
22. Position of the American Dietetic Association, Phytochemicals and functional foods, *J Am Diet Assoc* 95:493–496, 1995.
23. *Potential effects of congressional welfare reform legislation on family income,* Washington, DC, 1996, Urban Institute.
24. Preston SH: The next hundred years: children will pay, *New York Times Magazine* September 29, 1996.
25. Ray PH: The emerging culture, *American Demographics* 29–33, 56, 1997.

26. Reich R: New work is the way out for labor, *Philadelphia Enquirer,* September 6, 1993.

27. Simopolous AP: Diet and gene interactions, *Food Technology* 51:66–69, 1997.

28. Simopolous AP: Genetic variation and nutrition. Part 1. Population differences due to single gene defects and population differences in multifactorial diseases due to polygenic defects, *Nutrition Today* 30:157–167, 1995.

29. Simopolous AP: Genetic variation and nutrition. Part 2. Genetic variation, nutrition and chronic diseases, *Nutrition Today* 30:194–206, 1995.

30. Thomas PF, Earl R, editors: *Opportunities in the nutrition and food sciences: research challenges and the next generation of investigators,* Washington, DC, 1994, National Academy Press.

31. Wagner CG: Womens preferred futures, *The Futurist* May/June 1997, pp. 1–11.

32. Ware JE Jr, Bayliss MS, Rogers WH, et al: Differences in 4-year health outcomes for elderly and poor chronically-ill patients treated in HMO and fee-for-service systems: results from the Medical Outcomes Study, *JAMA* 276:1039–1047, 1996.

33. Woolf SH, Jonas S, Lawrence RS: *Health promotion and disease prevention in clinical practice,* Baltimore, MD, 1996, Williams & Williams.

THE EXPERTS SPEAK

SIX-POINT PLAN TO CREATIVELY MOVE COMMUNITY NUTRITION PROFESSIONALS INTO THE TWENTY-FIRST CENTURY

ANITA L. OWEN, MA, RD AND
PATRICIA L. SPLETT, PHD, RD

We stand at the dawn of a new era, one with rapidly changing technological, economic, and social environments. Community nutrition professionals will be faced with unlimited opportunities and enormous challenges as we move into the twenty-first century. With the new century ahead, how can we cope with the convulsive changes? How will we practice in this environment? We have developed a six-point plan to creatively move community nutrition professionals into the next century. This plan can be a blueprint not only for surviving but for thriving in a changing world.

No century in human history has experienced so many social transformations and such radical changes as the twentieth century. In just the last decade, we have seen stunning technological innovations, unprecedented economic opportunity, surprising political reform, a health care revolution, and great cultural rebirth.

When the steam engine first appeared in eighteenth-century Britain, no one dreamed that the curious contraption was part of a sweeping transformation now known as the "Industrial Revolution." But today we have little doubt that computers and telecommunications have brought a new revolution and that this new transformation will affect human life more profoundly than its predecessor. Now more change happens in a decade than occurred in an entire century in times past. And the tempo of change promises to get even faster because of rapid development of communications technology.

Another profound change we are experiencing is the health care revolution. Ultimately, we're told that the new system should provide all appropriate care in a seamless continuum. The way this system will grow and develop has important implications for how we practice as community nutrition professionals.

In the early 1980s, the impacts of lifestyle, environment, and biology, including genetics, on health were raised to a level of importance equal to that of the health care delivery system. Appreciation of these factors will be accelerated to new heights in the next century. One vivid example of an enormous change is the field of genetics. By the year 2005, scientists expect the Human Genome Project to complete the genetic mapping of man. Almost no human disease will be untouched by the knowledge gained. It is predicted that screening of infants at birth will be used to tell if the person will be at high risk for cardiovascular disease, diabetes, cancer, and a whole host of other diseases later in life. As community nutrition professionals, we will be counseling people about preventing these diseases based on their individual genetic profiles. This is just one example to highlight that we must be ready for change. We could wait and let others define our practice or we can be proactive and shape the role of the community nutrition professional in the twenty-first century. We choose the latter, and we believe it is possible using the following plan.

SIX-POINT PLAN TO CREATIVELY MOVE COMMUNITY NUTRITION PROFESSIONALS INTO THE TWENTY-FIRST CENTURY

I Preserve and Enhance the Greatest Asset You Have—"You"

With the dizzying array of communications that we encounter daily, both personal and professional, how do we anchor our lives to reach our goals yet deal effectively with a very complex world? As we struggle with this question, there may be some straightforward advice from Stephen Covey to assist us. His book *The Seven Habits of Highly Effective People* is considered the personal leadership handbook of the decade. Covey developed the "Seven Habits" after studying hundreds of books and essays on "success" published since 1776.[1] He indicated that the works published the last fifty years looked superficial—filled with what he calls "social band-aids" and gimmicks to improve your personality. In contrast, the literature of the first 150 years—the writings of Ben Franklin and Abe Lincoln—was based on character and talked about values such as *integrity, courage,* and *patience.* Covey based his book on these. The character ethic taught that there are basic principles of effective living and that people can experience true success and enduring happiness only as they learn and integrate these principles into their basic character. As we look at lifestyles, we need to keep in mind that each of us strive for effectiveness in our careers and personal life. Effectiveness comes when there is a balance between the desired results and the ability to produce these results. As community nutrition professionals, it will be helpful to apply the "Seven Habits" to your professional and personal lives (chapter 13). The seven habits include: be proactive; begin with the end in mind; put first things first; think win win; seek first to understand, this means listening; synthesize; and sharpen the saw.

To maintain balance in life we must regularly consider the four dimensions of self-renewal. These are

- *Physical:* exercise, nutrition, and stress management
- *Social/emotional:* service, empathy, synergy, and intrinsic security
- *Spiritual:* values clarification and commitment and meditation
- *Mental:* reading, visualizing, planning, and writing.

After you've looked at self-renewal and balance in your life, its time to look at yourself as objectively as possible. This can be done by taking an inventory of your strengths and needs. Develop short- and long-term goals to reach your full potential, then make a plan to accomplish those goals and implement it day by day. It has been said that everyone wants to change humanity, but nobody wants to change himself. Thus, we must begin with ourselves if progress is going to be made.

II Think in the Future Tense: What Skills Are Needed?

When I (Anita) was browsing in a bookstore in the Gatwick Airport in London, I was fortunate to find a book entitled *Thinking in the Future Tense* by Jennifer James (Simon & Schuster, 1996). It is a timely and hopeful book because it shows how to get a jump on change. These concepts are fully developed in this chapter. The way we think is the key to leadership skills for a new era. James indicated that we stand in a vortex of technologic, economic, demographic, and cultural change. Are we to deny it, resist it, or accept the fact that we too must change? She states that the best way to do this is to develop the ability to "think in the future tense." James indicates that the eight skills needed to know what the future looks like are *have perspective* by keeping our eyes and minds open to the forces of change as they affect our lives and work. Follow the societal and public health *trends* that are described in chapter 21. *Gain cultural knowledge* about our society (chapter 18), *be flexible,* and *have vision. Energy* is needed to do more with less, and we need to *use our intelligence* to take advantage of new and emerging technologies. Finally, we need *global values* to appreciate the richness of all cultures. These eight skills are the basic building blocks for understanding and adapting to change.

III Travel in Cyberspace: Use Major Technological Innovations

Computer applications have emerged as a viable means of gathering and disseminating nutrition information. Both stand-alone and on-line applications are being used to provide information and training in nutrition interventions for the public and professionals. While the use of on-line communications applications such as electronic mail (e-mail), electronic discussion groups, and list-serves (an interactive mailing list that distributes information to a large number of people simultaneously) are just emerging as important tools among community nutrition professionals, the exponential growth of Internet and the World Wide Web are making these technologies more and more accessible. If we are looking for success in the twenty-first century, we have to be comfortable in cyberspace, we cannot be among the electronically impaired.

IV Create the Future: Become an Active Participant in Health Care Reform

We need to understand how the new world of managed care will affect public health and where the interface will be most effective. This concept has not been fully explored to date. As managed care moves out of the hospital and into the community, knowledge of how to assess a community's health needs will be vital. Community nutrition professionals are well trained in community and nutrition assessment and can be an important resource in this area. New roles and responsibilities will evolve from the new health care, and the community nutrition professional must be an active participant in defining those new roles and responsibilities.

V Speak Out: Become an Advocate for Vulnerable Groups

The community nutrition professional has a responsibility to reach out to those populations that are at highest risk and lack the economic, political, physical, or linguistic ability to assert their own needs and interests. Social environmental factors that marginalize people and contribute to nutritional vulnerability include poverty, unemployment and underemployment, deficits in education and job skills, illiteracy, inability to speak English, cultural barriers, homelessness, hunger, chronic diseases such as AIDS, physical and mental disabilities, and geographic isolation. People experiencing these situations need other caring and committed professionals to reach out to them and to create systems that are accessible and appropriate, and to advocate for social change to deal with underlying causes for these conditions. Community nutrition professional must speak out on the nature and extent of problems that place their community and people within the community at risk. And they must join with political leaders and other concerned citizens to develop long-term approaches to underlying economic and social issues. These complex social issues require the concerted efforts of all those who are concerned with the quality of life in the community. Advocacy must be integral to the work of community nutrition professionals.

VI Use the Other Side of Your Brain: Be Creative

The biggest obstacle to creativity may be the belief that we can't do it. We become so accustomed to rules that we think they exist even when they don't! We can make creativity a part of everyday existence in private life and on the job. It takes retraining to break noncreative habits, specifically, the dominant left-brain tendency to rely entirely on logic and systematic approaches, while ignoring intuition and feelings. In his book, *Escape from the Maze,* James M. Higgins developed nine steps to personal creativity:[2]

- *Accept your innate creativity:* Try consciously to use your imagination and intuition.
- *Unlearn how not to be creative:* Start breaking the habits of predictable thinking you learned in school.
- *Expand your problem-solving style:* Whether you rely more on information or intuition, try the opposite.
- *Use creativity techniques:* There are hundreds of these, such as brain-storming, mindmapping, and storyboarding.
- *Get more in tune with your right brain:* For example, practice thinking more in pictures, not just in words and numbers.
- *Learn when to think:* Drowsiness and vigorous exercise both help to turn off the mind's internal censor.
- *Think in new ways:* Look for solutions in unfamiliar places. Don't rely on standard techniques only.
- *Face up to the complexity:* Some problems have no simple answers, but experience can make them easier to face.
- *Keep a record of your creativity:* Keep a notebook, cards, or tape recorder handy to preserve your fresh ideas.

The six-point plan can be an invaluable tool to those seeking to move forward, embrace change, and create their own tomorrows. It has been said that "life leaps like a geyser for those who drill through the rock of inertia." Let's start drilling—the twenty-first century awaits!

REFERENCES

1. Covey SR: *The 7 habits of highly effective people: powerful lessons in personal change.* NY 1989, p. 67, Simon & Schuster.
2. Higgins JG: *Escape from the maze,* New Management Publishing, p. 13, Nov. 1996, Winter Park, Florida.

TERMS USED IN MANAGED CARE

capitation A per-member, monthly payment to a provider that covers contracted services and is paid in advance of their delivery. A provider agrees to provide specified services to members for this fixed predetermined payment for the specified length of time, regardless of how many times the member uses the services. The rate can be fixed for all members or it can be adjusted for the age and sex of each member, based on actuarial projections of medical utilization. Capitation is the opposite of fee-for-service.

continuum of care An integrated delivery system that provides its patients with access to all services needed for health care in a highly integrated manner, allowing the patient to move to different sites and services in the system with strong continuity of care.

co-payment The amount the Medicare or insurance beneficiary or managed care enrollee must pay for a procedure or visit.

fee-for-service Traditional reimbursement in which the provider is paid according to the service performed. This is the reimbursement system used by conventional indemnity insurers.

gatekeeper One who screens patients seeking medical care to eliminate costly or needless referral to specialists for diagnosis and management. The gatekeeper is responsible for the administration of the member's treatment; he or she coordinates and authorizes all medical services, laboratory studies, specialty referrals, and hospitalizations.

HEDIS Health Care Employer Data and Information Set. Employers use HEDIS measures as a "report card" to rate health plan quality against regional or national norms, using specific performance measures designed by the National Committee for Quality Assurance.

integrated delivery system (IDS) A group of hospital systems, medical groups, and HMOs or insurance companies that form a network for the purpose of coordinating the continuum of care, eliminating redundant services, and developing comprehensive medical information systems under a single management system. The goal is the delivery of health care in a seamless system.

managed care Provision of health care in which access, cost, and quality are controlled by direct intervention before or during service. Programs rely on primary care physicians to manage patient care and control costs, encourage the use of case managers to plan and accelerate high-cost care when it is necessary, and promote arrangements between payer and providers to minimize health care costs whenever possible. The goal is a comprehensive system where patients get medically necessary care in the most cost-effective manner while maintaining quality and member satisfaction.

mandated benefits Health benefits that health care plans are required by state or federal law to provide to members.

outcomes management A process to manage the clinical outcomes of enrolles to increase patient and payer satisfaction while holding down costs. Outcomes management leads to practice guides and critical care pathways.

primary care Health services, including preventive care, provided by a family practitioner, pediatrician, internist, or obstetrician/gynecologist or their designee, in an ambulatory setting.

utilization review A process of monitoring the quality and necessity of medical services provided to discourage unnecessary and inappropriate care on treatment regimens.

NUTRITION CARE
DEFINITIONS AND DESCRIPTIONS

nutrition care A comprehensive array of food and nutrition services delivered to persons in the health care system to promote health, manage disease, and support rehabilitation and palliation. Nutrition services at the individual level include screening, and as indicated, assessment, intervention planning and implementation, referral, and follow-up. In institutional settings (hospitals, long-term care facilities, hospices), provision of foods tailored to meet needs of the patient or resident is also considered part of nutrition care.

nutrition screening The process of identifying characteristics known to be associated with nutrition problems. The purpose of screening is to identify persons who may be at nutritional risk and require further assessment. Nutrition screening can be done by a health care team member or community nutrition professional.

nutrition assessment In-depth review and analysis of a person's medical and diet history, laboratory values, and anthropometric measurements to verify nutritional risk or malnutrition and identify underlying causes so that appropriate nutrition intervention, tailored to the needs of the individual, can be planned and initiated. Nutrition assessment can be done by trained members of the health care team, especially dietitians.

NUTRITION INTERVENTION PLANNING AND IMPLEMENTATION

When a predisposing condition, risk factor(s), compromised nutritional status, or altered metabolic or physiologic state indicating the need for nutrition intervention is identified, a specific nutrition plan is developed for the individual. The plan identifies the appropriate intervention by type and amount (e.g., number of counseling visits) and includes specific objectives and a time frame.

Types of Nutrition Intervention

• **nutrition education and anticipatory guidance** Basic information related to food choices to maintain adequate nutrition and health. Examples include general information to a mother of a young infant about future introduction of solids and a reminder to a young adult about choosing fast foods that are lower in fat.

• **nutrition counseling** Working with an individual (or caretaker) to enable him or her to successfully modify eating practices to be consistent with a nutrition prescription. Nutrition counseling is usually provided by a registered dietitian or other community nutrition professional.

• **nutrition prescription or diet modification** Specific changes in one or more components of dietary intake to meet health promotion or disease management goals. Examples include 1,500-calorie diet to foster weight reduction, diabetic diet plan to control blood glucose and support normal growth and development of teen with type I diabetes, protein restricted diet for renal failure patient, and oral nutrition supplements to restore nutritional status of elderly resident in long-term care.

• **nutrition support** Delivery of nutrient needs enterally via a tube into the gastrointestinal tract or parenterally via intravenous infusion. Nutrition support is generally planned and implemented by a team including physician, dietitian, pharmacist, and nurse.

referral If the individual has inadequate physical, mental, and/or economic capability to manage the nutritional aspects of his or her intervention plan, a referral may be initiated to other health care or social service professionals, to food or economic assistance programs, or to other resources in the health care system or the community to support the achievement of nutrition care goals.

follow-up Later contact with the patient is necessary to assess the progress of the intervention, make adjustments if needed, and document the outcomes of the nutrition intervention. Follow-up may be done directly by the nutrition professional or by other care providers in the system. Procedures for a follow-up should be part of practice guidelines and critical care pathways.

documentation and reporting Standard process and outcomes indicators specific to the type of care rendered and/or the disease or condition of the patient should be documented for each provider-patient encounter. Summary information should be useful to other care providers, be in a form that is easily communicated across settings in the continuum of care, and facilitate continuity of nutrition care over time and across settings.

The American Dietetic Association uses the term medical nutrition therapy to summarize the above processes. Their definition follows.

medical nutrition therapy Medical nutrition therapy involves the assessment of the nutritional status of patients with a condition, illness, or injury that puts them at risk. This includes review and analysis of medical and diet history, laboratory values, and anthropometric measurements. Based on the assessment, nutrition modalities most appropriate to manage the condition or treat the illness or injury are initiated and include the following:

- Diet modification and counseling leading to the development of a personal diet plan to achieve nutritional goals and desired health outcomes.

- Specialized nutrition therapies including supplementation with medical foods for those unable to obtain adequate nutrients through food intake only, enteral nutrition delivered via tube feeding into the gastrointestinal tract for those unable to ingest or digest food, and parenteral nutrition delivered via intravenous infusion for those unable to absorb nutrients.

RESOURCES FOR FURTHER INFORMATION

Internet Sites for Congress

Many are interconnected, with a "pointer" to other agencies. Some systems, such as the Library of Congress, are often overcrowded, so don't be surprised if your connection is denied.

House addresses: A file servicer offers general information and directories, including the e-mail addresses to House members that have them. Type: gopher://gopher.house.gov

Senate addresses: The file server is similar to the House. Type: gopher://ftp.senate.gov

Library of Congress: Offers access to LOCIS system for tracking status of federal legislation and library catalog. Also includes directories of recent library exhibits, print and photographic archives. Type: gopher://marvel.loc.gov. Telnet locis.loc.gov

General Accounting Office: A listing of new reports from GAO. Type: telnet cap.gwu.edu (Login: guest, password: visitor; commands "go federal" or "go gao")

GOVERNMENT PUBLICATIONS

Government Printing Office (GPO): Publishes the *Congressional Directory, Congressional Record, Federal Register,* congressional bills, reports, hearings, and various other federal publications related to food and nutrition policy. Order by title or document number from GPO by calling 202–783–3228 or writing Superintendent of Documents, Attention: Inquiries, U.S. Government Printing Office, Washington, DC 20402.

House and Senate documents: For copies of House and Senate bills and documents such as committee reports and public laws, send a letter with request, accompanied by self-addressed, large, stamped envelope:

The Senate Document Room
Hart Senate Office Building, Room B-04
Washington DC 20515

The House Document Room
226 House Annex I
Washington DC 20515

INFORMATION ON CONGRESS AND FEDERAL LEGISLATION

Almanac of American Politics (Macmillan): A complete listing of biographical sketches of congressional member's voting records, interest group ratings, and election percentages.

Congressional Directory (GPO): A complete directory of all government offices, congressional committees, and executive and judicial branch offices.

The U.S. Congress Handbooks (I & II): Complete directories that identify members of Congress, their committees, and staff, as well as cabinet members. Features special articles and key phone numbers (source: The U.S. Congress Handbook, McLean, VA 22101).

Congressional Handbook: Annual directory of members of Congress (source: U.S. Chamber of Commerce, Legislative Action Department, 1615 H Street, NW, Washington, DC 20062).

Congress and Health: An Introduction to the Legislative Process and Its Key Participants (source: National Health Council, New York).

Congressional Insight Handbook: An Information Guide to the U.S. House of Representatives (source: Public Affairs Dept., National Association of Manufacturers, Washington, DC 20004–1703).

Congressional Quarterly Publications (Congressional Quarterly Inc., 1414 22d Street, NW, Washington, DC 20037):

Congressional Monitor: A weekly newsletter summarizing events in Congress, the White House, and the Supreme Court.

Congressional Record Scanner: A synopsis of the Congressional Record published daily when Congress is in session.

Campaign Practices Reports and Guide: A biweekly newsletter reporting on all significant campaign finance regulations, news, and trends.

Congressional Insight: A weekly newsletter analyzing the pressures, people, and politics that shape Capitol Hill decisions.

Congress in Print: A weekly notice that lists current published congressional documents.

The CQ Quarterly: A publication that summarizes current issues, organizes reference materials, and provides a bibliography of sources for further research.

The Congressional Record (GPO): A verbatim account of happenings on the Senate and House floors and scheduled committee meetings; issued daily when Congress is in session.

Congressional Yellow Book: A directory of Congress staff updated four times a year (source: The Washington Monitor, Inc., Washington, DC 20004).

ORGANIZATIONS INVOLVED WITH DOMESTIC FOOD AND NUTRITION POLICY

Name and address	Phone e-mail	FAX web site
SPECIAL INTEREST GROUPS		

Bread for the World,
    1100 Wayne Avenue, Suite 1000, Silver Spring, MD
	301–608–2400
	    bread@igc.apc.org
		301–608–2400
		    http://www.bread.org

Public Voice for Food and Health Policy, 1101 14th Street NW, Suite 710, Washington, DC	202–371–1840	202–371–1910
Nutrition Legislative News, P.O. Box 75035, Washington, DC 20013	202–488–8879	

Second Harvest,
    116 South Michigan Avenue, Suite 4,
    Chicago, IL 60603
	312–263–2303	

Urban Institute,
    2100 M Street NW, 5th Floor,
    Washington, DC 20037
	202–833–7200	

PROFESSIONAL ASSOCIATIONS		
American Dietetic Association, Office of Government Affairs, 1225 Eye Street NW, Suite 1250, Washington, DC 20005	202–371–0500	202–371–0840
American Association of Family and Consumer Sciences, 1555 King Street, Alexandria, VA 22314	703–706–4600	703–706–4663

American Society for Nutritional Sciences and American
    Society for Clinical Nutrition
    9650 Rockville Pike, Bethesda, MD 20014
	301–530–7050	301–571–1892

American Public Health Association, 1015 18th Street NW, Washington, DC 20036	202–789–5600	202–789–5661
American School Food Service Association, 1600 Duke Street NW, Alexandria, VA 22314	703–739–3900	703–739–3915
Society for Nutrition Education 7101 Wisconsin Avenue, Suite 901, Bethesda, MD 20814	800–235–6690	
VOLUNTARY HEALTH ORGANIZATIONS		

American Cancer Society, Office of Government Affairs,
    316 Pennsylvania Avenue SE, Suite 200,
    Washington, DC 20003
	202–546–4011	202–546–1682

American Heart Association, Office of Government Affairs,
    1150 Connecticut Avenue NW, Suite 819,
    Washington, DC 20036
	202–822–9380	202–822–9883

National Foundation of the March of Dimes,
    Office of Government Affairs, 1725 K Street, NW,
    Washington, DC 20036
	202–659–1800	202–296–2964

TRADE ASSOCIATIONS		
American Meat Institute, 1700 North Moore Street, Arlington, Va 22209	703–841–2400	703–527–0938

Food Marketing Institute,
    800 Connecticut Avenue NW, Suite 500,
    Washington, DC 20006
	202–429–8236	202–429–4549

International Life Sciences Institute/Nutrition Foundation, 1126 16th Street NW, Suite 111, Washington, DC 20036	202–659–0789	202–659–8654
National Dairy Council, 6300 North River Road, Rosemont, IL 60018	708–803–2077	

Name and address	Phone e-mail	FAX web site
National Academy of Sciences/Institute of Medicine, Food and Nutrition Board, 2101 Constitution Avenue NW, Washington, DC 20037	202–334–2000	202–334–2316
United Fresh Fruit and Vegetable Association, 727 North Washington Street, Alexandria, VA 22314	703–836–3410	703–836–2049
GOVERNMENT AGENCIES		
U.S. Department of Agriculture (USDA), 12th and Independence Avenue SW, Washington, DC 20250	202–720–3631 gopher.esusda.gov	202–720–5437 http://web.fie.com/web/ fed/agr
Extension Service (ES), 14th and Independence, Jamie Whitten Building, Room 338A, Washington, DC 20250	202–720–3377 gopher.esusda.gov	202–720-3945
Food and Consumer Services (FCS), 2101 Park Center Office, room 308, Alexandria, VA 22302	703–305–2062	703–305-2908
FCS Home Page URL Center for Nutrition Policy and Promotion Home Page: URL "Team Nutrition" Home Page: URL		http://www.usda.gov/fcs http://www.usda.gov/fcs/ cnpp.html http://www.usda.gov/fcs/ team.htm
Food Safety and Inspection Service, 4911 South Agriculture Building, Washington, DC 20250	202–720–7025	202–690–4437
Food and Nutrition Information Center (FNIC), National Agricultural Library, 10301 Baltimore Boulevard, Room 304, Beltsville, MD 20705	301–504–5414 gopher.nalusda.gov	301–504–6409
U.S. Department of Health and Human Services (DHHS), 200 Independence Avenue SW, Washington, DC 20201	202–619–0257 gopher.os.dhhs.gov	202–619-3363 http://ww.os.dhhs.gov
Food and Drug Administration (FDA), Center for Food Safety and Applied Nutrition, Room 4405B Federal Building, 200 C Street SW, Washington, DC 20204	202–205–4168	202–205–5295 http://www/fda/gov/ opacom/hpnews.html
National Institutes of Health (NIH), 9000 Rockville, Pike, Bethesda, MD 20892	301–496–4461	301–496–0017
National Center for Health Statistics (NCHS), 6525 Belcrest Road, Hyattsville, MD 20782	301–436–8500	
Office of Disease Prevention and Health Promotion (ODPHP), 2131 Switzer Building, 330 C Street SW, Washington, DC 20201	202–205–9007	202–205–9478
Centers for Disease Control and Prevention, 1600 Clifton Road, Atlanta, GA 30333	770–488–7510	770–488–7593

SELECTED PHYSICAL SIGNS OF MALNUTRITION

Organ system	Sign
Hair	*Lack of luster (P).* The hair is dull and dry. Effects of scalp disease and use of oil and other substances on the hair, and exposure to salt water and hot sun must be taken into account. *Thin and sparse (P).* The hair may become fine and silky in texture and cover the scalp less abundantly or completely than usual. In some ethnic groups with normally curly hair, malnutrition may produce pathological straightness. *Dyspigmentation (P).* The hair shows a distinct lightening of the normal color (black to dark brown to light brown to red-brown, etc.). Local practices, such as dyeing the hair, as well as effects of salt water, sunshine, and the use of oil and other substances should be considered. *Easy pluckability (P, Z, F).* A small tuft or clump of hair can be easily and painlessly pulled out of the scalp. Other changes, such as those listed above, are commonly present.
Face	*Diffuse depigmentation (P).* This occurs in dark-skinned individuals in severe protein-calorie malnutrition. Pallor associated with anemia may exaggerate the appearance of this condition. *Nasolabial dyssbacea (B).* This yellow, greasy appearance is produced by plugging of the ducts of enlarged sebaceous glands by sebum.
Eyes	*Conjunctival xerosis (A).* Dryness, thickening, and lack of luster of the bulbar conjunctiva of the exposed part of the eyeball. *Bitot's spots (A).* Well-demarcated, superficially dry, white-gray foamy plaques usually located lateral to the cornea in both eyes. *Corneal xerosis (A).* Hazy or opaque appearance of cornea. *Keratomalcia (A).* Softening of cornea. *Corneal vascularization (R).* Invasion of periphery of cornea with fine capillary blood vessels. Usually secondary to chronic irritative or inflammatory process.
Lips	*Angular stomatitis (R).* Excoriated lesions and fissuring at angles of the mouth. *Cheilosis (B).* Reddening, swelling, ulceration of lips.
Tongue	*Atrophic papillae (I).* Atrophy of filiform papillae (tastebuds), leaving tongue with smoother or slick appearance.
Gums	*Spongy, bleeding (C).* Swelling of gingival tissue between teeth, which may bleed on slight pressure.
Skin	*Xerosis (Z, F).* Generalized dryness with desquamation of superficial layers. *Follicular hyperkeratosis (A).* Hypertrophy of the corneous layer of skin surrounding the hair follicles, with formation of plaques. *Petechiae (C, K).* Small hemorrhagic spots in skin or mucous membranes. *Pellarous dermatosis (N).* Symmetrical, clearly demarcated, hyperpigmented areas of skin most commonly located on body regions exposed to sunlight. *Flaky-paint dermatosis (P).* Symmetrical hyperpigmented patches of skin that desquamate, leaving hypopigmented skin.
Nails	*Koilonychia (I).* Spoon-shaped deformity of fingernails of both hands in older children and adults.
Musculoskeletal system	*Frontal or parietal bossing. (D).* Localized thickening of these bones in skull. *Epiphyseal enlargement (C, D).* Enlargement of ends of long bones, especially noted in radius and ulna at the wrist. *Beading of ribs (D).* Symmetrical nodular enlargement of costochondral junctions in ribs. Comparable to epiphyseal enlargement noted in wrists.

Note: Letters in parentheses refer to deficiencies in the following nutrients: A = vitamin A, B = vitamin B complex, C = vitamin C, D = vitamin D, F = essential fatty acids, I = iron, K = vitamin K, N = niacin, P = protein, R = riboflavin, T = thiamine, Z = zinc.
Source: From Owen GM. Physical examination as an assessment tool. In Simko M, Cowell C, Gillbride, J, editors, *Nutrition Assessment: A Comprehensive Guide for Planning Intervention,* 2nd edition, Rockville, MD, 1995. Reprinted with permission of Aspen Publishers, Inc.

RESOURCES FOR NUTRITION EDUCATION AND COUNSELING

American Association of Retired Persons (AARP)
601 East Street, NW
Washington, DC 20049
Tel: 202–872–4700

American Dental Association
211 East Chicago Avenue
Chicago, IL 60611
Fax: 312–440–2500

American Dietetic Association
216 West Jackson Boulevard, Suite 800
Chicago, IL 60606–6995
Tel: 312–899–0040

American Geriatrics Society
770 Lexington Avenue, Number 300
New York, NY 10021
Tel: 212–308–1412
Fax: 212–832–8646

American Physical Therapy Association
1111 North Fairfax Street
Alexandria, VA 22314

American Speech Language–Hearing Association
1081 Rockville Pike
Rockville, MD 20852
Tel: 800–638–8255 or 301–897–5700
Fax: 301–571–0457

Arthritis Foundation
1314 Spring Street NW
Atlanta, GA 30309
Tel: 404–872–7100

Elder Care Locator
Tel: 800–677–1116

National Council on the Aging, Inc.
Health Promotion Institute
409 Third Street SW
Washington, DC 20024
Tel: 202–479–1200
Fax: 202–479–0735

National Meals on Wheels Foundation
2675 44th Street SW, Suite 305
Grand Rapids, MI 49509
Tel: 800–999–6262

National Osteoporosis Foundation
1150 17th Street NW, Suite 500
Washington, DC 20037

Nutrition Screening Initiative
1010 Wisconsin Avenue, NW, Suite 800
Washington, DC 20007

National Policy and Resource Center
   on Nutrition and Aging
Florida International University
Building OE200
Miami, FL 33199
Tel: 305–348–1517
Fax: 305–348–1518

Local services in your community:
   City or County Health Department
   Hospital Nutrition Services
   Local Senior Centers
   Local Mental Health Centers
   Local Affiliates of National Organizations
   Local Area Agency on Aging
   USDA Cooperative Extension Service

MAKING SENSE OF SCIENTIFIC RESEARCH ABOUT DIET AND HEALTH
A PAPER OF THE FOOD AND NUTRITION SCIENCE ALLIANCE

The Food and Nutrition Science Alliance (FANSA) is a partnership of four professional societies who have joined forces to speak with one voice on food and nutrition issues. Member organizations are The American Dietetic Association, The American Society for Clinical Nutrition Inc., the American Society for Nutritional Sciences, and the Institute of Food Technologists.

Principal Authors: Jeanne P. Goldberg, PhD., R.D., Jill M. Shuman, M.S., R.D., E.L.S.

Beta carotene; a nugget of nutritional gold[1]
(10/92)

All that glitters is not beta-carotene[2]
(2/9/94)

New benefit from beta-carotene[3]
(5/95)

Beta no more[4]
(1/19/96)

These four headlines appeared in prominent magazines, newspapers, and journals between 1992 and 1996, prompting consumer confusion and frustration. Given the contradictions in the headlines, people need more information to make sense of conflicting scientific research about diet and health.

Surveys show that Americans obtain more news about food safety and nutrition from the news media than from health care providers. The Center for Media and Public Affairs in Washington, DC, analyzed three months of news coverage (May–July 1995) from 37 local and national news outlets. The Center found that although the media frequently featured stories about research findings, the stories often omitted details that would allow readers to determine the relevance of the study results to their own lives. Few reports, for example, described the study's design, study conditions, or the statistical significance of the results. These omissions do a grave injustice to the study, because study design is critical to the interpretation of the results.

News stories that include information about study design offer readers more insight into the study's results, but reporters rarely have the luxury of time or space to provide in-depth explanations of the various types of studies. Stories that put a single study into a larger context, by including results of other studies investigating similar questions, are also especially informative. Understanding the process of scientific inquiry, including the types of study design, helps people make sense of science news.

STUDY DESIGN

Researchers commonly use three approaches to investigate health questions: epidemiologic studies, basic laboratory-based research, and clinical trials. Each type of study can yield useful information, but each also has its own set of limitations. Scientists generally refrain from drawing conclusions about the cause of a disease until a body of evidence supported by studies in all three categories, points to similar factors.

Epidemiologic Studies

Say, for example, researchers seek to identify the relationship between diet and heart disease. They may begin with epidemiologic studies, which help to determine the incidence and distribution of diseases in populations. There are several types of epidemiologic studies, including cross-sectional, case-control, and cohort. Using a cross-sectional study, researchers might measure the incidence of heart disease in men between 50 and 55 years of age in the United States, Japan and France. Say the incidence is higher in the United States. It would be premature, however, to conclude that living in the United States caused heart disease. Further study would be needed to determine why the incidence differs among countries. A case-control study might look at two groups of U.S. men—one group of 50 to 55 year olds with heart disease, and one without. Researchers could try to identify the factors from each group's past that differentiate the "case" participants from the "control" ones. Several factors may be identified. For example, the men with heart disease might report having consumed more red meat, exercised less, and driven bigger cars over the past 30 years. One limitation to this type of study is that it relies on participants' accurate recollection of their behavior long since past. Again, more studies would be needed before establishing whether any of the identified factors could be causally linked to heart disease. Researchers then might opt to gather information from a different perspective, this time using a cohort study. In this type of study, researchers identify one or more groups of participants, starting, for example, with men between the ages of 20 and 25. In this prospective study, researchers follow the men over time, periodically asking participants what they eat and how much they exercise, then note who gets heart disease and who does not. A limitation to this and all observational epidemiologic investigations is that researchers cannot control all of the variables, including behavioral and environmental changes, that may influence development or prevention of the disease and confound the study observations.

All three of these studies help researchers narrow down the list of plausible causes by demonstrating possible associations between diet or environmental factors and a particular disease. Epidemiologic studies cannot prove cause and effect, but they can help researchers formulate better questions to pursue through other types of studies.

Basic Research

Basic research is conducted in a laboratory under conditions that strictly control extraneous factors that could affect the results. Experiments might be done in a test tube, with animals, or in isolated systems using cells or tissues. Basic research often explores what is happening at the tissue, cellular or molecular level. It is an excellent way to determine the effects of a particular factor, such as a nutrient or a drug, under precisely controlled conditions.

For example, in one study two identical groups of mice might be fed either a diet high in saturated fat or a control diet that differed from the test diet in only the aspect under study (in this case, low in saturated fat). Any differences in growth, disease development, or nutritional status that emerged between the two groups might then be attributed to the difference between the two diets. The benefit of basic research is the ability to control all the conditions of the experiment except the variable being studied. Results of the basic research studies often may point out a need for more research. The drawback to basic research is that what happens under experimental circumstances may not mirror the complex situation of people's lives. In other words, the results of tests conducted in test tubes or on animals are not necessarily applicable to people and the way they live. That's why scientists make use of another important research tool—the clinical trial.

Clinical Trials

Clinical trials are research studies involving people who have agreed to follow a specific regimen. As with basic research studies, the best clinical trials are also rigorously controlled. Subjects are selected according to defined criteria. Studies often include at least one experimental or treatment group and control group. The experimental group receives a new drug, diet or treatment and the control group receives either an inactive (placebo) or an existing treatment. In one of the strongest study designs, the subjects are assigned randomly to treatment and control groups, helping to ensure that the final results are as unbiased as possible. Whenever possible, a clinical trial should be "blinded," meaning that no subject knows whether he or she is receiving the treatment or control. In a double-blinded study, the researchers don't know either until the study is over.

The overwhelming advantage of well-designed clinical trials lies in the random assignment of people to treatment and control groups, which is the only method capable of controlling for both known and unknown factors that may confound the results. Furthermore, the results of clinical studies may have more direct implications for human health than the results of basic research involving animals or test tubes.

On the other hand, sometimes the study groups are not representative of the population, making it difficult to generalize findings. In addition, clinical and ethical considerations limit the type of treatment that may be given to people. Tests to determine the maximum safe and effective dose of a nutrient, for example, can be problematic because it would be unethical to give people doses that may cause harm.

Researchers must be careful to design studies so as not to introduce bias. Suppose researchers decide to administer an experimental drug to one group and a placebo to another group. This is a blind study, so neither group knows if it is receiving the drug or placebo, but the researchers tell everyone that the drug causes a side effect, say, dry mouth. Once the people in the treatment group experience dry mouth, they know they are on the drug, the blind is broken, and the study is biased.

BUILDING A BODY OF EVIDENCE

Science is an evolutionary process. Any conclusion drawn from a single study should be viewed as preliminary. Additional studies add to the previous body of knowledge, answering some questions and posing new ones. It is important to remember that research results need to be interpreted, and that scientists' interpretations of the results of one study or a group of studies can vary. Furthermore, the meaning of data for a population may differ from the meaning of data for an individual, especially in the case of data from epidemiologic studies.

In the field of nutrition, scientists already have accumulated a strong body of evidence that supports sound advice for healthy Americans. That advice is articulated in the Dietary Guidelines for Americans and the Food Guide Pyramid, and states: "For good health, eat a variety of foods. Balance the energy from the food you eat with physical activity. Maintain or improve your weight. Choose a diet with plenty of grain products, vegetables and fruits; low in fat, saturated fat and cholesterol; and moderate in sugars, salt and sodium. And if you drink alcoholic beverages, do so in moderation." Many scientific studies about diet and health continue to support the conclusions that have led to these guidelines.

KEY SCIENTIFIC TERMS

Some words and phrases mean different things to scientists and non-scientists. Here's a list of terms and what they mean when scientists use them.

Associated with means there may be a connection, a co-occurrence more frequent than can be explained by mere coincidence, but a cause is not proven.

Double the risk is a useful phrase if the original risk is known. If, for example, the original risk is one in a million, the double risk is still low at 1 in 500,000. By comparison, there is much more cause for concern if a 1 in 100 risk doubles to 1 in 50.

Probability means the chance that an event will occur. Probability can be high or low; it does not mean certainty.

Statistically Significant (sometimes written just "significant") implies that there is a very low probability of having obtained the observed results if there is in fact no real effect or association.

Survival is not the same as cure. Survival rates describe the proportion of people with a specific disease or condition who are still alive after a given period.

FURTHER READING

Angell M, Kassirer JP. Clinical research—What should the public believe? *New England Journal of Medicine,* July 21, 1994, p. 189–190.

Reading Between the Headlines. *Food Insight,* September/October 1993.

Schmitz A. Food News Blues. *Health,* November 1991.

Understanding Risk: Tricky Business. *Harvard Health Letter,* October 1994.

Why do those #&*?@! experts keep changing their minds? *University of Berkeley Wellness Letter,* February 1995.

REFERENCES

1. *Better Homes and Gardens,* October 1992, p. 64–66.
2. *Journal of the American Medical Association* (JAMA), Feb. 9, 1994, p. 1455–1456.
3. *Prevention,* May 1995, p. 53–4.
4. *Time,* Jan. 29, 1996, p. 66.

INDEX

RECOMMENDED LEVELS FOR INDIVIDUAL INTAKE OF NUTRIENTS (as of May 1998)

Life-Stage Group	Protein (g)	Fat-soluble vitamins				Water-soluble vitamins			
		A (μgRE)	D (μg)[a]	E (mg TE)	K (μg)	C (mg)	B$_1$ (mg)	B$_2$ (mg)	Niacin (mg NE)
Infants (mo)									
0–5	13	375	5*	3	5	30	0.2*	0.3*	2*
6–11	14	375	5*	4	10	35	0.3*	0.4*	3*
Children (yr)									
1–3	16	400	5*	6	15	40	**0.5**	**0.5**	**6**
4–8	24	500	5*	7	20	45	**0.6**	**0.6**	**8**
Males (yr)									
9–13	45	1,000	5*	10	45	50	**0.9**	**0.9**	**12**
14–18	59	1,000	5*	10	65	60	**1.2**	**1.3**	**16**
19–30	58	1,000	5*	10	70	60	**1.2**	**1.3**	**16**
31–50	63	1,000	5*	10	80	60	**1.2**	**1.3**	**16**
51–70	63	1,000	10*	10	80	60	**1.2**	**1.3**	**16**
>70	63	1,000	15*	10	80	60	**1.2**	**1.3**	**16**
Females (yr)									
9–13	46	800	5*	8	45	50	**0.9**	**0.9**	**12**
14–18	44	800	5*	8	55	60	**1.0**	**1.0**	**14**
19–30	46	800	5*	8	60	60	**1.1**	**1.1**	**14**
31–50	50	800	5*	8	65	60	**1.1**	**1.1**	**14**
51–70	50	800	10*	8	65	60	**1.1**	**1.1**	**14**
>70	50	800	15*	8	65	60	**1.1**	**1.1**	**14**
Pregnancy									
<19	60	800	5*	10	65	70	**1.4**	**1.4**	**18**
19–50	60	800	5*	10	65	70	**1.4**	**1.4**	**18**
Lactation									
<19	65	1,300	5*	12	65	95	**1.5**	**1.6**	**17**
19–50	65	1,200	5*	12	65	95	**1.5**	**1.6**	**17**

Note: This table presents 1989 RDAs in ordinary type, 1997–1998 RDAs in bold type, and 1997–1998 AIs (Adequate Intake) in ordinary type followed by an asterisk (*). RDAs and AIs may both be used as goals for individual intake. RDAs are set to meet the needs of almost all (97 to 98 percent) healthy individuals in a group. For healthy breastfed infants, the AI is the mean intake. The AI for other life stage groups is believed to cover their needs, but lack of data or certainty in the data prevent clear specification of this coverage. [There are differences between the 1989 RDAs and the 1997/1998 recommended levels for individual intake of nutrients with respect to methods of derivation and age-groupings. However, space does not allow separate tables for the 1997/1998 recommended levels for individual intake of nutrients. Accordingly, the authors devised this table to summarize currently available data. It is not an official document developed or approved by the Food and Nutrition Board].

RE, retinol equivalent: 1RE = 1 μg retinol or 6 μg β carotene; TE, α-tocopherol equivalents;:1 mg d α-tocopherol = 1 α-TE; NE, niacin equivalent = 1 mg niacin or 60 mg dietary tryptophan.

[a] As cholecalciferol: 10 μg cholecalciferol = 400 IU of vitamin D

[b] As dietary folate equivalents (DFE). 1 DFE = 1 μg food folate = 0.6 μg of folic acid (from fortified food or supplement) consumed with food = 0.5 μg of synthetic (supplemental) folic acid taken on an empty stomach.